Practical Neuroangiography

Practical Neuroangiography

Pearse Morris, M.B., B.Ch.

Interventional Neuroradiologist
Massachusetts General Hospital
Consultant Interventional Neuroradiologist
Brigham and Women's Hospital
Assistant Professor of Radiology
Boston University
Boston, Massachusetts

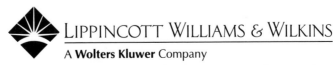

LIPPINCOTT WILLIAMS & WILKINS
A **Wolters Kluwer** Company
Philadelphia • Baltimore • New York • London
Buenos Aires • Hong Kong • Sydney • Tokyo

Editor: Charles W. Mitchell
Associate Managing Editor: Grace E. Miller
Production Coordinator: Felecia R. Weber
Designer: Dan Pfisterer
Illustration Planner: Lorraine Wrzosek
Cover Designer: Tom Scheuerman
Typesetter: Maryland Composition Co., Inc.
Printer: R. R. Donnelley & Sons Company
Digitized Illustrations: Maryland Composition
Binder: R. R. Donnelley & Sons Company

351 West Camden Street
Baltimore, Maryland 21201-2436 USA

Rose Tree Corporate Center
1400 North Providence Road
Building II, Suite 5025
Media, Pennsylvania 19063-2043 USA

Accurate indications, adverse reactions and dosage schedules for drugs are provided in
this book, but it is possible that they may change. The reader is urged to review the package
information data of the manufacturers of the medications mentioned.

Printed in the United States of America

Library of Congress Cataloging-in-Publication Data

Morris, Pearse.
    Practical neuroangiography / Pearse Morris.
        p.   cm.
    Includes bibliographical references and index.
    ISBN 0-683-30020-2
    1. Brain—Blood-vessels—Radiography.   2. Spinal cord—Blood
-vessels—Radiograph.   I. Title.
    [DNLM: 1. Cerebral Angiography.   2. Cerebral Arteries—anatomy &
histology.   3. Cerebrovascular Disorders—radiography. WL 141
M877p   1997]
RC386.6.A54M67   1997
616.8′107572—dc21
DNLM/DLC
for Library of Congress   97-3874
                                                                            CIP

*The publishers have made every effort to trace the copyright holders for borrowed material.
If they have inadvertently overlooked any, they will be pleased to make the necessary
arrangements at the first opportunity.*

To purchase additional copies of this book, call our customer service department at **(800)
638-0672** or fax orders to **(800) 447-8438**. For other book services, including chapter reprints
and large quantity sales, ask for the Special Sales department.

Canadian customers should call **(800) 268-4178**, or fax **(905) 470-6780**. For all other calls
originating outside of the United States, please call **(410) 528-4223** or fax us at **(410) 528-
8550**.

Visit Williams & Wilkins on the Internet: http/www.wwilkins.com or contact our customer service department at **custserv@wwilkins.com.** Williams & Wilkins customer service
representatives are available from 8:30 am to 6:00 pm, EST, Monday through Friday, for
telephone access.

                                                                99 00 01
                                                    3 4 5 6 7 8 9 10

Dedicated with love to Viki, Tristan, and Viveca

Preface

The purpose of this book is to help the reader become a more competent neuroangiographer. It was created to provide a complete and concise introduction to neuroangiography and neurovascular diseases for radiology residents, a more comprehensive review for diagnostic and interventional neuroradiology fellows, and a modern perspective to readers who trained in the past. Physicians in the related fields of neurology and neurosurgery, with whom we make clinical decisions, will also find much here that is useful.

I hope that this book will save the reader a great deal of time. I endeavored to include a range of knowledge, references, practical hints, and lessons that would otherwise be time-consuming to research or acquire. It is the book that I wish had been available at the start of my fellowship. The emphasis throughout is on practicality, concision, and safety.

The past 20 years have brought great changes to the practice of neuroradiology. MRI and CT have supplanted the use of angiography and pneumoencephalography for evaluation of masses and other structural lesions of the central nervous system. In tandem with these changes, interventional neuroradiology has become a dominant force in the management of neurovascular and other diseases. Increasingly, the modern mission of cerebral angiography is not simply diagnostic, but instead requires the acquisition of critical data needed for decisions on how to manage patients surgically or endovascularly. Technical and anatomic discussions in the following chapters reflect this new responsibility of the neuroangiographer.

Moreover, the field of interventional neuroradiology is gathering momentum; emergency procedures are being expected of neuroradiologists who have not had such experience. The final chapters introduce the reader to fundamental interventional principles and common emergency procedures.

Pearse Morris, M.B.

Acknowledgments

This book would not have been possible without the dedicated efforts of a large number of individuals involved in the clinical care of patients at Massachusetts General Hospital, Brigham and Women's Hospital, Massachusetts Eye and Ear Infirmary, and Boston Medical Center. I thank the staffs of the Interventional and Diagnostic Neuroradiology sections, the Neurosurgery and Neurology services, the nurses of the Intensive Care Units and neurosurgical floors, and the Anesthesia departments, all of whom contributed to the care of the patients described in the following chapters. In particular, I want to thank the technologists, nurses, and fellows of the Massachusetts General Hospital neurointerventional service for their unending commitment to clinical duty and patient care. I would also like to thank F. Huang-Hellinger, MD, PhD, R. Budzik, MD, B.J. Stallmeyer, MD, PhD, and L. Niklason, PhD, for their assistance in reviewing the manuscript.

Without the encouragement of my parents and parents-in-law and the support of my wife and our children, this project could not have been completed.

Pearse Morris, M.B.

Contents

PART I / TECHNIQUES AND SAFETY

"Avoir toujours un grand soin pour éviter l'entrée de l'air"

—Egas Moniz

Introduction

EGAS MONIZ (1874–1955)

António Caetano de Abreu Freire was born on November 29, 1874, in Avanca, Portugal. During his political pamphleteering days while a student at the University of Coimbra, he took a pen-name of a legendary Portuguese hero, Égas Moniz, which he continued to use throughout his life. He graduated from medical school in 1899. Following studies in Bordeaux and Paris under Babinski, Pierre Marie, and Dejérine, he assumed the Chair of Neurology in Lisbon in 1911, a position he held until his retirement in 1944. He had a full and interesting life, devoting much of his energy in later years to non-medical literary pursuits. It is said that he once fought a duel. In addition to his medical work, he had an active political career, serving as Portugal's Minister for Foreign Affairs, Ambassador to Spain, and as Chairman of the Portuguese delegation to the Paris Peace Conference after World War I, Portugal having been an allied combatant in the later stages of the war.

For his pioneering work of 1936 in describing the effects of prefrontal leukotomy in psychotic patients, he was awarded the Nobel Prize in medicine in 1949; but his remarkable life is better remembered now for his description of the first cerebral angiographic studies in human subjects.

Within months of Karl Roentgen's discovery of x-rays, an angiographic study of an amputated arm was conducted successfully in Vienna using Teichmann's mixture of lime, mercuric sulfide, and petroleum (1). Building on this and on the work of other pioneers of peripheral angiography, Moniz and his colleagues, Almeida Dias and Almeida Lima, undertook a series of animal and human experiments in 1926, out of which grew the early techniques of cerebral angiography. His initial presentation of this work was at the Société de Neurologie in Paris on July 7, 1927, where he described two series of patients (2).

The first six patients, all chronically ill with diagnoses of general paralysis of the insane, post-encephalitic parkinsonism, or brain tumors, were injected directly into the internal carotid artery with a 70% solution of strontium bromide. Mechanical problems with coordination of the injection and the radiographic exposure resulted in no images with contrast being obtained in the first five patients. A Horner's syndrome from perivascular extravasation of contrast developed in two patients, and a transient aphasia developed in one patient. As part of the surgical exposure of the carotid artery in the sixth patient, the internal carotid artery was ligated for 2 minutes to better synchronize the contrast bolus with the radiographic exposure. A successful series of four angiographic images was obtained on this patient, a 48-year-old post-encephalitic parkinsonian. Ironically, the images demonstrated a thromboembolic complication of the procedure with progressive occlusion of the anterior circulation. The unnamed patient died 8 hours later.

The second series of three patients, injected with 22–25% sodium iodide solution, had fewer complications. Successful images were obtained in the third patient, a 20-year-old man with a diagnosis of a hypophyseal tumor causing a Frölich-Babinski syndrome. The angiographic images demonstrated mass-effect with displacement of the anterior cerebral artery and middle cerebral artery by the tumor. It was the capacity of this imaging technique to demonstrate the effects of tumors and masses in the intracranial cavity that would become the prime focus of clinical neuroangiography for the following decades.

Although the original presentation by Moniz has many aspects that appear quaint by modern standards—the unregulated toleration of severe complications, the absence of any reference to consent by the patients involved, and the cursory investigation of toxicity of the contrast agents used—the body of work that he presented in 1927 is an impressive testimony to his inventive mind. His calculations of the concentration of agent necessary for visibility on film, allowing for dilution by the rapidly flowing blood of the internal carotid artery, were soundly based on a similar series of experiments performed on animals and cadavers. Out of a total of nine patients, he had successfully obtained useful angiographic images on only two, one set of which demonstrated a fatal complication of the procedure. Nevertheless, he was aware that some of the failures of the initial experiments lay with the x-ray equipment that was available to him, exposures of 0.25-sec duration, being too long for his purposes. He immediately foresaw the future potential of cerebral angiography for tumor characterization using stereoscopic exposures and rapid-sequence cinematographically recorded injections. His paper also shows his ability to learn quickly from mistakes and his early acknowledgment of the need for technical improvements aimed at image quality and patient safety.

THOROTRAST

Between 1927 and 1931, Moniz continued to use sodium iodide in solutions of 25–30%. In 1931, he switched to

Thorotrast, a 25% colloidal solution of thorium 232 dioxide. Despite escalating qualms over the safety of Thorotrast, this agent continued in worldwide radiologic use until after World War II, as a local or systemic contrast agent that could be imaged in virtually every body cavity. However, its use in the 1930s for cerebral angiography was associated with a high rate of thrombotic complications in the brain, as high as 60% in post-mortem surgical cases (3). Local perivascular extravasation of Thorotrast in the neck was a common problem with abscess or granuloma formation after the procedure (Figs. 1.1, 1.2). For those patients who survived the procedure, Thorotrast became an albatross around their necks in later life. Procedure-related morbidity and mortality continued to follow some of these patients for years (Figs. 1.3, 1.4, 1.5). Thorotrast, an -particle emitter with a physical half-life of 1.41×10^{10} years and a biologic half-life of 500 years (4), was sequestered particularly by the marrow, spleen, and liver. High rates of malignant complications ensued in these target

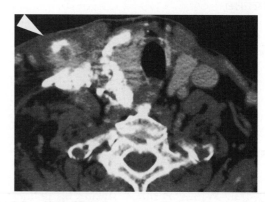

Figure 1.2. Neck CT of the same patient as Figure 1.1 (obtained on a previous admission). High attenuation Thorotrast has dissected through the soft tissue planes of the neck and was evident in the upper mediastinum on lower images (not shown). The patient's cutaneous sinus was at approximately the level marked by the arrowhead.

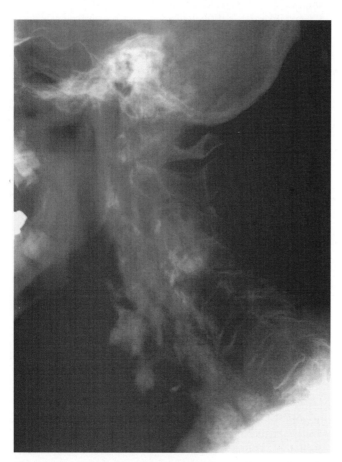

Figure 1.1. Lateral neck radiograph of a 74-year-old man who underwent carotid angiography with Thorotrast in 1946 for investigation of headaches. No specific diagnosis was made at that time. The procedure was complicated by extravasation of Thorotrast around the right carotid artery. Since that time, he has had recurrent problems with a chronically draining sinus on the right side of his neck and has had chemotherapy for lymphoma. The patient's presentation 50 years after the initial angiogram was related to a sentinel bleed from his neck sinus. The bleeding was witnessed only by the patient, but was described as being sufficient to soak a large towel with blood.

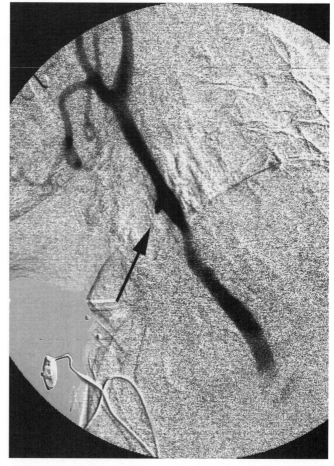

Figure 1.3. Right common carotid artery arteriography in the lateral plane demonstrates a pseudoaneurysm **(arrow)** of the common carotid artery below the bifurcation, close to the sinus tract. There is prominent subtraction artifact over the artery due to the density of the thorotrast.

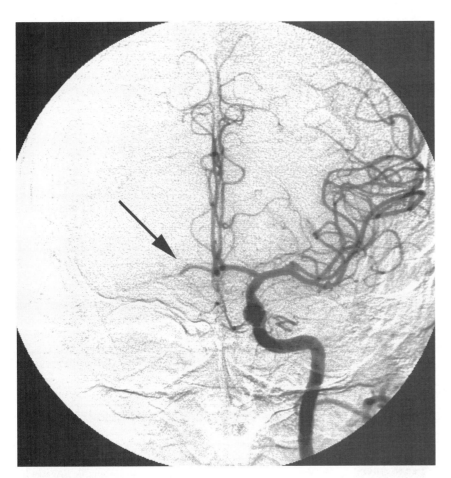

Figure 1.4. Left common carotid arteriography demonstrates prompt cross-filling to the right anterior cerebral artery circulation via the anterior communicating artery. Additionally, the A1 segment on the right **(arrow)** is robust, indicating a capacity to supply the middle cerebral artery circulation on the right via collateral flow.

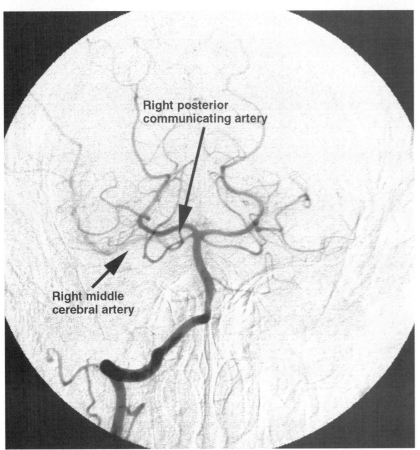

Right posterior
communicating artery

Right middle
cerebral artery

Figure 1.5. A shallow Townes projection of the right vertebral artery injection. The right posterior communicating artery is moderate in size and opacifies the right middle cerebral artery territory. Due to previous surgical scarring and induration around the sinus, surgical repair of the artery was not thought favorable. The patient tolerated emergency balloon occlusion of the right internal carotid artery and common carotid artery. He was discharged neurologically intact with no further bleeding from the site.

organs, as well as in the neck and mediastinum adjacent to the sites of extravasation, or where it was retained in body cavities, e.g., the paranasal sinuses. By the time its use was discontinued around 1950–54, it had been administered for a variety of radiologic procedures to tens of thousands of patients, possibly more than a million (5, 6). The fraction of these who had intravascular administration is not known.

Follow-up studies of Thorotrast patients from Denmark (7), Germany (8, 9), Portugal (10), Japan (11), and other countries indicate a high rate of delayed malignant disease attributable to this agent. Systemic administration of Thorotrast (15–40 ml for a typical cerebral study) has been estimated to cause a cumulative red marrow dose of 1.34–2.7 Gy (134–270 rads) or more. Subsequent malignancies particularly included tumors of the hepatobiliary system, which had a 200-fold increase in risk above baseline in the German study, and radiation-related leukemia (i.e., non-CLL types) (8) with a 10-fold increase in risk (4), in addition to other malignancies.

If the estimate of the number of patients placed at risk from Thorotrast administration is even remotely accurate, then the magnitude of this historical disaster becomes difficult to encompass. It is frequently said that until the mid-20th century, the practice of medicine killed more patients than it helped. Unfortunately, this may be true where the use of Thorotrast is concerned, and particularly so in reference to its use in neuroangiography. During the 1930s and 1940s, it is unlikely that a seriously ill patient could be cured based on information gathered from a neuroangiographic procedure alone.

From these inauspicious beginnings, the field of neuroangiography has endured. Although the standards of equipment, material, and radiographic technique are superior today than could have been foreseen in 1927, it nevertheless behoves us to bear in mind that the same overarching potential for disaster, as experienced by Moniz' patients, still exists today in every neuroangiographic procedure.

REFERENCES

1. Hascheck E, Lindenthal O. Ein Beitrag zur praktischen Verwethung der Photographie nach Röntgen. Wien Klin Wochenschr 1896;9(4):63–64.
2. Moniz E. L'encéphalographie artérielle, son importance dans la localisation des tumeurs cérébrales. Revue Neurologique 1927;2:72–90.
3. Eckström G, Lindren A. Gehirnschädingungen nach cerebraler Angiographie mit Thorotrast. Z für Neurochir 1938;4:227. Cited by Bonnal J, et Legré J. L'angiographie Cérébrale. Paris: Masson et Cie., 1958.
4. Andersson M, Carstensen B, Visfeldt J. Leukemia and other related hematological disorders among Danish patients exposed to Thorotrast. Radiation Res 1993;134:224–233.
5. Abbatt JD. History of the use and toxicity of Thorotrast. Environ Res 1979;18:6–12.
6. Falk H, Telles NC, Ishak KG, et al. Epidemiology of thorotrast-induced hepatic angiosarcoma in the United States. Environ Res 1979;18:65–73.
7. Andersson M, Storm HH. Cancer incidence among Danish Thorotrast-exposed Patients. J Natl Cancer Inst 1991;84:1318–1325.
8. Van Kaick G, Muth H, Kaul A, et al. Report on the German Thorotrast Study. Strahlentherapie 1986;80(suppl):114–118.
9. Van Kaick G, Wesch H, Luhrs H, et al. Neoplastic diseases induced by chronic alpha-irradiation-epidemiological, biophysical, and clinical results of the German Thorotrast study. J Rad Res (Tokyo) 1991;32 (suppl 2):20–33.
10. Da Silva Horta J, da Silva Horta ME, Cayolla de Motta L, et al. Malignancies in Portuguese thorotrast patients. Health Phys 1978;35:137–151.
11. Mori T, Kumatori T, Kato Y, et al. Present status of the medical study on thorotrast administered patients in Japan. Strahlentherapie (Sonderb) 1986;80(suppl):123–135.

CHAPTER 2

Performing a Cerebral or Spinal Arteriogram

REVIEWING PREVIOUS STUDIES

Before embarking on a cerebral or spinal angiogram, it is necessary to review all the relevant imaging studies available. Pertinent images should be mounted on a viewing box, preferably in the angiography suite, for inspection during the case. The importance of this prelusive step cannot be overemphasized. Prior review of the patient's studies will ensure familiarity with the particular clinical problem in hand and will help to avoid omissions during the study or confusion about laterality or location of the abnormality.

PATIENT EXAMINATION

In the course of obtaining consent from the patient, a focused neurologic examination by the neuroradiologist, documented in the patient's chart, is a worthwhile expenditure of 5 or 10 minutes. This examination should dwell on the patient's known or suspected neurologic deficits. It should also include a baseline evaluation of those functions most likely to deteriorate in the event of angiographic misadventure. Therefore, a quick evaluation of the patient's mental status, memory, orientation, language, visual fields and lower cranial nerve function, motor power, gait, and gross coordination should be *de rigueur* during all consent interviews. An adverse event in the course of an angiographic examination is rare. However, calls to the nursing floor to evaluate a patient with minor complaints of headache or apparent change in mental state after an angiogram are common and can be dealt with quickly for having previously documented the baseline condition of the patient. Such complaints are usually trivial in nature. However, a complaint of headache and a focal neurological deficit that may be new after a cerebral angiogram can evolve into a time-consuming process, which could have been avoided.

Similarly, baseline evaluation and marking of the peripheral pulses, using a Doppler device if necessary, will help to avoid unnecessary consumption of time afterwards. Prompt recognition of deterioration of a pulse can expedite a consultation with vascular surgery for suspected iliac or femoral artery dissection. On the other hand, a poor pulse obtained after an angiogram without a prior evaluation is an open-ended question.

Patients should remove all jewelry and dental prostheses before the case begins. Such devices, when left in place, have a way of projecting precisely on the area of abnormality, and their removal from the patient during the case, with a catheter already in the internal carotid or vertebral arteries, is not a benign or convenient interruption.

PLANNING THE ANGIOGRAPHIC STUDY

Having become acquainted with the patient and his/her medical status during the consent process, it is helpful while the patient is being prepared to plan how and in what order to study the cerebral vessels. By this advance consideration, a much improved study can be obtained. These technical improvements may be difficult to think of once the case gets under way, when one's mind becomes preoccupied with the techniques of vessel selection and catheter flushing.

Advance planning can help to avoid a multitude of problems in most aspects of a study. These include giving consideration to which side should be used for the arterial puncture, need for an arterial sheath, size of catheter and sheath system, type of contrast, and whether an aortic arch injection is necessary before selecting the great vessels. Familiarity with difficulties encountered by other angiographers in previous angiograms of a particular patient will help in making some of these decisions. For example, an agitated hemiplegic patient will undergo a safer test if:

- There is anticipation of the appropriate level of sedation or anesthesia to be used, including any need for airway protection or intubation.
- The arterial puncture is made on the plegic side so as to have the site of arterial repair on the side that will be least prone to motion during recovery.

Based on such considerations, it is possible to avoid previously encountered or otherwise predictable obstacles. Familiarity with any known history of carotid bifurcation disease will prompt extra caution in wire-manipulation while selecting the common carotid artery and will remind one to consider performing a run centered on the neck with the appropriate measuring devices in place.

The first vessel to be injected should be that most likely to demonstrate the suspected pathologic lesion. With this in mind a coin, ball-bearing, or other reference measurement device should be applied to the sides of the head or neck during preparation in anticipation of the first run. The filming rate may also be a factor to consider in advance, particularly if the abnormality in question is an arteriovenous malformation or other high-flow lesion. Moreover, advance planning will help to avoid omissions on the venous end of an injection such as using a field which is too confined or cutting off filming of the run prematurely. Try to think of what possible information the referring physician may need on a particular patient. For example, if the patient has a condition or tumor with a propensity to invade veins or dural sinuses, these structures must be visualized and evaluated in the course of the examination. Visualization of the jugular veins of the neck may require continuing the run longer than would seem intuitively obvious, particularly if an obstruction is segmental. Cut film technique should be remembered when a question of intracranial vasculitis has been raised in the clinical history.

Omission of an external carotid artery injection is a common oversight in cerebral angiographic studies. Most often, this short-falling only becomes apparent long after the study, when discussion of surgical options for an identified lesion turns to the alternative of external-to-internal bypass procedures. To avoid the retrospective embarrassment of having one's work so criticized, one should anticipate questions about the external carotid circulation where bypass procedures or the possibility of involvement of the external carotid artery with disease states might be considered:

- Occlusive diseases such as Moya-Moya disease, intracranial or extracranial dissections.
- Giant intracranial or otherwise inoperable aneurysms. A bypass procedure with subsequent surgical or endovascular occlusion of the parent vessel might be considered in certain difficult circumstances.
- Serpentine or dysplastic aneurysms of the middle cerebral artery.
- Cavernous aneurysms.
- Brain arteriovenous malformations when the AVM extends to the surface of the brain, and particularly when there has been prior infraction of the dura by a surgical procedure increasing the likelihood of dural-pial anastomoses.
- Dural vascular disease as a possible cause of subarachnoid hemorrhage. This should be considered particularly for patients with subarachnoid hemorrhage who have a higher likelihood of having incurred recent dural sinus thrombosis with recanalization and establishment of a dural arteriovenous malformation, e.g., post-partum subarachnoid hemorrhage.

CATHETERS, MEASUREMENTS, AND MATERIALS

Catheter outer diameters are measured in the French system, inner diameters are measured in inches, percutaneous needles are measured in a Gauge system, and embolization coils are measured in millimeters. There is not an easy way to correlate all of these measurement systems except to work consistently with a proven set of instruments. Generally, the disparity of the systems of mensuration in use is of little significance, but it is possible for practical problems to arise. One must avoid in particular the following situations:

Having punctured an artery with a small bore needle, one then discovers that the wire on the table is too large in caliber.

Having passed a wire successfully into the femoral ar-

tery, one might discover that the wire is too pliable to support passage of a dilator into a scarred groin-site.

One may spend hours trying to catheterize a particular vessel, only to realize that an embolic device will not fit through the hub or tip of the introducer catheter. Variability in manufacturing specifications for hand-made devices such as catheters is considerable. Coaxial insertion of a particular device might work well in one situation but fail in another. Therefore, testing the compatibility of devices before insertion into the patient is a good habit.

Catheter tips are tapered or untapered. Untapered catheters can be inserted only through a sheath. Catheters of 4 or 5 French size are the standard for diagnostic neuro-angiography. A 5 French cerebral catheter has an outer diameter (OD) of 0.066 inches, with an inner diameter (ID) up to .050 inches. Most 5 French catheters accept an 0.038'' guiding wire, but are usually so obturated by a wire of this size that continuous flushing of the catheter around the wire is not adequate. Some large ID 5 French catheters can be used for coaxial introduction of a microcatheter during a neurointerventional procedure. However, the inner lumen is usually so constrained by the coaxial device that injections of contrast through the remaining lumen of the catheter are suboptimal. Therefore a larger size guiding catheter, 6–9 French, is preferable in most instances for coaxial procedures.

For spinal diagnostic cases a series of 5.7 French spinal HS-1 and HS-2 catheters is available with inner diameters which accept an 0.025'' guide-wire. A recurved 5 French Mikaelsson catheter, available in variable lengths, is a little more difficult to use but can be an extremely effective spinal catheter for diagnostic or coaxial interventional cases. A 5.7 French Mikaelsson catheter with a fine, distal taper which takes an 0.025 guide wire, is also available for diagnostic spinal angiography. Spinal interventional cases requiring co-axial insertion of a microcatheter can be performed with a 6.5 French series of HS-1 or HS-2 spinal catheters, or with a 5 or 5.3 French Mikaelsson or Shepherd's Hook series of catheters.

The gauge system for measuring needle sizes can be simplified by remembering that the number refers to how many needles of that size, placed side by side, make an inch. For example, an 18G needle (the standard size for adults) measures 1/18'' in diameter. The only major caveat regarding needle size is that it is usually necessary to switch to a 19G needle for the arterial puncture when planning to use a 4 Fr catheter without a sheath. The needle puncture from an 18G will often cause excessive oozing of blood around a 4 Fr catheter during the case.

Catheters for cerebral angiography are made in a variety of pre-formed shapes and sizes. Most angiographers stick to a standard repertoire of 2 or 3 diagnostic catheters from the many available. The best catheter overall is probably the one with which one has greatest familiarity and practice. Difficult situations are usually most easily solved by working with one's standard catheter rather than one with an exotic unfamiliar curve. Catheters for cerebral angiography vary in length between 90 cm and 110 cm.

Guide-wires must therefore measure in the range of 145 cm−160 cm. A guide-wire of standard length for use below the diaphragm may not give enough wire for selecting difficult cranial vessels. Microcatheters usually measure approximately 150 cm and microwires 175 cm or longer.

Torquability or capacity to respond to steering by the angiographer is an imperative characteristic for cerebral catheters. This quality is achieved through braiding in the construction of the catheter and the use of proprietary polymers and blending techniques.

CONTRAST

Because of the expense of non-ionic contrast preparations, there is a strong and reasonable incentive to use ionic-type contrast in as many diagnostic examinations as possible. Nevertheless, non-ionic contrast is used exclusively, or almost so, in many hospitals for cerebral angiography. However, for diagnostic purposes the evidence in favor of using non-ionic preparations is marginal. Comparison studies between ionic and non-ionic preparations during cerebral angiography demonstrate a similar rate of neurological complications (1−7). Studies of systemic use of contrast, however, demonstrate that non-ionic preparations appear to be slightly safer and have a lower rate of allergic complications (8, 9).

Certainly non-ionic preparations should be used for neuroangiographic studies (10) in the setting of:

a previous history of contrast reaction
asthma
severe allergies
diabetes mellitus
sickle-cell anemia
renal impairment
cardiac failure
current condition, e.g. tumor or ischemic disease, which could involve a compromised blood-brain barrier and, therefore, a greater vulnerability to the higher neurotoxicity and osmolality of ionic agents (11)
anticipation of selective external carotid artery injections
spinal angiography
neurointerventional procedures

Non-ionic contrast agents are denominated according to the content of organic iodine per ml, e.g. Omnipaque® 300 contains 647 mg of iohexol/ml, equivalent to 300 mg of organic iodine per ml. Ionic contrast agents are denominated according to the weight per volume percentage of iodine-containing salt solution, e.g. Conray® 60 contains 60% iothalamate meglumine, 600 mg per ml, equivalent to 282 mg of organically bound iodine per ml.

An ionic preparation denominated 60 is therefore the approximate equivalent of a non-ionic preparation denominated 300 in terms of iodine concentration and vessel opacification. These two particular concentrations have been the standard for cerebral angiography for many years. The improved performance of modern image-intensifiers in digital imaging allows one to consider use of a

Table 2.1
Minimization of Contrast Load

The total dose of iodine needed for a particular cerebral angiogram can be reduced by 50% or more by using the following guidelines:

- Using lower strength contrast where possible, e.g., 200 strength non-ionic instead of 300 with a modern image intensifier system.
- Careful planning of injections and fields of view to avoid a need for repeated injections.
- Elimination of unnecessary runs, e.g., aortic arch injections require 30−50 cc of contrast for a diagnostic yield so low that an aortogram is usually not warranted as a routine part of a cerebral angiogram (12).
- Using contrast syringes on the table filled half-and-half with contrast and saline. Diluted contrast is adequately imaged on modern digital equipment to allow reduction of contrast used for catheter navigation and test-injections by 50%.
- Improving technique of road-map acquisition; most road-map systems respond better to a smaller volume staccato-burst of contrast (3 cc−5 cc) than to a slow 10 cc infusion. A shorter roadmap acquisition will also eliminate artifact from respiratory motion.
- Minimizing use of hand-injections for unnecessary road-maps. For instance, it is usually possible to navigate vessels from the aortic arch in young patients without using road-maps.
- Preloading the dead-space of the catheter system with half-strength contrast and then pushing it with saline for roadmap acquisition. This technique is important in children and patients with renal failure where use of road-mapping should be kept to a minimum (or avoided completely), due to the burden of additional contrast which it adds to the study.
- Aspirating contrast from the dead-space of the catheter system at the completion of each run before resuming flush. This and the previous measure can save 4−5 cc of contrast per injection, which can make a critical difference in a child during a study with multiple injections.

lower concentration of contrast for cerebral angiography. Ionic 43% preparations or non-ionic 180−200 preparations provide adequate vessel opacification on modern machines, with the advantage of a lower iodine total dose and a lower osmolality challenge to the blood-brain barrier (see Tables 2.1 and 2.2). Lower strength contrast has the additional advantage of a lower viscosity compared with preparations of higher concentration. This is a factor for consideration in microcatheter injections either by hand or by power-injector. With 0.018″ microcatheters, and particularly with 0.010″ microcatheters, there is a discernible difference between contrast preparations in the ease of bolus delivery during digital runs.

It is important to remember to switch to 300 or 60% preparations when performing cut-film studies. Generally, lower strength contrast is not adequate for cut-film angiography. However, it is more important still to recall that contrast strengths above those of ionic 60% or non-ionic 320 are contraindicated in cerebral angiography. See Table 2.2 for calculation of maximum tolerable dose of contrast in a well-hydrated patient.

ARTERIAL PUNCTURE AND SHEATH PLACEMENT

The arterial puncture must be made with a view to hemostasis after completion of the study. Therefore, the angle

Table 2.2
Commonly Used Contrast Agents for Cerebral Angiography

Name	Solution (mg/ml)	Osmolality (mOsmol/kg water)[a]	Viscosity (centipoise at 37 C)[b]	Iodine Content (mgI/ml)
Conray® 43 iothalamate meglumine	430	1,000	2	202
Conray® 60 iothalamate meglumine	600	1,400	4	282
Hypaque® 60 diatrizoate meglumine	600	1,415	4.12	282
Isovue® 200 iopamidol	408	413	2.0	200
Isovue® 300 iopamidol	612	524	4.7	300
Omnipaque® 180 iohexol	388	408	2.0	180
Omnipaque® 300 iohexol	647	672	6.3	300
Optiray® 240 ioversol	509	502	3.0	240
Optiray® 300 ioversol	636	651	5.5	300

Formula: Maximum Tolerable Contrast Dose

$$\frac{\text{Weight kg} \times 5}{\text{Serum Creatinine mg/dL}} = \text{tolerable volume of 300 non-ionic contrast (or equivalent)}$$

Example: A 75-kg adult patient who is well hydrated with a serum creatinine of 1.5 mg/dL would tolerate an approximate total dose of 250 ml of ionic 60% or non-ionic 300 preparations, equivalent to 70.5 g and 75 g of iodine respectively. If using the lower concentrations of 43% or ionic 200 preparations, these equivalent doses calculate to an allowable volume of 349 ml and 375 ml respectively. These volumes assume that the patient is adequately hydrated and that no other prevailing medical condition is present. The total volume may be extended in cases where the entire duration of contrast administration is prolonged over many hours such as during an interventional procedure. This formula functions as a useful rule of thumb, but probably errs on the conservative side. In adult patients with normal renal function, total doses of non-ionic 300 contrast between 400 and 800 ml are frequently used in long interventional cases with no adverse effect (13). The pharmacokinetics of intravascular contrast materials are described as having an -phase (distribution) and an   half-life of approximately 30 minutes, and a   phase (elimination) with a   half-life of 1.5±2 hours in a patient with normal renal function and adequate hydration. Therefore, after 2 hours in a patient with normal renal function about half of the contrast administered will have been excreted allowing a commensurate recalculation of the maximum tolerable dose. In the setting of renal impairment the   half-life becomes prolonged up to days in duration.

[a] Normal human plasma osmolality = 282±295 mOsm/kg water.

[b] Viscosity of water is approximately 1 centipoise (cp) and that of static human blood at 37 C is about 3.5 cp.

of insertion of the 18G needle is approximately a 45 angle to the skin in a line on a plane with the direction of the artery and in a site which allows compression against a bone afterwards. The easiest site is at the common femoral artery on the right side (Figure 2.1). The most critical procedure in gaining access to the artery is the passing of the wire, which runs the risk of intimal or medial dissection. Therefore, a wire with a J-curve may be the safest. Consideration must be given to the size of wire required. For instance, some smaller sheaths come with a prepackaged 0.025″ wire. This is usually adequate to give support to the dilator of a sheath. However in a patient with copious tissue or scarring in the groin, such a slight wire will not support a dilator or catheter as it advances. Without being able to pass even a small dilator over such a thin wire, it cannot then be exchanged for a stiffer wire without losing arterial access. Where such difficulties are anticipated the wire of choice to support insertion of a sheath should be at least an 0.035″. Where the arterial puncture is being made through an arterial graft of prosthetic material, an even stiffer wire such as an 0.038″ Amplatz wire should be inserted initially (see Table 2.3).

Wiping the wire clean of blood and clot between successive passes of the dilators, the arterial site is progressively dilated to allow smooth passage of the sheath dilator/obturator and finally of the sheath itself (Figures 2.2, 2.3). The sheath is hooked up to flush, the dilator is removed with the wire, and the sheath is sutured or otherwise secured in position (Figure 2.4). If a tapered catheter is

Table 2.3
When to Consider a Sheath

For a small expense in time incurred in setting up a second flush-line, inserting and suturing a sheath in place, the advantage gained can make the difference between a smooth completion of a study and an impossible struggle. It should be considered at any time during a study when severe difficulties are being encountered or unacceptable oozing at the arterial site is developing. Placement of a sheath at such a stage is more of an interruption to the study and therefore prospective placement of a sheath can be well worthwhile, particularly in the following circumstances:

- Any patient in whom previous technical difficulties were encountered during angiography especially with vessel selection
- Any patient with multiple previous angiograms or any other reason to suspect scarring in the groin
- Where catheter exchanges are anticipated
- Elderly (65 years), chronically hypertensive, or other patients with suspected or known atherosclerotic disease
- With vascular prosthetic grafts sheaths are imperative lest the graft tear the catheter during manipulation
- Anticoagulated patients in whom one may leave the sheath in place temporarily
- Intraoperative studies, axillary punctures, or other circumstances where one anticipates working under cramped or restricted physical circumstances

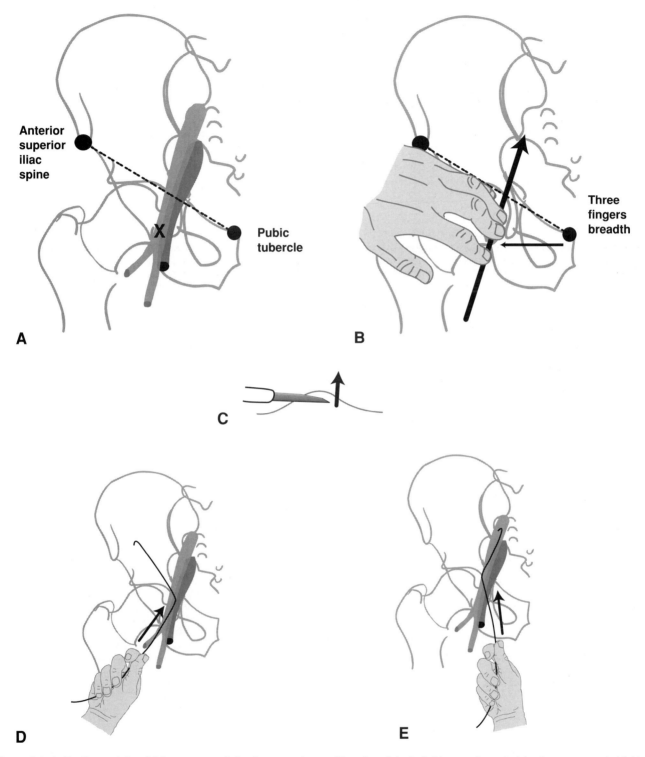

Figure 2.1. A–E *Femoral Arterial Puncture.* A line between the anterior superior iliac spine and the pubic tubercle corresponds with the inguinal ligament **(A)**. In an adult patient a puncture site 3 finger-breadths below this line along the pulse of the artery provides a useful guide **(arrow in B)**. From here, a needle thrust at 45° towards the umbilicus will usually find a lie in a position suitable for compression against bone after the case (x in A). When making a skin incision in a very thin patient or child, it is possible to nick the underlying artery.

Therefore, it is desirable to make an incision into a suspended fold of skin with the sharp edge of the blade pointed up **(C)**. Among the diffi-culties encountered in passing a wire retrogradely into the femoral artery is the possibility of selecting the circumflex iliac artery **(D)**. With a J-wire this problem can be circumvented by counterintuitively direct-ing the wire towards the offending artery. The J-curve against the arterial wall will bounce the wire medially and up towards the external iliac artery **(E)**.

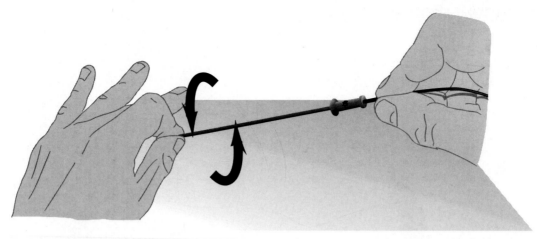

Figure 2.2. *Dilator Advancement.* Advancing a dilator, catheter, or sheath should be a smooth process requiring a minimum of tension. For larger sheaths it is advisable to prepare the artery with successive passes of smaller caliber dilators. A dilator or catheter can be passed less traumatically by spinning the device in an anticlockwise fashion as one advances slowly. The assisting hand is holding the wire with a degree of tension sufficient to straighten it but not withdraw it from the body. It is helpful for this hand to hold the wire away from drapes and tubings which might impair the spinning motion of the advancing hand. When using a shorter wire, such as those prepackaged with the sheath, it is vitally important for the assisting hand to follow the hub of the dilator towards the groin once the artery has been entered. If not, there is a strong risk of the sharp dilator advancing over the wire into the iliac artery and perforating the vessel.

Figure 2.3. *Wire Straightening.* Mandrel wires can be straightened by gripping tightly and stretching the wire. This can be done by using the 4th and 5th digits to fix the wire tightly against the palm and extending the thumb and forefinger. Dots indicate points of pressure. Alternatively, interweaving the wire-shaft between the 3rd and 4th can improve traction.

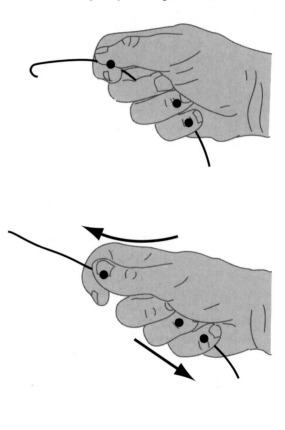

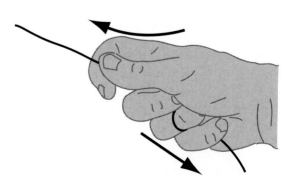

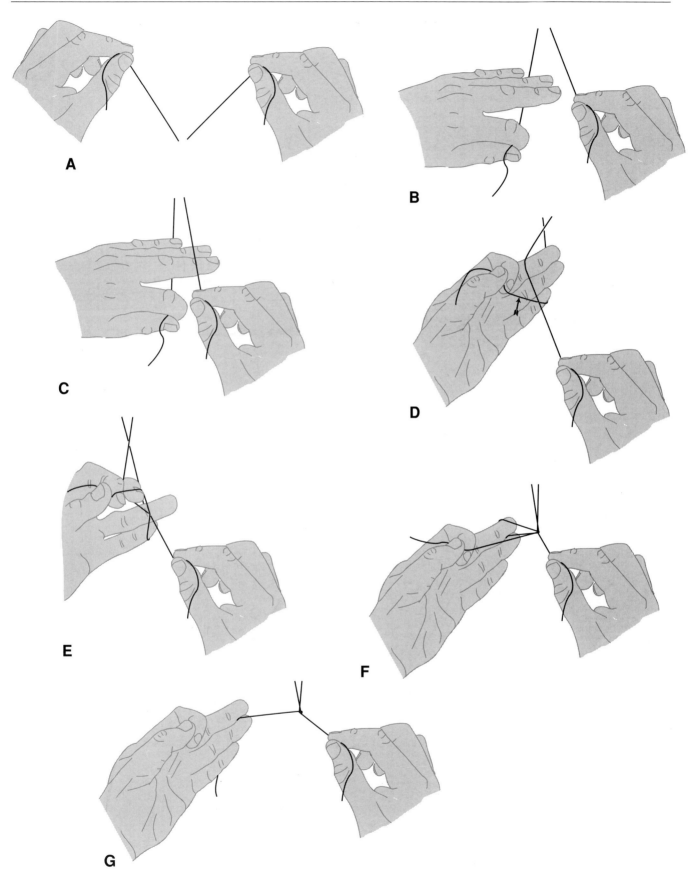

Figure 2.4. *Single Hand Suture.* A silk suture to secure the sheath in place should be inserted in such a fashion as to eliminate play of the sheath within the artery during manipulation of the catheter. A loose sheath working back and forth within the lumen has a greater probability of dissecting the intima or expanding the arteriotomy site with bleeding around the sheath.

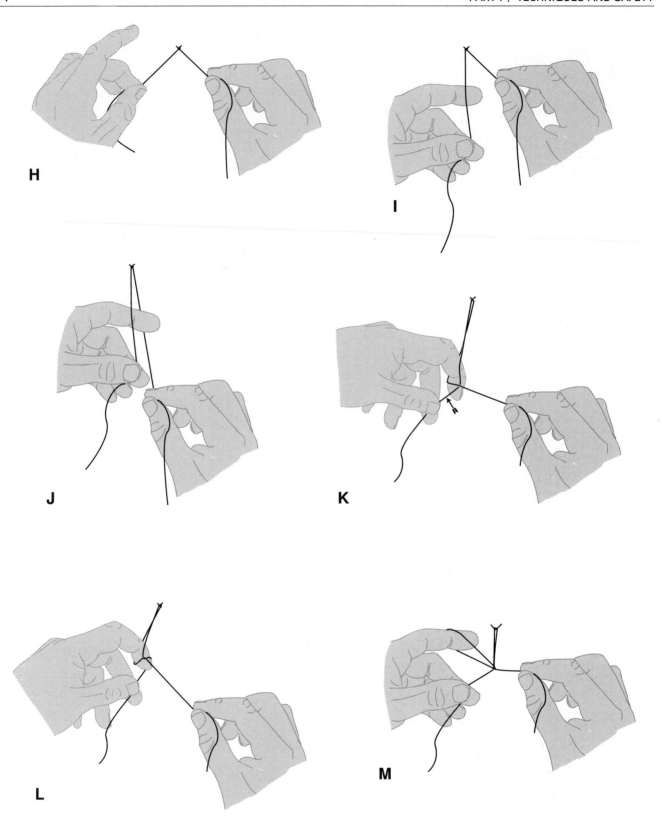

Figure 2.4. *(continued)*

being passed directly into the arterial site, the same procedure is followed, except that a 5 Fr catheter does not usually require prior dilation of the arterial site, unless scarring is present. In both instances—passage of the sheath and catheter—the arterial site is wiped clean of accumulated clot prior to passage of the tip to prevent intrusion of thrombus into the arterial tree or into the tip of the catheter. While passing the catheter or dilator a spinning motion of the advancing hand helps to twist the device into the artery smoothly and minimizes trauma to the arterial wall. Slight tension on the wire provided by an assistant helps this passage.

Difficulty with passing a dilator or sheath over the wire should prompt a pause to evaluate the tip of the device lest it should have become damaged during the attempted insertion. Examine the tip carefully. It is common to find that the plastic sheath fitted over the dilator has developed a small tear or irregularity which would possibly lacerate the vessel wall if it were forced through the arterial puncture site.

AORTIC ARCH NAVIGATION

With the tip of wire leading, the catheter is advanced from the groin to the descending thoracic aorta. The wire is removed and wiped clean. In the majority of patients a J-wire or any curved wire will advance all the way from the groin to the aortic-arch without fluoroscopic monitoring in the pelvis and abdomen. If difficulties are anticipated, or if the patient has known atherosclerotic or aortic aneurysmal disease, then it is safer to monitor the progress of the wire. When particular difficulties are encountered in the iliac arteries or if they appear noticeably tortuous, it

may be a good idea to insert a longer sheath, e.g. 24'' length, to straighten out the vascular route between the groin and the aortic arch. Similarly, when navigating a catheter in the arch one may notice an absence of corresponding motion between the catheter tip on the fluoroscopic image and one's hands. This usually means that the catheter has become wrung, and most often the site of kinking is at the groin or in the tortuous iliac arteries (Figure 2.5). Great care is needed at this point to unwring the catheter slightly and withdraw it partially from the body until the damaged section is out. Then a wire can be passed to secure arterial access and a long sheath inserted.

After the catheter has been placed in the descending aorta and the wire removed, the catheter is aspirated vigorously to clear bubbles, clots, and thrombogenic debris collected as it traversed the subcutaneous tissues of the groin. The catheter is then placed on continuous heparinized flush. For the first clearing of the catheter after insertion, a more forceful pursuit of surprisingly tenacious bubbles within the catheter is prudent. The hydrostatic pressure transmitted down the catheter from the aortic arch which allows back-bleeding to occur is frequently not adequate to overcome the adhesive qualities of clots and bubbles in the catheter. An assertive tapping of one's finger on the catheter-hub and particularly at junctions such as stopcocks etc. will often evoke an otherwise undetected shower of bubbles from the catheter. This is most common after the initial insertion of a new catheter but can be seen with surprising frequency during the case after wire-removal or other manipulations.

Once positioned in the proximal descending aorta, the angiographer rotates the catheter until the tip is facing

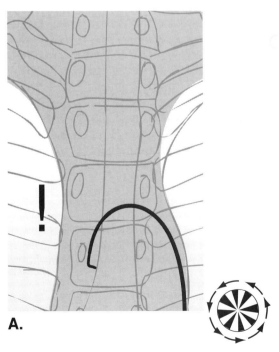

A.

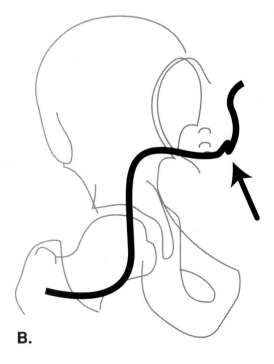

B.

Figure 2.5. *Catheter in the Aorta is not Responding: Danger of Catheter Kinking.* The catheter-tip is not responding to repeated torquing motions at the groin **(A).** Check for backflow and kinking. Beware

of the danger of tearing the catheter or femoral artery when a tight kink **(arrow)** is present. Remove the catheter over a wire and place a long sheath to straighten out the iliac system.

Figure 2.6. *Catheter Manipulation.* The catheter is steered at the groin-site by the left hand. The remainder of the catheter is kept straight outside the body to reduce counter-torque. The right hand is used to make the outside catheter move in unison with the inside catheter. The motion of the left hand should be a fine, delicate spinning motion between thumb and forefinger. It is not performed by flexion/extension of the wrist or elbow. It should be executed with the finesse suited to trying to pick a lock rather than the force used to turn the ignition-key of a car.

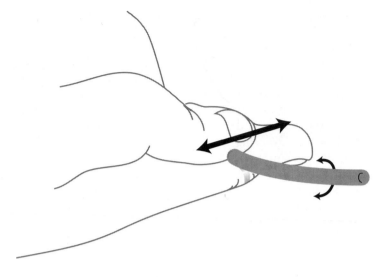

anteriorly towards the image intensifier, and the catheter is advanced over the aortic arch (Figures 2.6, 2.7). A position facing anteriorly translates into an inferior direction as the catheter is advanced over the arch. The catheter responds best to anti-clockwise rotation by a delicate, smooth spinning with the left hand at the skin entrance, and with the right hand moving in synchrony at the catheter-hub. The outwardly visible catheter should be kept straight to eliminate accumulation of counter-torque outside the body and to prevent any inadvertent jumps of the wire inside the body when the catheter is advanced.

Having traversed the aortic arch with the catheter-tip pointing down, the major vessels are selected by gently dragging the catheter back with the tip pointed up. With the tip of the catheter pointing towards the patient's head, it is pulled back until a small flick indicates that the brachiocephalic artery is engaged (Figure 2.8).

CATHETER FLUSHING

Catheters can be flushed either by using a continuous irrigation system, a variety of which are available, or by intermittently double-flushing the catheter with syringes every 90 seconds. When using the double-flush syringe method, it is important that the entire length of the catheter be aspirated vigorously with the first syringe, the contents of which are then discarded, before clearing the catheter forwards with fresh heparinized saline.

Using any of the systems for continuous irrigation with heparinized saline helps to free one's mind and hands from the responsibility of keeping the catheter clear of blood and allows one to concentrate on other aspects of the study. However, if not thoroughly cleared of air-bubbles before the procedure and vigilantly monitored during the procedure, the supposed safety of continuous irrigation may become an illusion. Misused or neglected continuous flush systems have the potential for great calamity. There are different systems of tubing and adapters available for providing a constant stream of heparinized flush

(4,000–6,000 units/L) using either a pressurized bag or an electronically driven pump. Depending on how these connect to the catheter it may be possible using a hemostatic valve on a Y-adapter or manifold to continue the flush while the wire is being manipulated (Figures 2.9, 2.10, 2.11, 2.12). This system has theoretical advantages over a system where flow of flush must be interrupted to allow insertion of the wire.

There are significant risks inherent to use of a continuous irrigation system:

Firstly, all systems of continuous irrigation carry a risk of complication if one fails to resume flow after each hand-injection or run by neglecting to reopen the stopcock immediately. A generous rate of flow of flush (150cc–200cc minimum per hour) is imperative, bearing in mind that a typical catheter may have a total volume of 4–5 cc. With blood refluxed back to the valve, it will take at least 60 drops or 240 microdrops in a drip-chamber system to clear the catheter thoroughly from proximal to distal end. This does not make allowance for laminar flow with stasis of dependent blood in the catheter.

When using a pressurized bag system, the rate of forward flow is very finely balanced between one which allows adequate irrigation and one which generates a turbulent jet in the chamber, allowing bubbles to enter the tubing. Furthermore, it is easy to intuitively overestimate the actual volume of saline being advanced per minute when using a microdrop system. When acquainting oneself with such a system, it is useful to prime the tubing with saline and allow it to run at what one perceives as an adequate rate. Then attach a dry catheter to the system. The duration of time before one sees saline emerge from the catheter tip is usually surprisingly long and represents the same time that stagnant blood will sit in the catheter after each wire-exchange at that rate of flush.

With a Tuohy-Borst valve system which allows continued flow of flush during wire manipulation, it is important to realize that the rate of forward flow will be compromised by insertion of a wire into a standard catheter. Back-flow

1. Tip is pointing posteriorly. Movement is discordant.

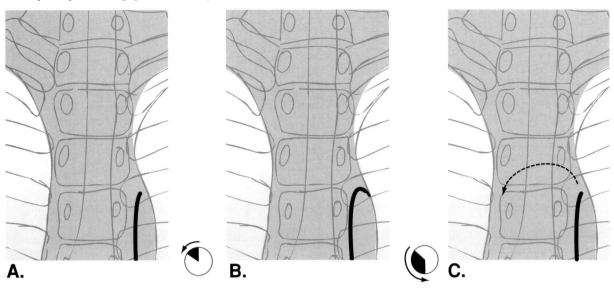

2. Tip is pointing anteriorly. Movement is concordant.

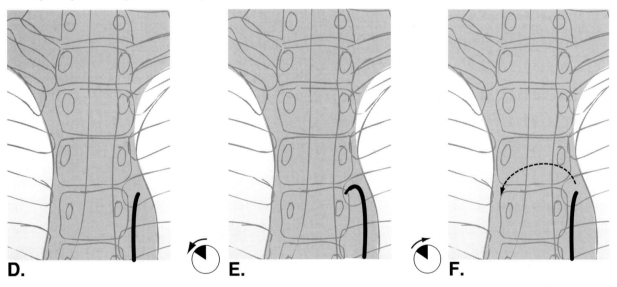

Figure 2.7. A–F *Turning the Catheter Anteriorly in the Aorta.* To minimize the time that one has an obturating wire within the catheter, it is preferable to steer the catheter, if possible, to the brachiocephalic artery and select its ostium before using a wire. Most aortas will allow a hockey-stick or curved catheter to cross smoothly. To do this the tip of the catheter needs to avoid being selected on the way over by the left subclavian and left common carotid arteries. By starting in the descending aorta with the catheter-tip pointed anteriorly and pushing straight in, the catheter will sweep across the arch with the tip pointed down.

Because the fluoroscopic image is two dimensional, it can be difficult to discern whether the tip is pointing anteriorly or posteriorly. By forming a hypothesis or assumption about the position of a randomly placed catheter and testing that assumption with an anticlockwise motion, the true position of the catheter can be perceived, and a correction applied.

1. The catheter tip position is unknown. Assume that it is facing anteriorly **(A).** A 30 ±45 anticlockwise spin causes the tip to elongate towards the patient's left **(B),** which is discordant with an anterior position. Therefore, the tip was in fact facing posteriorly. The anticlockwise motion is then continued until a 180 turn from the original position is achieved **(C).** The catheter is then pushed over the arch.

2. The catheter tip position is unknown. Assume that it is facing anteriorly **(D).** An anticlockwise spin evokes elongation of the tip to the patient's right, concordant with an anterior position **(E).** Reverse the applied spin to regain an anterior position **(F)** and push the catheter over.

The same logic is used to achieve a posteriorly directed catheter-position when performing spinal angiography.

Figure 2.8. A–D *Selecting the Great Vessels: Establishing a Stable Catheter Address in the Left Common Carotid Artery.* **(A)** The catheter is advanced over the aortic arch by keeping the tip pointed inferiorly. This avoids trauma to the intima of the arch, and it prevents the catheter tip from becoming trapped by vessel ostia on the way over. **(B)** A 180° spin of the catheter in the ascending arch places the tip in a vertical upright position. The catheter is gently pulled back. Usually this motion will select the brachiocephalic artery with a discernible jump and straightening of the catheter, except in the most difficult circumstances. **(C)** Pulling back from the brachiocephalic artery in a precisely vertical tip position will often cause the catheter to jump past the left common carotid artery and into the left subclavian artery. To avoid this problem, as one pulls back the catheter from the brachiocephalic artery, spin the catheter 15–30° anticlockwise to make it point slightly anteriorly. This will select the anteriorly disposed left common carotid artery more effectively. **(D)** To stabilize the catheter in this position while one prepares the wire, it is necessary to reverse the spin to the vertical position. Apply the same measure of clockwise spin to point the catheter directly into the artery and to maintain its purchase on this vessel.

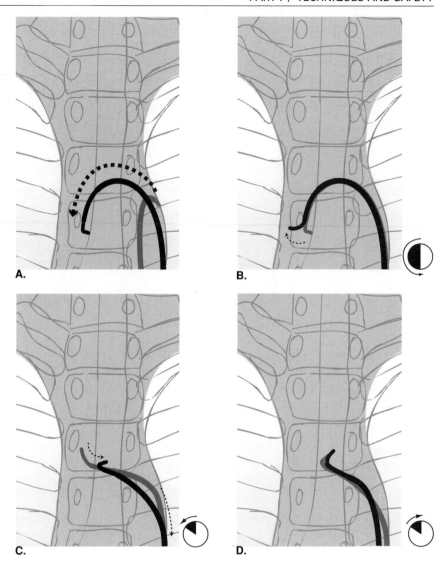

A.

B.

C.

D.

Figure 2.9. A–H *Priming a Flush Line with a Pressure-Bag System.* **(A)** A liter bag of fluid from which all residual gas has been removed and to which 4,000 to 6,000 units of heparin has been added is prepared. The chamber of the pressure-line is plugged into the bag. The distal clamp of the pressure-line, i.e. the end on the sterile field, is tightly closed. **(B)** The line is pinched tightly by an assistant, and the chamber is squeezed to allow inflow from the bag to fill the chamber about one third of capacity **(C)**. **(D)** When the bubbles from the inside of the chamber have all been flicked away from the inner surface of the chamber, the hand pinching the line lets go slowly. Fluid will advance into the proximal part of the line from the chamber. Without having pinched the line before filling the chamber, pinching the chamber would cause a back-and-forth movement of bubbles within the line which would make a bubble-free column of fluid difficult to attain.

(E) With a clear, bubble-free column of fluid in the proximal part

of the line, pressure is smoothly inflated into the bag to 300 mm Hg. This must be done with sufficient speed to allow timely completion of the task but not so fast that a jet of turbulent bubbles is generated in the chamber **(G)**. This would cause bubbles to advance into the tubing. Inflation causes the air within the chamber to be compressed. A minimal volume of air is necessary to allow visualization of the drip within the chamber. Therefore it is necessary not to overfill the chamber with fluid before the compression. Hence the recommendation for filling the chamber to only a third of its volume in B.

(F) The distal control-clamp of the pressure-tubing (on the sterile field) is used to advance air followed by the column of fluid all the way through the system. The line is rechecked carefully for bubbles. The control clamp must be moved to check beneath for hidden bubbles **(H)**. The line must be pinched distally to allow this. All bubbles must be flicked forward to the end of the line.

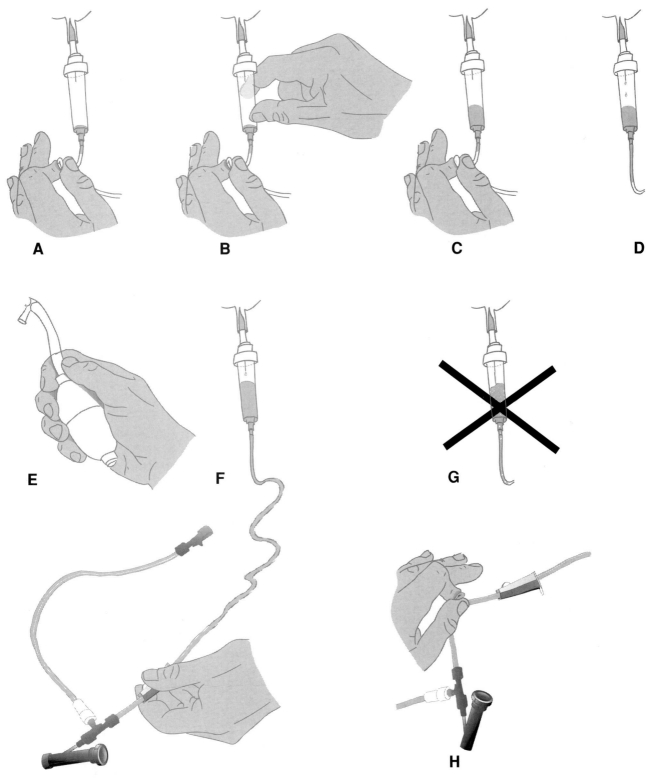

Figure 2.9. *(continued)*   If a bubble is adherent to the tubing along its mid-section or near the chamber, it is often very difficult and tedious to clear it by flicking the tubing all the way to the end. Rather, it is easier to clear the whole tubing anew by:
- establishing a moderately brisk rate of flow in the tubing,
- Having an assistant suspend the chamber upside down to allow 2±3 cm of air to enter the tubing and then let it down carefully. This

clean column of air with the pursuing meniscus will clear all the microbubbles along the tubing.
- Before the new column of air hits the control clampÐhaving less viscosity than flush, this air will rush through the clamp generating turbulence in the chamberÐpinch the tubing distally, pull the clamp back proximal to the column of air, reclamp tightly, and then resume flow.

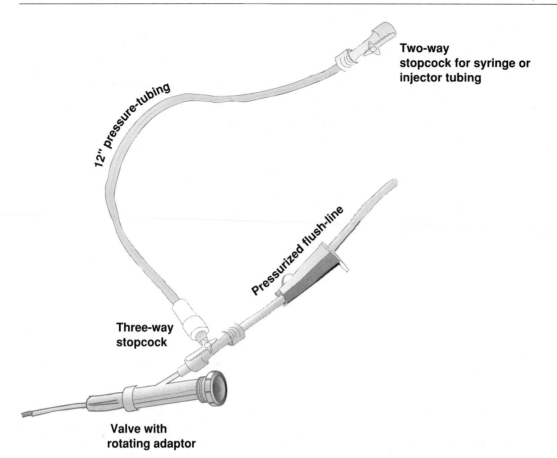

Two-way stopcock for syringe or injector tubing

12″ pressure-tubing

Pressurized flush-line

Three-way stopcock

Valve with rotating adaptor

Figure 2.10. *Y-valve Set-up for Continuous Flush.* A commonly used system for continuous irrigation of flush is illustrated. A pressurized flush line enters a Tuohy-Borst Y-adapter via a 3 way stopcock. The other hub of the 3 way stopcock can be used to attach syringes directly, but it is much more convenient to attach a short, flexible pressure-line. In this way the catheter is unlikely to be disturbed by motion at the hub when attaching syringes etc. A two-way stopcock at the end of the 12″ side-arm can be added to provide a convenient site for attaching syringes or the tubing from the power-injector.

A rotating adapter at the site of attachment of the system to the catheter assures that the catheter can pivot independently of the tubing system. This avoids disturbance of the catheter by tension in the tubing.

Figure 2.11. *Clear All Bubbles from the Tubing Carefully.* The Y-adapter and side-arm must be vigorously cleared of bubbles before the case starts. This can be done by flushing vigorously with a 20 ml syringe before attaching the pressure line, and by then tapping for residual bubbles while a brisk rate of flow runs.

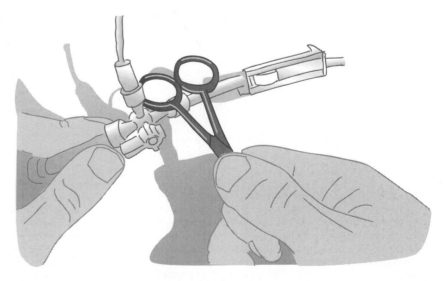

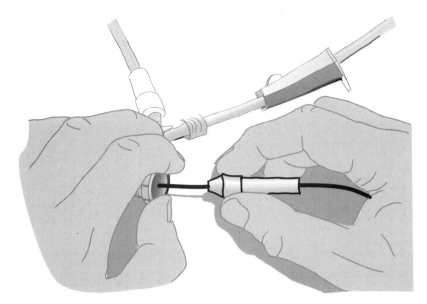

Figure 2.12. *Torque Device Position.* For most precise control of the wire, the torque device should be close to the hub of the valve. If not controlled from this position, torque applied to the wire is typically expended as a slewing of the wire outside the catheter with unpredictable transmission of movement to the wire-tip. During wire manipulation the valve is sufficiently tight that backbleeding from the catheter does not occur. In this manner, flush continues to be directed into the catheter around the wire.

of blood into the catheter to the level of the adapter is inevitable when one opens the valve to insert a wire or other device. Insertion of an obturating wire into the blood filled catheter worsens the stagnation and increases the risk of thrombus formation. To prevent this from happening, allow the catheter to flush ahead of the wire by halting the advance of the wire before it obturates the catheter and by tightening the hemostatic valve. A few seconds of pause is observed to allow a column of fresh flush to precede the wire into the catheter (Figures 2.13). Then as the wire is being advanced the valve is adjusted to allow sealed manipulation of the wire while diverting flush into the catheter.

Leaving the hemostatic valve inadvertently unsealed after removing the wire poses the risk of air being withdrawn into the system while a syringe or injector are being attached, and a large bolus of air could be injected intracerebrally by an inattentive hand. For this reason a check of the valve is a mandatory automatic component of the routine whenever a syringe or injector are being attached and drawn back.

Constant vigilance by the operators and assistant staff towards the catheter flush line is necessary to avoid inadvertent closure of the flush-line after arteriographic runs or hand-injections. Electronic pumps carry the advantage of allowing an automatic alarm system to sound when the flush is turned off. Systems operated by pressure bags can be manually adjusted and evaluated at a glance more easily by the angiographer, but without an alarm system they have to be monitored all the more closely. A flash-light trained on the drip-chamber is a useful aid. The pressure gauge should be monitored intermittently during the case to detect spontaneous deflation of the pressure bag.

An additional safety note with reference to the pressure-bag system is necessary. Most plastic saline bags have 10–20 cc of air within when supplied from the manufacturer. This air should be evacuated from the bag via a needle at the time of insertion of heparin. The reason for this is that the gravitationally dependent saline contents of the bag may expend during the course of a long case, and, if undetected, the residual volume of air may then be forced into the flush line with the potential for causing a massive air-embolism. The prefatory aspiration of air from the bag and insertion of heparin should be done using a needle not larger than a 19G or 20G. A hole in the rubber seal of the bag larger than this size frequently leaks when pressurized to 300 mm Hg.

Meticulous table-technique in all aspects of syringe handling is necessary to avoid generation or introduction of bubbles into the catheter (Figures 2.14, 2.15, 2.16, 2.17). Backflow of blood into the catheter and stasis during wire-manipulation should be minimized (Figure 2.18, 2.19, 2.20, 2.21, 2.22).

HEPARIN AND PROTAMINE SULPHATE REVERSAL

When systemic heparinization is used during a diagnostic or interventional procedure, the effectiveness of the dose can be most easily monitored by checking the activated coagulation time (ACT) with a Hemochron System (International Technidyne Corp., Edison, NJ) in the angiography suite. An ACT level of 1.5 to 2.5 times the baseline value is desired (14). Usually, a heparin bolus of 3,000 to 5,000 units (60 U/kg) is used for adults. The ACT is then checked 5–10 minutes later. For long cases, checking of the ACT and hourly maintenance doses of heparin are necessary. Heparinization is commonly used as a routine precaution in children during transfemoral neuroangiographic procedures to reduce the likelihood of arterial occlusion at the puncture site.

When immediate reversal of heparinization is required at the end of the procedure, a dose of protamine sulphate delivered carefully over 10 minutes can be given. The dose can be calculated as 10 mg of protamine sulphate per 1,000 units of active heparin still circulating, using 1.5–2 hours

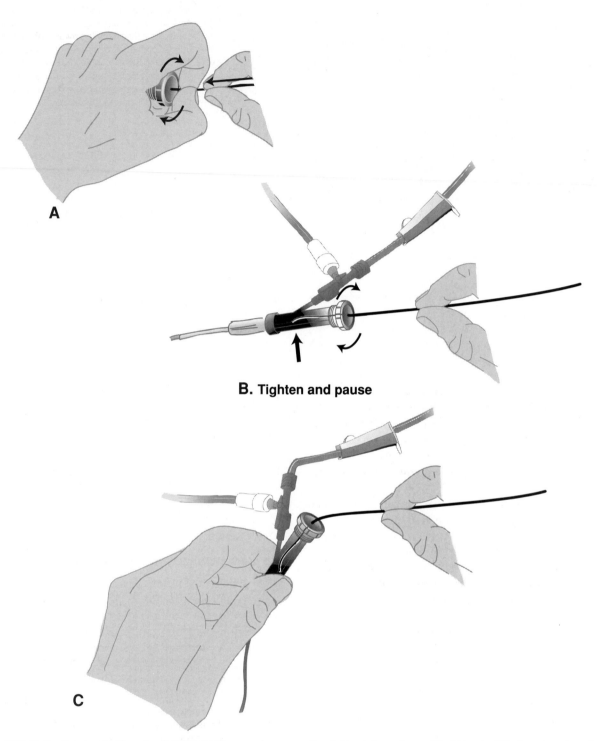

Figure 2.13. A–C *Pausing to Allow the Catheter to Clear.* Insertion of a wire or coaxial microcatheter through the valve is inevitably going to allow some backbleeding into the catheter and adapter **(A).** To promote clearing of the catheter before advancing the wire, seal the valve when the wire-tip is inside the adapter **(arrow in B).** This allows diversion of all flush into the catheter ahead of the wire.

Gravitational dependence **(C)** of blood within the adapter can be used to clear the backwater area of the adapter too.

Notice that the stopcock is inadvertently illustrated in the closed position. If one chooses to use a flush-system that does not have an electronic alarm-system, checking the status of the flush line at the chamber has to be a continuous task throughout the case.

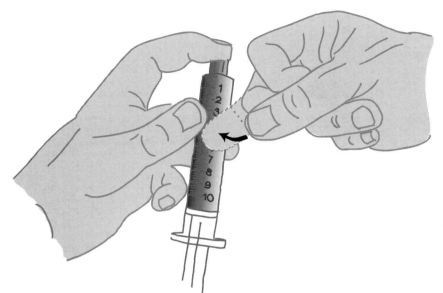

Figure 2.14. *Clearing Bubbles from Syringe to Avoid Eye-Splashes.* After filling the syringe with contrast smoothly so as not to generate bubbles, remaining air must be tapped to the top of the syringe and expelled by advancing the meniscus. To prevent eye-splashing, the syringe tip should be covered as illustrated. This allows one to be forceful in one's efforts to eliminate all bubbles.

as an approximate half-life of heparin. The ACT can be rechecked prior to removal of the arterial sheath to assure correction of coagulation.

CATHETER POSITIONING

Fluid dynamics at the interaction of the jet of contrast emerging from the catheter tip with the flow patterns of the catheterized vessel have an important bearing on some of the risks of angiography (Figures 2.23, 2.24). The patterns of flow in the major cranial vessels may dwell on a spectrum between a state of near laminar flow on one end and various degrees of disturbed flow approaching turbulence on the other (16, 17). These patterns depend on the contour of bifurcations, turns of adjacent vessels, the presence of stenotic lesions, or the distance from the aorta. For the purposes of an angiographic study the injected bolus of contrast needs to disturb the laminar pattern of flow in the vessel enough to opacify the lumen and its territory completely. To accomplish this necessary dispersion of contrast within the vessel lumen, i.e. to prevent slipstreaming of the contrast, the velocity of flow from the catheter must significantly exceed that in the vessel. Furthermore, the streamlines of the catheter jet distal to the catheter tip must be divergent (18).

A simple formula can calculate the average velocity (U) of contrast exiting the catheter tip:

$$U_{average} = \frac{Q}{R^2}$$

where Q is the volume of injection per second and R is the radius of the catheter at its exit. However, flow within the catheter, as in any long cylindrical tube, has a parabolic velocity gradient whereby peripheral flow is slower than that at the center. Mabon et al. (18) have taken the peak velocity at the center of the catheter lumen to approach $2U_{average}$. With a catheter of a 4 to 6 French size commonly used in diagnostic neuroangiography, $U_{average}$ may exceed 900 cm–1,200 cm/sec for an 8–10 ml/sec injection. The shear forces on the intimal wall generated by a jet of this magnitude depend greatly on the angle of incidence. They also depend strongly on the distance between the catheter tip and the wall of the vessel. Mabon et al. (18) calculated that with the catheter direction parallel to the axis of the flow within the vessel, injection rates of this magnitude are theoretically capable of producing shear stresses of 2,000 dynes/cm² over a 2 cm segment of vessel wall and more focal mural shear stresses as high as 5,000 dynes/cm². For comparison, reference ranges of normal physiologic stress are approximately 50 dynes/cm². Animal data indicate that high velocity flow over periods as short as one hour with shear stresses of approximately 380 dynes/cm² can produce intimal cell loss, cellular fragmentation, and endothelial stripping of the aorta of dogs (19).

Given these experimental results, it is clear that considerable care is necessary in catheter positioning in reference to the curvature of the vessel. Extreme care is necessary in situations where a number of injections in a single vessel might be anticipated when interrogating a particular lesion. The shear stress on the vessel wall from a standard injection rate may be sufficient to dislodge atheromatous plaques from the walls, causing distal emboli. Injection sites should therefore be selected away from any atheromatous irregularity seen on the roadmap images. Similarly, vulnerability of the intima to shear forces may be amplified by the presence of wire-related or catheter-induced spasm, and a tiny intimal tear could then be aggravated to a full-blown dissection by an immediately adjacent injection.

In order to minimize trauma to the intima of the catheterized vessel, it is desirable to position the catheter so that its distal curve conforms to that of a similar curve in the surrounding vessel. This avoids a situation in which an injection might be made directly against an intimal wall

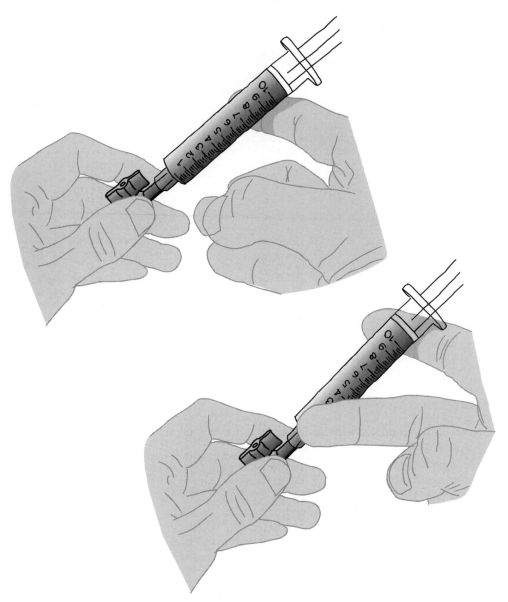

Figure 2.15. *Tap Vigorously to Remove Trapped Bubbles.* After attaching a syringe, meniscus to meniscus, the region of the hub is tapped vigorously to remove adherent bubbles. Notice that the 2 way stopcock is open to allow backflow. Backflow is important to indicate that there is not occlusion of the catheter tip. Active backflow also improves one's sensitivity to hidden bubbles. Bubbles adherent to the inner surface of the syringe should also be cleared.

where the considerable kinetic force of the jet is transformed to pressure. Although there are theoretical data which imply that shear forces on the intima may be less with an injection perpendicular to the intima rather than parallel, the risks of a subintimal injection argue against such considerations. Usually the common carotid artery in adults is sufficiently capacious that concern about catheter-positioning is less acute than during more selective injections. In the internal carotid artery and vertebral artery such positioning is important.

Depending on the size and appearance of the vertebral artery, two catheter positions are used most commonly. A low position at C6 prior to the vessel entering the foramen transversarium has the advantage of minimizing wire or catheter manipulation within this critical vessel. A high position at C2, at the laterally directed curve of the artery, favors a compatibility between the shape of the catheter and the 90° lateral turn of the vessel. Furthermore, an injection at this higher level has a greater chance of refluxing the contralateral vertebral artery to opacify the contralateral posterior inferior cerebellar artery. If successful, this obviates the need to select the contralateral vertebral artery. It also offers the theoretical advantage of performing an injection distal to the site of potential origin of the artery of cervical enlargement (anterior spinal artery), the argument being that an angiographic occlusion of the vertebral artery in the high cervical region is likely to be less damaging if supply to the anterior spinal artery

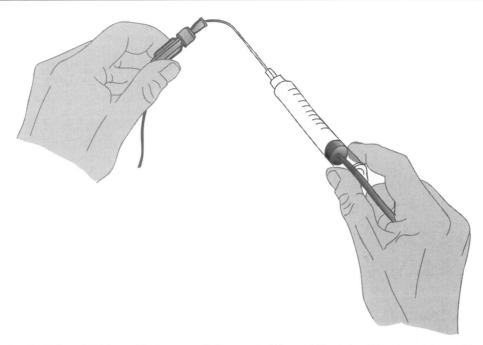

Figure 2.16. *Clearing the Hub and Raising a Meniscus.* Before attaching a syringe or tubing to a catheter or stopcock, all bubbles and blood should be cleared thoroughly. A flush-syringe with a dilator stump or I.V. catheter can be used effectively for this purpose.

is maintained. When the vertebral artery is extremely tortuous, hypoplastic, or otherwise unfavorable in appearance for catheterization, a very proximal engagement, if possible, of the vessel origin with just the tip of the catheter and a long, slow injection with a 1 second rise will be more effective in opacification than a subclavian artery injection.

In the internal carotid artery, a position of the catheter at the lower edge of C2 is usually most favorable. Alternatively, any position where the catheter-curve conforms itself to the cervical loop(s) of the artery can be used. When making repeated injections in a single vessel, it may be prudent to shift the catheter position slightly between runs, the better to disperse the effect of maximal intimal stresses over a larger area.

A linear rise of the injection rate between 0.2 ml and 1 ml over the first second is probably also a worthwhile routine precaution for all injections to minimize the effects of shear on the intima. It will introduce the jet of contrast as a crescendo rather than as a staccato, and will allow some relatively gradual displacement of the catheter away from an adjacent intimal surface before the full force of the jet is introduced. It also attenuates any whipping effect on the catheter which might displace it from a tenuous position, such as a proximally engaged vertebral artery.

A theoretical source of intimal damage during catheter injections in the major cranial vessels is the Venturi effect, by which the contrast-jet may cause infolding or collapse of the arterial walls distal to the catheter tip. Doumanian and Amplatz (20) described this phenomenon at high injection-rates in dogs where collapse of the vessel-wall was so severe that the jet of fluid sliced the infolded vessel wall.

With clinical injection rates, particularly in adult veins or occasionally in the pliable arteries of children, this phenomenon is seen in a more benign form. Because of the high rate of inflow from the aorta to the major cranial vessels, this phenomenon is unlikely to be seen during cerebral angiography. However, it could become a factor if blood-flow were dampened proximally, such as might happen if one were to catheterize a vessel distal to a critical stenosis or if the catheter were to become clamped by a focus of concentric mural spasm.

DO NOT ADVANCE THE CATHETER ALL THE WAY TO THE WIRE-TIP

An intimal dissection most likely is initiated by the tip of a wire being inadvertently forced into a subintimal position. This is probably more likely to occur if the catheter tip is pushed almost to the end of the wire, causing the wire-tip to lose its flexibility. If the catheter is then pushed over the end of the embedded wire, a small intimal tear will be amplified into a dissection.

Therefore, always allow the distal wire to retain its flexibility by keeping the catheter-position short.

CHECKING CATHETER POSITION

Immediately after selecting a vessel, particularly a critical vessel such as the internal carotid or vertebral arteries, the wire is removed carefully. Attention during wire-withdrawal is directed initially to the catheter tip and assuring that withdrawal of the wire does not have a detrimental effect on the catheter position. A bobbing motion in time with the cardiac cycle transmitted from the aortic arch

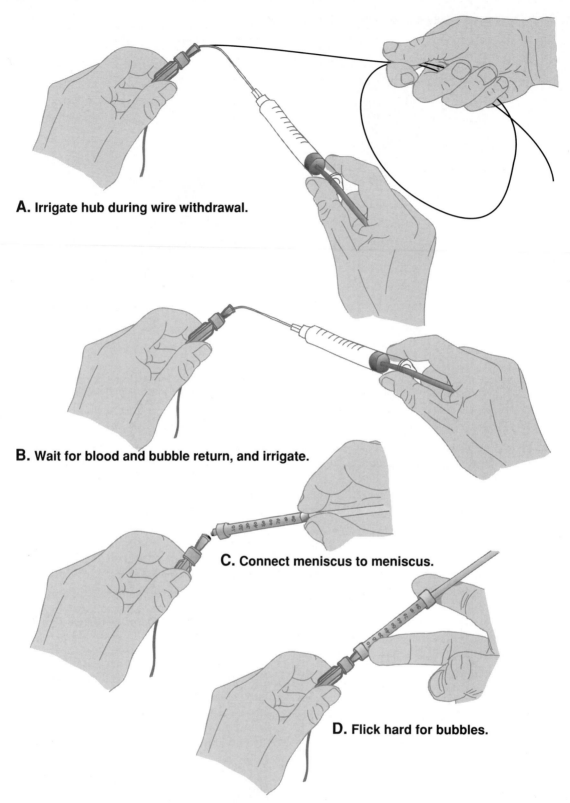

A. Irrigate hub during wire withdrawal.

B. Wait for blood and bubble return, and irrigate.

C. Connect meniscus to meniscus.

D. Flick hard for bubbles.

Figure 2.17. A–D *Microcatheter Clearing.* **(A)** As one withdraws a wire from a microcatheter, there is a negative pressure generated within which causes implosive generation of bubbles within the lumen around the wire. Furthermore, air may be suctioned into the microcatheter from the hub. One can see this happen; as the wire is withdrawn, the fluid meniscus drops and disappears. To minimize this effect and to keep the inside of the microcatheter wet with heparinized flush, the meniscus in the hub is replenished by a stream of flush from a syringe with a stump of a dilator or angiocatheter attached. This also helps to clean the wire, which is wiped by the assistant's left hand (not illustrated here) as it is withdrawn.

(B) When the wire is out, wait for blood and bubble return and irrigate until it appears that no more bubbles are returning. If no return is seen, the microcatheter may need to be withdrawn slightly or suction with a syringe until one sees free-flowing blood. If these maneuvers are not immediately successful, the microcatheter should be assumed to be clotted or kinked, both very perilous events. The microcatheter should be removed immediately.

(C) Connect the syringe to the hub, meniscus to meniscus, and flick hard **(D)** for bubbles before injecting.

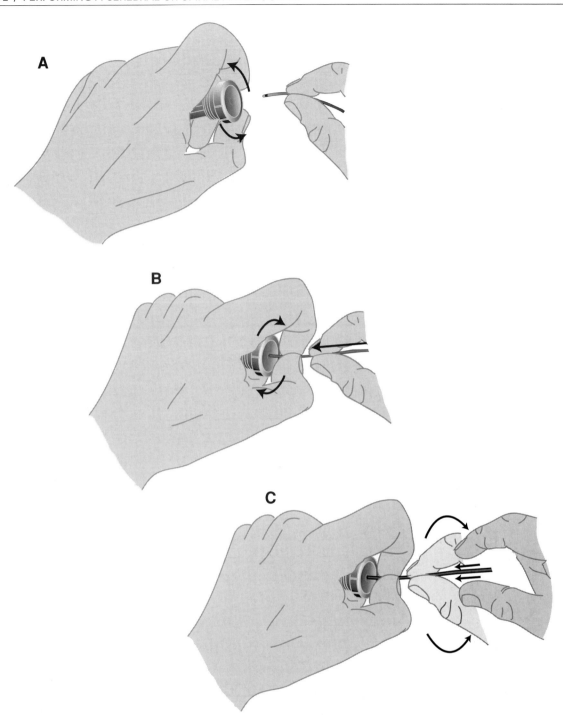

Figure 2.18. A–C *Coaxial Insertion of Micro Device or Wire through the Tuohy-Borst Valve.* Slippery hydrophilic wires and microcatheters can be difficult to insert into a Tuohy-Borst valve. It is necessary to perform this motion quickly and with minimal opening of the valve, so as to reduce backflow into the catheter and blood loss. **(A)** The Y-adapter is cradled firmly by the higher digits and heel of the left hand. In one motion the left thumb and fore-finger begin to loosen the valve, while the right hand presents the wire or microcatheter tip to the valve and presses it right into the valve. In this fashion, the wire-tip will slip through the valve as soon as enough space is available. Upon witnessing this, the left hand begins to retighten the valve **(B)** by using the volar surfaces of the proximal thumb and forefinger in a rotational motion, while the palmar surfaces of the thumb and forefinger more distally clamp the microcatheter. After tightening the valve, pause to clear the catheter.

Therefore, the process effectively becomes one of the right hand feeding the microcatheter to the left hand, with passage into the valve being secondary. The reason for this is that hydrophilic wires, balloons, microcatheters etc. which are wet become very difficult to control and will slip back and forth within the valve, unless the left hand pinions them in position while the pushing right hand readjusts itself **(C).**

If one is advancing a microcatheter in this fashion without a supporting microwire within, it is very important that the assistant should be injecting flush into the hub of the microcatheter all the while, to keep it from becoming clotted with blood during this process.

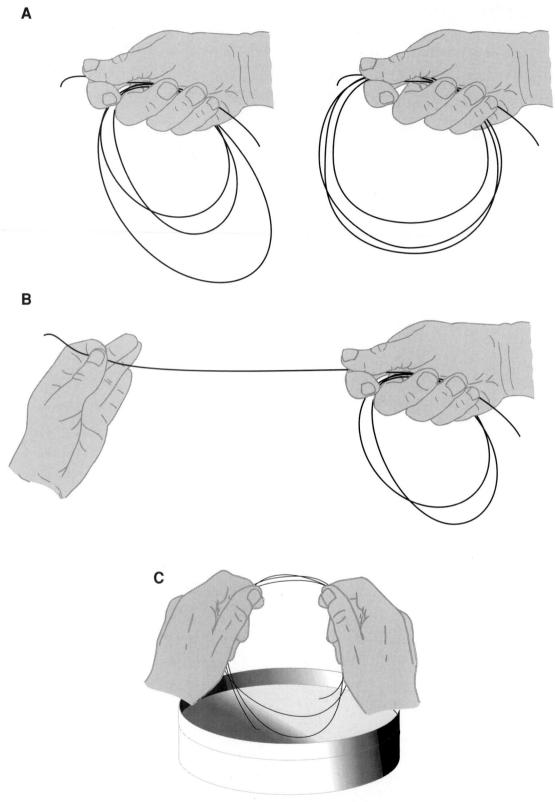

A

B

C

Figure 2.19. A–C *Wire Handling.* Tense wires and microwires can be difficult to control with one hand. The right hand must function as both a reservoir for redundant loops and as a dispenser for paying out wire loop-by-loop. With a little practice, this becomes easy to manage. The right hand functions as two units **(A):**

    1. thumb and forefinger,
    2. higher digits and palm.

One unit must always keep control of the redundant set of loops. Therefore, as the higher digits open to release or gather a loop, the thumb and forefinger must be closed around the coils.

(C) To keep control over the wire, it may be placed under a towel or, in the case of hydrophilic wires, in a basin of flush. To prevent a loop from springing free and becoming contaminated, keep a two-handed grip on the loops and slide them into the basin. It is preferable to always place the wire in the same position, e.g. running clockwise to the torque-handle which is placed at 2 o'clock in the basin. In this fashion, removal of the wire from the basin is a more predictable process.

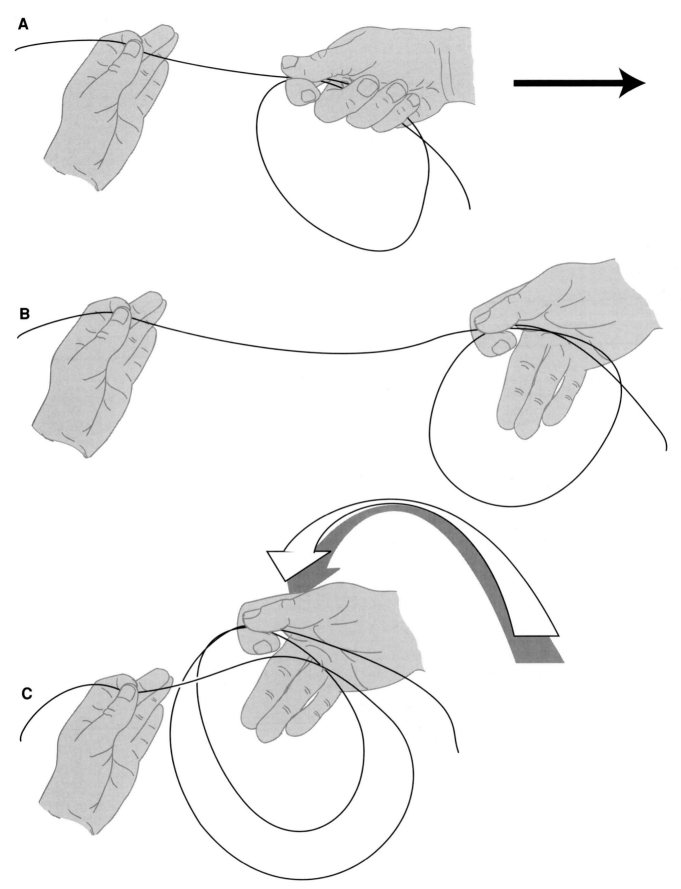

Figure 2.20. A–C *Wire Withdrawal.* The trick to controlling a wire as one gathers its loops is to use the thumb and forefinger of the right hand to keep the loops under control **(B)** while the higher digits open to receive a new loop. The sweep must be away from oneself, collecting the new loop on the returning part of the arc.

Figure 2.21. *Microwire Shaping.* Microwires can be shaped easily by dragging the tip across one's finger under pressure of a shaping rod. The pressure needed for this is extremely light. Overshaped microwires are very difficult to straighten. The radius of curvature of the induced shape is related to the length of wire drawn over the rod and to the force applied.

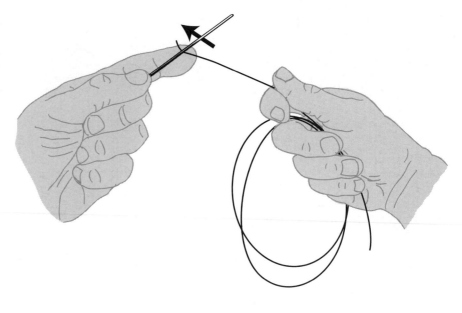

Figure 2.22. *Make a Plane from the Palmar Regions of the Fingers.* By limiting degrees of freedom of small objects, such as balloons or microcoils, one's control over them, e.g. when threading a delicate device, is much improved. By confining them to a working plane devised from the higher digits, manipulation becomes infinitely more controllable.

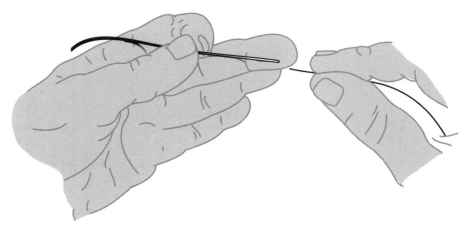

along the catheter indicates that it has not become wedged in a vessel turn or area of spasm (Figures 2.25, 2.26, 2.27). Attention during the latter part of the wire-withdrawal is focused on the fluid meniscus in the hub of the catheter or fluid behavior in the Y-adapter. A suctioning of fluid into the catheter or a sucking sound as the wire emerges indicates the presence of a vacuum in the catheter because the catheter tip is against the arterial wall or clamped by tight spasm. Although one's immediate reflex, on hearing this sinister sound, is to pull down the catheter, it is vitally important to *turn off the continuous flush line first,* particularly if the hemostatic valve is tight. Otherwise upon resumption of flow when the catheter-tip is free, the pressurized flush will push the generated bubbles in the catheter into the artery. After switching off the flush, slowly pull down the catheter, checking under fluoroscopy if necessary to monitor the catheter-tip, until back-flow is seen at the catheter hub. Suction the catheter to remove remaining air and resume flush.

If the wire has been removed uneventfully from the catheter, the routine is to backbleed the catheter for approximately 5–10 seconds while tapping vigorously for

bubbles, and then resume forward flush by tightening the hemostatic valve or reopening the flush line of the manifold. Before hooking up to the injector for a run, recheck the catheter position and check for spasm. This is best done with a subtracted mask on which small hand-injections can be made to test flow in the vessel and to confirm that the catheter curve still conforms to the artery.

Before doing an angiographic run of any of the cranial vessels, it is very important to assess run-off first (Figures 2.28, 2.29). This avoids the dangers of injecting into a vessel which is atretic distally, e.g. a vertebral artery ending in a posterior inferior cerebellar artery, or injecting into a vessel with a dissection, critical aneurysm, or pseudoaneurysm in which a standard injection-rate could conceivably exacerbate the problem. Alternatively, a vessel feeding a vascular malformation may need a higher rate of flow.

After positioning for the run and checking run-off, the catheter is connected to the injector. This is tightly sealed and checked carefully for bubbles with assertive tapping of the junction points as the assistant draws back until blood emerges freely from the catheter without bubbles. This is then pushed forward to clear the catheter and to prime it

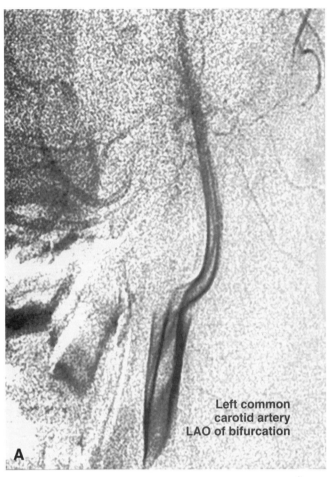

Left common
carotid artery
LAO of bifurcation

Figure 2.23. A–B *Streaming of Flow.*   **(A)** A left common carotid artery demonstrates how the slow trickle of contrast at the end of the injection opacifies the streaming vortices of flow around the common carotid bifurcation.

(B) A lateral view of a basilar artery aneurysm demonstrates a lucent circumferential layer within the aneurysm and within the upper basilar artery (arrows). This represents the unmixed blood from the non-injected vertebral artery. This also extends into the right posterior communicating artery (arrowheads), enlarged in this 64-year-old female with a right frontal arteriovenous malformation (not shown).

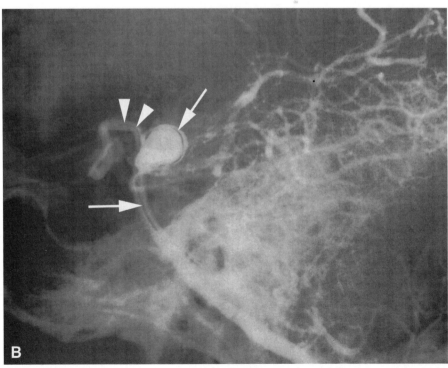

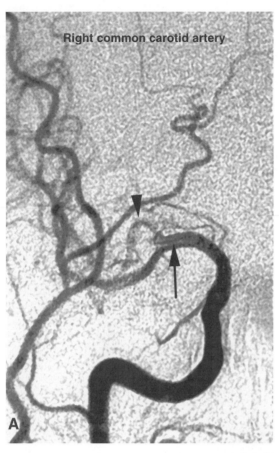

Right common carotid artery

A

Figure 2.24. A–B **(A)** A right common carotid artery injection shows streaming of unopacified blood in the main stem of the right middle cerebral artery (arrow) with poor opacification of the superiorly directed branch (arrowhead). Notice that the timing of the external carotid artery circulation is ahead of the internal carotid artery, another reflection of a hemodynamic problem.

(B) The left common carotid artery injection in the same patient gives a complementary view wherein the lucent streaming in the right middle cerebral artery now derives from the unopacified right carotid inflow.

Conclusion: there is an unusual hemodynamic phenomenon present causing the left internal carotid artery to provide more flow to the right hemisphere than the right internal carotid artery. Therefore, even without knowing that this patient had a critical right internal carotid artery stenosis (off screen), one could deduce the presence of such an obstruction to flow. This deduction is corroborated by the appearance of the external carotid artery in A. Catheter induced spasm or a dissection could give the same hemodynamic appearance.

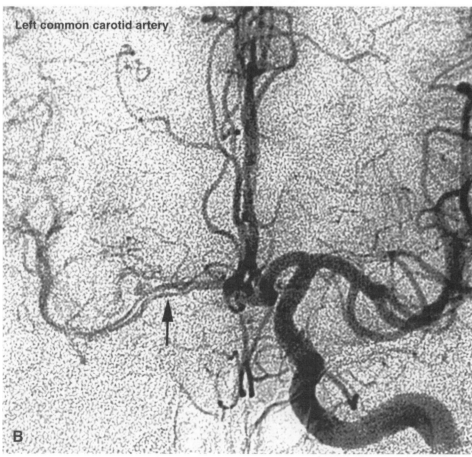

Left common carotid artery

B

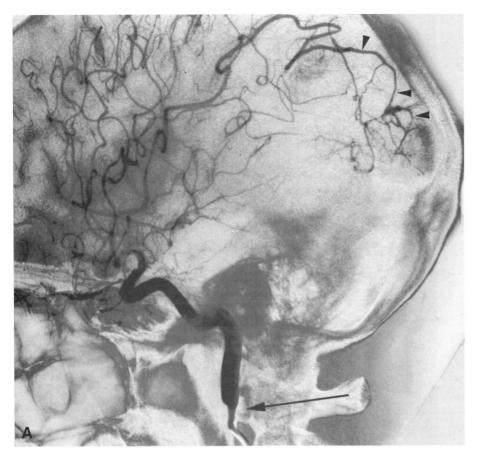

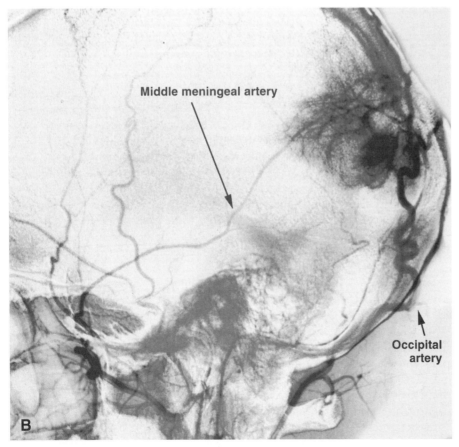

Figure 2.25. A, B *Hemodynamic Effects of Catheter Induced Vasospasm during Evaluation of Extra-axial Hemangiopericytoma.* A right internal carotid artery injection lateral plane **(A)** in a 34 year old patient with a hemangiopericytoma of the right occipital region. There is spasm around the catheter tip (arrow). An image in the late arterial phase demonstrates a stagnant column of contrast in the cervicalÐcavernous internal carotid artery. One may deduce the observation of stagnation from the fact that the main stems of the anterior cerebral artery and middle cerebral artery ipsilaterally are being washed out (diluted) through collateral channels. A branch of the middle cerebral artery has been parasitized by the tumor **(arrowheads).** This tumor has a vascular pattern more disorganized and irregular than vascular meningiomas, better seen through opacification of the occipital artery and middle meningeal artery in the external carotid artery injection **(B).**

Figure 2.26. *Hemodynamic Effects of Catheter-Induced Arterial Spasm.* A left internal carotid artery injection inadvertently performed in the presence of moderately severe spasm. The hemodynamic effects of spasm are evident in the appearance of prominent reflux into the external carotid artery branches. Moreover, the A1 segment is poorly opacified even though it appears to be of robust proportions. This represents a hemodynamic effect, not an occlusion of the A1 segment. Bi-directional flow can be confirmed by looking at sequential images.

This is potentially significant as an event such as this could prevent visualization of an aneurysm of the anterior communicating artery complex, particularly if the spasm were relieved by the time the contralateral carotid artery was studied.

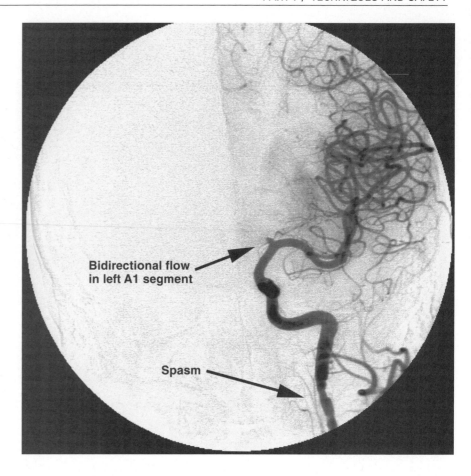

with contrast. With microcatheters, or when the guiding-catheter is in a small vessel, it is better not to have the assistant draw back towards the power-injector after the hook-up. This will induce spasm or occlude the catheter. In these circumstances have the assistant maintain forward flow during and after the hook-up. Clear, audible instructions must therefore be communicated at all times to the assisting staff during the hook-up in terms of the desired direction of contrast flow. A final check of contrast run-off in the head can be done at this point by watching under fluoroscopy while the assistant advances the injector. It is not rare to discover at this point that the cervical carotid or upper vertebral artery are represented by a stagnant column of contrast due to the unsuspected development of spasm.

SPASM AROUND THE CATHETER TIP

In most instances withdrawal of the catheter from the vessel will relieve the irritation to the vessel within a few minutes. Before reflexly pulling down the catheter, however, it is worth pausing for just a moment to ask oneself how long the catheter has been in this position and is it possible that this spasm has been present unknown for more than a minute or two? If this is the case then it is probably worthwhile to aspirate vigorously 10–20 ml from the catheter before pulling it down lest some thrombus should have formed around the tip or in the vessel distal to it. Even in

the event of severe spasm, formation of thrombus will be infinitely less likely if a generous flow rate of flush has been in place.

WIRE MANIPULATION AND GREAT VESSEL CATHETERIZATION

Catheters and wires possess complementary behavioral characteristics which can be used to steer into the distal vascular tree from the remote vantage of the common femoral artery. Modern techniques of manufacture allow refinement of these instruments such that the wires and catheters each have a multi-segmental composition, providing the theoretical versatility of being able to take advantage of a greater array of behavioral traits in a given team of instruments.

While these refinements are undoubtedly propitious, they compel the angiographer to a greater analysis of instrument behavior whenever severe navigational difficulties are encountered. Specifically, when having difficulties in catheterization of a particular vessel, the precise point of failure in the system of instruments then in hand must be identified before an intelligent modification or replacement of an instrument can be countenanced (Figures 2.30, 2.31, 2.32, 2.33, 2.34, 2.35). Exculpatory accounts that the vessels were "too tortuous" can be avoided by analyzing the precise reason for failure of the current instruments. Tortuous vessels certainly are a major problem in elderly

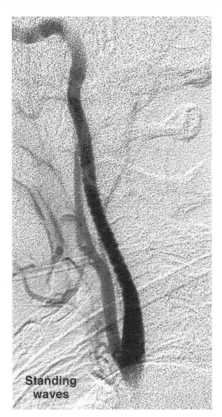

Figure 2.27. Standing waves, a transient phenomenon related to the contrast injection, have a more regular corrugated appearance than mural spasm. They do not compromise the vessel lumen significantly.

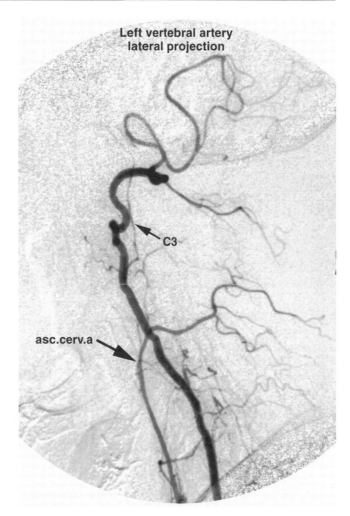

Figure 2.28. *Importance of Testing Vessel Run-off before Performing Power-Injections.* Before doing full volume power injections into the cerebral vessels, it is very important to assess for catheter related spasm or dissection. Assessing run-off in the head is also vitally important. The possibility that a catheterized vertebral artery ends in a posterior inferior cerebellar artery should always be considered, as demonstrated here. The C3 anastomotic branch of the left vertebral artery is marked as is the ascending cervical artery (asc. cerv. a.). The ascending cervical artery is directed posteriorly to assume the territory more commonly associated with the deep cervical artery.

A full-volume injection into a hypoplastic vertebral system such as this could have severe consequences.

or hypertensive patients but they exercise this effect in different ways.

Most problems with vessel catheterization fall into a few categories:

1. Vessel Identification and Selection with the Catheter Tip

Most frequently, a problem with vessel-selection lies with catheter positioning in the aortic arch. The tip must be pointing directly into the vessel and usually must be pulled back and perched on the closest rim of the ostium (i.e. closest to the angiographer's control). This allows the most direct route of access to the target artery. When a particular vessel or its residual stump following pathologic occlusion is not seen at all, one must consider the possibility of anomalous vessel origins. The most commonly encountered anomalies include a common ostium or trunk for the brachiocephalic and left common carotid arteries, an aortic arch origin of the left vertebral artery, and an aberrant right subclavian artery.

The ostium of a left vertebral artery arising directly from the aortic arch can be frequently difficult to find with a catheter tip; the catheter commonly jumps from the left common carotid artery to the left subclavian artery as one withdraws. If one suspects that a left vertebral artery is arising from the aortic arch, its ostium can be sometimes

found by rotating the catheter tip clockwise from the left subclavian artery while advancing slightly.

2. Proximal Tortuosity of the Vessel Impairing Preliminary Navigation by the Wire

When the vessel has been identified but the wire will not advance sufficiently and collapses into the aorta, then a number of possibilities should be considered. If, in fact, a tortuous vessel is at fault, then straightening the vessel with a sustained inhalation on the part of the patient, turning the patient's head, or small repeated coughs by the patient as the wire advances, can frequently be helpful (Figures 2.30, 2.31). Failing this, a more pliable wire may succeed

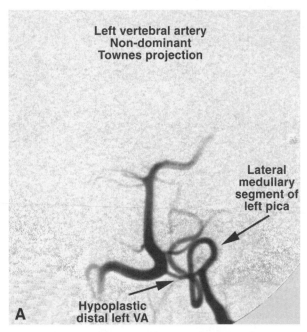

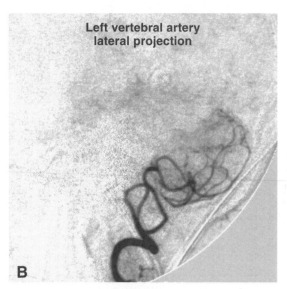

Figure 2.29. A, B *Injection of a Distally Hypoplastic Vertebral Artery.* **(A)** A non-dominant left vertebral artery was inadvertently injected. Fortunately, there was sufficient outlet through the hypoplastic distal intradural left vertebral artery. The patient tolerated the injection. However, in such instances, unless unusual circumstances prevail, the right vertebral artery should be injected. If it should be necessary to study the posterior circulation through a hypoplastic vertebral artery such as this, the injection should be performed by hand.

(B) However, the patient developed prolonged spasm of the proximal left vertebral artery with the appearance of a persistent, non-diluting column of contrast extending through the territory of the left vertebral artery. Notice that the remainder of the posterior fossa opacified in A, has already passed its venous phase. The catheter should be pulled down immediately. A roadmap image could then be obtained from the left subclavian artery to rule out an intimal dissection.

in navigating the tortuous segment; it may not, however, be sufficiently robust to support the subsequent advance of the catheter. Consideration should be given to this potential problem before calling for such a wire. A wire with a pliable, distal long taper but a stiffer proximal shaft can be an excellent compromise. For example, the long-taper stiff-shaft Terumo wire has an excellent combination of a pliable distal tip, which can engage a tortuous system, and a proximal segment, which resists deformity within the aorta as one applies forward tension to the catheter.

3. Proximal Tortuosity of the Vessel Impairing Advancement of the Catheter Over the Wire

If the distal vessel can be navigated with the wire in hand but the catheter cannot be advanced over it, then maneuvers on the part of the patient to straighten the course of the vessel as mentioned above may be of assistance.

Additionally, it may be necessary to anchor the wire more distally than usual, usually in the external carotid artery tree, to allow sufficient support for the catheter (Figure 2.30). Generally, the tip of a steerable wire, pointing anteriorly in the common carotid artery, will select the external carotid artery as it advances and will soon thereafter give a characteristic turn as it finds the linguo-facial artery. Using this deflection as a guide that the internal carotid artery has been avoided, the wire can be advanced still further into the distal external carotid artery. In pa-

tients for whom some particular concern about using this technique exists, such in suspected carotid bifurcation disease, a lateral road-map can illuminate potential hazards. If the vessel selection is precarious, one may wish to work in the AP plane with a road-map centered on the aortic arch. In this case, it is possible with most biplane systems to acquire a road-map in the AP plane centered on the aortic arch, and then move the table to center on the neck and acquire a road-map in the lateral plane. The two road-maps can be alternately recentered as needed using some incidental land-mark, such as dental prosthetic material or EKG leads, etc., when switching from one view to another.

After advancing the wire as far distally as one considers safe, the catheter can then be advanced slowly. The previously described patient maneuvers can be employed as needed. Some experienced angiographers use a *vibrato* motion of the hand to advance the catheter slowly in such a situation, others move the catheter very slowly in time with the cardiac cycle. On occasion, a smooth spinning of the catheter as one slowly puts more forward tension behind the catheter's advance can be extremely helpful. Probably the common denominator in all such techniques is a reduction of friction between the catheter and the vessel wall on the outside and with the wire on the inside. Hydrophillically coated catheters and microcatheters are designed to take advantage of a lower friction coefficient with the surrounding vessel during navigation. The cost

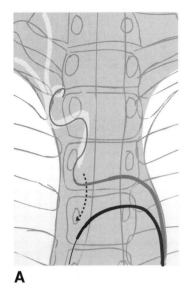

A

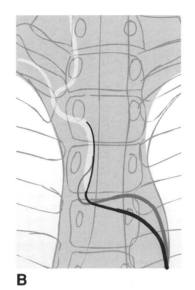

B

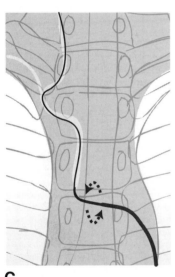

C

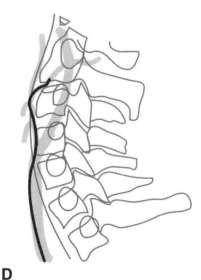

D

Figure 2.30. A–D *Difficult Brachiocephalic Catheterization.* To improve one's chances of selecting a tortuous brachiocephalic artery and right common carotid artery, pull back the catheter to the proximal rim of the vessel and have the patient take a sustained inhalation **(B).** This will straighten the course between the descending aorta and the neck enough to make a critical difference. It may be necessary to use a long taper pliable wire.

Advance the wire as far as possible in the external carotid artery system to improve one's purchase, particularly if one is using a pliable wire. Consider using a lateral roadmap, obtained by injecting below in the vessel ostium **(D).** This will ensure against selecting the internal carotid artery inadvertently.

Allow the patient to regain a breath. Request another sustained inhalation, but do not delay because the wire will have been in the catheter for some time now.

Spin the catheter as you advance **(C).** This will reduce friction between the catheter and the vessel wall, and between the catheter and the wire. If the catheter becomes stuck on a particular curve, ask the patient to cough, if one is completely certain that the wire is in the external carotid artery.

---

associated with such reduced friction is a lower stability of the catheter when the final position has been gained.

4. Tortuosity of the Aortic Arch Causing Redundant Loops in the Catheter

Tortuosity of a capacious aortic arch is a difficulty which can simulate many of the obstacles described above. It may prevent advancement of the wire or of the entire system, and should be thought of whenever an advancing motion of the catheter at the groin is not met with a corresponding advance of the catheter-tip on the fluoroscope. It is a common phenomenon during microcatheter advancement. Any insertion of a given length of microcatheter which is not met with a corresponding advance of the microcatheter tip should prompt consideration that a loop is prolapsing in the neck, or that the microcatheter is pushing the off-screen main catheter into the aorta. Clearly, in these

situations the vascular tree is consuming catheter length somewhere, and this is usually in the aortic arch.

A similar phenomenon can be seen with diffuse aneurysmal disease of the abdominal aorta. In this situation, the ever-increasing curvature and tension of the catheter-wire system in the redundant aorta adversely affects the angle with which the catheter addresses the great vessel, culminating in collapse of the whole system into the ascending aorta. Therefore, this may cause one to think erroneously that the problem lies in tortuosity of the proximal cephalic vessel preventing navigation of the wire or catheter.

The solution to this problem is to straighten the system proximally as much as possible. This can be done by moving to a stiffer 7 French catheter, or by using a stiffer wire. Moving to a larger catheter is probably the more economical and effective maneuver because a 5 French catheter is very likely to continue being problematic in such a difficult

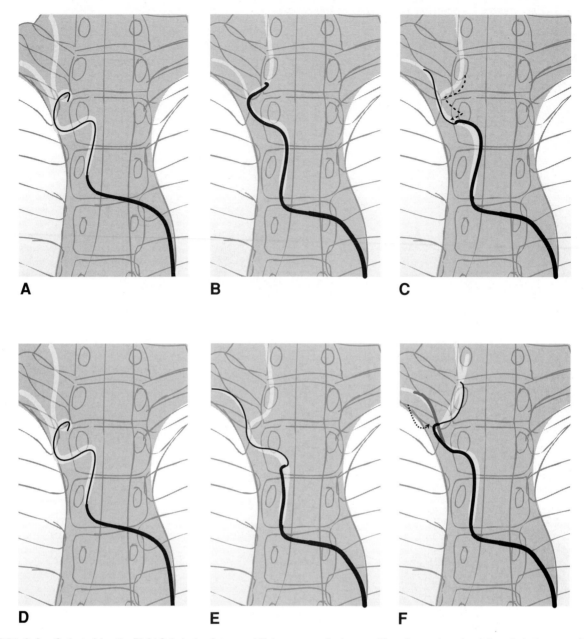

A   **B**   **C**

D   **E**   **F**

Figure 2.31. A–L *Catheterizing the Right Subclavian Artery and Right Vertebral Artery I & II.*   If it is not possible to select the right subclavian artery directly from the aortic arch, then a number of possibilities might be considered.

(A) The right common carotid artery is selected and the catheter is advanced into it. The wire is withdrawn to the catheter shaft. The catheter is then torqued to point to the patient's right **(B),** and withdrawn slowly towards the brachiocephalic artery. A slight kick of the catheter will be seen when the subclavian ostium is reached **(C),** and the wire can be advanced. In a tortuous system, a catheter with a wire inside is less likely to prolapse back into the aorta as one retracts to search for a proximal vessel. A catheter with a sharper angle at its tip can make a crucial difference in searching for an elusive right subclavian artery; a Headhunter or Davis A1 catheter can both be excellent in this situation.

Occasionally, it may be possible to spiral the wire within the brachiocephalic artery to select the right subclavian artery. If an apparently correct position is maintained by the catheter, but it keeps selecting right common carotid artery, then rotating the catheter to a counterintuitive position may allow the wire to bounce into the right subclavian artery **(E).** In all these situations, it is very easy to lose one's position in the right subclavian artery as one retracts in searching for the right

vertebral artery. Therefore, when the right subclavian artery has been selected distally, remove the wire, clean the catheter, and make a roadmap from a distal position in the right subclavian artery, aiming to opacify the right vertebral artery by reflux. Then advance a supporting wire all the way to the catheter tip again before starting to retract to the right vertebral artery. The presence of a supporting wire will diminish the risk of collapsing the catheter out of the right subclavian artery. Notice that the wire in the vertebral artery **(F)** courses medial to the projected course of the common carotid artery, although it starts laterally. Confusion about the right vertebral artery versus the right common carotid artery when a wire has been passed can occur. Obliquing the intensifier may help; a vertebral wire will follow the course of the foramina transversaria. Having the patient swallow may help too; a carotid wire should move with swallowing.

For particularly difficult right subclavian arteries, there is often not an easy answer. The most difficult cases are those in which the right subclavian artery pursues a vertically inferior course from a tortuous brachiocephalic artery **(G, H).** In these patients, the only possible solution is to find precisely the correct angle and select it with whatever curved catheters or wires one can obtain. A 30 RAO road-map is often extremely helpful in showing the way. A catheter such as a Headhunter with a more extreme curve than a standard hockey-stick is sometimes

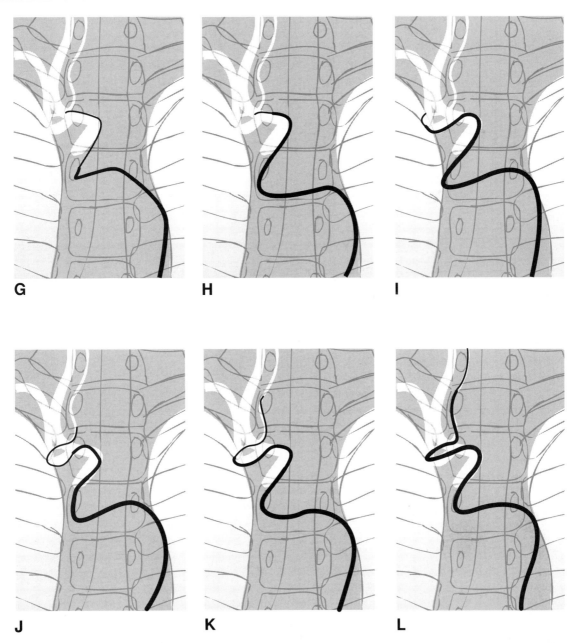

Figure 2.31. A–L *(continued).* very good at finding the correct angle and at selecting the right vertebral artery subsequently **(I).** A Davis catheter usually has a tighter curve than a Berenstein catheter and frequently has the critical edge for directing a wire around a difficult ostium. A curved Bentson wire may emerge from the catheter into the brachiocephalic artery with the correct angle to select the right vertebral artery. A sustained inhalation by the patient will often straighten the proximal vessels to allow passage of a catheter or wire in an otherwise impossibly tortuous situation.

Note that the roadmap image of the vertebral artery has been illustrated as running medial to the course of the tortuous right common carotid artery. This is a point over which some confusion can occur.

aorta. When the wire-catheter system is advanced into the carotid artery from the arch, an inevitable degree of forward tension is present due to the physical forces necessary to coerce it to such a position. A relatively stiff wire used to get to this position will resist deformity from accumulated tension. In contrast, an unsupported catheter does not have this capacity to resist tension. If the wire is removed from the system without having first adjusted for the accumulated tension, then the catheter will inevitably uncoil itself within the capacious aorta, causing a retraction of the tip in the carotid artery and possibly prolapse into the arch. Therefore, after advancing the wire-catheter system of a piece into the great vessel of choice, it is necessary to retract the system to straighten the course of the catheter before removing the wire.

The apparently "spontaneous" retraction of the catheter from the carotid or subclavian vessels due to accumulated tension after removal of the wire is precisely the

1. In the left subclavian artery

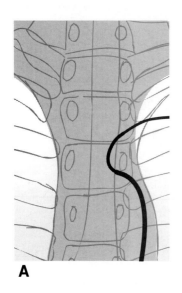

A

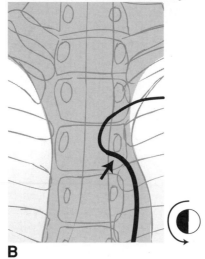

B

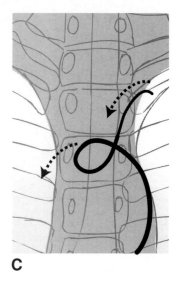

C

2. In a capacious aortic arch

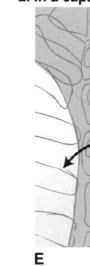

D

E

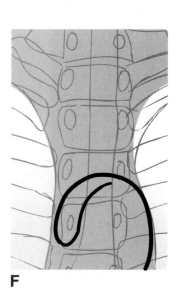

F

3. Off the aortic valve

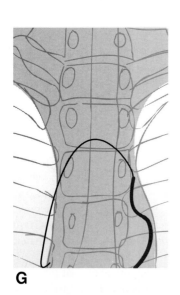

G

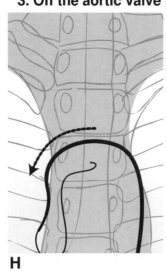

H

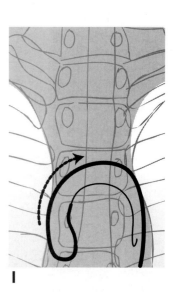

I

opposite of the usual behavior of wire-guided microcatheters, but derives from the same phenomenon. With microcatheters there is a similar accumulation of tension during the advance, but the friction of the microwire within the microcatheter functions as a brace. A microcatheter with accumulated tension is usually confined proximally by the introducing catheter and distally by a narrow arterial tree. Therefore, the confined microcatheter system can only more in one direction, i.e. forwards. When the microwire is removed the microcatheter is more free to expend its tension by advancing forward, which it frequently does in considerable degree. Unless the same careful retraction and straightening of the wire-catheter system is used with microcatheter manipulation, severe intracranial complications can ensue from an uncontrolled microcatheter acting like an harpoon against a vessel or aneurysm wall.

On the other hand, removing tension from a microcatheter-microwire system by retraction, if overdone, can result in loss of hard won access to a distal vessel. Using movement of the radio-opaque microcatheter tip is not a sufficiently sensitive signal. Usually, elasticity of the microcatheter is such that when the tip finally begins to move back it will do so in excessive degree. It is often more efficacious to monitor for changes in a visible loop of the wire within the microcatheter proximally. As one retracts the system, the proximal loops shift to adjust to loss of redundancy. The microwire can then be withdrawn with a diminished risk of forward motion. In any intracranial position, but particularly critical situations, e.g. near an intracranial aneurysm, one should monitor the microcatheter tip closely as the wire is being withdrawn to detect any change in position (Figure 2.36).

Another danger to consider during wire-removal is the hazard of the catheter becoming kinked and occluded at a point of sharp curvature as the supporting wire is removed. This is a potentially disastrous event which can be difficult to recognize as it frequently occurs outside of the field-of-view, e.g. at the distal tip of the guiding catheter in the case of coaxial microcatheters, or high in the aortic arch in the case of guiding catheters. Most commonly, absence of back-flow from a catheter is an indication that the distal

tip is apposed against a vessel wall. Back-flow can be restored by slight retraction of the catheter. However, in a difficult aortic arch the possibility of catheter kinking should be kept in mind. This is an extremely dangerous situation because blood in the distal catheter already stagnant from a prolonged catheterization quickly thromboses and may propagate itself into the arterial tree.

Finally, it must be acknowledged that some vessels are defiant to catheterization. A recurved catheter shape, such as a Simmons type of catheter, while giving less maneuverability and flexibility in superselection of carotid branches, proves indispensable in certain patients, and is, nonetheless, an excellent way to accomplish a diagnostic study under difficult circumstances (Figures 2.32, 2.33, 2.34, 2.35).

A Note on Exchange-Length Wires

Great pains should be taken to avoid, if at all possible, use of exchange-length wires in cerebral angiography. During interventional procedures the use of exchange-wires may be unavoidable, but they should probably be used only when the patient has been heparinized and when the tip of the wire is in the external carotid artery circulation. Over the wire exchanges done in the aortic arch should be performed with the tip of the exchange-wire in the descending aorta, distal to the cephalic vessels. A catheter-exchange over a 350 cm wire is a time-consuming procedure no matter how smoothly it is accomplished. Even though the outer, visible portion of the wire may appear clean after being wiped, the new catheter being inserted has the opportunity to shave accumulated debris, platelets and thrombus from the exchange-wire over its full length. This debris is then free to fall from the catheter tip after removal of the exchange wire and has been the cause of many severe embolic complications in the cerebral circulation.

SPINAL ANGIOGRAPHY

Indications

Spinal angiography is used to evaluate certain vascular diseases, or to identify the origins of the spinal arteries prior

---

Figure 2.32. A–I *Reforming a Simmons Curve.* 1. Reforming in the Left Subclavian Artery. Generally the unformed catheter-tip will seek the ostium of the left subclavian artery without difficulty. A dirigible wire, such as a Terumo wire, or a soft curved wire, such as a Bentson, can be used to navigate the Simmons catheter tip into the subclavian artery past the vertebral artery **(A).**

This wire can be withdrawn into the main shaft of the catheter proximal to the curve **(arrow in B)**. Better yet, the wire can be removed and the stiff end of the Bentson wire advanced to this point, but no further, to support the catheter-shaft. The next step is to create drag on the tip of the catheter by torquing it in the aorta, and then pushing it into the ascending arch. The success of this technique depends on having the curved section of the Simmons catheter barely in the subclavian artery so that it becomes the fulcrum of rotation when

torque is applied. If the curved section is too far into the left subclavian artery, it cannot reform and the catheter will become pushed further out the artery.

2. In a Capacious Aortic Arch

In a capacious aortic arch, a 7 French Simmons catheter tapered to a 5 French tip, will reform itself if one can create enough drag on the tip by torquing and then pushing. This maneuver can be assisted by placing a wire within the shaft of the catheter, as in B, for additional support.

3. Off the Aortic Valve

A 3-J wire pushed over the arch and curved off the aortic valve so that its tip is pushed as far back across the arch as possible will usually work **(H).** Any concerns about aortic valvular disease or coronary artery disease should preclude use of this technique.

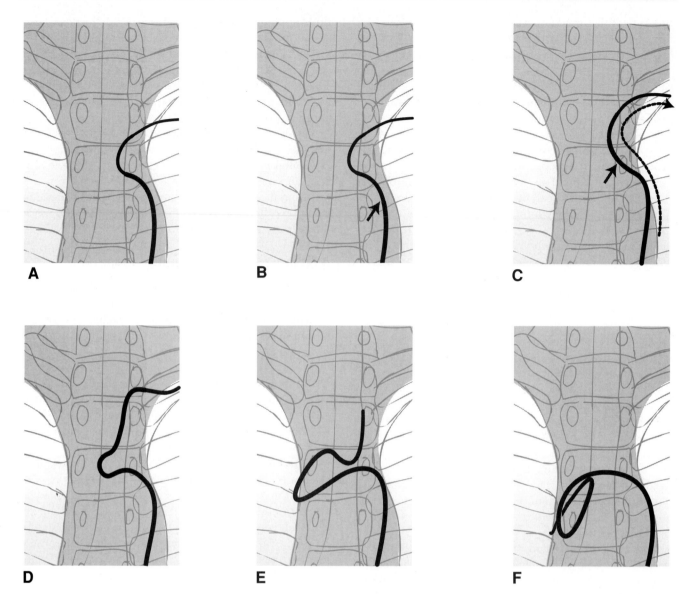

Figure 2.33. A–F *Avoid Forming a Knot with a Simmons Catheter.* One of the numerous ways in which it is possible to form a knot with a Simmons catheter is during reformation of the catheter in the left subclavian artery. If insufficient torque or incorrect positioning is applied to the catheter, it may simply advance into the subclavian artery. This may happen by having the supporting wire too proximal in the catheter **(arrow in B).** By advancing the catheter further, a new fulcrum point becomes established. By pushing further, the catheter eventually folds on itself, giving the appearance of a Simmons curve.

When this false loop is pushed over the aortic arch, it may drag the true curve out of the left subclavian artery. The true curve may then reform itself but does so pointing in the wrong direction. At this point, the criss-crossing segments of the Simmons catheter have the capacity to interweave and form a knot. If this happens, do not drag on the catheter and tighten the knot. Instead, push the catheter in as far as possible to the most capacious segment of the aorta, and straighten out the loops with a stiff wire.

to spinal surgery. Alternatively, the study may be necessary to evaluate lesions of the spine or vertebral column in the setting of a presurgical evaluation or embolization. When a complete spinal angiogram is required to search for a possible dural arteriovenous malformation or fistula, then the study must evaluate the entire dural vasculature from the foramen magnum to the sacrum without omission (See Table 2.4). Spinal dural arteriovenous malformations are notoriously elusive unless a technically adequate injection is made directly into the affected pedicle. Furthermore, dural arteriovenous malformations of the spine may pres-

ent with conal symptoms or myelographic findings quite remote from the site of the fistula. Except for knowing that spinal dural arteriovenous malformations are more likely to be found in the thoracic and lumbar spine than in the cervical area, there is no *a priori* way of focusing a spinal angiogram for this disease. A spinal angiogram in which "most" of the vessels were injected would be the equivalent of a cerebral angiogram for aneurysm detection in which "most" of the cerebral vessels were visualized.

Spinal tumors and intramedullary arteriovenous malformations, on the other hand, are often more defined

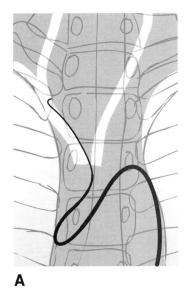

A

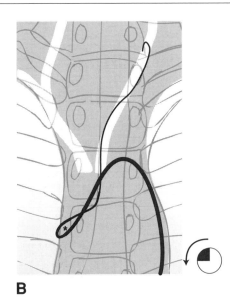

B

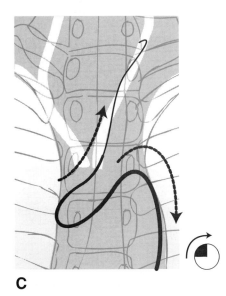

C

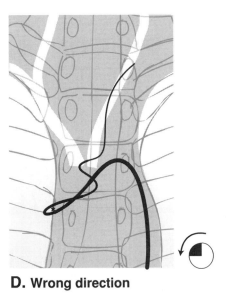

D. Wrong direction

Figure 2.34. A–D *Selecting the Left Common Carotid Artery with a Simmons Type Curve.* Generally, a reformed Simmons catheter and Bentson wire will seek the brachiocephalic artery without difficulty **(A)**. Remember that to advance the Simmons catheter up the carotid, it must be retracted at the groin. It is safer and more effective to always lead the Simmons catheter with a soft wire.

The left common carotid artery may be more difficult to select than the brachiocephalic. By remembering that the left common carotid artery frequently has an anterior disposition at its ostium relative to the brachiocephalic artery, one sees why rotating the catheter tip anteriorly (anticlockwise) is necessary **(B).** However, in older patients the degree to which this is necessary is often surprising, so that the catheter may look like it is criss-crossing itself, lost somewhere in the ascending aorta **(B).** It is necessary to use an extreme anterior position in some patients to avoid selecting the brachiocephalic artery again as one advances the Bentson wire **(B).**

When the artery has been found by the wire, the Simmons catheter is retracted at the groin to advance it into the left common carotid artery. It may or may not open out the crossed loop in the aortic arch as it does so. Given the propensity of the Simmons catheter to knot on itself, it is better to undo the anterior turn that one has used to select the left carotid **(C).** The closed loop (*) at the turn of the Simmons catheter should begin to enlarge and open if one is turning the correct way to straighten the attitude of the catheter.

In **(D)** the Simmons has been turned the wrong way (more anticlockwise) causing the closed loop to tighten (*), and the twisted catheter is obstructing its own advance up the left common carotid artery.

with respect to suspected location prior to undertaking an angiogram. Even in a limited examination, it is nevertheless worthwhile to consider extending the study until the next neighboring uninvolved anterior spinal artery is visualized. The locations of the anterior and posterior spinal arteries are a particular concern in all situations where embolization of the paraspinal vessels is being considered.

Anesthesia during Spinal Arteriography

Because many of the critical vessels of interest during a spinal arteriogram are of such small size, the quality of images can be significantly degraded by a slight amount of motion or respiratory artifact. Most spinal angiograms are long procedures and it is difficult for patients to remain absolutely still during that time. Depending on the indications for the study, a spinal angiogram can be focused on a known lesion or area, or may require a diagnostic evaluation of the entire spinal axis. In either event, the procedure is invariably tedious for the patient and is best done under general anesthesia, if possible. The main purpose of this is to avoid obtaining a technically inadequate study due to motion artifact. Furthermore, under general anesthesia, respirations can be suspended for the duration of each angiographic run, eliminating respiratory artifact. Occasionally when embolization is considered for a known focal lesion in a particularly cooperative patient, the study can be performed with a lighter degree of anesthesia.

Figure 2.35. *Selecting a Bovine Origin Left Common Carotid Artery with a Simmons Type Curve.* This technique is similar to selecting a difficult, anteriorly inclined left common carotid artery with a Simmons catheter, except everything is done to a greater extreme and without leaving the brachiocephalic artery. The Simmons catheter is torqued 180 to completely reverse direction in the distal brachiocephalic artery. This is called a ``scissors maneuver'' because of the form of the catheter at this point **(B)**. It is then pushed in at the groin to retract it in the brachiocephalic artery. With some persistence and by keeping the very tip of the catheter pointing to the patient's left side, the left common carotid artery is selected with a Bentson wire **(C)**. In this situation, correction of the Simmons position must be an exact reversal of the previous torquing maneuver. Otherwise, the wire and catheter will be wrapped around one another.

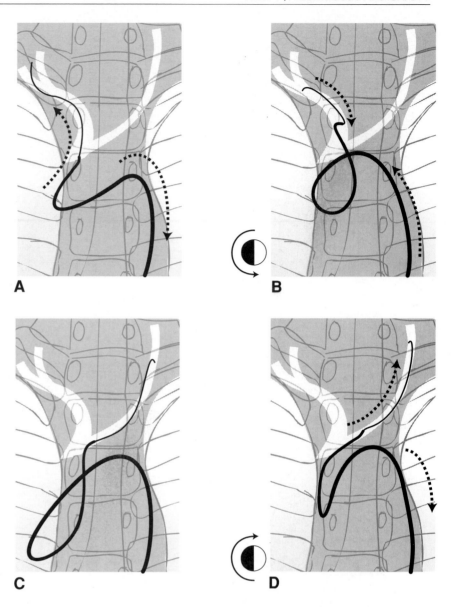

Technical Considerations in Spinal Arteriography

Spinal angiography, being something of a major undertaking for all involved, must be done with an eye to technical perfection (Figure 2.37, 2.38) in order to dispel subsequent considerations of whether the study might need to be repeated because of perceived errors or omissions.

Enumerating the vertebral bodies is the first task in a complete or focused spinal study, in order to avoid miscommunication about anatomic levels. The number of rib-bearing vertebrae must be counted under the fluoroscope and collated with the number of lumbar type bodies. In situations of an indeterminate configuration, an arbitrary decision on a system of nomenclature should be established and explicitly described in the report of the case, e.g. ``There are eleven rib-bearing vertebrae which for the purposes of this study will be numbered T1 to T11, and 5 non-rib bearing vertebrae which will be numbered L1 to L5,'' etc.

Patient positioning is the next consideration. Spinal angiography, in the thoracic and lumbar regions, is done using AP fluoroscopy only. It is important for the purposes of identifying the posterior and anterior spinal arteries that the imaging plane be precise. Therefore, the fluoroscope is positioned for all runs such that the spinal processes are aligned half-way between the spinal pedicles. When a degree of rotational scoliosis is present an adjustment of the fluoroscope may be necessary between different levels of the spine.

Minimization of the contrast volume from the very beginning of the study is critical (See Table 2.1). While it may not be apparent as a potential problem in the initial phase of a complete spinal angiogram, later technical difficulties can provoke a cumulative total dose of contrast well in excess of 400 ml–500 ml on a routine basis. Standard precautionary measures, such as hydration of the patient before, during, and after the procedure with close monitoring of urine output, are therefore important.

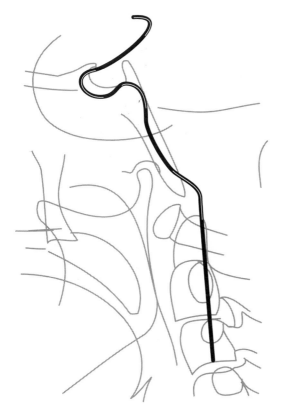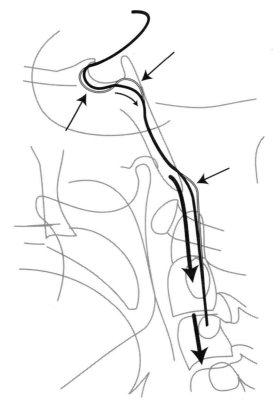

Figure 2.36. *Removal of Forward Tension from the Microcatheter prior to Wire-Removal.* In order to pull back a sufficient quantity of microwire and microcatheter (together) to reduce forward tension but not lose the position of the catheter tip, watch the proximal loops of the system for motion **(arrows)**. When the loop closest to the tip begins to move, all the tension has been removed.

Table 2.4
Vessels Required for a Complete Spinal Angiogram

Vertebral arteries
External carotid arteries
Thyrocervical trunks
Costocervical trunks (including the superior intercostal artery)
Supreme intercostal arteries (usually T2±T4)
Segmental arteries from T4 to L3 (or L4 if present)
Median sacral artery (midline from the aortic bifurcation)
Lateral sacral arteries (from the internal iliac arteries)

Vessel Selection During Spinal Angiography

The segmental vessels of the spinal column change orientation as one ascends the aorta. Frequently one has to make allowance for this change by exchanging catheters during the procedure.

1. Lumbar segmental arteries are more likely than their thoracic counterparts to have a conjoined pedicle giving rise to both the left and right branches.

2. Lumbar bony pedicles and segmental arteries are more widely spaced from their superior and inferior neighbors than are their counterparts in the thoracic spine.

3. Lumbar vascular pedicles take origin from the aorta with an inferiorly directed or horizontal course. This pattern changes slowly as one ascends the aorta to a more superiorly directed course. The supreme intercostal artery (variable in territory but frequently including T2, T3, and T4) is directed with a sharply superior angle from the aorta.

4. The diameter of the descending thoracic aorta is greater than that in the lumbar region. The implication of this anatomic tapering is that different constraints are placed on the catheter in these two regions by the walls of the aorta. Therefore, the behavior of a particular catheter may be quite different in various locations.

During vessel selection, it is necessary for obvious reasons to be familiar with the anterior-posterior orientation of one's catheter within the aorta, the arterial pedicles of the spine being posterior, or postero-medial in the thoracic aorta. Because the pattern of the arterial pedicles changes only slightly from one level to another, it is most helpful to select the vessels in a *sequential, systematic manner,* taking precautions not to miss any vessel or become confused about enumeration. The intercostal arteries run along the inferior surface of the correspondingly numbered rib. The technologist or nurse should have a *spinal angiography work-sheet* for recording the numbers and identifications of all the runs, so that one can tell at a glance whether all the vessels have been found, and, if not, which pedicles remain to be studied.

Taking a cue from the attitude of the catheter at the

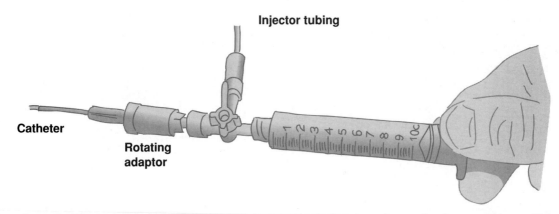

Figure 2.37. *Set-up For Diagnostic Spinal Angiography.* For diagnostic spinal angiography, a continuous flush system would generate too much dead space and, thus, excessive waste of contrast load with each injection. A three way stopcock and a swivel adapter attached to the syringe and catheter provide an efficient means of rapidly searching for the next vessel and immediately toggling from syringe to injector tubing for the run. For coaxial spinal manipulations, a continuous flush system is used during interventional procedures.

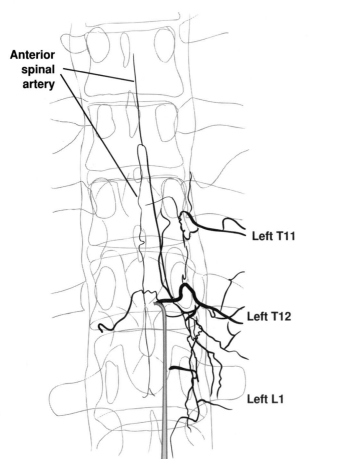

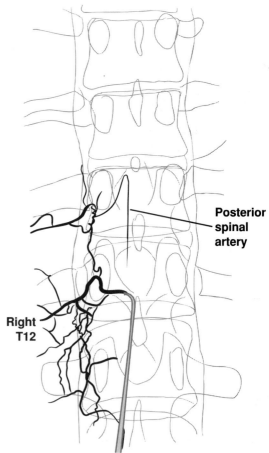

Figure 2.38. *Anterior and Posterior Spinal Arteries.* In selecting the spinal arterial pedicles, it is necessary to know whether one's catheter is pointing anteriorly or posteriorly, as described in Figure 2.7. The posterior processes of the vertebrae are aligned exactly in the middle. In this manner, the precisely midline course of the anterior spinal artery can be discerned from the paramedian course of the posterior spinal artery.

vessel ostium at one level, those of the next level up or down can be divined fairly accurately, thus minimizing contrast use in blind searching. Vessel ostia, in the absence of vertebral anomalies such as hemi-vertebrae, tend to be extremely reliable in their alignment in the left-right and cranio-caudad directions. If a particular vessel cannot be seen at all after a prolonged search of the appropriate area, the possibility that it might be occluded or congenitally hypoplastic should be considered by looking at the contiguous levels. Prominent filling of the vessels of that territory through collateral channels without evidence of washout from the unselected vessel is adequate reassurance that the missing vessel need not be pursued further.

A variety of catheter shapes are manufactured for spinal angiography. The change in orientation of the vascular pedicles from an inferior or horizontal slant in the lumbar region to a superior inclination in the upper thoracic region is the factor which tends to be most significant in determining the optimal choice for a change of catheter shapes. Inferiorly pointing catheters such as the HS-1 are better suited in the lower aorta, while superiorly directed catheters such as the H-1-H may be more suited for the thoracic region. A particularly capacious aorta, requiring a catheter with an ample secondary curve which can span the diameter of the aorta, e.g. HS-2 or Mikaelsson, is another factor to consider when a stable position cannot be achieved.

There is a certain knack to stabilizing the catheter tip in the segmental artery once the ostium is selected. The catheter tip must be coaxed a little further into the vessel than it will spontaneously purchase of its own accord. By twisting the catheter tip a little further to the side of the pedicle in question, combined with a gentle forward push in the case of the HS-1 or H-1-H catheters, a subtle degree of tension can be established in the catheter which will hold it in position for the subsequent run. Alternatively, with a recurved type of spinal catheter, such as the Mikaelsson shape, slight downward tension on the catheter is assistant towards a similar end. The final step to maintaining catheter position during the injection is to assure that the external segment of the catheter, hindered by tubing and drapes outside the body, does not have a degree of counter-torque which might undo the hold that the catheter-tip has on the artery. Therefore, stabilization of the outer catheter is necessary to avoid ejection of the catheter tip from the artery as contrast is injected. A linear rise to introduce the injection can be very helpful as well.

In particularly difficult pedicles which can be seen on roadmapping but which are repugnant to catheterization, some further options can be considered. A soft wire might be steerable into a stable position more distally in the pedicle; this can then be used to advance the catheter further into the artery. Failing this, a road-map image can be used to steer a wire-directed microcatheter coaxially into the pedicle, through which a run can be accomplished.

INTRAOPERATIVE ANGIOGRAPHY

Depending on the preferences of the neurosurgeon, intraoperative angiography immediately after clip placement may be requested to assist with difficult intracranial aneurysms, particularly those in the paraclinoidal area. Technically, these can be difficult angiographic procedures. It is often necessary to work in a cramped position at the patient's left groin, the television monitor may be some meters distant and behind various pieces of draped equipment, and movement of the portable fluoroscope is hampered by the paraphernalia of the sterile surgical field. The following points make the process easier:

- The surgical team must procure and remember to use a radiolucent head-holder for the surgical table at the beginning of the case. They must also remember to include the groin in the preparation of the sterile surgical field during draping. To avoid loss of time gaining arterial access to the femoral artery after the clip has been applied to the aneurysm, it is advantageous to have placed a sheath in the femoral artery on a slowly-flowing irrigation system (2,000 units of heparin/L) at the beginning of the surgical procedure. Therefore, should the aneurysm clip be causing an unexpected problem, the delay until discovery by angiography is minimized.
- Use high density (300 non-ionic) contrast for maximal visibility on the portable fluoroscope. Additionally, catheters are available with tips impregnated with high density material. The margin of increased visibility afforded by these catheters on portable fluoroscopy units is considerable.
- Vessel selection is considerably more difficult in the operating room. A Simmons type catheter with an accompanying Bentson wire frequently proves a more efficient combination under such circumstances.

Under operating-room circumstances, hand-injections of the common carotid arteries are technically adequate. Common carotid selection and injection is safer than trying to select the internal carotid artery under trying and potentially dangerous circumstances.

The utility of intraoperative and postoperative angiography has been confirmed in a number of studies. MacDonald et al. (21) found a 20% incidence of unexpected significant findings in patients who had undergone surgical clipping of aneurysms. These findings included residual aneurysm at the clipped site, other unrecognized aneurysms, or vessel occlusions. The utility of intraoperative angiography was studied by Derdeyn et al. (22) who found that surgical technique was altered in 11%–12% of cases in a large series, based on information gathered from the angiogram. A similar rate of clip repositioning was reported in a prospective study by Alexander et al. (23). However, they and other authors observe that intraoperative angiography does not emulate the quality of conventional studies, and that postoperative conventional arteriography may still be necessary in certain cases.

INJECTION RATES

Visualization of an artery during an angiogram requires that injected contrast be the equivalent of approximately 30% of the volume of flowing blood. Therefore, larger arteries and vessels with faster flow will require faster injections. Immediately after cessation of the injection, a pro-

Table 2.5
Suggested Injection Rates

Vessel	Linear Rise (sec)	Rate (ml/sec)	Total Volume (ml)
Common carotid head run	0±0.2	7±10	10±14
Common carotid neck run for carotid bifurcation disease	0±0.2	4±6	6±8
Common carotid for AVM	0±0.2	10	12±14
Internal carotid	0±0.5	4±8	6±10
Internal carotid with acutely ruptured aneurysm and acute SAH (may by better done with common carotid injection or hand-injections to reduce risk of rupturing the aneurysm)	0.2±0.5	3±6	6±8
Internal carotid when attempting to evaluate collateral flow (normal sized vessel)	0.2	8±10	10
Internal carotid for a large AVM	0±0.5	8±10	10±14
External carotid proximal to facial artery	0±0.2	3	6±9
Distal external carotid	0±0.2	2	4±6
Vertebral artery with adequate distal run-off (reduce rates or do hand-injections for acute SAH)	0.5±1.0	4±5	8±10
Vertebral artery for AVM	0.5±1.0	5	10±12
Subclavian artery with sphygmomanometer cuff inflated for visualization of the vertebral artery circulation.	0±0.2	8±10	14±16
Costocervical and thyrocervical trunks	0±0.2	2	4±6
Facial, lingual, occipital, ascending pharyngeal arteries	0±0.2	2±3	4±6
Aortic arch	0	20±30	30±50
Intercostal, lumbar arteries	0±0.5	1±2	4
Internal Iliac arteries	0	6±10	10±12

The figures are approximate guidelines for rates and volume of injections in adults. In older children and adolescents the figures can be reduced approximately 40%. With cut-film the figures can be increased approximately 10±15%. Although 43% or 180±200 strength contrast is adequate for modern digital imaging, 60% or 300±320 strength contrast is necessary for cut-film imaging.

In the setting of acute subarachnoid hemorrhage due to ruptured aneurysms, many experienced neuroradiologists perform common carotid artery injections rather than selective internal carotid artery injections, or use hand-injection techniques rather than power-injections, to avoid imposing critical non-physiological stresses on a recently ruptured vessel (See Chapter 3).

For standard 5 French catheter injections the injector is set at 300 psi. For aortic arch injections with a pig-tail catheter, a setting of 1,000 psi or the maximal tolerance of the catheter is used; for microcatheters outside the intracranial circulation, 450 psi. For microcatheters intracranially use hand-injections.

cess of dilution begins such that opacification of the veins is less pronounced than that of the arteries. For this reason, in disease states where a foremost interest lies in the status of the venous system, consideration may be given to placing emphasis on a longer injection rate with a higher total volume than one might normally use.

Deciding on the rate of injection for a particular vessel depends on the caliber of the vessel, rate of flow, distal run-off, and catheter position. A useful rule of thumb suggests that when using a 10 cc syringe on a catheter with 0.038″ inner diameter, a forceful hand-injection is the equivalent of 5 cc per second. Therefore, when testing for catheter position, reflux with a hand-injection made in this fashion would indicate that a rate of less than 5 cc per second should be considered (see Table 2.5). A linear rise or graded introduction of the injection into the vessel runs the theoretical risk of diluting the leading edge of the contrast bolus, but generally such an effect cannot be identified as a significant factor on the final images. Therefore a linear rise is a good precaution, particularly in precarious or unstable catheter positions, to prevent sudden whipping of the catheter from the vessel, or in positions where the catheter does not conform to the vessel.

MAGNIFICATION ERRORS

Precise measurement of size is important for treatment decisions regarding aneurysms and arteriovenous malfor-mations. During endovascular treatment of intracranial aneurysms it is necessary to know the dimensions of the aneurysm lumen in order to choose the correct coil-size for building the initial frame-work. For arteriovenous malformations, estimations of volume and area have an important bearing on treatment decisions, because the expected efficacy of radiosurgery is based on the volume of arteriovenous malformation being irradiated. Arteriovenous malformations with a maximal linear diameter of 1.2 cm (24) or volume less than 4 cm^3 (25) have demonstrated complete obliteration following stereotactic radiosurgery in 80%–90% of cases at two-year follow-up.

There are two major factors which cause significant magnification errors in calculation of lesion size based on externally applied markers such as coins and grids, or internal references such as the known diameter of a catheter tip. The relative position of the markers and lesion along the central ray generates an inherent error of geometric magnification. The latter is compounded by error related to relative position away from the central axis of the beam where the divergent nature of the beam amplifies the error of measurement. Linear measurements calculated without correcting for these factors are subject to errors of 13% or greater, meaning that when such linear measurements are used to calculate area or volume, the error factor may be as great as 25%–40% (26).

To correct for magnification error on angiographic images, greater accuracy can be attained by using sizing markers placed on both sides of the head and correcting for geometric magnification, assuming that the lesion is in the central beam and in the center of the head. This is the most elementary of solutions and is probably the most commonly used. Alternatively, still greater correction can be had by partially correcting for divergence of the beam and a non-central position of the lesion, as described in the formula given by Horton (27).

Different formulae are used to calculate the volume of an arteriovenous malformation based on the linear dimensions in three planes. A simple calculation of the volume of an assumed spherical contour is sometimes used:

$$volume = \frac{a \times b \times c}{2}$$

Brown et al. (28) calculated the volume of an arteriovenous malformation as an elongated sphere:

$$volume = \frac{4\ (s/2)^3}{3} + \frac{s^2 \cdot (L\text{-}s)}{4}$$

where s is the smallest and L the largest diameter of the arteriovenous malformation.

VIEW SET-UP AND ANEURYSM EVALUATION

There are factors to consider in setting up a field of view for an angiographic run. It is important to maximize the quality of images by extracting the optimal amount of information from each injection. This involves both a careful positioning of the patient's head in the fluoroscopic field, and an adjustment of the center and diameter of view according to the situation. Modern angiographic rooms provide a degree of flexibility with magnification, collimation, and angulation which was not possible with cut-film angiography, and it is important to use this versatility to maximal advantage. Best images can often be obtained by thinking in advance of what particular information is necessary from each injection, particularly those that are peculiar to this patient's lesion or diagnosis. Tumors obstructing or invading venous sinuses, dural sinus thromboses, collateral flow through various routes, etc. may all require special consideration or deviations from the routine set-up. For example, with parasagittal meningiomas it is often difficult to see whether the superior sagittal sinus is completely occluded because adjacent bridging veins are superimposed. A steep cranio-caudad angulation with slight obliquity can be very helpful in this circumstance.

Carotid Artery Standard Views

Standard internal carotid artery views require orthogonal PA and lateral images of the supratentorial space which include the inner table of the skull (Figure 2.39). The lateral view can be straightened by using the orbital roofs or the external auditory meati as guides to eliminate lateral skew. PA obliquity can be finely tuned by observing the asymmetry of the linea innominata on the lateral aspects of the orbits. The degree of cranio-caudad angulation on the initial PA view can have a strong influence on some areas which may be of interest. This can be assessed during set-up by gauging the relationship of the supra-orbital rims to the petrous ridges. By placing the supraorbital rims down onto the petrous ridges or lower, one might obtain an excellent view of the main stems of the A1 and M1 segments with elimination of bone-subtraction artifact from the supraorbital rims. This can be useful in evaluating intracranial vasospasm or an aneurysm at the origin of a lenticulostriate branch of the M1 segment. However, a view in this position superimposes the supraclinoid internal carotid artery on the horizontal segment of the cavernous internal carotid artery.

Vertebral Artery Standard Views

Usually a vertebral artery lateral view does not require visualization of the whole head unless filling of the posterior communicating arteries to the anterior circulation is of particular interest. Therefore, to improve image quality one should aim to fill the entire fluoroscopic screen with the vertebro-basilar circulation. Because of the possibility of the posterior inferior cerebellar artery taking origin from below the foramen magnum, usually a field-of-view down to C1 or C2 is helpful.

The anterior view of the vertebral artery injection is usually done as a Townes projection. This can be conceptualized as peering over the tip of the clivus down into the foramen magnum. This view demonstrates the branches of the posterior circulation at the cost of superimposing these vessels on one another and of foreshortening the view of the basilar artery itself. To evaluate the trunk of the basilar artery or aneurysms of the basilar tip, a Townes view is usually not the optimal view, unless the aneurysm is projecting due posteriorly. For these locations, craniocaudad angulation towards a Caldwell or Waters projection is usually more informative.

Aneurysm Neck and Profile

With digital subtraction angiography, most sensitive angiographic detection of aneurysms can be performed at the computer monitor where contrast and density can be manipulated for each image. It is very important not to overlook this because the final printed images will contain only a fraction of all the data collected during an angiographic examination.

For consideration of endovascular treatment of intracranial aneurysms a primary item of information is the configuration of the aneurysm neck in relationship to the parent vessel. Therefore, while there is always an onus to minimize the number of angiographic runs in a particular vessel, it is also important to finish the study with some understanding of this particular aspect of the aneurysm architecture. Rotational angiography has the capacity to eliminate much of the guess-work involved in choosing the correct projection, but even this technique requires that a decision be made on the optimal head position during the run.

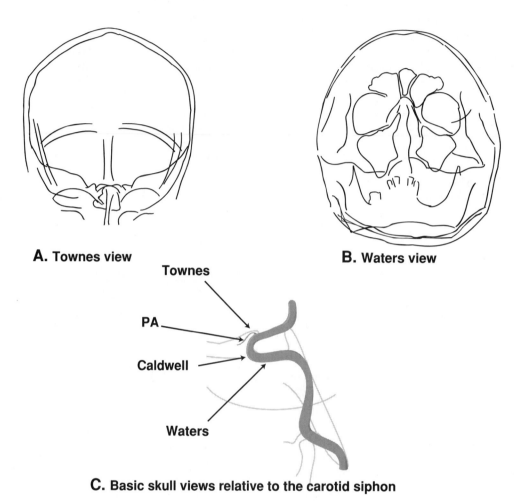

A. Townes view

B. Waters view

C. Basic skull views relative to the carotid siphon

Figure 2.39. *Basic Skull Views.* The frontal view of the skull can be simplified into a decision about where one wishes to place the supraorbital rims in reference to the petrous ridges.

The Townes view **(A)** places the orbital rims low in the field, so that one is looking into the posterior fossa from a superior vantage. This is the standard initial view for the posterior fossa in the frontal plane.

The Waters view **(B)** places the petrous ridges low in the field. For the posterior circulation, a Waters view is frequently helpful for evaluating the basilar artery trunk or basilar tip aneurysms, particularly those which point anteriorly. For the carotid circulation, a Waters view, in combination with obliquity, is very useful for teasing apart the loops of the internal carotid artery and determining the morphology of aneurysms of the siphon.

The PA view **(D)** places the petrous ridges between the mid-equator of the orbits and as high up as behind the orbital rims. As a standard view of the internal carotid artery, this view usually provides the best overall combined view of the siphon and intracranial circulation. More angulation towards a Townes, i.e. superimposing the orbital rims on the petrous ridges, improves the evaluation of the A1 and M1 seg-

ments by eliminating subtraction artifact from the orbital rims, but at the cost of superimposing elements of the carotid siphon. Angulation in the other direction to superimpose the petrous ridges on the orbital floor, i.e. a Caldwell projection, improves the evaluation of the siphon but at the cost of foreshortening the supraclinoidal segment **(C).** The latter projection, i.e. superimposition of orbital floor and petrous ridges, combined with ipsilateral obliquity of the image intensifier, gives an excellent transorbital view of the middle cerebral artery division pattern.

In the lateral view **(E),** the most easily discerned landmarks on a fluoroscopic image are the orbital roofs. If necessary the patient's head can be tilted to align these guides. Alternatively, superimposition of the external auditory meati can be a guide, although these landmarks are less easily followed on fluoroscopic images. Skewing the lateral view, i.e. elevating one orbital roof in reference to another, can be extremely helpful in evaluation of paraclinoidal aneurysms. During evaluation of paraclinoidal aneurysms the internal carotid artery contour on the lateral projection can be conceptualized as the brow of a hill over which one is attempting to gain the optimal view of an aneurysm.

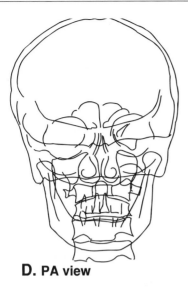

D. PA view

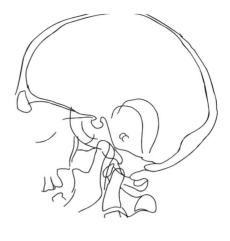

E. Lateral view

Figure 2.39. *(continued)*

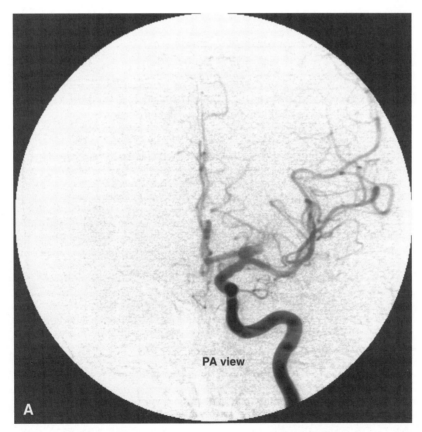

PA view

A

Figure 2.40. A–C *Aneurysm Evaluation I.* **(A)** PA view of an unruptured aneurysm projecting over the left internal carotid artery bifurcation in a 43 year female. There is a double density of contrast along the medial aspect of the aneurysm suggesting that this is something other than a straight-forward bifurcation aneurysm. The lateral view **(B)** shows that the aneurysm (arrow) is clearly distal to the anterior choroidal artery (arrowhead), but its precise point of origin is still difficult to discern.

By hypothesizing that this aneurysm is lying along the anterior aspect of the supraclinoidal segment, a view which foreshortens this segment of artery, separating it from the superiorly directed aneurysm

should be helpful, i.e. inclining the frontal view towards a Caldwell view. To remove superimposition of the aneurysm on the A1 segment, it was decided to foreshorten this segment too by using a 30 RAO projection **(C).** This combination resulted in an excellent demonstration of the aneurysm neck arising from the proximal A1 segment. An LAO inclination might have worked well too, but the M1 segment would probably then have superimposed on the neck, obscuring the true origin of the aneurysm. Notice the lobulation of the aneurysm dome projecting to the patient's left. This suggests that the aneurysm may be undergoing a phase of expansion.

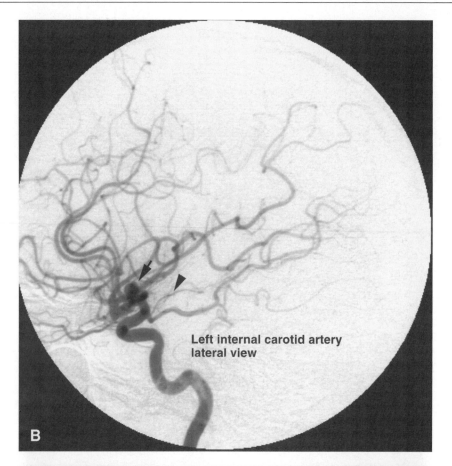

Left internal carotid artery
lateral view

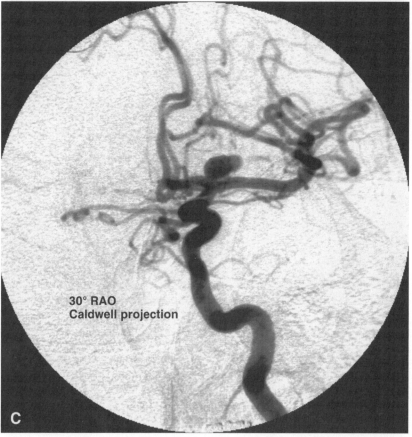

30° RAO
Caldwell projection

Figure 2.40.   *(continued)*

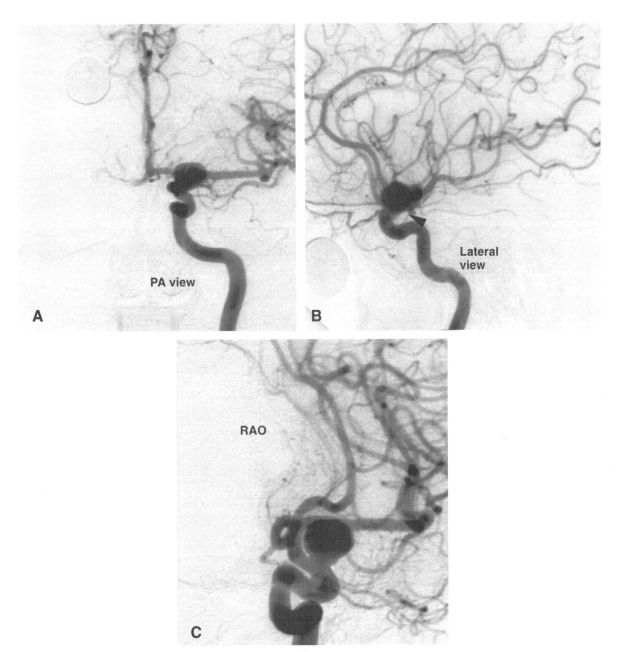

Figure 2.41. A–C *Aneurysm Evaluation II.*   A PA **(A)** and lateral view **(B)** of an aneurysm of the supraclinoidal segment demonstrates a 10 mm aneurysm which appears to project laterally and superiorly from the internal carotid artery. A 3 mm aneurysm (arrowhead) is seen near the expected origin of the posterior communicating artery on the lateral view.

In this case, an LAO frontal view would superimpose the aneurysm dome and the distal supraclinoidal internal carotid artery. An RAO view with no change in cranio-caudad angulation would improve the profile of the aneurysm, but some superimposition of the lower aneurysm, the supraclinoidal internal carotid artery, and the middle cerebral artery would occur. To avoid this, an RAO angulation with inclination towards a Townes view **(C)** makes a profile or brow of the superolateral aspect of the internal carotid artery, giving an excellent view of the aneurysm neck.

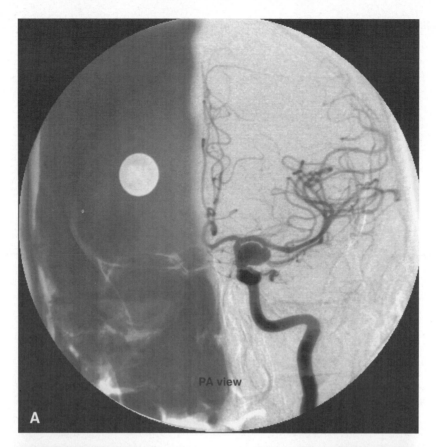

PA view

A

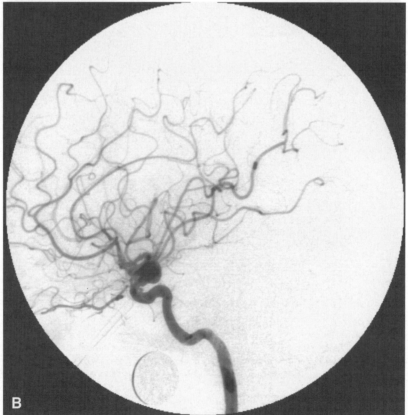

B

Figure 2.42. A–D *Aneurysm Evaluation III.*   PA **(A)** and lateral **(B)** views of an unruptured, lobulated supraclinoidal carotid aneurysm in a 35-year-old female. This was thought initially to project from the supero-lateral aspect of the internal carotid artery, and an RAO view, similar to the technique of Figure 2.42, was obtained **(C)**. Coin marker = 18 mm.

However, persistent superimposition of the internal carotid artery and the aneurysm on this view indicated that the aneurysm was lying behind (under) the carotid artery. An LAO transorbital **(D)** view confirms the posterolateral disposition of the aneurysm.

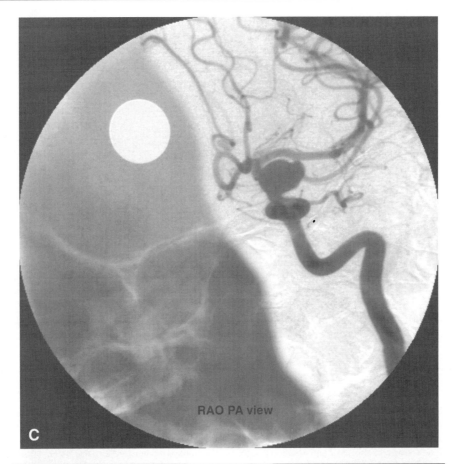

C   RAO PA view

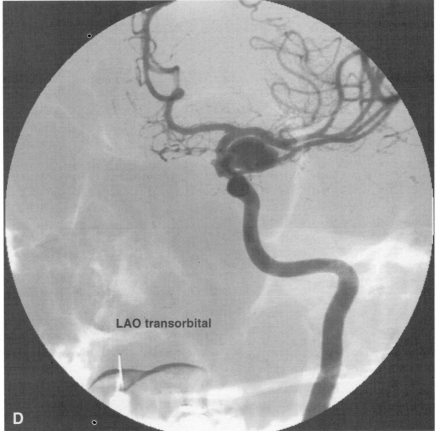

D   LAO transorbital

Figure 2.42. *(continued)*

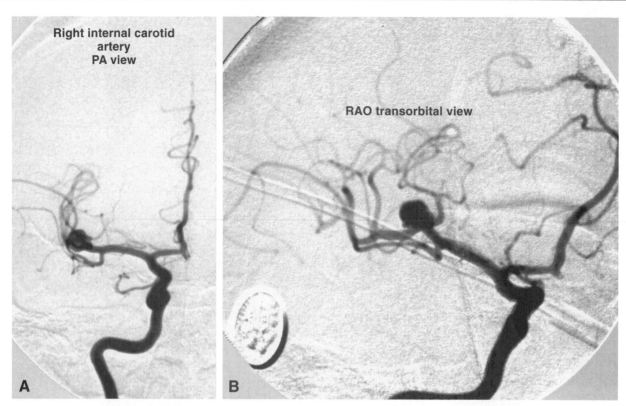

Figure 2.43. A, B *Aneurysm Evaluation IV.*   A PA view of the left internal carotid artery demonstrates a lobulated 9 mm aneurysm of the right middle cerebral artery (coin marker = 18 mm uncorrected). By placing the petrous ridges lower in the field and rotating to an RAO projection, a view evaluating the aneurysm in reference to the bifurcation of the middle cerebral artery was obtained. In this particular case, it could be argued that the supplemental view was not necessary. However, it is potentially important before surgery to know if an aneurysm in this location involves a segment of one of the divisions. Had such been the case, an eca-ica bypass might be a consideration.

Certain views are typically helpful for aneurysms in specific locations (29). However, each patient's anatomy varies considerably and each aneurysm is prone to have peculiarities which confound standard views. When difficulties are encountered it is usually necessary to resort to improvised projections to achieve the most helpful view. These can be achieved by constructing a hypothesis in one's mind of the aneurysm morphology and the parent artery based on the initial set of orthogonal views. A projection can then be established by a combination of equipment rotation and repositioning of the patient's head to test one's hypothesis (Figures 2.40, 2.41, 2.42, 2.43, 2.44, 2.45). The information from this run will either confirm the hypothesis or will give data to construct a more informed conjecture.

ANTERIOR COMMUNICATING ARTERY COMPLEX ANEURYSMS

The anterior communicating artery complex is frequently the most difficult site to interrogate definitively at angiography. Most commonly an anterior communicating artery aneurysm projects along the extended line of thrust of the dominant A1 segment. Therefore, an ipsilateral anterior oblique view (25 –35), i.e. perpendicular to the dominant

A1 segment, should optimize the profile of the aneurysm as the A2 segment bevels away superiorly, leaving an unobstructed view of the anteriorly projecting aneurysm. Particular consideration may be necessary for a multilobulated anterior communicating artery aneurysm in which a lobule projects posteriorly. This can be difficult to visualize during surgery and sometimes results in a clipping procedure leaving a residual lobe. A base view of the anterior communicating artery can be most helpful to evaluate this type of aneurysm. A base view is also very helpful for a situation where an obliquely oriented dysplastic anterior communicating artery simulates an aneurysm.

POSTERIOR COMMUNICATING ARTERY ANEURYSMS

A steep ipsilateral obliquity (55) is usually in a good range for optimizing one's view of the posterior communicating artery neck. Magnification views to evaluate superimposed turns of the posterior communicating artery or infundibula are often necessary. A fetal posterior communicating artery will often have a more lateral origin on the posterior wall of the internal carotid artery compared with a more medial origin and course of a non-fetal posterior communicating artery. Occasionally, retrograde filling of a suspicious posterior communicating artery dilatation can be promoted by compression of the ipsilateral carotid artery during vertebral artery injections. This maneuver can be particularly helpful in the setting of large dysplastic aneurysms the precise origin of which can be difficult to discern.

MIDDLE CEREBRAL ARTERY ANEURYSMS

The configuration of the middle cerebral artery is very variable. Ipsilateral transorbital oblique views such that one looks at the bifurcation or trifurcation without overlying petrous bone can be helpful, i.e. place the petrous ridge along the inferior orbital rim. A submento-vertex or base view of the head may also be very helpful for aneurysms in this location. A roadmap mask with a test hand-injection may help to fine-tune positioning in this and other locations.

VERTEBROBASILAR ANEURYSMS

For aneurysms or suspicious densities at the origin of the posterior inferior cerebellar artery, an ipsilateral oblique view angled 35–45 can be helpful. At the tip of the basilar artery, optimal views of the neck of the aneurysm must also try to identify the location of thalamoperforator arteries. The initial lateral view will be a guide in terms of whether the aneurysm is projecting anteriorly or posteriorly. An AP view perpendicular to the main axis of the aneurysm can then be assayed. Additional points of information which a neurosurgeon may wish to consider include the bifurcation angle of the basilar artery and the position of the neck of the aneurysm in relationship to the dorsum sellae. In the setting of a low basilar artery bifurcation with an acute angle, an aneurysm neck low behind the sella and flanked on either side by ascending P1 segments can present significant surgical problems in choice of approach.

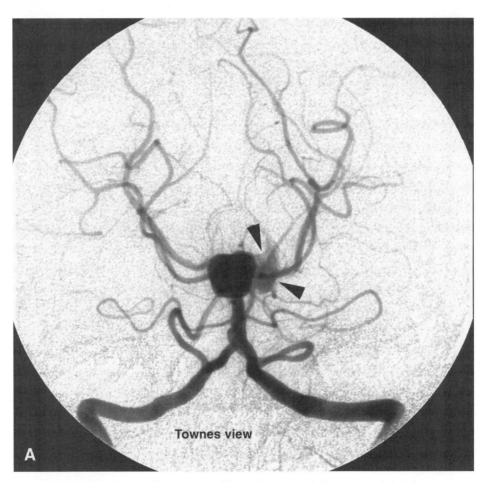

Townes view

A

Figure 2.44. A–C *Aneurysm Evaluation V.* A Townes view **(A)** of a complex, ruptured basilar tip aneurysm in a 65-year-old patient presenting with Grade IV subarachnoid hemorrhage. There is a large, irregular daughter sac or pseudoaneurysm **(arrowheads)** projecting to the left side of the main aneurysm. The main aneurysm dome superimposes on the foreshortened basilar artery. A lateral view (not shown) demonstrated that the aneurysm projected anteriorly. In the course of evaluation of the patient for endovascular coil therapy, successive Caldwell **(B)** and Water's views **(C)** rotate the neck of the aneurysm into profile, separating it from the P1 segments.

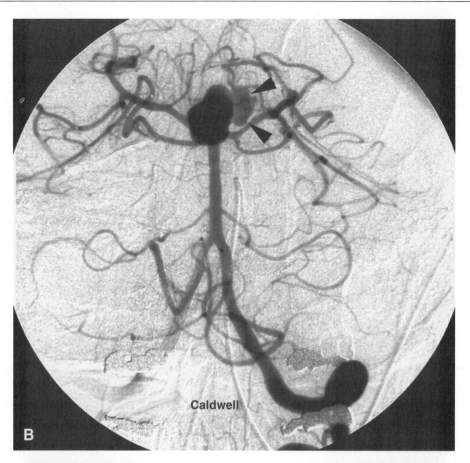

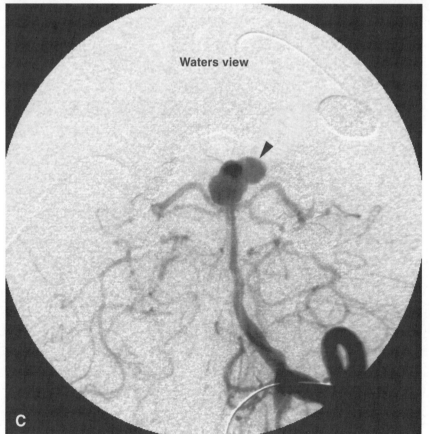

Figure 2.44. *(continued)*

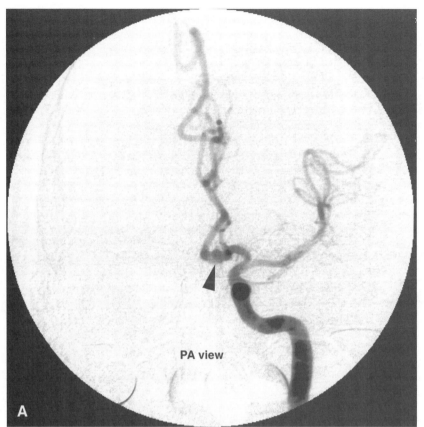

PA view

A

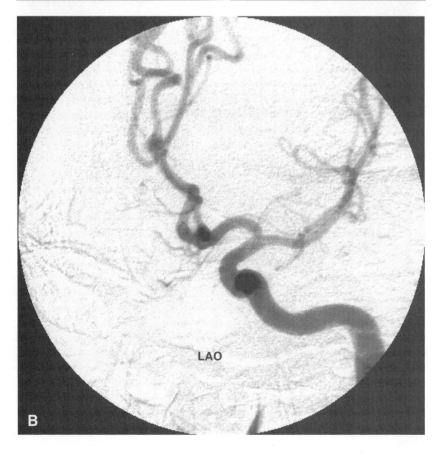

LAO

B

Figure 2.45. A–D *Aneurysm Evaluation VI.* A left internal carotid artery injection **(A)** in a 34-year-old patient with a right hemispheric arteriovenous malformation demonstrates enlargement of the right distal anterior cerebral artery filling via a suspiciously bulbous anterior communicating artery **(arrowhead).** A standard LAO projection **(B)** to evaluate the anterior communicating artery failed to clarify.

Figure 2.45. *(continued).* Considering the possibility of an aneurysm projecting posteriorly, an RAO projection was obtained **(C)** but was suboptimally positioned to exclude the possibility of an aneurysm completely. A base view **(D)** confirmed that the anterior communicating artery was enlarged and sinuous (arrow). However, no aneurysm was present.

It is important to minimize the number of injections made into the internal carotid artery or vertebral artery. However, in circumstances such as this the patient would probably have been subjected to an unnecessary craniotomy if an erroneous conclusion had been reached during the angiogram.

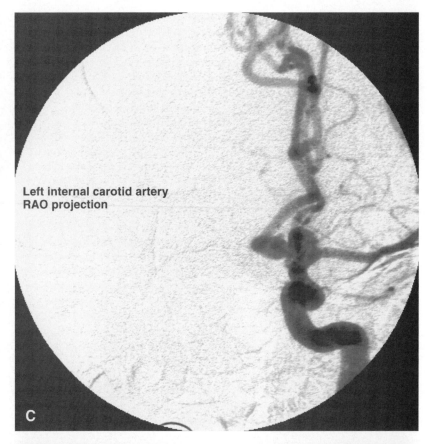

Left internal carotid artery
RAO projection

C

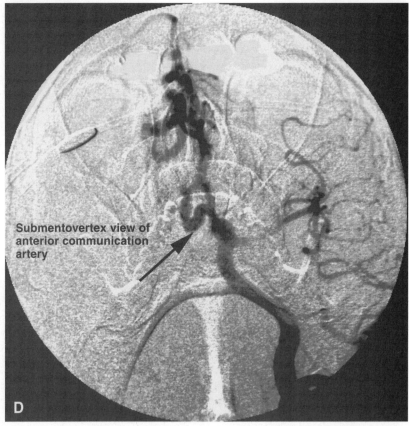

Submentovertex view of
anterior communication
artery

D

REFERENCES

1. Skalpe IO, Lundervold A, Tjøstad K. Complications of cerebral angiography. Comparing Metrizamide (Amipaque) and Meglumine Metrizoate (Isopaque Cerebral). Neuroradiology 1980; 19:67–71.

2. Bird CR, Drayer BP, Velaj R, et al. Safety of contrast media in cerebral angiography: iopamidol vs. methylglucamine iothalamate. AJNR Am J Neuroradiol 1984;5:801–803.

3. Bryan RN, Miller SL, Roehm JO, Weatherall PT. Neuroangiography with iohexol. AJNR Am J Neuroradiol 1983;4:344–346.

4. Pelz D, Fox AJ, Vinuela F. Clinical trial of iohexol vs. Conray 60 for cerebral angiography. AJNR Am J Neuroradiol 1984;5: 565–568.

5. Kido DK, Potts DG, Bryan RN, et al. Iohexol in cerebral angiography: multicenter clinical trial. Invest Radiol 1985;20(suppl 1):S55-S57.

6. Lovencic M, Jakovac I, Klanfar Z. Iohexol versus meglumine-Ca-metrizoate in cerebral angiography: a randomized double blind cross-over study. Acta Radiol Suppl (Stockh) 1986;369: 521–523.

7. Pelz DM, Fox AJ, Vinuela F, Lylyk P. A comparison of iopamidol and iohexol in cerebral angiography. AJNR Am J Neuroradiol 1988;9:1163–1166

8. Wolf GL, Arenson RL, Cross AP. A prospective trial of ionic vs. nonionic contrast agents in routine clinical practice: comparison of adverse effects. AJR 1989;152:939–944.

9. Katayama H, Yamaguchi K, Kozuka T, Takashima T, Seez P, Matsuura K. Adverse reactions to ionic and nonionic contrast media. Radiology 1990;175:621–628.

10. Latchaw RE. The use of nonionic contrast agents in neuroangiography. A review of the literature and recommendations for clinical use. Invest Radiol 1993; 28(Suppl 5):S55-S59.

11. Velaj R, Drayer B, Albright R, Fram E. Comparative neurotoxicity of angiographic contrast media. Neurology 1985;35: 1290–1298.

12. Caplan LR, Wolpert SM. Angiography in patients with occlusive cerebrovascular disease: Views of a stroke neurologist and neuroradiologist. AJNR Am J Neuroradiol 1991;12:593–601.

13. Rosovsky MA, Rusinek H, Berenstein A, Basak S, Setton A, Nelson PK. High-dose administration of nonionic contrast media: a retrospective review. Radiology 1996;200:119–122.

14. Cipolle J, Seifert RD, Neilan BA, et al. Heparin kinetics; variables related to disposition and dosage. Clin Pharmacol Ther 1981; 29:387–393.

15. Fujii Y, Takeuchi S, Koike T, et al. Heparin administration and monitoring for neuroangiography. Am J Neuroradiol AJNR 1994;15:51–54.

16. Kerber CW, Liebsch D. Flow dynamics for radiologists. II. Practical considerations in the live human. AJNR Am J Neuroradiol 1994;15:1076–1086.

17. Kerber CW, Liebsch D. Flow dynamics for radiologists. I. Basic principles of fluid flow. AJNR Am J Neuroradiol 1994;15: 1065–1075.

18. Mabon RF, Soder PD, Carpenter WA, Giddens DP. Fluid dynamics in cerebral angiography. Radiology 1978;128:669–676.

19. Fry DL. Acute vascular endothelial changes associated with increased blood velocity gradients. Circulation Research 1968;22: 165–197.

20. Doumanian HO, Amplatz K. Vascular jet collapse in selective angiocardiography. Radiology 1967;100:346–352.

21. MacDonald RL, Wallace C, Kestle JRW. Role of angiography following aneurysm surgery. J Neurosurg 1993;79:826–832.

22. Derdeyn CP, Moran CJ, Cross DT, Grubb RL, Dacey RG. Intraoperative digital subtraction angiography: a review of 112 consecutive examinations. Am J Neuroradiol AJNR 1995;16: 307–318.

23. Alexander TD, MacDonald RL, Weir B, Kowalczuk A. Intraoperative angiographic in cerebral aneurysm surgery: a prospective study in 100 craniotomies. Neurosurgery 1996;39:10–18.

24. Betti O, Munari C, Rosler R. Stereotactic radiosurgery with the linear accelerator: treatment of arteriovenous malformations. Neurosurgery 1989;24:311–321.

25. Lunsford LD, Konziolka D, Flickinger JC, et al. Stereotactic radiosurgery for arteriovenous malformations of the brain. J Neurosurg 1991;75:512–524.

26. Elisevich K, Cunningham IA, Assis L. Size estimation and magnification error in radiographic imaging: implications for classification of arteriovenous malformations. Am J Neuroradiol AJNR 1995;16:531–538.

27. Horton JA. Sizing rings: a simple technique for measuring intracranial lesions. Am J Neuroradiol AJNR 1995;16:1449–1451.

28. Brown RD, Wiebers DO, Forbes G, et al. The natural history of unruptured intracranial arteriovenous malformations. J Neurosurg 1988;68:352–357.

29. Lin JP, Kricheff II. Angiographic investigation of cerebral aneurysms. Technical aspects. Radiology 1972:105:69–76.

CHAPTER 3

Complications of Cerebral Angiography

If the indications for cerebral angiography have been clearly considered in advance, then the risk should be a minute fraction of that posed to a patient by not having the study. Nevertheless, complications of cerebral angiography include the possibility of killing the patient or permanently destroying a life. For this reason, it is important to be constantly aware of the potential for complications during cerebral angiography in all patients. Many serious complications of angiography are made worse by the effects of continuing the study, oblivious to a developing problem. If some complications cannot be anticipated and avoided, then early detection of problems is the most effective means of controlling their gravity (Figs. 3.1, 3.2, 3.3). This applies most particularly in the angiography suite. Anticipation of potential or imminent problems is also a feature of pre-angiographic evaluation of the patient and of post-angiographic care.

NEUROLOGIC COMPLICATIONS OF CEREBRAL ANGIOGRAPHY

Recent studies of complications of cerebral angiography, based on clinically evident neurologic complications arising within 24–72 hours of transfemoral cerebral angiography, report an overall incidence of approximately 0.5–4% (1–10). The majority of these events are transient with permanent neurologic deficits persisting in only 0.1–0.5% of patients in most such studies, or as many as 1.2% in the asymptomatic carotid artery stenosis (ACAS) study (10).

Some studies contain a bias in that they consider neurologic events to be angiographic complications only if they appeared to be related to the angiogram in the opinion of the investigator. Faught et al. (11), Earnest et al. (4), and Olivecrona (12) avoided this bias by including all neurologic deteriorations occurring within 24 hours of a cerebral arteriogram. They found neurologic deterioration rates of approximately 9–12% for all neurologic events and 5% for permanent events in patients referred for evaluation of recent ischemic disease. Many of the recorded complications were exacerbations of previous conditions. Earnest et al. (4) have speculated that compromise of cerebral blood flow in this group of patients may be a final common pathway for many of these complications. Likely causes include inadequate hydration or normalization of blood-pressure before the angiogram in patients for whom cerebral circulation is dependent on a hypertensive baseline state. On the other hand, consideration must be given to the rate of spontaneous disease-related, rather than pro-

cedure-related, events in this population over a similar period. Baum et al. (13) studied a group of patients whose angiographic examinations were canceled, and who demonstrated a similar incidence of clinical events in the time period that would have been considered in evaluation of post-angiographic complications.

Variable features among studies of complications after cerebral angiography include the patient population and diseases, referral characteristics of the institution, whether the study took place at a teaching hospital, the changing practice of radiology depending on the year of the study, and whether the post-angiographic evaluation was done by a radiologist or a neurologist. Risk factors for clinically evident neurologic complications in the first 24 hours after cerebral angiography include:

- Patients who are referred because of stroke or transient ischemic attacks (9)
- Patients whose angiograms demonstrate greater than 50–70% stenotic disease of the cerebral vessels (7, 9, 11)
- Patients older than age 70 (4, 9)
- Patients whose angiograms require a higher volume of contrast (4, 6, 9)
- Patients whose angiograms last more than 60–90 minutes or require multiple catheters (3, 6, 9)
- Patients with systemic hypertension or renal impairment (4, 6)
- Patients referred for subarachnoid hemorrhage or who are immediately postoperative (2, 4)

The risk of cerebral angiography performed by trainees at teaching hospitals has been examined by a number of studies (1, 3, 5, 14). McIvor et al. (14) and Mani et al. (2) concluded that difficulty in catheter manipulation by inexperienced radiologists was a risk factor for the examination taking more time, possibly in turn creating a higher likelihood of neurologic complications. However, institutional differences in terms of patient populations probably have a stronger effect on the nature and risk of complications. Some studies report on large patient groups (1,000) in whom death rates between 0% and 0.1% were recorded in the 24 hours after angiography. Upon reflection, patient groups comprised of a substantial proportion of cases presenting with acute subarachnoid hemorrhage could not be expected to do so well during a 24-hour period of observation even without an angiogram. This implies that selection bias may have a large influence on the conclusions of some studies.

A conclusion that all cerebral angiographic examinations are associated with a rate of neurologic complications in the range of 1–3% may be misleading. First, neurologic

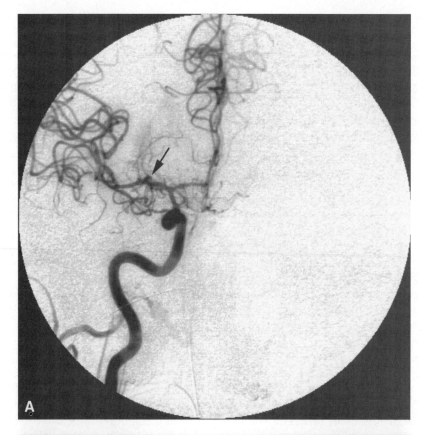

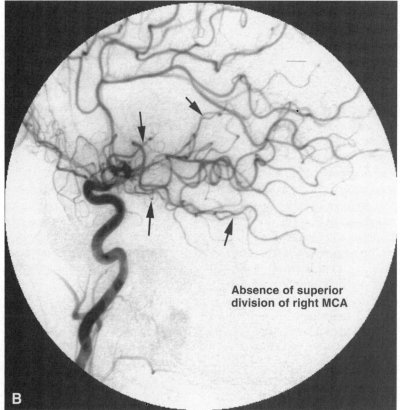

**Absence of superior
division of right MCA**

Figure 3.1. A–D Importance of prompt recognition of complications. A 65-year-old male undergoing angiographic evaluation of a posterior fossa dural arteriovenous malformation. A right internal carotid artery PA injection **(A)** demonstrates a stump-like density **(arrow in A)** off the middle cerebral artery. Although there appears to be an adequate number of middle cerebral artery branches on the PA view, the lateral view **(B)** demonstrates a lucency in the window formed under the pericallosal branch of the anterior cerebral artery due to occlusion of the superior division of the right middle cerebral artery. The branches of the inferior division are present **(arrows in B)**. This represents a procedural complication probably due to thrombus formation in the catheter. The patient was heparinized immediately, and the systolic blood pressure was elevated to 160 mm Hg.

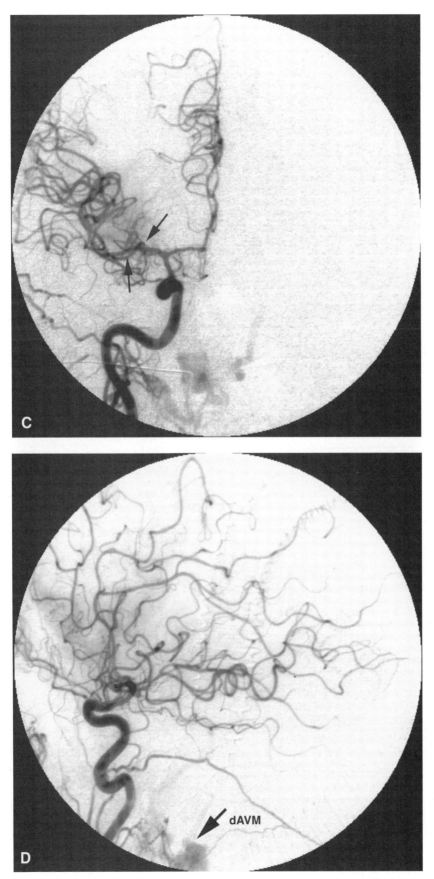

Figure 3.1. *(continued)* A common carotid arteriogram **(C and D)** done minutes later in anticipation of emergency thrombolysis demonstrated reopening of the superior division **(arrow in C).** Compare the lateral appearance after reopening **(D)** with the appearance during occlusion **(B),** demonstrating the sensitivity of the lateral view to branch occlusion of the middle cerebral artery. The patient recovered from this complication without clinical or imaging evidence of a related deficit. Pathologic opacification of veins in the posterior fossa is seen due to the dural arteriovenous malformation (dAVM) in the region of the foramen magnum.

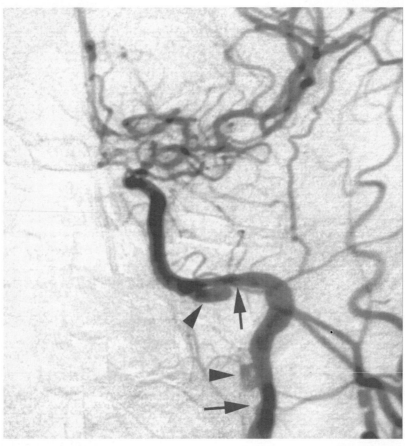

Figure 3.2. *Catheter-related dissection.* A left common carotid artery injection in 45-year-old female with grade IV subarachnoid hemorrhage and severe intracranial spasm of the left M1 and A1 segments. Irregular narrowing (arrows) of the cervical and petrous internal carotid artery, with pseudoaneurysm or pouch formation (arrowheads), is present. This complicated dissection was probably initiated by a previous angiographic procedure, and subsequently aggravated by episodes of paroxysmal hypertension experienced by the patient. Having seen a dissection on this side, one should be all the more concerned about whether one is present on the other side. This was, in fact, the case with this patient. It is important to consider the possibility of a covert dissection in all patients who have recently undergone angiography. High quality road-map images should be obtained before selecting the internal carotid artery or vertebral artery in these patients. This precaution carries obvious benefits for the patient and angiographer.

complications may not be clinically evident during a bedside examination. Dagirmanjian et al. (15) have demonstrated that Doppler sonography detects an average of more than 70 microembolic events per patient during cerebral angiography, without clinical evidence of a deficit. Although the authors described these events as clinically benign, rigorous neuropsychologic testing might be necessary to substantiate this. The incidence of small embolic infarcts occasionally seen on T2-weighted or diffusion-weighted MRI after cerebral angiography is unknown, but these events do come to attention occasionally. Presumably these clinically silent events are more common than the published complication rates that are based on clinically evident events. Gabrielsen (16) has commented that complication rates at many institutions are probably substantially higher than those quoted in medical journals, pointing out that a diminution of the workload in cerebral angiography implies that trainee and practicing neuroradiologists now gain less expertise than 20 years ago.

Emboli to the brain during cerebral angiography may represent dislodged atheromatous material, thrombus from the catheter, or air-bubbles. That these events may be clinically silent in many instances does not necessarily imply that they are benign. A retrospective review of medical records on cardiac surgery patients, for instance, might reveal a complication rate of 3.4% for altered mental state and 1% for stroke, but prospective investigation of higher motor and cognitive functioning detects transient and persistent neurologic and intellectual dysfunction rates considerably higher (17–20).

Terminal arteriolar or capillary focal dilatations measuring 10–40 m in diameter resulting from air or fat microemboli during aortography and cardiac bypass surgery can be identified at autopsy (21). These are of sufficient quantity that they could cause psychomotor dysfunction without necessarily giving histologic evidence of adjacent tissue ischemia. The importance of emboli of this size can be emphasized when one recalls that gelfoam powder of particle size 60 m can be used in tumor embolization when end-vessel penetration and tumor necrosis are intended. Animal experiments and clinical experience in divers with air-embolism to the brain suggest that a small volume of air can be tolerated and will pass quickly through the pial capillary bed without causing cerebral dysfunction. With higher volumes, bubbles become trapped in the pial arterioles, which then dilate with rapid onset of decline in cerebral function (22). Similarly, scuba divers who have suffered decompression illness or air-embolisms demonstrate MRI and CT focal deficits and problems with neuropsychologic testing indicating the focal ischemic effects of gas-bubbles in the cerebral circulation (23, 24). Cerebral air-embolism after angiography can occasionally be documented with CT (25), but its incidence and the degree to which it can occur without injury to the patient are not known.

The number of air-emboli to the brain during cardiac surgery correlates with the degree of postoperative cognitive deficit (26), and it is therefore important to eliminate or minimize this risk during cerebral angiography. Markus et al. (27) have demonstrated that Doppler recorded events in the human middle cerebral artery, probably representing microemboli of air during cerebral angiography, are similar to those seen in sheep experiments. The authors (27) found that with higher density non-ionic contrast (340 mg/ml) the likelihood of detecting air-emboli in the contrast could be reduced significantly by allowing the syringe of high density contrast to stand for a few minutes. This phenomenon of slow clearance of air from the high-density contrast was not seen with lower strength contrast (140 mg/ml) or saline that had been allowed to stand for a few minutes. Markus et al. (27) commented that one possible explanation for this could be that vigorous suction necessary for drawing up a syringe of higher viscosity contrast might be responsible for introducing more microbubbles. The same authors reported also that air-bubbles are more likely to be introduced by a rapid injection than a slow one. Speculative conclusion, in the absence of evidence to the contrary, would suggest that slow filling of contrast syringes during angiography might be a prudent precaution, as well as meticulously clearing any adherent bubbles from the inside of the syringe or catheter-hub prior to injections.

A practical consideration in reference to anesthetic gases and the risk of introducing bubbles via an angiographic catheter deserves attention. Bubbles of room-air inadvertently introduced into the blood stream where the concentration of nitrous oxide is high during general anesthesia are theoretically likely to expand considerably as the partial pressure of nitrous oxide gas inside the bubbles equalizes with the surrounding blood. For this reason, anesthetic agents other than nitrous oxide gas are preferable during neuroangiographic procedures.

TRANSIENT GLOBAL AMNESIA AND CORTICAL BLINDNESS AS COMPLICATIONS OF CEREBRAL ANGIOGRAPHY

Neurologic complications of cerebral angiography other than those clearly related to hemispheric ischemia may occasionally be seen and are usually transient in nature. Some patients have been reported with abrupt onset of transient global amnesia after cerebral angiography (28, 29). This has been ascribed to an effect on the posterior circulation with particular reference to the medial temporal lobes. Some cases of amnesia may be related to previously diagnosed temporal lobe epilepsy, whereas others are seen in patients with atherosclerotic vertebro-basilar disease (29). Transient global amnesia after cerebral angiography usually occurs in the absence of other neurologic signs, and patients invariably recover without specific intervention within 24 hours. It can occur after use of ionic and non-ionic contrast. The possibilities of atheromatous emboli and particulate contamination of contrast have been mooted as possible explanations. Jackson et al. (30) reported an anomalous 17% incidence of transient global amnesia after vertebrobasilar angiography in a particular group of patients studied over a 24-month period. This transpired to be related to a faulty contrast warming cabinet that resulted in contrast being injected at a temperature higher than that of the body. The authors concluded that intracranial vasospasm was the explanation for their observation of transient global amnesia. The same authors included a case of transient cortical blindness within this group of patients. A migrainous phenomenon to explain these events seems plausible (31, 32). Similar but lesser transient symptoms such as subjective perceptions of visual scintillations, with or without associated headache, can occasionally be reported after angiography and presumably happen through the same mechanism.

A case of bilateral sensorineural hearing loss after vertebrobasilar angiography, recovering within 24 hours, has been reported by Matsuoka et al. (33). These authors treated the patient empirically with high doses of methylprednisolone and ascribed the complication to bilateral anoxia of the cochlea. Transient involuntary leg movement (monoballismus) was reported in five patients during anterior and posterior circulation cerebral angiography by Komiyama et al. (34). They speculated that transient hemispheric or brainstem ischemia might be the etiology. A direct neurotoxic effect of contrast has also been proposed to explain some of these events, more likely to occur in situations in which the blood-brain barrier has been compromised. Studdard et al. (35) reported a case of temporary cortical blindness associated with persistence of contrast stain in the occipital visual area, and they proposed a direct toxic effect of the contrast on the brain in a patient with poor renal function.

ANEURYSMAL RUPTURE DURING ANGIOGRAPHY

Probably the most severe neurologic event that can occur during cerebral angiography is rebleeding of a freshly ruptured aneurysm, associated with a mortality of at least 79% (36) . For many years, it was thought that rebleeding during angiography was coincidental because it was believed there was no evidence of an increase of intra-carotid or intracranial pressure during angiographic injections (37,

38). However, the high prevalence of transient opacification of intracerebral vessels through the communicating arteries during angiography would seem to argue that intracranial transmission of a substantial pressure wave is commonplace (Fig. 3.4). More modern studies (39–41) have demonstrated under laboratory conditions that although an intracarotid contrast injection may cause a reflex bradycardia and mild hypotension, there is an initial 1–2 second period of elevated intracarotid pressure, which declines over approximately 2–10 seconds. Nornes et al. (42) have confirmed with Doppler sonography a biphasic pattern of middle cerebral artery flow-velocity during angiography. In the setting of an aneurysm with a recently perforated wall secured only by fresh clot and hematoma, power-injections of standard rates accompanied by an increase in intravascular pressure at the level of the circle of Willis could be responsible for inducing rehemorrhage.

Koenig et al. (43) reported on ten cases of aneurysmal rupture during angiography and reviewed the literature. They observed a 100% mortality rate in their patients, and thought that this high rate (in excess of the 41–46% mortality observed with aneurysmal rerupture under other circumstances) was, at least in part, related to extravasation of hyperosmolar contrast around and into the brain. Moreover, they advised that consideration be given to a reduction in contrast injection-rates to about 4 cc per sec in patients with recent subarachnoid hemorrhage. In the setting of vasospasm or elevated intracranial pressure such a rate should give adequate arterial opacification and reduce the risk to the fragile aneurysm. Komiyama et al. (36) conducted an extensive review and found a 79% mortality associated with aneurysmal rupture during angiography. This event occurred in approximately 3% of all patients referred for angiography because of acute subarachnoid

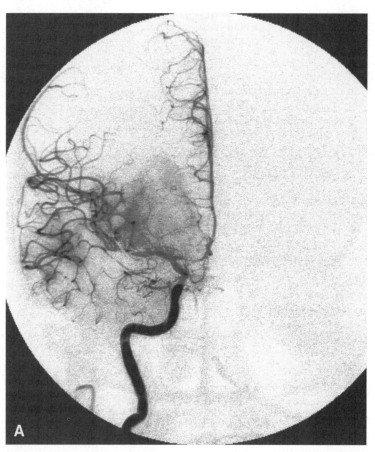

Figure 3.3. A–D Dangers of intracranial microcatheter manipulation without heparinization. A 54-year-old female with grade III subarachnoid hemorrhage underwent an operation for a right middle cerebral artery bifurcation aneurysm. Severe spasm was noted in the operating room and treated with topical application of papaverine. Still under general anesthesia, a CT demonstrated evidence of a right middle cerebral artery superior division infarct. She was then brought to angiography for intraarterial papaverine therapy for vasospasm. The initial run **(A)** demonstrated patency of the mainstem of the right middle cerebral artery, but some distal branches of the middle cerebral artery were slow to fill. Because of her immediately postoperative status, heparin was not administered. A microcatheter was passed without difficulty to the right supraclinoid internal carotid artery, and 100 mg of papaverine infused. A run then demonstrated occlusion of the distal middle cerebral artery stem **(arrow in B)** and filling defects in the pericallosal and callosomarginal artery **(arrowheads in C)**. Notice how the main catheter in B has assumed an unfavorable position, needing adjustment. With administration of a bolus of heparin and elevation of blood-pressure, the embolus occluding the right middle cerebral artery broke up. Flow was much improved on a subsequent run **(D)**. Had flow not resumed, administration of thrombolysis would probably have been necessary. However, the risks of thrombolysis in a patient 3 hours after a craniotomy with an established infarct would have been considerable.

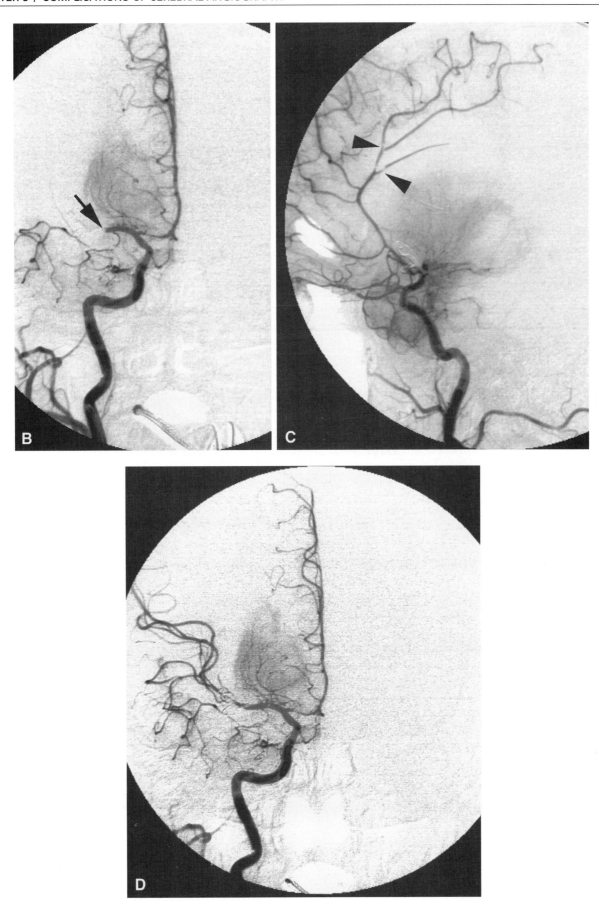

Figure 3.3. *(continued)*

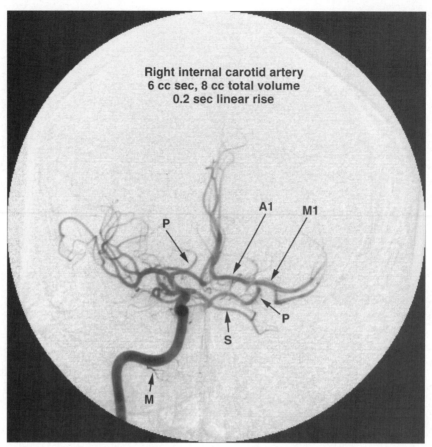

Right internal carotid artery
6 cc sec, 8 cc total volume
0.2 sec linear rise

Figure 3.4. Non-physiologic hemodynamic effects of internal carotid artery injections. A 27-year-old male patient presenting with dural sinus thrombosis after multiple systemic diseases, complicating an underlying diagnosis of AIDS. A 6 ml/sec × 1.3 sec injection in the cervical right internal carotid artery opacifies the entire anterior and posterior circle of Willis, in the absence of occlusive arterial disease elsewhere. The superior cerebellar arteries are visualized bilaterally (S), as are the posterior cerebral arteries (P). Notice the persistent mandibulo-vidian artery from the right petrous internal carotid artery (M). With a slightly different angulation of the intensifier, one can see how the A1 and P1 segments can be directly superimposed on a frontal projection such as this. Therefore when an internal carotid artery injection opacifies the contralateral posterior cerebral artery in this manner, it can be sometimes easy to misinterpret it as the contralateral A1 and M1 segments.

hemorrhage. Particular features of this group of patients were that most such angiographic bleeds occurred on day 0 after the initial subarachnoid hemorrhage and were more likely to be observed when cerebral angiography was undertaken within 6 hours of the initial bleed. Teal et al. (44) have commented that a test-injection by hand can occasionally be more provocative to a constrained vascular tree than injections made with the power-injector, indicating that extreme caution should be exercised in this maneuver too. One of the cases reported by Koenig et al. (43) ruptured in this manner during a hand-injection. Saitoh et al. (45) reported a rerupture rate for aneurysms of approximately 5% during angiography done within 6 hours of the initial bleed. However, they and other authors do not believe that this small increase in risk warrants a policy of delaying the cerebral angiogram.

An intraprocedural rupture may not always be seen on the angiographic images (Fig. 3.5). The only warning may be changes in the patient's vital signs, subjective complaints, and a deterioration in neurologic status, which should be monitored after each angiographic run. With more extreme extravasation, subtle persistence of contrast on the images or frank opacification of the subarachnoid space and ventricles may occur. With a sudden increase in intracranial pressure, diminished run-off of contrast in the internal carotid artery may be seen. When stagnation of contrast in the internal carotid artery is seen, one may first think of an occluding embolus, but sudden sustained elevation of intracranial pressure can cause similar stagnation and poor run-off of contrast. Severe bradycardia or diminished cardiac output can give a similar fluoroscopic appearance. Nornes (46) reported data on the changes in internal carotid artery blood flow and pressure associated with intraoperative aneurysmal rupture. There is an initial increase in flow proportional to the amount of leakage from the aneurysm, followed by a marked reduction in flow with end-diastolic flow arrest or diastolic flow-reversal. Angiographically this pressure flux has been seen with intra-procedural aneurysm rupture as a diminished or stagnant run-off of contrast from the internal carotid artery.

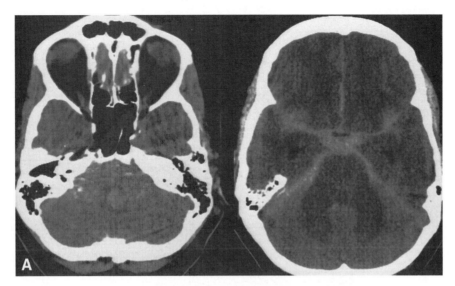

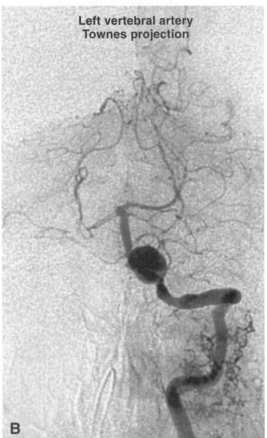

Figure 3.5. A–C *Aneurysm rupture during angiography.* A 64-year-old female presenting with grade IV subarachnoid hemorrhage. A preangiographic CT **(A)** demonstrates extensive cisternal hemorrhage, dilatation of the temporal horns, and a mass-like rounded density within the IVth ventricle. An injection was performed in the left vertebral artery **(B),** demonstrating a rounded aneurysm projecting in the midline posterior to the vertebro-basilar junction. The patient immediately became hypertensive with drainage of fresh blood from the ventriculostomy. A non-subtracted image of the head from late in the run **(C)** demonstrates contrast layering in the occipital horns and IIIrd ventricle following intraventricular rupture of the posterior fossa aneurysm. (Case courtesy of R. Klufas MD, Boston.)

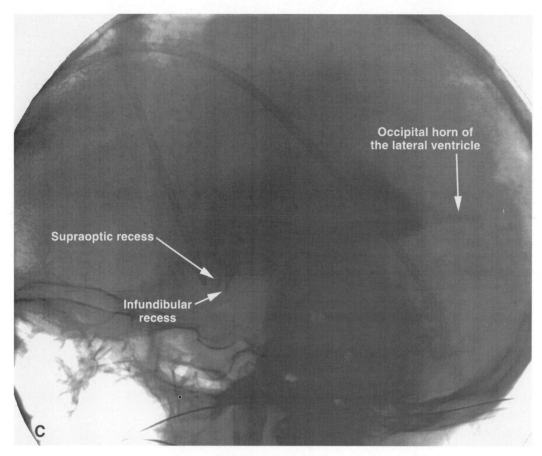

Figure 3.5. *(continued)*

Similar concerns for the status of the aneurysm and the potential for rebleeding should prompt concern about fluctuations in systemic blood pressure during intubation of the patient. This may occur if general anesthesia is being induced for an endovascular procedure or if patient agitation requires general anesthesia.

NONNEUROLOGIC COMPLICATIONS OF CEREBRAL ANGIOGRAPHY

Nonneurological complications predominantly include hematoma formation at the arterial puncture site. The risk of a significant hematoma is reported at approximately 6.9–10.7% (6, 12) for femoral puncture sites. Higher hematoma rates for carotid and axillary/brachial sites have been reported at 25.3% and 15.7% respectively (12), although Kerber et al. (47) reported a hematoma rate of only 6% for axillary puncture sites and a 1% complication rate of axillary artery thrombosis. Local complications during and after transbrachial punctures using a 4 French catheter have been reported ranging from 2.1–44% (48, 49). However, the pulse is more difficult to control in the axillary and brachial areas during compression, and these sites are more likely to be problematic than the femoral.

The risk of hematoma formation probably is influenced by a number of factors including increased age of the patient, cooperation of the patient, size of sheath or catheter

used, and the presence of atherosclerotic disease. Thomson and Thomson (5) found that almost all puncture site hematomata occurred in patients older than age 60. Dion et al. (6) reported that patients older than age 70 had a hematoma rate of 18% after transfemoral cerebral angiography, of whom one third needed fluid replacement or surgical repair.

Femoral artery pseudoaneurysms are rare after neuro-angiographic studies with an incidence of approximately 0.05–0.55% (50). In the event of an iliac artery dissection during an angiographic study, during the subsequent management, if possible, an angiographic image of the dissection should be obtained and pull-down pressures above and below the dissection should be recorded.

Other non-neurologic complications of cerebral angiography with an incidence of less than 1–2% (6, 12), but which constitute serious problems, include myocardial infarction, cardiac arrest, angina pectoris, and allergic reactions. Minor complications include nausea or vomiting, benign bradycardia or extrasystoles, fainting, paresthesia in the leg due to nerve infiltration with local anesthetic, or delayed hematoma formation after discharge home.

Premedication for Contrast Reaction

With a patient for whom the possibility of complications such as an allergic reaction require special consideration, extra precautions are necessary. These include more specific discussion of the risks with the patient. Additionally, premedication with corticosteroids, diphenhydramine, and cimetidine in patients with histories of previous allergic reaction is required (51–53).

Patients with a previous episode of anaphylactoid reaction to contrast have a risk of approximately 17–35% of a similar reaction on subsequent re-exposure (54–56). Yocum et al. (51) found that a high-risk group of patients, so categorized on the basis of previous contrast reaction, had an 18.3% incidence of repeat reaction with intravenous or intraarterial administration of contrast. Prior administration of diphenhydramine 50 mg IV reduced the rate of minor reactions in that study to 4.2%. Using a pretreatment regimen of prednisone 50 mg PO every 6 hours for three doses ending 1 hour before the procedure and diphenhydramine 50 mg IM 1 hour before the procedure, Greenberger et al. (52) demonstrated a reduction in rate of severe reaction in a high risk group of patients to 0.3%. The incidence of mild reactions was reduced to 7.1%. For emergency patients, with whom a delay in the study for extended premedication is not possible, the authors recommended hydrocortisone 200 mg IV stat and repeated every 4 hours during the procedure. Lasser et al. (53) found that pretreatment with methylprednisolone 32 mg PO during the 24 hours before an angiogram and repeated 2 hours before the procedure resulted in a detectable reduction in rates of adverse reaction in all patients. In addition to steroid doses equivalent to these studies, most departments also recommend cimetidine 300 mg usually given parenterally with diphenhydramine 50 mg, before or at the start of a procedure. For high risk patients precautionary notification of the anesthesiology staff before the case gets started is good to ensure that assistance will be promptly available if airway problems develop. For these patients the case should not get under way without having one or preferably two large bore IV access sites established.

HYDRATION AND DIABETIC PATIENTS

Adequate hydration of all patients particularly those with borderline or established renal impairment is important in the hours before the procedure when the patient is being kept NPO (no food or liquid by mouth). An IV line running at 80–120 ml/hr will prevent the patient from becoming dehydrated during the period of waiting.

Diabetic patients on NPO status will require modification of their insulin dose. Usually elimination of their short-acting insulin dose and administration of half of their longer-acting dose on the morning of the procedure will suffice, with a sliding scale for the remainder of the day after the procedure. Type II diabetic patients should be questioned carefully to ensure that they have not been taking metformin or other contraindicated substance before the procedure (57).

PROCEDURAL DETECTION OF COMPLICATIONS

It is easy to focus one's attention entirely on the angiographic images and on considerations of technique during the procedure and to neglect to monitor the patient's neurologic status for important changes. Attaching the patient to monitoring devices for vital signs and O2 saturation is obviously an essential preparatory step, particularly where use of sedative agents during the procedure is anticipated. These devices can lull one into a sense of security that the patient is being monitored in every necessary way. However, this can be a mistake as the monitors and angiographic images do not always reveal problems that have arisen. This can be particularly true with sedated or intubated patients in whom one might be inclined to assume a status quo because of the absence of any volunteered complaints. Intermittent checks of extremity strength, language function, level of consciousness, or pupil symmetry are important for the early detection of hemispheric events or alteration in intracerebral pressure. In patients with subarachnoid hemorrhage who have a ventriculostomy in place, the ICP should be monitored closely. A routine check of all major parameters should be done after every intracerebral run; without these checks a lapse of 30–40 minutes may occur before an important change in the patient's status is detected.

POST-PROCEDURAL PATIENT CARE

Patients should leave the angiography suite with a preliminary chart-note indicating the procedure performed, the technique used, and the relevant clinical findings. There should also be a lucid set of orders for patient immobilization, groin and pulse precautions, and intravenous fluids to continue over the following 4–8 hours. Contingency orders for changes in neurologic status or other complications should include a telephone number at which the nurse taking care of the patient can contact the radiology team and/or the referral physician. Most of the problems that arise in this time are minor. They include mild headache, hypotension from the effects of medication and prolonged fasting, or groin hematoma problems due to failure of the patient to comply with instructions. Many of these can be avoided with intravenous hydration or PRN medication orders for headache, nausea, vomiting, etc. as a routine component of the post-angiogram paperwork.

Outpatients who are being discharged home on the same day should be given explicit instructions, as should their family members, on groin-care after they return home. It is probably a good idea to demonstrate to them where and how exactly to compress the groin site in the event rebleeding. Advice to recline in the car seat, to avoid of strenuous activity for 24 hours, and on proper care of the groin puncture site are all routinely included with these instructions.

REFERENCES

1. Mani RL, Eisenberg RL. Complications of catheter cerebral angiography: analysis of 5000 procedures. I. Criteria and incidence. Am J Radiol 1978;131:861–865.
2. Mani RL, Eisenberg RL. Complications of catheter cerebral angiography: analysis of 5000 procedures. II: relation of compli-

cation rates to clinical and arteriography diagnoses. Am J Radiol 1978;13:867–869.

3. Mani RL, Eisenberg RL. Complications of catheter cerebral angiography: analysis of 5000 procedures. III: assessment of arteries injected, contrast medium used, duration of procedure, and age of patient. Am J Radiol 1978;131:871–874.

4. Earnest F, Forbes G, Sandok BA, et al. Complications of cerebral angiography: prospective assessment of risk. Am J Radiol 1984;142:247–253.

5. Thomson KR, Thomson SMcA. Complications of cerebral angiography in a teaching hospital. Austral Radiol 1986;30:206–208.

6. Dion JE, Gates PC, Fox AJ, et al. Clinical events following neuroangiography: a prospective study. Stroke 1987;18:997–1004.

7. Hankey GJ, Warlow CP, Molyneux AJ. Complications of cerebral angiography for patients with mild carotid territory ischaemia being considered of carotid endarterectomy. J Neurol Neurosurg Psychiatr 1990;53:542–548.

8. Warnock NG, Gandhi MR, Bergvall U, et al. Complications of intraarterial digital subtraction angiography in patients investigated for cerebral vascular disease. Br J Radiol 1993;66:855–858.

9. Heiserman JE, Dean BL, Hodak JA, et al. Neurologic complications of cerebral angiography. Am J Neuroradiol 1994;15:1401–1407.

10. Executive Committee for the Asymptomatic Carotid Atherosclerosis Study. Endarterectomy for Asymptomatic Carotid Artery Stenosis. JAMA 1995;273:1421–1428.

11. Faught E, Trader SD, Hanna GR. Cerebral complications of angiography for transient ischemia and stroke: prediction of risk. Neurology 1979;29:4-15.

12. Olivecrona H. Complications of cerebral angiography. Neuroradiology 1977;14:175–181.

13. Baum S, Stein GN, Kuroda KK. Complications of "no arteriography." Radiology 1966;86:835–838.

14. McIvor J, Steiner TJ, Perkin GD, et al. Neurological morbidity of arch and carotid angiography in cerebrovascular disease. The influence of contrast medium and radiologist. Br J Radiol 1987;60:117–122.

15. Dagirmanjian A, Davis DA, Rothfus WE, et al. Silent cerebral microemboli occurring during carotid angiography: frequency as determined with Doppler sonography. Am J Neuroradiol 1993;161:1037–1040.

16. Gabrielsen TO. Commentary; Neurological complications of cerebral angiography. Am J Neuroradiol 1994;15:1408–1411.

17. Shaw PJ, Bates D, Cartlidge NEF, et al. Early intellectual dysfunction following coronary bypass surgery. Q J Med 1986;58:59–68.

18. Sotaniemi KA, Mononen H, Hokkanen TE. Long term cerebral outcome after open heart surgery: a five year neuropsychological follow-up study. Stroke 1986;17:410–416.

19. Smith PL, Treasure T, Newman SP, et al. Cerebral consequences of cardiopulmonary bypass. Lancet 1986;1 (8485):823–825.

20. Shaw PJ, Bates D, Cartlidge NE, et al. Long-term intellectual dysfunction following coronary bypass graft surgery: a six month follow-up study. Q J Med 1987;62:259–268.

21. Moody DM, Bell MA, Challa VR, et al. Brain microemboli during cardiac surgery or aortography. Ann Neurol 1990;28:477–486.

22. Helps SC, Meyer-Witting M, Reilly PL, et al. Increasing doses of intracarotid air and cerebral blood flow in rabbits. Stroke 1990;21:1340–1345.

23. Greer HD, Massey EW. Neurologic injury from undersea diving. Neurologic Clinics 1992;10:1031–1045.

24. Warren LP, Djang WT, Moon RE, et al. Neuroimaging of scuba diving injuries to the CNS. Am J Neuroradiol 1988;9:933–938.

25. Voorhies RM, Fraser RAR. Cerebral air embolism occurring at angiography and diagnosed by computerized tomography. J Neurosurg 1984;60:177–178.

26. Pugsley W, Klinger L, Paschalis C, et al. The impact of microemboli during cardiopulmonary bypass on neuropsychological functioning. Stroke 1994;25:1393–1399.

27. Markus H, Loh A, Israel D, et al. Microscopic air embolism during cerebral angiography and strategies for its avoidance. Lancet 1993;341:783–787.

28. Wales LR, Nov AA. Transient global amnesia: complications of cerebral angiography. Am J Neuroradiol 1981;2:275–277.

29. Pexman JHW, Coates RK. Amnesia after femorocerebral angiography. Am J Neuroradiol 1983;4:979–983.

30. Jackson A, Stewart G, Wood A, et al. Transient global amnesia and cortical blindness after vertebral angiography: Further evidence for the role of arterial spasm. Am J Neuroradiol 1995;16:955–959.

31. Juni J, Morera J, Lainez JM, et al. Transient global amnesia after cerebral angiography with iohexol. Neuroradiology 1992;34:141–143.

32. Giang DW, Kido DK. Transient global amnesia associated with cerebral angiography performed with use of iopamidol. Radiology 1989;172:195–196.

33. Matsuoka A, Shitara T, Okamoto M, et al. Transient deafness with iopamidol following angiography. Acta Oto-Laryngologica-Suppl. 1994;514:78–80.

34. Komiyama M, Yasui T, Izumi T. Transient involuntary movement of the leg (monoballismus) during cerebral angiography. Am J Neuroradiol 1995;16:1942–1945.

35. Studdard W, Davis D, Young S. Cortical blindness after cerebral angiography. J Neurosurg 1981;54:240–244.

36. Komiyama M, Tamura K, Nagata Y, et al. Aneurysmal Rupture during angiography. Neurosurgery 1993;33:798–803.

37. Bakay L, Sweet WH. Cervical and intracranial intra-arterial pressures with and without vascular occlusion. Surg Gynecol Obstet 1952;95:67–75.

38. Greitz T. A radiological study of the brain circulation by rapid serial angiography of the carotid artery. Acta Radiol (suppl) 1956;140:21–33.

39. Lin JPT, Kricheff II, Chase NE. Blood pressure changes during retrograde brachial angiography. Radiology 1964;83:640–646.

40. Hayakawa K, Okuno Y, Miyazawa T, et al. The decrease of intracarotid pressure following carotid angiography. Invest Radiol 1994;29:S96-S98.

41. Saitoh H, Hayakawa K, Nishimura K, et al. Intracarotid blood pressure changes during contrast medium injection. Am J Neuroradiol 1996;17:51–54.

42. Nornes H, Sorteberg W, Nakstad P, et al. Haemodynamic aspects of clinical cerebral angiography. Concurrent two vessel monitoring using transcranial Doppler ultrasound. Acta Neurochir 1990;105:89–97.

43. Koenig GH, Marshall WH, Poole GJ, et al. Rupture of intracranial aneurysms during cerebral angiography: Report of ten cases and review of the literature. Neurosurgery 1979;5:314–324.

44. Teal JS, Wade PJ, Bergeron RT, et al. Ventricular opacification during carotid angiography secondary to rupture of intracranial aneurysm. Radiology 1973;106:581–583.

45. Saitoh H, Hayakawa K, Nishimura K, et al. Rerupture of cerebral aneurysms during angiography. Am J Neuroradiol 1995;16:539–542.

46. Nornes H. Cerebral arterial flow dynamics during aneurysm haemorrhage. Acta Neurochir 1978;41:39–48.
47. Kerber C, Mani RL, Bank WO, et al. Selective cerebral angiography through the axillary artery. Neuroradiology 1975;10:131–135.
48. Uchino A. Local complications in transbrachial cerebral angiography using the 4-F catheter. Neurolo Med Chir (Tokyo) 1991;31:647–649.
49. Millward SF. Letter to the editor: Routine transbrachial angiography. Radiology 1989;172:577.
50. Coley BD, Roberts AC, Fellmeth BD, et al. Postangiographic femoral artery pseudoaneurysms: Further experience with US-guided compression repair. Radiology 1995;194:307–311.
51. Yocum MW, Heller AM, Abels RI. Efficacy of intravenous pretesting and antihistamine prophylaxis in radiocontrast media-sensitive patients. J Allergy Clin Immunol 1978;62:309–313.
52. Greenberger PA, Patterson R, Simon R, et al. Pretreatment of high-risk patients requiring radiographic contrast media studies. J Allergy Clin Immunol 1981;67:185–187.
53. Lasser EC, Berry CC, Mishkin MM, et al. Pretreatment with corticosteroids to prevent adverse reactions to non-ionic contrast media. AJR 1994;162:523–526.
54. Witten DM, Hirsch FD, Hartman GW. Acute reactions to urographic contrast media: Incidence, clinical characteristics and relationship to history of hypersensitivity states. Am J Roentgenol 1973;119:832–840.
55. Shehadi WH. Adverse reactions to intravascularly administered contrast media: A comprehensive study based on a prospective survey. Am J Roentgenol 1975;127:145–152.
56. Fischer HW, Doust VL. An evaluation of pretesting in the problem of serious and fatal reactions to excretory urography. Radiology 1972;103:497–501.
57. Dachman AH. New contraindications to intravascular iodinated contrast material (letter). Radiology 1995;195:545.

CHAPTER 4

Radiation Risks and Safety

The quantity of risk associated with radiation exposure of patients and medical personnel during diagnostic angiographic procedures is not known precisely. The risk is probably very small.

An extensive body of epidemiologic and other evidence demonstrates that radiation exposures far in excess of those used for diagnostic procedures are associated with an increased incidence of delayed malignancy. Other delayed side effects of radiation include growth retardation, lenticular opacities, premature atherosclerotic vascular disease, and mental retardation after in utero exposure. These data emerge from studies of populations intentionally or inadvertently exposed to significant doses of radiation. These studies include the following:

• Patients with ankylosing spondylitis treated with x-irradiation
• Patients exposed to thorotrast
• Children with thymic enlargement or tinea capitis who were treated with high doses of local radiation
• Uranium miners
• Radium dial painters
• Military personnel exposed during weapons testing maneuvers
• Survivors of the Hiroshima and Nagasaki bombings
• Victims of the Chernobyl disaster

From studies of exposed populations, data have been collected to give an estimate of the relationship between high radiation doses and biologic effect, with particular emphasis on carcinogenesis. Various regressions of the dose-risk curve down to radiation levels relevant to diagnostic and interventional neuroangiography can be performed based on certain assumptions. The gravity of the conclusions arising from these extrapolations depends on the assumptions made about the lower end of this curve; some assumptions about the curve suggest a higher risk than do others.

Perception of Risk from Radiation

The uncertainty of the degree of risk involved with radiation exposures during neuroangiographic procedures frequently serves only to amplify the anxiety surrounding this question. Unfortunately, it can be overlooked that the risk involved is diminutive. Popular imagination has a strong tendency to underestimate the risks involved with banal activities or events and to overestimate the dangers posed by the exotic or rare (1). Botulism, lightening-strikes, and nuclear reactor accidents may rank highly in surveys of popular anxieties, whereas the risks of highway driving, smoking, or of a sedentary life-style are overlooked. For

similar reasons, most readers would probably overestimate the answers to the following questions:

Q. Estimates of the acute death-tolls at Hiroshima and Nagasaki range as high as 140,000 and 70,000 respectively in the initial days and weeks following the bombings. What percentage of the casualties died from radiation-related injuries (2)?

Q. A 1950 National Census in Japan identified approximately 159,000 survivors of the Hiroshima bombing and 125,000 from Nagasaki. How many of the survivors have since died from radiation-related leukemia?

Q. Among the survivors from Nagasaki and Hiroshima who died of cancer, to what extent is their malignant disease attributable to exposure to radiation?

Radiation exposure and its associated dangers have the capacity to provoke alarm. It is easy to become intimidated by having to deal with units of measurement that do not have an intuitive meaning in the domain of human experience. Perception of risk by the public and the legal community may assume a reality and magnitude of its own, which varies with the degree of risk suggested by scientific data.

To place the nature of risk from radiation in an understandable context, one must first consider that the number of known fatal malignancies following gamma or x-irradiation is small compared with more common fatal diseases. This does not trivialize the serious risks from radiation exposure, but places the risk in a relative context. Concrete comparisons are probably the best medium to demonstrate that, having been exposed to diagnostic or interventional levels of radiation, a radiation-related malignancy is a highly unlikely prospect.

Intuitive bias would probably lead most to believe that among atomic bomb survivors, epidemiologic studies should show a massive number of radiation-related malignancies. In fact, although the relative risks of malignancy are high, the absolute numbers are surprisingly low. It is estimated that an exposure of 1 Gy increases the risk of leukemia by a factor of 5.2 (2). To present the risk in a less alarming manner, one might point out that the average exposure of Japanese survivors has been estimated at 0.25 Gy. Of the Japanese survivors enrolled in the Life Span Study (i.e., approximately one third of the total number of survivors) 37,800 had died by 1990. When one takes expected rates of cancer into account in a similar nonexposed population, the number of excess cancer deaths related to radiation within this group is approximately 430

(3, 4). The number of radiation-related leukemia cases in the same study had reached 290 by 1987 (5). Stated otherwise, approximately 59% of those survivors who died from leukemia and 8% of the survivors who died from other malignancies did so from a radiation-related cancer (2). Some of these victims received whole body doses of up to 5 Gy (500 rad). Recent data, however, on atomic bomb-survivors indicate that a detectable risk of leukemia or lymphoma can be found in groups with exposures as low as 0.5 Gy (50 rad) (6). Although the retrospective dosimetry estimates of the gamma and neutron fluxes involved have been revised periodically, doses involved in these studies are not remotely approached by diagnostic neuroangiographic procedures.

Similarly, the absolute numbers of cases of radiation-related leukemia and other malignancies are very small in follow-up studies of other exposed populations. All of the studies that attempt to demonstrate a carcinogenic effect from whole body doses of under 0.05 Gy are of a design and size that make them vulnerable to statistical inconsistencies or methodologic oversights (3, 7). Studies of human subjects in this dose range with positive findings have, on occasion, demonstrated an increased risk of malignancy in small populations. For instance, a follow-up study in 1983 (8) of the 1957 "Smoky" bomb test-site in Nevada demonstrated an almost four times increased incidence of some forms of leukemia in military personnel exposed to an average of 10 mGy (1 rad) whole-body dose. There was no evidence of increased mortality from any other form of cancer. With reference to leukemia, this positive result translates to an extreme risk at variance with the relatively lower observed rates of leukemia in Japanese atomic-bomb survivor studies or with risks associated with background radiation (7). The authors, Caldwell et al. (8) concluded that "this one positive finding may be either attributable to chance or the result of an unknown combination of factors . . . this conclusion cannot be generalized." However, the Nevada test-site or other similar events have entered media folklore as evidence of the severe risks of radiation exposure (9).

Epidemiologic studies of atomic bomb survivors and other groups exposed to high levels of radiation (50 rad) have demonstrated a clear relationship between exposure and the subsequent risk of malignancy, particularly leukemia (excluding CLL) and carcinoma of lung, ovary, thyroid, stomach, and breast (3). Exposure levels below this range, which would be of interest in evaluating possible risks to patients and medical personnel from neuroangiographic procedures, cannot be studied directly because of methodologic difficulties and because of the enormous number of subjects that such a study would require.

Dose-Response Curve

An extrapolation of the dose-risk curve below the 100 rad range can be performed in a linear, quadratic, or linear-quadratic manner (Fig. 4.1).

With a linear curve, the risk of malignancy is directly

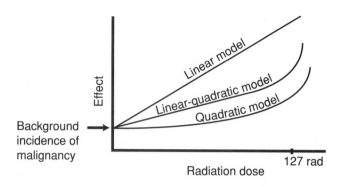

Figure 4.1. *Dose-response curve.* Common mathematical models for induction of radiation-related tumors are represented. At zero exposure a baseline rate of cancer is still present due to the background rates of disease.

proportional to the exposure. At the lower end of the curve, the number of radiation-related tumors is obscured by the incidence of spontaneous malignancies in a given population.

A quadratic curve assumes that the risk is proportional to the square of the dose and gives a curve that increases steeply with increasing doses.

Alternatively, a linear-quadratic curve, in which a linear curve at lower doses gives way to a quadratic curve at higher doses, appears to be a more likely model based on animal studies and on data from atomic bomb survivors. Solid tumors and leukemia have demonstrated different dose-response curves. Furthermore, a different temporal sequence is seen for various tumors after radiation. The excess incidence of leukemia becomes apparent after 2 years and peaks at approximately 6 years, whereas the incidence of solid tumors may not peak until 15–20 years after exposure. A linear-quadratic curve is now most favored for describing the likely risk of most forms of carcinogenesis after radiation exposure. According to Brown (10), the curve inflection point, where it makes a transition from linear to quadratic in form, is determined by the density of DNA in the genome. This means that for mammalian tissue, the curve changes from linear to quadratic at approximately the 127 rad point. Below this level, much of the evidence is either disputed or conjectural, and the measure of risk from an exposure of 10 rad or less is still unknown.

Radiobiology

The adverse effects of x-rays on tissue are related to a transfer of energy to the tissue by indirect ionization. With x-rays in the diagnostic range, the two processes involved, which result in ionization, are the photoelectric effect and the Compton effect. Approximately 5% of x-rays in the diagnostic range undergo coherent scattering. This process is not important for transfer of energy because only a change of direction of the x-ray photon takes place, without a change in energy and without ionization. Coherent scattering contributes a little to film fogging.

In the photoelectric process, an incident photon interacts with and loses *all* of its energy to a K, L, or M shell electron, which is then ejected from its orbit. The ejected electron becomes a "photoelectron." The ejected electron is replaced in its shell by an electron from an outer orbit, which releases "characteristic radiation" as it moves to the inner, more tightly bound position.

In the Compton effect, the incident photon of the x-ray beam loses *part* of its energy to an outer electron, which is ejected from its orbit. The ejected electron is referred to as the "recoil electron." The x-ray photon continues in a deflected direction with a commensurately reduced energy.

The ionizing effect of radiation in the diagnostic range is mediated by the photoelectrons and recoil electrons. They result in the formation of free radicals in tissue, which may then interact with other cellular components, particularly with DNA and RNA.

The probability of a photoelectric interaction between a photon and an atom is proportional to the third power of the atomic number of the atom. A photoelectric interaction is more likely to occur with a lower energy photon than it is with a higher energy beam, provided that the photon energy is greater than the binding energy of the electron. The photoelectric effect is therefore likely to occur with photons in the lower energy range of a diagnostic beam. The photoelectric effect is also likely to occur in tissue that contains atoms with a higher atomic number, such as calcium or iodine. Therefore, photoelectric interactions are good for image quality in that they give a high contrast between soft tissue and bone or between soft tissue and iodinated contrast. However, because the photoelectric effect results in *all* of an incident photon's energy being deposited in the patient, the absorbed radiation dose to the patient tends to be higher when the photoelectric effect is dominant. Therefore, to reduce patient exposure, it is desirable to keep the kV setting as high as possible while maintaining adequate image contrast.

Compton interactions, on the other hand, are responsible for the scatter radiation to operating personnel involved in a fluoroscopy procedure. In the diagnostic range, most of the energy of the incident photon is retained by the photon, and very little is transferred to the recoil electron. The practical implication of this is that scatter radiation emanating from a patient is almost as energetic as the photons of the primary beam. For instance, a 75 keV photon deflected by 90 has an energy of 66 keV; when deflected by 180 the energy level is still a considerable 58 keV (11). Therefore the scatter beam, which can be conceptualized as having its center at the skin entrance site on the patient, must be taken to represent a potentially serious source of radiation to operating personnel.

Stochastic and Deterministic Effects of Radiation

The detrimental effects of human radiation exposure are divided into genetic (placing future generations at risk) and somatic (affecting the exposed individual). Somatic effects can be broadly classified into those related to the local tissue effects of radiation exposure (epilation, skin erythema, necrosis, retrolenticular opacities, etc.) and carcinogenic effects.

Somatic carcinogenic side effects and genetic effects of radiation probably occur through common pathways involving free-radical damage to DNA. The risks of these effects are sometimes termed stochastic, i.e., they are best described in terms of probability. Although they are more likely to happen with increasingly higher exposures, the severity of the effect, if it happens, is not dose-related. Stochastic effects are considered to be possible at all levels of exposure, i.e., they do not have a threshold level. In other words, a radiation-related malignancy is more likely to occur after a higher level of exposure, but may occur after a low exposure too. The net effect to the victim is the same in either instance.

Non-stochastic effects, sometimes called deterministic, are dose-related and affect the exposed tissue. They involve acute or chronic complications such as epilation, ulceration, fibrosis, or lenticular opacities. Usually, they are not seen below a certain critical or threshold level of exposure.

The genetic effects of radiation exposure are probably less significant than the somatic effects. Radiation effects on the genetic material of circulating lymphocytes can be detected with exposures as low as 0.1 Sv (10 rem). Such changes have been used following the Chernobyl disaster to estimate exposures retrospectively in rescue-workers. However, a detectable genetic effect of radiation exposure in subsequent generations after the atomic bombings at Hiroshima and Nagasaki has been elusive. These effects are thought to be small enough to be obscured by the background noise of spontaneous mutational phenomena (3, 4).

Tumor initiation after radiation exposure is the focus of most concern in evaluating the risks of radiation and is probably due to DNA point-mutations, base-pair deletions, or translocations. It is not known what factors may place a particular individual at risk for such critical events. Patients with some genetic disorders such as xeroderma pigmentosum and ataxia-teleangiectasia are more sensitive to the carcinogenic effects of radiation than other members of the general population. Children exposed to fallout contamination after nuclear accidents are more at risk than adults for malignancies such as leukemia and thyroid neoplasia. Children treated with radiation therapy for retinoblastoma also appear to have a higher susceptibility to radiation-induced tumors than do other children or adults treated similarly for other types of tumors.

Promotional effects on tumor genesis may also be important, and these may be independent of radiation exposure. Tumor promotion may involve such factors as the hormonal or dietary status of the patient. For instance, breast tumors after fluoroscopic exposure of the chest in female children are not seen until maturity, indicating that the initiated cell(s) may remain latent until triggered by other stimuli (12).

EXPOSURE QUANTIFICATION AND RADIATION "DOSE"

Quantification of radiation needs to take into account a number of factors including the intensity of the source, the nature and energy of the source, and the area or particular organs of the patient exposed to the source. A lexicon of terms exists to describe the units of measurement for these variable factors. The most meaningful of these units is the "effective dose" (H_E). Calculating the effective dose for a radiographic procedure gives a number in standardized units, which allows comparison between different procedures and permits correlation with probability scales from reference data. The following sections explain the derivation of the effective dose.

Quantification of Beam Intensity

Beam intensity is quantified by measuring the ionization charge induced by an x-ray beam in a given mass of air. This unit is the roentgen (R), which is defined as 0.000258 coulomb per kilogram of air. It is a measurement of intensity that is independent of any biologic effects of the beam or the presence of tissue in the field. Modern angiography suites are frequently equipped with ionization chambers attached to the exit portals of the tubes. They measure the intensity of the exiting beam and give a reading expressed in roentgens per minute. By using this reading and by calculating the attenuation of the beam between the ionization chamber and the patient, estimations of patient exposure can be reached.

Quantification of Energy Deposition in Tissue ("Dose")

The "dose" of radiation to a person or a volume of tissue is a concept that can have different meanings. A purely physical notion of what constitutes a dose of radiation is the quantity of energy transferred to the tissue by the beam. Energy absorbed by tissue from an x-ray beam in the diagnostic range is measured in rad or gray (Gy). A Gy is defined as an absorbed dose causing a deposition of 1 joule of energy in each kilogram of absorbing tissue. A Gy is the same as 100 rad. A rad, the older unit being phased out but still used in the clinical vernacular, was defined as the deposition of 100 ergs per gram of tissue.

Depending on the rate at which they deposit energy in tissue per unit of distance traversed (keV/micron), radiation beams are described as either low linear energy transfer (LET) or high LET. Compared with particulate emissions, which have a strong capacity to induce ionization, x-rays in the diagnostic range are considered low LET. Exposure to 1 roentgen of beam intensity in the diagnostic range results in an energy deposition of almost 1 rad, approximately 93 ergs/g. Consequently, the terms roentgen

and rad are frequently used interchangeably in the diagnostic range.

To comply with new standards but to facilitate thinking is units of rad, many publications use the unit centigray (cGy), which is the same as a rad. Absorbed doses are usually cited in a temporal reference (e.g., rad/min or Gy/h).

Quantification of Biologic Responsiveness to Radiation: Dose Equivalence H_T

Units such as the gray or rad deal with purely physical parameters. To approach a more meaningful concept of "dose," account must be taken of the biologic effects of these measurable physical quantities. A Gy or 100 rad of exposure may have different effects on the tissue substrate in question depending on the nature of the radiation source and on the vulnerability to radiation of that particular tissue type. To take this variable response into account, it becomes necessary to devise a quantity to measure the biologic equivalence of specified exposures. This explains the acronymic derivation of the unit devised for this purpose, the rem-roentgen equivalent man. The international unit now in use for expressing the biologic equivalence of radiation dose is the sievert (Sv). A sievert is equal to 100 rem.

Estimates of biologic dose equivalence, i.e., the "dose equivalent (H_T)," represented by sieverts or rems are calculated by multiplying the physical dose (Gy or rad) by a weighting factor W_R.

The weighting factor (W_R) is determined by the type and energy of the radiation source. A relative weighting factor, W_R (Q in older literature), is assigned to various radiation types to generate a scale, which reflects the biologic effectiveness of exposure to different sources. Alpha particles have a W_R of 20, while photon sources have a W_R of 1. An exposure of 1 rad to a source with a W_R of 1 gives a dose equivalent of 1 rem. Hence in the diagnostic X-ray range, where W_R is always 1, rem and rad or Sievert and Gy are interchangeable.

When a tissue is exposed to different types of radiation, separate calculations using correspondingly varied values for W_R are conducted for each type of radiation involved. These numbers are summed to give the total dose equivalent (H_T) for that tissue.

Partial Body Exposure: Effective Dose Equivalent or Effective Dose (H_E)

How is risk to the whole person calculated when only part of the body is exposed to the radiation source? It would seem cogent, for instance, that a certain level of partial body irradiation must represent as great a risk of carcinogenesis as would some lower degree of whole body irradiation. Moreover, partial body irradiation involving the thyroid gland or gonads is more dangerous than irradiation involving the extremities only.

To generate a calculation based on partial body exposure, the ICRP introduced the effective dose equivalent (H_E), now termed the effective dose, which is also measured in Sieverts.

Various tissues are assigned weighting factors depending on their respective sensitivities to radiation. For instance, thyroid tissue is assigned a tissue weighting factor (W_T) of 0.05 in the 1990 recommendations of the ICRP (13, 14, 15). An equivalent dose (H_T) to the thyroid of 8 mSv could then be calculated to 8 mSv $\times$ 0.05 = 0.4 mSv effective dose (H_E). In other words, an equivalent dose of 8 mSv confined to the thyroid gland represents the same risk to the individual as if the whole body had received a dose of 0.4 mSv.

To calculate the entire risk to an individual from a quantified exposure, the effective doses for all the critical organs involved are summed to give a number, the total effective dose (H_E). This number can be compared with known quantities and risk-tables. For instance, the effective annual dose from background radiation exposure is approximately 2.5–5.0 mSv depending on altitude and geological variables. This is a useful number to remember as a reference point for interpreting H_E values; it gives one a scale of reference to grapple in a meaningful way with doses involved in medical procedures. A chest x-ray has an effective dose of 0.08 mSv, a CT of the head 1.11 mSv, or a barium enema 4.06 mSv (16).

Other units of measurement that one might encounter frequently include the *entrance skin dose* and the *dose-area-product* (DAP). The entrance skin dose represents the dose experienced by the skin at the point of beam entry to the body. The dose area product is the product of the entrance skin dose and the area of skin in the primary beam.

STUDIES OF X-RAY EPILATION FOR TINEA CAPITIS

From among the epidemiologic and follow-up studies of populations exposed to radiation, the most relevant to diagnostic and interventional cerebral angiography are those of children exposed in the 1940s and 1950s for treatment of *tinea capitis*. Children typically aged 6–8 years were given exposures of 300–400 roentgens or more to the scalp. The treatment was administered in single dose or in divided sessions over a period of 5 days to induce hair loss. New hair grew after approximately 6 weeks. This form of treatment ended in 1958 by which time an estimated 200,000 children had been so treated worldwide (17).

The procedure was performed with a beam of 75–100 kV with or without an aluminum filter. Retrospective estimations of doses have been published (18, 19) indicating doses to the scalp of 450–850 rad, to the cranial marrow of 385 rad, and brain doses of 70–175 rad. The thyroid gland received a mean of 6.5 rad, the pituitary gland 49 rad, and the eye 47 rad (20).

Follow-up studies of over 2,000 children in the United States (21) and over 10,000 children in Israel (22) have been published periodically since that time. The former study from New York demonstrated higher rates of leukemia in the irradiated group (4 cases versus 1 in a control group), brain tumors (3 cases), parotid tumors, thyroid tumors, and skin malignancies in the irradiated field. There was also a higher rate of diverse psychiatric diagnoses among the irradiated group, at least in the U.S. study. The Israeli follow-up study (22) also demonstrated a slightly higher number of leukemia cases among the irradiated group (7 versus 5 expected), as well as statistically elevated rates of benign and malignant tumors of the head and neck, meninges, parotid, and thyroid gland. Although these observations on rates of delayed malignancy in the irradiated group appear to be valid and conform to the paradigm of radiation being a known risk factor for tumor formation, the incidence rates within this population nevertheless appear to be low. The significance of elevated rates of psychiatric diagnosis in the New York cohort is unknown.

The incidence of radiation-related malignancy in these studies is very low, whereas the radiation doses involved were considerably higher than those used during cerebral angiography. These studies more than any other offer some solid reassurance that the long-term risk of malignancy from angiographic procedures is vanishingly small, even in children.

Radiation Exposure during Neuroangiographic Procedures

Patient Exposure

Because radiation exposure during diagnostic neuroangiography involves both a small measure of real risk, and a potentially larger element of perceived risk, minimization of radiation exposure is important for the patient and the angiographer (Fig. 4.2). In a litigious society, the documentation of this minimization effort probably has more tangible benefits than the dose-reduction itself. There are a number of practical steps that one may follow to reduce the exposure to staff and patients (see Table 4.1).

For routine diagnostic neuroangiography, deterministic effects of radiation in the adult patient are not seen because the total skin-entrance dose usually falls far below the levels where concern about epilation (2–6 Gy) or lens opacification (approximately 2 Gy) might arise (23, 24). Therefore for diagnostic studies, the entrance skin dose is less important than the effective dose because the effects of radiation which warrant consideration lie in the stochastic domain. Comparison with other radiological procedures can be made by calculating the effective dose (H_E) for each type of procedure.

Studies of patient dosimetry report a range of dose estimates. Feygelman et al. (23, 25) estimated that a diagnostic cerebral angiogram using both cut-film and digital techniques involves an average H_E value of 10.6 mSv. This figure is equivalent to the dose from a nuclear brain scan using 1,000 MBq of Tc-99m gluconate or approximately 5–8 CT scans of the head. By using more recently published weighting factors (14), Russell and Fawcitt calculated that Feygelman's estimates would be reduced by 20% (26). In one of the most thorough of recent dosimetry

Figure 4.2. *Importance of collimation.* Even the most perfunctory nod to collimation can reduce exposure considerably. The DAP (dose-area-product) in **(B)** is reduced by a factor of 2.5 compared with **(A),** i.e., a reduction of 60%, assuming no change in tube output.

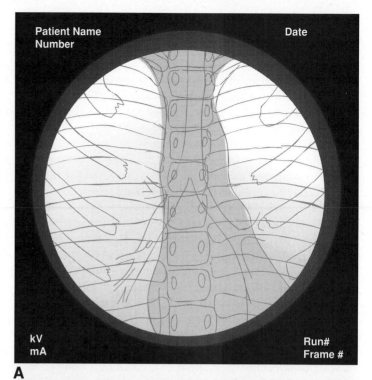

A

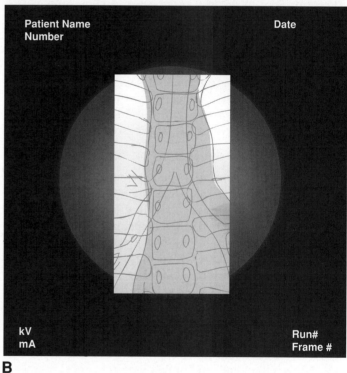

B

studies for four-vessel cerebral angiography using digital imaging and manual injection techniques, Marshall et al. (27) reported an average patient H$_E$ of approximately 3.6 mSv per study. Their findings indicate that patient dosimetry is approximately the same as in studies that used cut-film angiography (28), even though digital techniques involved twice the number of images.

The typical fraction of H$_E$ deriving from fluoroscopy rather than from filming during cerebral angiography varies. It depends on the difficulty of vessel selection and has been estimated at 22–67% of the total exposure (23, 27, 29). This represents a major component of the exposure involved in most such procedures. Therefore, sustained attention to eliminating unnecessary fluoroscopy time might contribute to a significant reduction in overall radiation exposure.

For long interventional procedures, deterministic effects from radiation exposure become a consideration in addition to the more concerning stochastic effects. It is not rare to see a patient who develops significant epilation and even erythema of the scalp at the site of maximal skin exposure after a long neuro-interventional procedure. Huda and Peters (24) calculated that a particular patient who had received a fractionated skin dose of 6.6 Gy during a long neurointerventional procedure (a dose that is at the highest end of the range of exposures used in this type of procedure) had an approximately 0.3% risk of carcinogenesis deriving from the procedure. Most neurointerventional cases involve exposures of less than 2 Gy (200 rad) skin entrance dose per plane. Kuwayama et al. (30) estimated that in long interventional cases in which total fluoroscopy time may be frequently in excess of 1–1.5 hours, the skin exposure to the patient would probably be of the same order as that used in the 1940s and 1950s for treatment of tinea capitis (discussed earlier).

Berthelsen and Cederblad (31) calculated that the H_E to patients undergoing embolization of a brain arteriovenous malformation ranges from 6 to 43 mSv. These results are considerably higher than the calculated H_E dose of 3.44 mSv for interventional neuroangiographic procedures reported by Bergeron et al. (32). The latter study noted that this lesser figure is similar to 1 year of natural background irradiation in North America, and estimated the stochastic risk of this exposure as one fatal cancer for every 5,814 procedures.

Personnel Exposure

As a rule of thumb, the radiation dose to the exposed areas of the angiographer can be calculated as between 1/100 to 1/1,000 (31, 33) that of the patient. This is a variable relationship depending on the set-up of a particular room and the angiographer's techniques and position.

Berthelsen and Cederblad (31) estimated that the H_E dose to the angiographer and assisting personnel ranges from 3 to 86 Sv per case or approximately 5 mSv per year, assuming a case-load of about 200 embolizations. A similar figure for an annual case-load of 120 coronary angiography procedures has been reported by Gustafsson and Lunderquist (34). This figure would represent an estimation of dose similar to that received from undergoing a barium enema (4.06 mSv) and a CT scan (1.11 mSv) each year, or the difference in cosmic radiation involved in living in Denver, Colorado (altitude 1,610 m) instead of at sea level for 17 years (3, 4).

These estimates of personnel exposure during neuroangiography are slightly higher than the mean annual H_E dose (measured under the collar) for general interventional radiologists. The annual effective dose for this group, approximately 3.16 mSv to 10.1 mSv, has been calculated to represent a risk of excess fatal cancer of approximately 1 per 10,000 careers (35). Niklason et al. (35) also emphasized the importance of wearing a thyroid collar during interventional cases by pointing out that a typical dose to the unshielded thyroid of the angiographer increases the calculated effective dose (H_E) by a factor of 2. In other words, wearing a thyroid collar cuts one's effective dose by half.

Marshall et al. (27) calculated the eye and left hand dose to the radiologist to be 14 Gy and 19 Gy respectively per case during diagnostic angiography. This is the equivalent of the cosmic radiation involved in a round-trip flight from Los Angeles to New York (36). Figures of double and quadruple these results have been reported by earlier studies (28, 37). Kuwayama et al. (31) (1994) reported left-hand exposures to personnel during embolization procedures between 0.05 mSv and 3.55 mSv. These figures involve differences between studies of at least one order of magnitude. It is probable that various measures of radiation protection, room design, and improvements in machine performance may explain some of the differences between these studies. Studies with lower reported dose rates (27) are more explicit in their discussion of protection measures. Kuwayama et al. (30) concluded that in the course of a busy year (170 cases), based on calculations on their most extreme cases, a neuroangiographer may exceed the annual recommended dose limits to the skin of the left hand (500 mSv/yr) and eye (150 mSv/yr). This study, like that of Berthelsen and Cederblad (31) was performed with the x-ray tube on the *right* side of the patient, i.e., in a position that gives the operator more backscatter exposure than if it were placed on the opposite side. Although this dose is unlikely to induce cataract formation over the course of a lifetime, Kuwayama et al. (30) recommended using lead glasses to protect one's eyes. Such protection is in the reader's interest because it gives the added assurance of preventing blood-splashes to the eye.

In terms of routinely quantifying or even approximately defining the risk of stochastic effects from low level radiation-exposure, the data are incomplete. Recommendations on upper limits of acceptable collective effective doses are intended to be applied at a population level and not for calculation of risks to particular individuals (33). Some stochastic risk is thought to exist at whole body entrance dose levels above 0.1 Gy (10 rad) and more certainly above 1 Gy (100 rad). Extrapolation of the probability curve below the 0.1 Gy mark rests on uncertainty. In the face of this uncertainty, the general admonition is to keep exposure "as low as reasonably achievable" (ALARA).

Radiation exposure to a particular patient undergoing a diagnostic or interventional procedure depends on some factors that are outside of the angiographer's apparent control but for which he/she may be expected to assume some legal responsibility. Given the increasing number of fluoroscopically guided interventional procedures being done, in the future some spontaneous malignancies may be blamed on these procedures. A written record of one's departmental conformity with nationally endorsed recommendations and of a periodic quality assurance program for equipment maintenance may be the best defense in such a situation.

Table 4.1
Reducing Radiation Exposure

Attention to the ongoing cumulative skin dose to a patient during a procedure can reduce skin-entrance doses during long cases by more than 50% (38).

- Minimize the use of radiographic and geometric magnification. Most modern units are equipped with three intensifier sizes. Radiation is minimized by working on the lowest magnification level and with as small a field as possible. Geometric magnification (increasing the distance from the patient to the intensifier) forces the tube to increase output to allow the intensifier sufficient exposure to generate an image. A visual check of the patient-to-intensifier distance at the beginning of the case and after each adjustment of position will improve oversight of this factor.
- Keep the field size as small as possible to reduce the dose-area-product and to reduce the level of backscatter to operating personnel. Collimate the field as much as possible at every opportunity (Fig. 4.2). This improves image quality by eliminating scatter.
- Eliminate the use of constant fluoroscopy during catheterization of the descending aorta and pelvis, or while engaged in other tasks that do not require fluoroscopy. Familiarity with a particular wire will allow one to insert it almost to the tip of the catheter before one needs to turn on fluoroscopy. A torque-handle as a landmark on the wire greatly helps in this technique if one knows where the handle was previously placed in reference to the catheter hub. This technique is particularly useful for microwire and coil-pusher manipulation.
- Keep a screen or distance between the operator and the point of maximal scatter. The source of maximal radiation to the angiographer is the point of skin entry of the beam. Therefore, when standing on the patient's right side, the lateral beam should be directed towards the operator into the left side of the patient's head. The image intensifier which receives only a small fraction of the total radiation output should be on the same side as the operator. The AP tube should be underneath the table.
- Reduce air-gap and minimize use of filters and screens between the patient and the intensifier; these will drive up the tube output.
- Keep the kV of the tube output as high as possible, preferably in the range 70±90 kV. These factors are usually set, however, by the automatic exposure control. This range will give adequate image contrast and improve the profile of the radiation curve by reducing the proportion of "soft" x-rays that contribute only to exposure and not to the image. Excessively high kV settings, on the other hand, lead to images with poor contrast, and cause an increase in personnel exposure.
- Keep the filming rate at 1.5±2 frames per second or less and use higher rates only when clearly needed. Keep the run duration short, e.g., an oblique magnification view of an aneurysm does not usually require a prolonged venous phase as this information will have been satisfactorily gathered on the initial AP and lateral view.
- Eliminate unnecessary fluoroscopy time on maneuvers that can be accomplished by sight. The fluoroscopy pedal should not be used to remind the angiographer that the lateral intensifier is too far out or that the patient's jewelry is still in place. After each adjustment of patient position or after selecting a new vessel, the selected magnification level and the position of the image intensifiers should be visually checked before pressing the fluoroscopy pedal. For instance, an approximate Townes position can be obtained by moving the AP unit or the patient's head. Then fluoroscopy can be used to fine-tune the position.
- Diligent use of radiation screening devices, aprons, rolling shields, ceiling mounted shields, and shields hanging from underneath the operating table are self-evident imperatives. At all times, these devices should be interposed between the operator and the skin entrance site on the patient.
- For prolonged exposure in a particular area of the patient, rotate the tube and intensifier during the case to spread the skin-dose over a larger area.

Practical Conclusions

The total duration of fluoroscopy depends on the nature of the case, but the angiographer can strive to reduce this time and other factors contributing to the total exposure considerably (Table 4.1). Modern biplane fluoroscopy units have an output range of 2–10 roentgens per minute as measured at table-top, depending on the fluoroscopy mode selected. This output can be trimmed somewhat by using modern sensitive image-intensifiers, but the cumulative output still translates into a typical skin entrance dose of 2–5 rad/min^{-1}. An hour of exposure in one plane can add up to a dose sufficient to induce temporary epilation (30), affecting possibly as many as 10% of patients who undergo interventional neuroradiologic procedures (38). Pulse-progressive fluoroscopy can reduce this entrance dose considerably (33).

A definitive conclusion on the risks posed to patients and angiographers from diagnostic and interventional procedures is not attainable using current data and statistical methods. It is overwhelmingly likely that the risk to the patient and operating personnel is very small, possibly infinitesimally small. The reader is strongly encouraged to prioritize the development of personal routines and habits for improved manipulation of those variables under his/her direct control, which will reduce this exposure.

REFERENCES

1. Lenihan J. The Good News about Radiation. 1st ed. Madison: Cogito Books, 1993.
2. Schull WJ. Effects of Atomic Radiation. A half-century of studies from Hiroshima and Nagasaki. 1st ed. New York: Wiley-Liss, 1995. (Page 12: Approximately 30% of the acute fatalities were due to the effects of radiation. Citing Oughterson AW, LeRoy GV, Liebow AA, et al. Medical Effects of Atomic Bombs. USAEC, Office of Technical Information, Technical Information Service, Oak Ridge, Tennessee, Report NNP-3041, Volume 6, 1951).
3. Mettler FA, Upton AC. Medical Effects of Ionizing Radiation. 2nd ed. Philadelphia: W.B. Saunders, 1995.
4. United Nations Scientific Committee on the Effects of Atomic Radiation (UNSCEAR): Sources and effects of ionizing radiation. Report to the General Assembly, Annex on Hereditary Effects, Vienna, 1993.
5. Preston DL, Kato H, Kopecky, et al. Studies of the mortality of A-bomb survivors. 8. Cancer mortality. Radiat Res 1987;111: 151–178.
6. Preston DL, Kusumi S, Tomonaga M, et al. Cancer incidence in atomic bomb survivors. Part III: Leukemia, lymphoma, and multiple myeloma, 1950–1987. Radiat Res 1994;137(suppl): S68-S97.
7. Webster EW. Garland Lecture. On the question of cancer induction by small x-ray doses. Am J Roentgenol 1981;137: 647–666.
8. Caldwell GG, Kelley D, Zack M, et al. Mortality and cancer frequency among military nuclear test (Smoky) participants, 1957 through 1979. JAMA 1983;250:620–624.
9. Johnson CJ. Cancer incidence in an area of radioactive fallout downwind from the Nevada Test Site. JAMA 1984;251:230–236.
10. Brown JM. The shape of the dose-response curve for radiation carcinogenesis. Extrapolation to low doses. Radiat Res 1977;71: 34–50.

11. Curry TS, Dowdey JE, Murray RC. Christensen's Physics of Diagnostic Radiology. 4th edition. Philadelphia, Lea and Febiger, 1990.

12. Moolgavkar SM. Hormones in multi-stage carcinogenesis. Cancer Surv 1986;5:635–648.

13. International Commission on Radiological Protection (ICRP). Recommendations of the International Commission on Radiological Protection. ICRP Publication 26, Pergamon Press, 1977.

14. International Commission on Radiological Protection (ICRP): Recommendations of the International Commission on Radiological Protection (ICRP publication 60). New York, Pergamon Press. Ann ICRP 1991;21:1-3.

15. International Commission on Radiological Protection Publication 60. The system of protection for proposed and continuing practices. Oxford, England: Pergamon Press. Ann ICRP 1990; 5 1990.

16. National Council on Radiation Protection and Measurements. Exposure of the U.S. population from Diagnostic Medical Radiation. Report No. 100, Bethesda, MD 1989.

17. Albert RE, Omram AR. Follow up study of patients treated by x-ray epilation for tinea capitis. I. Population characteristics, posttreatment illnesses, and mortality experience. Arch Environ Health 1968;17:899–918.

18. Schultz RJ, Albert RE. Follow-up study of patients treated by x-ray epilation for tinea capitis. III. Dose to organs of the head from the x-ray treatment of tinea capitis. Arch Environ Health 1968;17:935–950.

19. Werner A, Modan B, Davidoff D. Doses to brain, skull, and thyroid, following x-ray therapy for tinea capitis. Phys Med Biol 1968;13:247–258.

20. Harley NH, Albert RE, Shore RE, et al. Follow up study of patients treated by x-ray epilation for tinea capitis. Estimation of the dose to the thyroid and pituitary glands and other structures of the head and neck. Phys Med Biol 1976;21:631–642.

21. Shore RE, Albert RE, Pasternack BS. Follow up study of patients treated by x-ray epilation for tinea capitis. Arch Environ Health 1976; 31:17–24.

22. Modan B, Baidatz D, Mart H, et al. Radiation induced head and neck tumours. Lancet 1974:277–279.

23. Feygelman VM, Huda W, Peters KR. Effective dose equivalents to patients undergoing cerebral angiography. Am J Neuroradiol 1992;13:845–849.

24. Huda W, Peters KR. Radiation-induced temporary epilation after a neuroradiologically guided embolization procedure. Radiology 1994;193:642–644.

25. International Commission on Radiological Protection (ICRP). Recommendations of the International Commission on Radiological Protection. ICRP Publication 26, Pergamon Press, 1977.

26. Russell JGB, Fawcitt R. Commentary. New risks, new doses. AJNR Am J Neuroradiol 1992;13:850–852.

27. Marshall NW, Noble J, Faulkner K. Patient and staff dosimetry in neuroradiological procedures. Br J Radiol 1995;68:495–501.

28. Tryhus M, Mettler FA, Kelsey C. The radiologist and angiographic procedures: absorbed radiation dose. Invest Radiol 1987;22:747–750.

29. Plunkett MB, Gray JE, Kispert DB. Radiation exposure from conventional and digital subtraction angiography of cerebral vessels. Am J Neuroradiol 1986;7:665–668.

30. Kuwayama N, Takaku A, Endo S, et al. Radiation exposure in endovascular surgery of the head and neck. Am J Neuroradiol 1994;15: 1801–1808.

31. Berthelsen B, Cederblad A. Radiation doses to patients and personnel involved in embolization of intracerebral arteriovenous malformations. Acta Radiol 1991;32:492–497.

32. Bergeron P, Carrier R, Roy D, et al. Radiation doses in patients in Neurointerventional Procedures. Am J Neuroradiol 1994;15: 1809–1812.

33. Bushong SC. Commentary: Hazards Evaluation of Neuroangiographic Procedures. Am J Neuroradiol 1994;15:1813–1816.

34. Gustafsson M, Lunderquist A. Personnel exposure to radiation at some angiographic procedures. Radiology 1981;140:807.

35. Niklason LT, Marx MV, Chan HP. Interventional radiologists: Occupational radiation doses and risks. Radiology 1993;187: 729–733.

36. Wallace R. Measurements of the cosmic radiation dose in subsonic commercial aircraft compared to the city-pair dose calculation. Lawrence Berkley Report No. 1505, 1975. Cited by Mettler and Upton, 1995, p. 42.

37. Chopp M, Portnoy HD, Schurig R, et al. Clinical dosimetry during cerebral angiography. Neuroradiology 1980;20:79–81.

38. Norbash AM, Busick D, Marks MP. Techniques for reducing interventional neuroradiologic skin dose: tube position rotation, and supplemental beam filtration. Am J Neuroradiol 1996; 17:41–49.

PART II / ANATOMY

CHAPTER 5

Embryology of the Cranial Circulation

A rudimentary description of the embryonic origins of the cranial vessels will assist in understanding the variants and anomalies that may be seen during cerebral angiography. The terminology and nomenclature of embryologic literature can be very intimidating and obscurantist; however, the major events that describe the vascular embryology of the brain are simple to understand. Moreover, such an understanding, rather than a memorization of categorically distinct variants, will allow a flexibility in one's thinking about these anomalies. Archetypal variations are easily recognized in textbooks; for the interpretation of angiograms, however, it is necessary to realize that numerous intermediate anomalous states may coexist and are rarely, if ever, exactly similar in different cases. The following synopsis of the embryology of the cranial vasculature is based largely on the classic papers by E. D. Congdon (1) and D. H. Padget (2, 3, 4, 5).

PRIMITIVE AORTIC ARCHES

The embryologic development of the aortic arch and great vessels is described in two stages (1). A branchial stage (3–14 mm crown-rump length) corresponds with the arterial pattern seen in lower vertebrates, similar to that supplying the gill apparatus (*branchia* = *gill*). A post-branchial phase describes the evolution of the adult arterial pattern from the remnants of the branchial components.

The six pairs of primitive aortic arches—the existence of the 5th arches being inconstant or contentious—fill a developmental role in association with the development of the pharyngeal pouches (Fig. 5.1). This occurs by virtue of the initially cephalic location of the primitive heart and the interruption, by the pharyngeal structures, of the route between the ventral aortic sac and the dorsal paired aortae. To circumvent the pharyngeal pouches, the aortic outflow interdigitates between the pouches starting with the first set of aortic arches. As the cardiac structures migrate into the thorax, the primitive aorta is drawn caudally, so that the cephalically located aortic arches, being uneconomical in disposition, regress and are replaced by other successively forming and regressing sets of arches. Not all six pairs of arches are present at a single time, as represented by synoptic diagrams.

From a point of interest in the cephalic vessels, the major events in the post-branchial phase are:

- Regression of the left dorsal aorta between the third and fourth arches, such that the former becomes the source of the major carotid branches off the aortic arch (Fig. 5.1G).

- Derivation of the subclavian arteries from 6th intersegmental arteries, themselves branching from the fourth aortic arches bilaterally. The subclavian arteries assume the supply of the caudal end of the vertebral arterial network. This allows evolution of the most common adult configuration whereby the vertebral arteries, deriving from the 6th intersegmental arteries, enter the foramina transversaria of the C6 vertebral body (Fig. 5.1F).

- Attenuation of the right 4th aortic arch to a caliber commensurate with a role of supplying the right subclavian artery. The right 4th dorsal aorta regresses caudad to that point, leaving the adult right subclavian artery to derive supply from the brachiocephalic artery (a remnant of the third and fourth arches), except in instances of an aberrant right subclavian artery (Fig. 5.1H).

ARTERIAL EMBRYOLOGY

The cranial arterial vasculature in its adult form evolves in early fetal life through a number of simultaneous or overlapping steps. Primitive embryonic vessels without an adult derivative usually regress completely, but are of interest by virtue of occasional anomalous persistence. Their closure results in hemodynamic changes that contribute in part to the genesis of other permanent vessel derivatives from the embryonic plexi. These derivatives emerge with an economic regression of the otiose remaining plexal components. It is unlikely that a major anomaly or variant vessel could occur in complete isolation from the remainder of the cerebral vasculature because of the interdependent nature of the various steps. Anomalies associated with early events, e.g., failure of regression of the primitive maxillary or hypoglossal arteries, are more rarely seen than those with later events, e.g., persistence of a trigeminal artery or failure of normal diminution of the territory of the anterior choroidal artery.

Major variants of the cranial vasculature are important to recognize. They have a bearing on the risks of subsequent disorders related to anomalous hemodynamics, particularly aneurysm formation, and they need to be studied clearly prior to surgical or interventional procedures. The presence of carotid-basilar anomalous connections, for instance, would be of major significance in the planning of a Wada test in which inadvertent perfusion of the posterior fossa with sodium amytal could have disastrous consequences due to anesthesia of the brain-stem. Embolization of external carotid branches where the posterior inferior cerebellar artery takes origin from the ascending pharyngeal artery would similarly require special consideration.

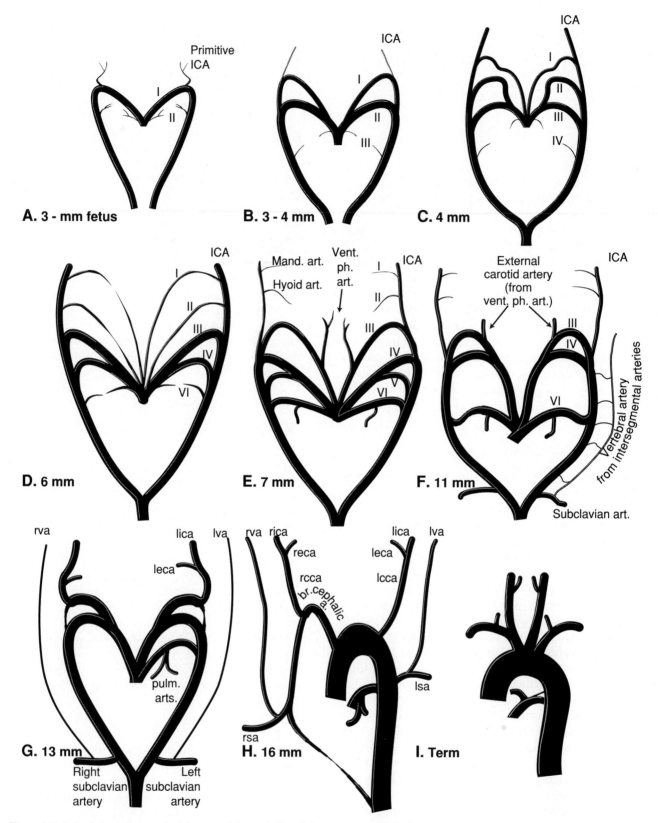

Figure 5.1. A–I Schematic unscaled diagram of the evolution of the embryonic aortic arches; ica = internal carotid artery; eca = external carotid artery; sa = subclavian artery; cca = common carotid artery; va = vertebral artery; vent. ph. art. = ventral pharyngeal artery; mand. art. = mandibular artery; Roman numerals = primitive aortic arches.

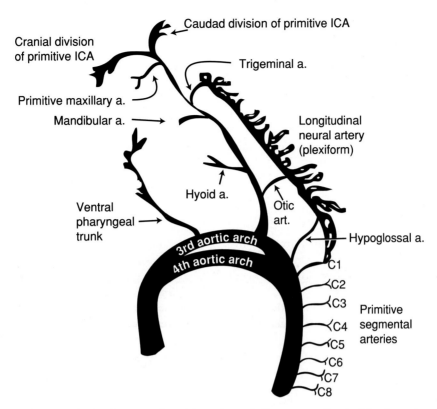

Figure 5.2. Embryologic development of cranial arteries at 4±6-mm stage. See text for discussion. Allowing for variability in timing between fetuses, parts of this diagram correlate with Figure 5.1E.

The same risks in varying degrees apply to minor variants depending on the situation in hand.

4-mm Fetal Stage

At the **4 mm fetal stage** the first and second aortic arches are involuting and their remnants, the *mandibular* and *hyoid arteries* respectively, become incorporated as branches of the third arch (Fig. 5.2). The third arch is the precursor of the internal and common carotid artery. The hyoid artery is discussed below.

The mandibular artery has a less complicated evolution than the hyoid artery, and, in Padget's opinion, is associated with the superficial petrosal nerve, thus represented in adult form by the artery of the Vidian canal. The mandibular artery is frequently seen in children, particularly in the setting of a hypervascular mass in the external carotid artery territory, such as a juvenile angiofibroma (6) or tonsillar hyperplasia (7).

The primitive internal carotid artery continues cephalad and gives a major anastomosis to the posterior circulation, the *primitive trigeminal artery*, at the level of the trigeminal ganglion. Further along its course, the primitive internal carotid artery gives a branch adjacent to Rathké's pouch, the *primitive maxillary artery*, which courses ventrally to the base of the optic vesicle. The primitive maxillary artery later regresses to assume a more mesial course and according to Padget does not commonly play a significant role in the evolution of the adult circle of Willis, being represented in adult form by the inferior hypophyseal artery. De la Torre and Netsky (8) ascribed a more important role to the primitive maxillary artery by comparing its development with that of the maxillo-carotid anastomosis in dogs, which connects the internal maxillary artery with the cavernous internal carotid artery. These authors argued that the primitive maxillary artery can be an important route of inter-carotid vascular supply in the event of prenatal carotid occlusion and that the primitive maxillary artery plays an important role in the evolution of dural and orbital supply. Most modern sources follow Padget's direction, with some debate over the exact identity and nomenclature of those few rare cases of trans-sellar or post-sellar reconstitutions of congenitally occluded internal carotid arteries (9–11).

The primitive internal carotid artery forms two divisions at its most cephalad branching-point:

- Cranial division (*the primitive anterior cerebral artery*) curves around and in front of the optic vesicle to reach the olfactory area;
- Caudal division (*precursor of the posterior communicating artery*) ends in the region of the developing mesencephalon.

Phylogenetic comparisons indicate that the cranial division of the internal carotid artery in humans is homologous with the medial olfactory artery in lower orders, such as fish and reptiles. This vessel is seen to evolve into the anterior cerebral artery as one ascends the phylogenetic hierarchy, implying that the anterior cerebral artery in humans is the direct embryonic continuation of the internal carotid artery, whereas the middle cerebral artery is a secondary branch of this vessel (12).

In the hindbrain area, the arterial vasculature consists initially in paired, separate, *longitudinal neural plexi* supplied cranially by the trigeminal artery and caudally by the first cervical artery. The caudal supply from the C1 segmental artery is supported by input from the *otic artery* at the level of the acoustic nerve and from the *primitive hypoglossal artery* at the level of the XIIth nerve. These latter two vessels are highly transient and regress early.

5–6-mm Fetal Stage

The first arch derivative, the mandibular artery, is diminishing in this stage, but the second arch derivative, the hyoid artery, continues to be robust and goes on to play an important role in the genesis of the middle meningeal artery and ophthalmic artery.

A vessel in the area ventral to the first two aortic arches, and which originates from the third arch, becomes prominent and is termed the *ventral pharyngeal artery* (1). This vessel is the precursor of much of the proximal external carotid artery vasculature (Fig. 5.3).

In the hindbrain, the caudal division of the internal carotid artery forms anastomoses with the cranial end of the bilateral—and as yet separate—longitudinal vascular plexi (*longitudinal neural arteries*). These anastomoses will form the posterior communicating artery, and as they emerge the trigeminal arteries begin to regress. During this stage, the *primitive (lateral) dorsal ophthalmic artery* originating from the proximal internal carotid artery is becoming identifiable. This is one of two embryonic sources of vascular supply to the developing eye discussed later.

7–12-mm Fetal Stage

The ventral pharyngeal system becomes more extensive; lingual and thyroidal branches are identifiable (Fig. 5.4). The ventral pharyngeal artery can be conceived of as the precursor of the lower or proximal external carotid artery. The upper portion of the external carotid artery evolves later from the hyoid artery.

In the posterior neck, longitudinal anastomoses between the cervical segmental arteries begin to fuse and form the longitudinally disposed vertebral arteries. Whereas they ultimately form a single dominant vessel, i.e., the primitive vertebral artery, ipsilateral parallel longitudinal vertebral

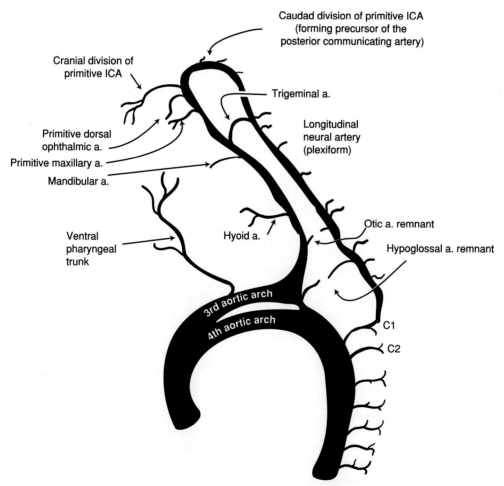

Figure 5.3. Embryologic development of cranial arteries at 5±7-mm stage. See text for discussion. Allowing for variability in timing between fetuses, parts of this diagram correlate with Figures 5.1E and 5.1F.

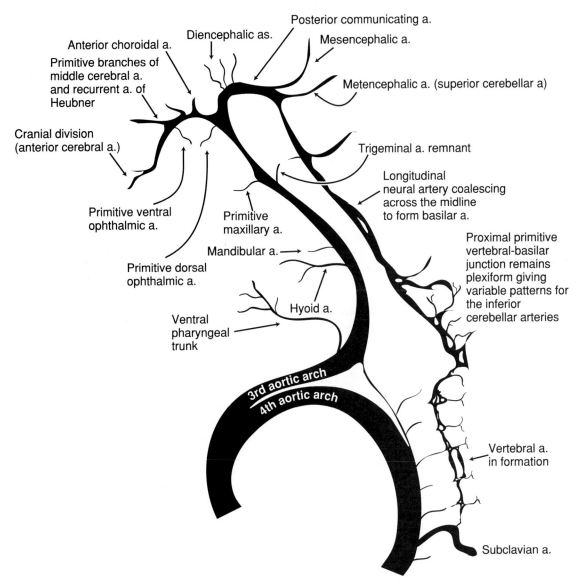

Figure 5.4. Embryologic development of cranial arteries at 9-mm stage. See text for discussion. This diagram correlate with parts of Figures 5.1F and 5.1G.

channels can persist, which explains the etiology of duplications of the vertebral arteries. More cephalad, the longitudinal neural arteries of the hindbrain are still separate from one another for the most part, but have begun to form prominent anastomoses across the midline.

The cranial division of the internal carotid artery (i.e., that part thought of in adult form as distal to the origin of the posterior communicating artery) can be identified giving a branch with prominent diencephalic supply, i.e., the primitive *anterior choroidal artery*. More distally the *middle cerebral artery* is first recognized as multiple twigs branching from the cranial division of the internal carotid artery (i.e., from the anterior cerebral artery). Coalescence of these twigs into a single branch to form the middle cerebral artery proper occurs later. Persistence of a twig separate from the middle cerebral artery trunk can explain

the anomaly of an accessory middle cerebral artery arising from the proximal anterior cerebral artery. A striate artery with a long phylogenetic history is consistently seen arising from the anterior cerebral artery at the level of the anterior communicating artery. It represents the *recurrent artery of Heubner* (12). This represents the supply of the anterior cerebral artery, well recognized in many lower species, to the medial and anterior parts of the palaeo-striatum.

The cranial division (anterior cerebral artery) also gives a branch, the *ventral (nasal) primitive ophthalmic artery*, directed towards the cranial and ventral parts of the optic plexus. By a process of anastomotic connections, the origin of the primitive ventral ophthalmic artery later migrates proximally from the anterior cerebral artery to the internal carotid artery to assume the paraclinoid location typically seen in adult life.

12–14-mm Fetal Stage

The development of the hyoid artery and, in particular, of its principal branch, the *stapedial artery,* shape the appearance of the distal external carotid artery circulation and middle meningeal artery. The fate of the stapedial artery also determines the nature, location, and extent of anastomotic connections between the middle meningeal artery and the ophthalmic artery (Fig. 5.5).

The arterial plexus supplying the eye coalesces into two main trunks at this stage. The dorsal ophthalmic artery gives a temporociliary artery supplying the caudodorsal aspect of the optic cup with a hyaloid branch (later to become the central retinal artery) to the fetal ocular cleft. The primitive ventral ophthalmic artery is still in the process of proximal migration and gives a common nasal-ciliary artery as its main trunk.

A plexiform anastomosis between the anterior cerebral arteries is identified at around this time which will evolve into the anterior communicating artery. When this plexus fails to regress into a single channel, the possibility of multiple variations, duplications, or fenestrations of the anterior communicating artery becomes evident.

16–18-mm Fetal Stage

Fate of the Stapedial Artery

The stapedial artery is now at the zenith of its development. The stapedial artery arises from what will become the proximal intracranial internal carotid artery and runs between the crura of the primitive stapes (Fig. 5.5). In most placental mammals, the stapedial artery is a dominant source of vascular supply to the non-neural structures of the face, orbit, and dermatocranium for at least some period of time during ontogeny. It may persist into adult life for some species, e.g., the European hedgehog (13). The fate of the stapedial artery in humans is to undergo a very proximal trunk regression in association with an annexation of its territories by the ventral pharyngeal trunk (external carotid artery) and by the ophthalmic artery.

The stapedial artery arises near the middle ear promontory and after supplying the back wall of the middle ear cavity, stapedius muscle, and mastoid region, it travels anterolaterally through the intercrural foramen towards the tympanic roof, anterior to the epitympanic recess (13, 14). It divides into a *superior (supraorbital) ramus and inferior (infraorbital) ramus.*

Infraorbital Ramus of the Stapedial Artery

The inferior ramus runs in company with the lesser superficial petrosal nerve and exits from the floor of the middle cranial fossa to the infratemporal fossa to support a large area of dermatocranial supply through its large *maxillomandibular branch*. This trunk forms prominent anastomoses with the ventral pharyngeal trunk (proximal external carotid artery), which therefore becomes the dominant supply to this territory when the stapedial artery undergoes proximal regression at the level of the middle ear. The segment of vessel representing the transcranial connection between the inferior ramus of the stapedial artery and the exocranial territory will reverse flow after this annexation and corresponds in adult life with the stem of the middle meningeal artery traversing the foramen spinosum. Proximal regression alone of the stapedial artery does not fully explain the assumption of the maxillo-mandibular territory by the external carotid artery because in cases of a persistent stapedial artery arising from the internal carotid artery, this extracranial territory is still supplied usually by the external carotid artery, except in extremely rare instances (15). When a persistent stapedial artery giving rise to the middle meningeal artery is present, however, or where the middle meningeal artery arises from another source such as the ophthalmic artery, the middle meningeal artery trunk does not breach the skull base in its usual form. In many such variants the foramen spinosum will be diminutive or absent (as is reportedly the case in 10% of natives of New Guinea [16]). The stem of the hyoid trunk and stapedial artery proximal to the point of regression becomes the carotico-tympanic branch of the internal carotid artery. The segment of the stapedial artery immediately distal to the point of regression will reverse flow after the annexation and corresponds with the tympanic branch of the middle meningeal artery in adult life (17).

Supraorbital Ramus of the Stapedial Artery

The superior (supraorbital) ramus of the stapedial artery supplies a large territory of the developing orbit and the primitive dural coverings of the brain. The dural supply is assumed by the external carotid artery when the stapedial artery regresses proximally and corresponds with the territory of the middle meningeal artery. The territory of the supraorbital ramus or artery in the region of the orbit undergoes further changes, which influence the development of the ophthalmic artery and its connections with

Figure 5.5. *Development of the hyoid-stapedial artery.* A schematic illustration of the hyoid-stapedial artery at its zenith (approximately 20-mm stage) is represented in the center. The maxillo-mandibular trunk exits from the primitive cranium via a route that will later represent the foramen spinosum (f.sp.). The maxillo-mandibular trunk is annexed by the ventral pharyngeal artery and becomes the distal external carotid artery. The hyoid artery regresses at the level of the stapes (st.). The stem of the infraorbital division reverses direction of flow through the foramen spinosum and becomes the trunk of the middle meningeal artery. The orbital branches of the supraorbital division are annexed in varying degrees by the ophthalmic artery. Numerous outcomes are possible in terms of the variability of vessel regressions necessary to achieve the ``normal state.'' Of the variants illustrated, **(D, G),** and **(H)** are extremely rare.

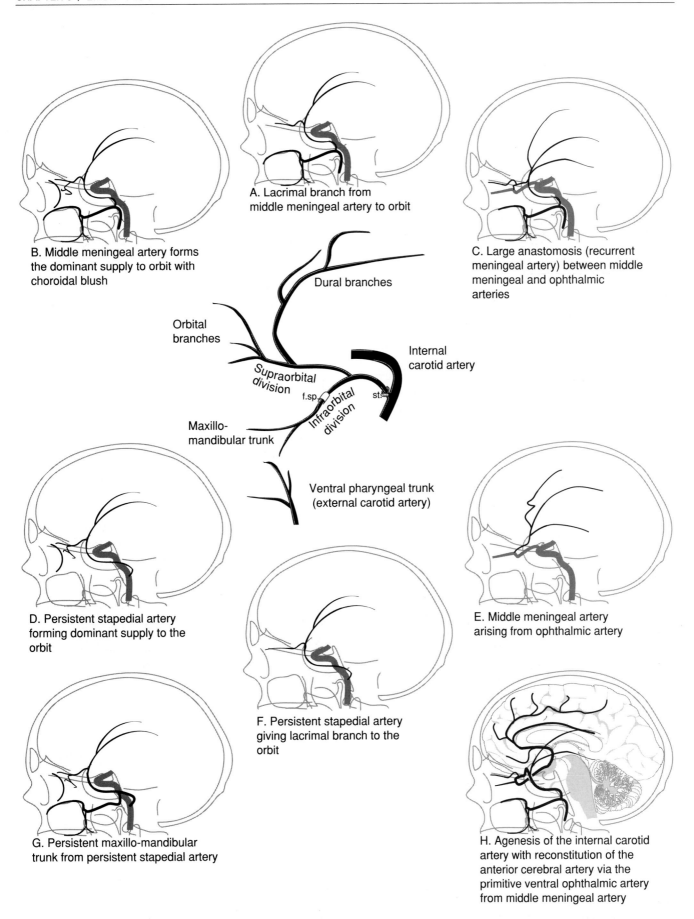

A. Lacrimal branch from middle meningeal artery to orbit

B. Middle meningeal artery forms the dominant supply to orbit with choroidal blush

C. Large anastomosis (recurrent meningeal artery) between middle meningeal and ophthalmic arteries

Dural branches

Orbital branches

Supraorbital division

Internal carotid artery

f.sp.

Infraorbital division

st.

Maxillo-mandibular trunk

Ventral pharyngeal trunk (external carotid artery)

D. Persistent stapedial artery forming dominant supply to the orbit

E. Middle meningeal artery arising from ophthalmic artery

F. Persistent stapedial artery giving lacrimal branch to the orbit

G. Persistent maxillo-mandibular trunk from persistent stapedial artery

H. Agenesis of the internal carotid artery with reconstitution of the anterior cerebral artery via the primitive ventral ophthalmic artery from middle meningeal artery

the middle meningeal artery territory. The orbital branch of the supraorbital artery divides as it enters the orbit into vessels that accompany the lacrimal, frontal, and nasociliary branches of the ophthalmic division of the trigeminal nerve.

Evolution of the Dorsal and Ventral Primitive Ophthalmic Arteries

At approximately the 18-mm stage, the ventral primitive ophthalmic artery (from the anterior cerebral artery) has gained the upper hand in dominance of supply to the optic apparatus, and the dorsal ophthalmic artery has begun to regress. By adult life the dorsal ophthalmic artery is usually represented by an anastomosis, the deep recurrent ophthalmic artery, between the ophthalmic artery and the inferolateral trunk of the cavernous internal carotid artery. When the dorsal ophthalmic artery persists or is the dominant vessel, the ophthalmic artery demonstrates a site of origin from the cavernous segment of the internal carotid artery.

The normal process of coalescence of the ventral and dorsal ophthalmic trunks and the orbital branches of the supraorbital artery results in a transient vascular anastomotic ring around the proximal optic nerve most consistently present in the 20–24 mm stage. Persistence of this ring in complete form may occasionally be seen in adults but is rare. Most commonly (85%), the ring regresses partially along its ventral aspect so that in adults the ophthalmic artery swings from beneath the nerve to curve around the lateral aspect of the nerve and crosses *over the nerve* to a medially directed course. In approximately 15% of instances, the dorsal part of the ring is the segment that recedes, in which case the artery crosses from lateral to medial *under the nerve* (See Chapter 8).

With reference to the anastomoses between the ophthalmic artery and supraorbital artery, various patterns may be seen. When the orbital branch of the supraorbital artery divides proximally within the middle cranial fossa, the sphenoid bone, which ossifies later, will allow more than one transosseous route for these vessels. Most commonly, the supraorbital artery (later to become the middle meningeal artery) connects with the ophthalmic artery through the superior orbital fissure via a proximal vessel called the *sphenoidal artery* or *recurrent meningeal artery* (18) or *orbital branch of the middle meningeal artery* (19). In approximately 50% of dissected specimens, there is an additional transosseous foramen (multiple in 5–15% of specimens) lateral to the superior orbital fissure, which allows anastomoses between the middle meningeal artery and the lacrimal division of the ophthalmic artery (20, 21). This foramen has been given various names including the *foramen meningo-orbitale* (19, 21), the *foramen of Hyrtl* (22), and the *cranio-orbital foramen* (20), and the vessel that traverses it is most commonly called the *meningo-lacrimal artery* (20). Variable points of regression in the genesis of the middle meningeal artery and the ophthalmic artery can therefore lead to anomalous states whereby the ophthalmic artery

gives rise to the middle meningeal artery or vice versa. Alternatively, the middle meningeal artery may be the dominant source of supply to the ophthalmic artery (the most common arrangement in some species such as the rabbit), or only the lacrimal area of the orbit may be supplied dominantly by the middle meningeal artery. The middle meningeal artery may connect proximally with the ophthalmic artery through the superior orbital fissure and distally through the foramen meningo-orbitale in the same dissection specimens, prompting Diamond (20) and other authors to deduce that these are separate entities and not variant courses of a single vessel. By recalling that the ventral primitive ophthalmic artery originally arises from the cranial division of the primitive internal carotid artery (i.e., the anterior cerebral artery), the highly unusual possibilities of the ophthalmic artery arising from the anterior cerebral artery (23) and of the anterior cerebral artery being supplied by the orbital branches of the middle meningeal artery can be explained (24) (Fig. 5.5H).

Evolution of the Posterior Circulation

Over a variable period of development between the 9-mm and 40-mm stages, the *basilar artery* is formed by a midline coalescence of transverse anastomoses between the paired longitudinal neural arteries. Numerous islands or interruptions of this midline fusion can be seen in the early stages but become fewer with time. When such an interruption persists into adult life, this constitutes a fenestration of the basilar artery. The paired neural arteries are themselves plexiform in appearance, and it is from this plexiform origin that the major branches of the basilar artery and distal vertebral artery evolve. Consequently, variability in the origins and course of the cerebellar arteries is commonly seen in adults, particularly those of the posterior inferior cerebellar artery and anterior inferior cerebellar artery, which form later than the superior cerebellar artery. For instance, a persistent remnant of the primitive trigeminal artery together with an anomalous pattern of regression of the longitudinal neural arterial plexus can combine to give an origin of the anterior inferior cerebellar artery or posterior inferior cerebellar artery from the internal carotid artery. The possibilities and combinations of variations are numerous.

As a general rule (12), origin of the posterior cerebral artery circulation switches from the internal carotid artery to the basilar artery with ascending phylogenetic rank. The form and pattern of the posterior cerebral artery becomes settled in human ontogeny later than that of the other major vessels. As part of the phylogenetic vacillation surrounding this process, variants, in which the posterior cerebral circulation derives from the anterior choroidal artery, internal carotid artery, and basilar artery, can be seen. Most commonly, a posterior cerebral artery arising from the internal carotid artery, predominantly or exclusively, is described as being of "fetal origin."

VENOUS EMBRYOLOGY

Padget's quotation of an earlier author (25) "there is no overstatement in Mall's picturesque comment that the history of the arteries is relatively simple when compared with the gyrations the veins undergo" summarizes the complexity of cranial venous embryology. However, the following points can be abstracted in the interests of simplification.

- Unlike the arteries that reach a form resembling the adult configuration at the 40-mm fetal stage, the veins do not reach such a semblance until the 80-mm stage or later. Evolution of the venous system continues into the post-natal period such that an infant may display sinuses or veins not usually seen in adults, e.g., the sphenobasal vein or various tentorial sinuses. Alternatively, connections or veins seen in adults may not be identifiable in infants, e.g., the cavernous sinus may not yet drain to the superior petrosal sinus, and the lateral mesencephalic vein may not be present at birth. Furthermore, when a prenatal vascular malformation is present, such as a Vein of Galen aneurysm or arteriovenous malformation, primitive venous channels or sinuses that normally regress before birth may be present giving the malformation a bizarre venous pattern with unfamiliar connections (26, 27).
- The adult midline superior sagittal sinus derives from a plexiform dural venous channel covering the telencephalon and diencephalon from which it receives pial-arachnoidal draining veins. The primitive dural plexus is initially connected laterally to other plexal components that will become the transverse sinus, sigmoid sinus, and the superficial and deep middle cerebral veins. With development of the telencephalon at a rate disproportionate to the rest of the brain, expansion posteriorly of the cerebral hemispheres results in a displacement and stretching of the arachnoidal veins posteriorly relative to their site of insertion into the superior sagittal sinus. According to Padget, this phenomenon explains the observation that many draining cortical veins of the cerebral hemispheres drain into the superior sagittal sinus *against* the direction of flow. Additionally, their derivation by a process of being drawn away from the sinus across the cortical surface explains why the major cortical draining veins of the cerebral hemisphere are *superficial* to the pial arteries, in contrast to the smaller pial veins, which lie *beneath* the arteries.
- The torcular Herophili evolves from a venous dural plexus and frequently has a configuration such that the superior sagittal sinus predominantly drains to the right side while the straight sinus may drain to the left. This and other asymmetries favoring accelerated development of the venous system on the right side were ascribed by Padget (4, 5) and Okudera (28) to the venous anatomy of the thorax in which venous drainage is more prompt from the right side, in contrast to the left, which is routed via the sinus venosus.
- The cavernous sinus and inferior petrosal sinus develop from the pro-otic sinus, which evolves in association with the venous drainage of the orbit. Initially it has no part in the venous drainage of intracranial structures, effectively being a rerouting of craniofacial drainage via an intracranial channel. Therefore, venous drainage of areas considered to be associated with the cavernous sinus and its related tributaries in the adult must have an alternative embryological pathway before connections to the cavernous sinus are established. These pathways are dural sinuses related to the primitive tentorium, which can some-

times persist into adulthood. When the sphenoparietal sinus, for instance, does not connect medially with the cavernous sinus, it may drain posteriorly via a tentorial sinus, sometimes called the "sphenobasal sinus," "sphenotemporal sinus," or "ophthalmomeningeal sinus," to the superior petrosal sinus or transverse sinus. Alternatively, transsphenoidal venous pathways via the foramen ovale or foramen of Vesalius may connect to the pterygoid plexus.
- The basal vein of Rosenthal is fragmented in its genesis and connects late to the Galenic system. It does not become recognizably formed until the 60-mm to 80-mm stage and represents the longitudinal confluence of primary pial channels seen in lower vertebrates, which correspond with telencephalic, diencephalic, mesencephalic, metencephalic, and myelencephalic veins. Its drainage is initially laterally (infratentorially) via a "trigeminal vein," corresponding with the superior petrosal sinus of adulthood, towards the tentorial sinuses. Drainage of the basal vein of Rosenthal primarily to the tentorial sinuses may be seen in adults. The lateral anastomotic mesencephalic vein is a post-natal structure.
- Variant or minor dural sinuses seen occasionally in adults, such as the occipital sinus (extending from the torcular Herophili inferiorly towards the foramen magnum) or the marginal sinus (surrounding the foramen magnum), may be typically prominent at birth and during childhood (28).

ENUMERATION OF THE CERVICAL SEGMENTAL ARTERIES

A potential point of confusion can arise in a discrepancy, which exists between the embryologic enumeration and angiographic descriptions of cervical branches of the vertebral artery. Angiographically, the nomenclature of the cervical branches of the vertebral artery corresponds with the enumeration of the cervical nerves. The C3 branch of the vertebral artery, for instance, emerges near the C3 nerve roots between the C2 and C3 vertebral bodies. A point of clarification made by Padget (3) is necessary when reading some of the embryologic literature relevant to this area.

The primitive arterial vessels that contribute to the formation of the vertebral artery are the *segmental arteries*, numbered for each of the eight embryonic somites that are formed in the neck, and numbered correspondingly with the cervical nerves, i.e., the first cervical segmental artery lies *above* the developing C1 vertebral body. As the process of development evolves, the segmental arteries become redesignated as the *intersegmental arteries* and the first cervical intersegmental artery is designated as the one emerging *below* the C1 vertebral body.

If the C1 intersegmental artery corresponds with what was earlier termed the C2 segmental artery, then what becomes of the earlier C1 segmental artery? To describe this vessel, comparative anatomists invoke the *proatlas*, which is a rudimentary vertebral structure in some animals intercalated between the atlas and the occipital bone. It is occasionally seen in man. The vessel in this area, i.e., the C1 segmental artery, which has been shuffled out of place in the renumbering scheme, is now designated the *proatlantal intersegmental artery.* Therefore, the etymology of this obscure term is explained when the rare anomaly of the proatlantal intersegmental artery is described. This occurs when the major contributor to vertebral artery flow is from the embryonic C1 segmental artery rather than from lower in the neck.

Other common and rare anomalous origins of the vertebral artery are explained by a similar process. A left vertebral origin directly from the aorta between the left common carotid artery and the left subclavian artery corresponds usually with a point of entry into the vertebral canal via the 4th foramen transversarium. Rare variants explained by the same process include origin of the left vertebral artery from the aorta *distal* to the origin of the left subclavian artery or from the thyrocervical or costocervical trunks.

REFERENCES

1. Congdon ED. Transformation of the aortic-arch system during the development of the human embryo. Contrib Embryol 1922; 14:47–110.
2. Padget DH. The development of the cranial arteries in the human embryo. Contrib Embryol 1948;32:205–262.
3. Padget DH. Designation of the embryonic intersegmental arteries in reference to the vertebral artery and subclavian stem. Anat Rec 1954;119:349–356.
4. Padget DH. The cranial venous system in man in reference to development, adult configuration, and relations to the arteries. Am J Anat 1956;98:307–355.
5. Padget DH. The development of the cranial venous system in man, from the viewpoint of comparative anatomy. Contrib Embryol 1957;36(247):80–140.
6. Davis KR. Embolization of epistaxis and juvenile nasopharyngeal angiofibromas. Am J Neuroradiol 1986;7:953–962.
7. Jinkins JR. The Vidian artery in childhood tonsillar hypertrophy. Am J Neuroradiol 1988;9:141–143.
8. De la Torre E, Netsky MG. Study of persistent primitive maxillary artery in human fetus: Some homologies of cranial arteries in man and dog. Am J Anat 1960;106:185–195.
9. Tracy PT. Unusual intercarotid anastomosis associated with anterior communicating artery aneurysm. Case report. J Neurosurg 1987;67:765–767.
10. Kishore PRS, Kaufman AB, Melichar FA. Intrasellar carotid anastomosis simulating pituitary microadenoma. Radiology 1979;132:381–383.
11. Smith RR, Kees CJ, Hogg ID. Agenesis of the internal carotid artery with an unusual primitive collateral. Case report. J Neurosurg 1972:37:460–462
12. Abbie AA. The morphology of the fore-brain arteries, with especial reference to the evolution of the basal ganglia. J Anat 1934; 68:28–470.
13. Wible JR. The eutherian stapedial artery: character analysis and implications for superordinal relationships. Zoological J Linnean Soc 1987;91:107–135.
14. Diamond MK. Homologies of the stapedial artery in Humans, with a reconstruction of the primitive stapedial artery configuration of Euprimates. Am J Phys Anthropol 1991b;84:433–462.
15. Rodesch G, Choi IS, Lasjaunias P. Complete persistence of the hyoido-stapedial artery in man. Case report. Intrapetrous origin of the maxillary artery from ICA. Surg Radiol Anat 1991;13: 63–65.
16. Lippert H, Pabst R. Arterial Variations in Man. München: J.F.Bergmann Verlag, 1985.
17. Steffen TN. Vascular anomalies of the middle ear. Laryngoscope 1968;78:171–197.
18. Lasjaunias P, Vignaud J, Hasso AN. Maxillary artery blood supply to the orbit: Normal and pathological aspects. Neuroradiology 1975;9:87–97.
19. Royle G. A groove in the lateral wall of the orbit. J Anat 1973; 115:461–465.
20. Diamond MK. Arterial homologies of the human orbit: a reappraisal. J Anat 1991;178:223–242.
21. Georgiu C, Cassell MD. The foramen meningo-orbitale and its relationship to the development of the ophthalmic artery. J Anat 1992;180:119–125.
22. Lasjaunias PL. Craniofacial and Upper Cervical Arteries: Functional Clinical and Angiographic Aspects. Baltimore: Williams & Wilkins, 1981.
23. Hassler W, Zentner J, Voigt K. Abnormal origin of the ophthalmic artery from the anterior cerebral artery: Neuroradiological and intraoperative findings. Neuroradiology 1989;21:85–87.
24. Lasjaunias P, Berenstein A. Arterial anatomy: introduction. In: Surgical Neuroangiography: Functional anatomy of Craniofacial Arteries. Berlin, Springer-Verlag, 1987;1:244.
25. Mall FP. On the development of the blood vessels of the brain in the human embryo. Am J Anat 1904;4:1–18.
26. Mullan S, Mojtahedi S, Johnson DL, et al. Cerebral venous malformation-arteriovenous malformation transition forms. J Neurosurg 1996b;85:9–13.
27. Mullan S, Mojtahedi S, Johnson DL, et al. Embryological basis of some aspects of cerebral vascular fistulas and malformations. J Neurosurg 1996;85:1–8.
28. Okudera T, Huang YP, Ohta T, et al. Development of posterior fossa dural sinuses, emissary veins, and jugular bulb: morphological and radiologic studies. Am J Neuroradiol 1994;15: 1871–1883.

CHAPTER 6

Aortic Arch

Cerebral angiography can usually be performed without the need for an aortic arch injection. Considering the time, effort, difficulty, and contrast load involved in a pigtail catheter injection in the ascending aorta, and then replacing that catheter with one suitable for selective angiography, the undertaking is usually not worthwhile on a routine basis (1). However, an arch aortogram may prove necessary in the setting of proximal great vessel stenosis, tortuosity, or anatomic variations. This can be accomplished with 30–50 ml of contrast. The best projection is usually 30–40 in a left anterior oblique projection. It should be considered prospectively in patients in whom proximal stenotic disease is suspected, particularly with cases such as subclavian steal phenomenon, or in patients with congenital heart disease. Additionally, during catheterizations that are proving exceptionally difficult, resorting to an arch aortogram can clarify the anatomy immediately.

The many possible variations of the aortic arch can prove a challenge for catheterization (Fig. 6.1). The most common variations, a bovine arch (Figs. 6.1B, 6.1C), origin of the left vertebral artery from the arch (Fig. 6.1H), and an aberrant right subclavian artery (Fig. 6.1K), can be quickly recognized and catheterized without an arch injection.

RIGHT AORTIC ARCH

This may be an incidental finding or may be associated with known congenital heart disease or a vascular ring. The descending aorta may be right or left sided. The branching pattern is described as mirror-image (Fig. 6.1M) (with a high associated rate of congenital heart disease) or non-mirror image (Fig. 6.1N) (with an aberrant left subclavian artery).

DOUBLE AORTIC ARCH

This has a variable anatomy. From an angiographic viewpoint, important factors include the relative size of the two arches, the side of descent, the position of the ductus arteriosus, and the possibility of atresia. Usually each arch will give off a common carotid artery and a subclavian artery (Figs. 6.1O, 6.1P).

BI-INNOMINATE ARTERY

This is a rare entity. The aortic arch has a symmetric appearance with each innominate artery giving a common carotid and subclavian artery (Fig. 6.1D).

ABERRANT RIGHT SUBCLAVIAN ARTERY

This is a common anomaly and has an association with Down's Syndrome. The term usually refers to origin of the right subclavian artery from a point distal to the left subclavian artery (Fig. 6.1K). The right vertebral artery will usually arise from the right subclavian artery. The aberrant right subclavian artery may arise from an aortic diverticulum (Kommerell) and pursues a retro-esophageal course. It can frequently be recognized by the unusual course taken by the wire and catheter from the thoracic aorta. However, be careful as such an appearance of the wire crossing the midline can also be seen with inadvertent catheterization of a right supreme intercostal artery.

With rarer forms of aberrant origin of the right subclavian artery from points more proximal in the aortic arch, the right vertebral artery may arise separately from the arch.

BICAROTID TRUNK

The right and left carotid arteries may share a common trunk. This is particularly likely in the setting of an aberrant origin of the right subclavian artery. In such instances, the left carotid artery may have a steep recurrent course making catheterization more difficult.

CAROTID BIFURCATION

The right common carotid artery is usually slightly shorter than the left. The carotid bifurcation is usually at the C3–C4 level but can occur from C2 down to T2 vertebral levels. From a practical point of view, the angle of the mandible is a useful landmark for initial placement of the tip of the wire during carotid catheterization. In more than 75% of patients, the internal carotid artery lies posterolateral to the external carotid trunk. This means that an ipsilateral anterior oblique projection will usually be the best view for evaluation of the carotid bifurcation in single-plane fluoroscopy rooms.

VERTEBRAL ARTERY VARIANTS

The vertebral artery is usually the first branch of the subclavian artery (Fig. 6.2). The level at which the vertebral artery enters the canal of the foramen transversarium is determined by which cervical intersegmental artery persists as the vertebral artery. In more than 95% of cases, the left vertebral artery enters the foramen transversarium at the C6 vertebral level. Alternative sites of entry will be seen in

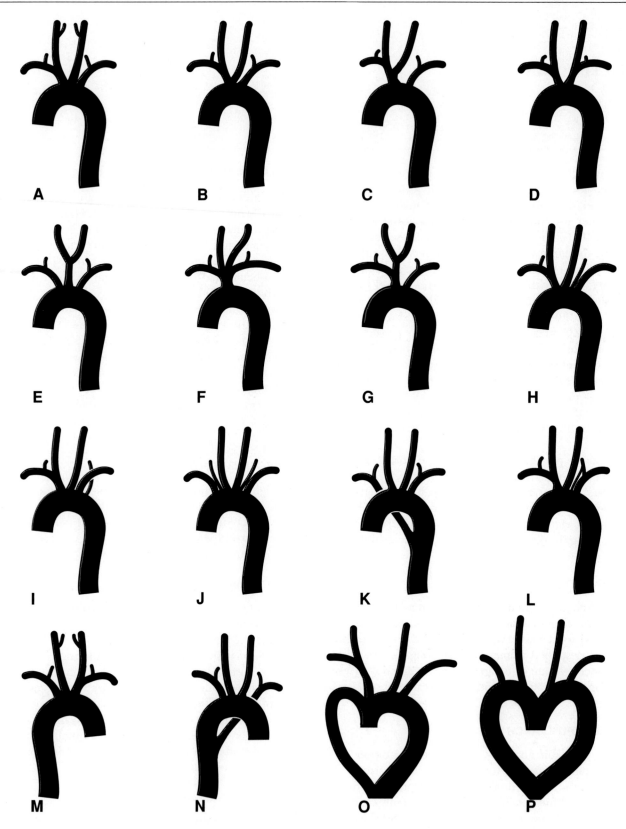

Figure 6.1. A–P Aortic arch variations and anomalies. Schematic illustration of the major groups of aortic anomalies.

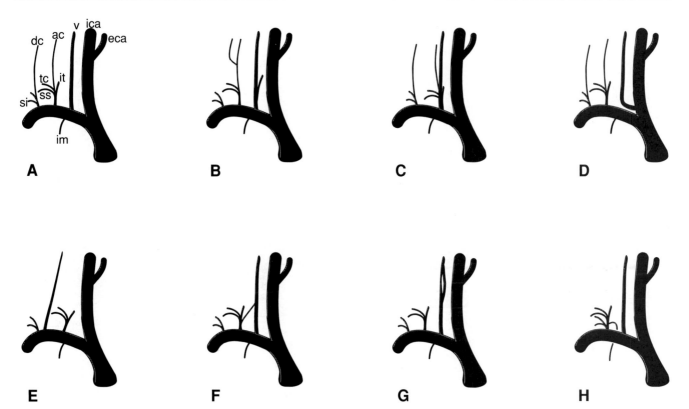

Figure 6.2. A–H Subclavian artery and cervical trunk variations. A schematic representation of the major variations of the branches of the proximal right subclavian artery of concern during neuroangiographic procedures is provided; ica = internal carotid artery; eca = external carotid artery; v = vertebral artery; it = inferior thyroidal artery; ac = ascending cervical artery; dc = deep cervical artery; tc = transverse cervical artery; ss = suprascapular artery; si = superior intercostal artery; im = internal mammary artery. Variant **(A)** represents the standard description in which the thyrocervical trunk and the costocervical trunk arise distal to the vertebral artery. In **(B),** the inferior thyroidal artery shares a common trunk with the vertebral artery, whereas the deep cervical territory is taken over by the ascending cervical artery. In **(C),** the vertebral artery is represented as a branch of the thyrocervical trunk. In **(D),** the vertebral artery arises from the proximal common carotid artery. The vertebral artery arises from the right subclavian artery distal to the thyrocervical trunk in **(E).** In **(F),** the vertebral artery has a duplicated origin, with a smaller distal limb arising from the thyrocervical trunk. In **(G),** the vertebral artery has a duplicated segment more distally. In **(H),** the thyrocervical and costocervical arteries share a common trunk.

cases of variant origin of the left vertebral artery. A left vertebral artery arising directly from the aortic arch usually enters the foramen at approximately the C4 level. With a proatlantal intersegmental origin of the vertebral artery from the internal carotid artery (proatlantal artery type I), origin of the vertebral artery from the internal carotid artery joining the usual course of the vertebral artery at C1 will be seen (2). With origin of the artery to the posterior fossa from the external carotid artery corresponding with the C2 level, this is termed a proatlantal type II artery. A less common variation is persistence of the C7 intersegmental artery entering the canal at the C7 level and giving an arch origin for the left vertebral artery distal to the left subclavian artery. With the exception of a C4 vertebral artery arising from the aortic arch, these variations are rare (see Chapter 12).

REFERENCES

1. Caplan LR, Wolpert SM. Angiography in patients with occlusive cerebrovascular disease: Views of a stroke neurologist and neuroradiologist. Am J Neuroradiol 1991;12:593–601.
2. Legré J, Tapias PL, Nardin JY, et al. Anastomose intersegmentaire carotide externe—vértébrale d'origine embryonnaire. J Neuroradiol 1980;7:97–104.
3. Lippert H, Pabst R. Arterial Variations in Man. München: J.F. Bergmann Verlag, 1985.

CHAPTER 7

The Circle of Willis

"By this kind of provision the Arteries about to enter the Brain are provided: yea, and the passages of the Veins, destined for the returning of the blood from thence, seem also to be disposed with a wonderful artifice. For when the anterior bosoms transfer their load into the two Laterals, which are the posterior, and they themselves end in the Jugular Veins, it is observed, that those latter bosoms have furrows or cavities insculped whereby they may settle or rest upon the hinder part of the Head; and when as either bosom, through a proper hole, being about to go into the Jugular Vein, slides out of the skull; nigh that hole, in the outward part of the Skull, a round and ample den is made hollow, and covered over by the extremity on either side of the same bosom, inlarged into a greater capacity, to the end, that the blood, whilst it slides forth out of the Head with a full torrent, should not rush into the Veins with too rapid and vertiginous an influx, and so make a forcible entry on the Heart it self, therefore it hath here a diversion large enough, in which estuating or boiling up, till a more free and open space may be granted to its course, it may be staid without any trouble. Certainly there can be nothing more artificial thought upon, and that can better argue the Providence of the great Creator, than this fit or convenient disposition of the blood in the brain, and without it, and the way of its reciprocation in divers Animals, accomodated to the necessity of every one. And lastly, in the dissection of Beasts, more miracles of the same nature happen, whereby shewing the Finger and Divine Workmanship of the Deity, a most strong and invincible Argument may be opposed to the most perverse Atheist."

[The Anatomy of the Brain. In: Dr. Willis's Practice of Physick, Being the Whole Works of that Renowned and Famous Physician. London: T. Dring, C. Harper, & T. Leigh, 1684; 60.]

The first description of the circle of Willis is credited to Dr. Thomas Willis who published his work in 1664 (1), written in Latin and illustrated by Sir Christopher Wren. Although a schema of the circle of Willis is easy to remember, there is enormous interindividual variation in the configuration of this arterial ring. Most intracranial saccular aneurysms occur on the circle of Willis or on the major branches close by. Of these, 82–85% occur anterior to a transverse line bisecting the posterior communicating arteries, with the single most common site being the region of the anterior communicating artery complex.

ANATOMIC RELATIONSHIP TO SURROUNDING STRUCTURES

The relationships of the circle of Willis and, particularly those of the anterior cerebral artery and anterior communicating artery to surrounding cisternal and neural structures can be more easily envisioned if it is remembered that the optic chiasm or nerves and the infundibulum are subtended anteriorly *through* the ring of the circle (Figs. 7.1, 7.2, 7.3). The image of the arterial circle as a crab reaching around the optic chiasm with its claws may help to recall this relationship. The optic apparatus enters this ring at an angle that sweeps from postero-superior to antero-inferior as the optic nerves make their way towards the optic canals. Optic nerve and chiasm displacement or compression with visual field deficits may be frequently seen with aneurysms of the anterior circle of Willis. In fact, Wildbrand's knee, the genu of nasal fibers, which loop into the posterior aspect of the contralateral optic nerve before continuing posteriorly in the optic tract, was described in 1915 (2) in the setting of optic nerve compression by an aneurysm. The relationship of the optic chiasm to the anterior communicating artery is then easily remembered, as is the way that it derives perforator feeders from the *inferior* aspect of the anterior communicating artery and A1 segments. The tight apposition of the optic tracts and the basal forebrain can be easily remembered and underscores that the anterior choroidal artery must travel posteromedially *under* the optic tract before turning laterally into the choroidal fissure. The optic tracts will therefore receive perforators from the medial and superior aspects of the anterior choroidal artery and posterior communicating artery below.

The posterior communicating artery usually joins the posterior cerebral artery in front of the midbrain by leaving the posteromedial aspect of the internal carotid artery and ascending posteriorly, superiorly, and slightly medially. The oculomotor nerve lying between the posterior cerebral artery and superior cerebellar artery is a fairly constant relationship; and therefore, it follows that the posterior communicating artery is usually superior or superomedial to the oculomotor nerve. Aneurysms in the region of the posterior communicating artery may present frequently with IIIrd nerve signs.

The position of the mamillary bodies in front of the midbrain allows one to recall that they are suspended above the posterior aspect of the ring of the circle of Willis. The posterior communicating artery sends between four and eight an-

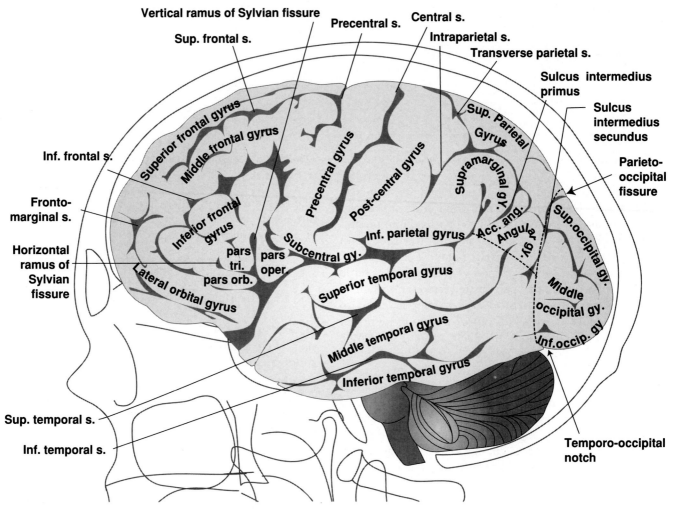

Figure 7.1. *Lateral view of brain.* Illustration of the lateral aspect of the brain used as a template in subsequent diagrams. S. = sulcus; Gy. = gyrus; Sup. = superior; Inf. = inferior; pars orb. = pars orbitalis; pars tri. = pars triangularis; pars oper. = pars opercularis; acc. ang. = accessory angular gyrus (variant).

terior perforating vessels superiorly towards the diencephalon. The sites of origin of these vessels are more frequently in the anterior half of the posterior communicating artery. The largest identifiable perforator in 80% of dissection specimens terminates between the mamillary bodies and the tuber cinereum. Therefore, this vessel is sometimes called the *premamillary artery* or *thalamotuberal artery* (3).

VARIATIONS IN THE CIRCLE OF WILLIS

The propensity of the circle of Willis for anomalies and variations is of interest in that the hemodynamic strains associated with these variations combined with defects in the media at vessel junctions predispose to aneurysm formation (Figs. 7.4, 7.5). Patients with aneurysms are more likely to have asymmetries or anomalies of the circle of Willis (4). Berry or saccular aneurysms form at a turn or curve in the artery, usually at a bifurcation point (5, 6). The impact of hemodynamic stresses on bifurcations in the formation of aneurysms is reflected in the observation

that aneurysms most often point in the direction in which flow would have traveled had its course not been deflected by the arterial wall. It is therefore cogent that in the setting of an anterior communicating artery aneurysm with asymmetry of the A1 segments, the aneurysm will point along the line of hemodynamic thrust from the dominant A1 segment. In this circumstance, the aneurysm will project anteriorly and away from the side of the dominant A1, a relationship that is the case in the majority of such aneurysms. Some degree of A1 asymmetry is found in the majority of anterior communicating artery aneurysms (7). Similarly, the effects of hemodynamic stresses contribute, at least in part, to the formation of aneurysms at the sites of variant vessel origins. Aneurysms are associated with anomalous vessels or in situations with higher than usual rates of flow. Aneurysms are seen more frequently than one would expect by coincidence in the setting of variant carotid-vertebrobasilar anastomoses, arterial feeders of arterio-venous malformations, or after occlusion of

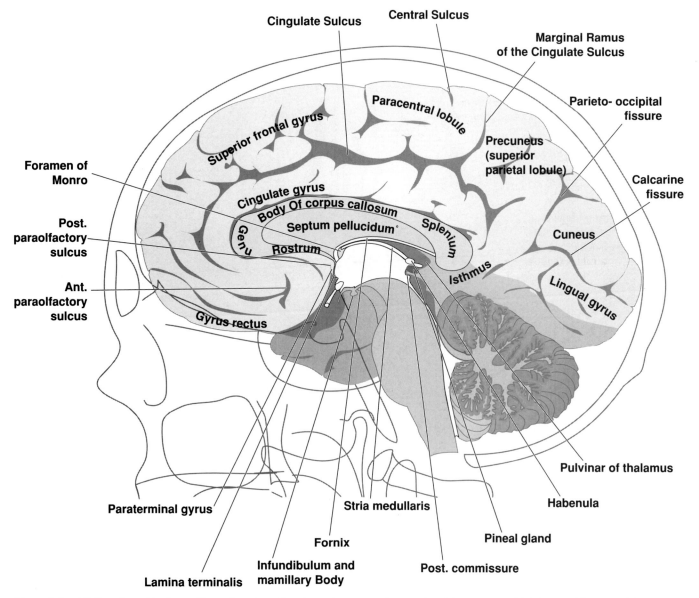

Figure 7.2. *Midline view of brain.* Illustration of median view of the brain used as a template in later diagrams. Notice in particular the marginal ramus of the cingulate sulcus. This defines the posterior margin of the paracentral lobule, providing a useful means of identifying the central sulcus on sagittal MRI images.

cranial vessels by balloon-closure, surgical ligation, or disease. For instance, an azygous anomaly of the anterior cerebral artery, seen in less than 1% of brains, is associated with a higher-than-usual rate of aneurysm formation (8–10).

Vessel Size

The circle of Willis is formed by a communication between the left and right carotid intracranial circulations at the anterior communicating artery and by bilateral communications between the carotid and vertebrobasilar circulations through the posterior communicating arteries. Because of the large number of embryologic steps involved in the evo-

lution of the circle (11) and of each of its many components, variations and anomalies are common. Of these, the most common are those related to size of individual segments. Variability in the circle of Willis is not chaotic but has an order that conforms to hemodynamic principles, replicated in mathematical models (12, 13). Therefore, for instance, an inverse relationship in size between the P1 segment of the posterior cerebral artery and the diameter of the posterior communicating artery is commonly seen. Similarly the anterior communicating artery tends to be largest in the setting of unilateral hypoplasia of an A1 segment. Hillen et al. (14, 15) demonstrated that the relationship curve of flow versus vessel diameter is steepest in the 0.5–2 mm range. This implies that compensatory hemodynamic effects can

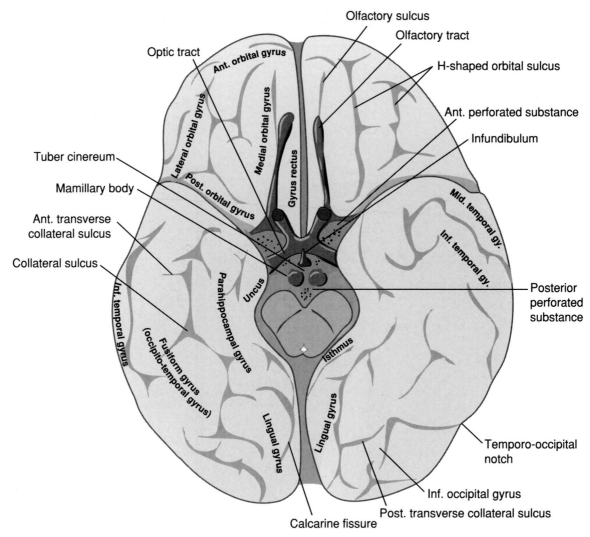

Optic tract

Ant. orbital gyrus

Olfactory sulcus

Olfactory tract

H-shaped orbital sulcus

Medial orbital gyrus

Ant. perforated substance

Lateral orbital gyrus

Infundibulum

Tuber cinereum

Post. orbital gyrus

Gyrus rectus

Mamillary body

Mid. temporal gy.

Ant. transverse
collateral sulcus

Inf. temporal gy.

Collateral sulcus

Uncus

Inf. temporal gyrus

Parahippocampal gyrus

Posterior
perforated
substance

Fusiform gyrus
(occipito-temporal
gyrus)

Isthmus

Lingual gyrus

Lingual gyrus

Temporo-occipital
notch

Inf. occipital gyrus

Post. transverse collateral sulcus

Calcarine fissure

Figure 7.3. *Base of brain.*   Illustration of the base view of the brain used in subsequent diagrams. Notice in particular the relationship of the anterior perforated substance to the olfactory tract. The lenticulo-striate arteries enter the base of the brain via the anterior perforated substance and are divided into medial and lateral groups by a line extended posteriorly along the lie of the olfactory tracts.

Figure 7.4. A–P *A–P. Circle of Willis variations and anomalies.* Schematic representation of most of the anomalies and variants discussed in the subsequent chapters. The view is from above; therefore the anatomic right is on the reader's right. aca = anterior cerebral artery; mca = middle cerebral artery; acha = anterior choroidal artery; pca = posterior cerebral artery; sca = superior cerebellar artery; aica = anterior inferior cerebellar artery; pica = posterior inferior cerebellar artery. **(A)** Symmetric pentagonal circle of robust components. **(B)** Hypoplastic posterior communicating arteries and anterior communicating artery. **(C)** Fenestration/duplication of the anterior communicating artery; duplication of the right superior cerebellar artery; left aica/pica artery; hypoplastic distal right vertebral artery; curve of the basilar artery is with the direction of inflow from the dominant vertebral artery. **(D)** Duplicated left middle cerebral artery from internal carotid artery; accessory right middle cerebral artery from A1 segment; fetal left posterior communicating artery coursing more laterally than usual, and related hypoplastic elongated left P1 segment; duplicated right superior cerebellar artery with upper branch arising from P1 segment; duplicated left anterior inferior cerebellar artery; extradural origin of right posterior inferior cerebellar artery. **(E)** Fenestrated anterior communicating artery with "triplicated A2"; right vertebral artery terminates in a posterior inferior cerebellar artery. **(F)** Hypoplasia of right A1 segment; left anterior choroidal artery arises from left middle cerebral artery; right anterior choroidal artery arises from right posterior communicating artery; low bifurcation of the basilar artery with common stem for right posterior cerebral artery and right superior cerebellar artery. **(G)** Complete absence of right A1 segment (rare); duplication of right anterior choroidal artery; low bifurcation of basilar artery. **(H)** Triplicated A2; low basilar artery bifurcation; fenestration of the basilar artery. **(I)** Bilateral fetal posterior communicating arteries; bilateral hypoplastic P1 segments; duplication of distal right vertebral artery. **(J)** Azygous anterior cerebral artery; dominant anterior choroidal artery supply to left hemisphere (duplication of posterior communicating artery). **(K)** Trigeminal artery variant with continuity of upper and lower basilar artery; ipsilateral fetal posterior communicating artery. **(L)** Trigeminal artery variant with discontinuity between upper basilar artery and lower basilar artery.

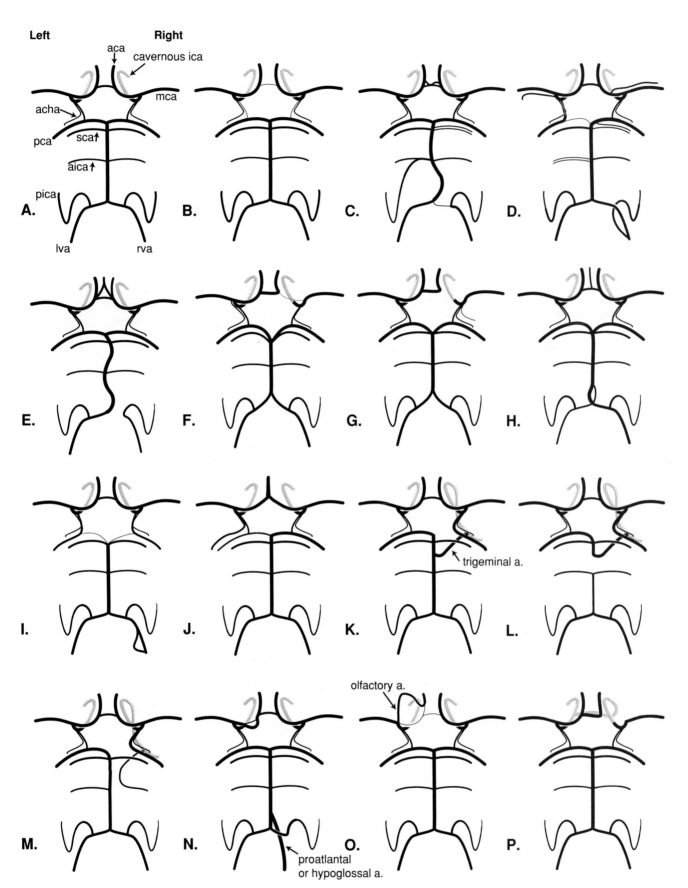

Figure 7.4. *(continued)*
(M) Trigeminal variant giving origin to right anterior inferior cerebellar artery; unrelated origin of right anterior choroidal artery from right posterior communicating artery. **(N)** Persistent carotid-vertebral circulation (proatlantal or hypoglossal artery); unrelated duplication of left A1 segment, the larger channel representing an infraoptic course. **(O)** Primitive olfactory artery giving dominant supply to anterior cerebral artery. **(P)** Agenesis of right internal carotid artery with reconstitution via cavernous branch from left internal carotid artery, most likely representing a persistent primitive maxillary artery.

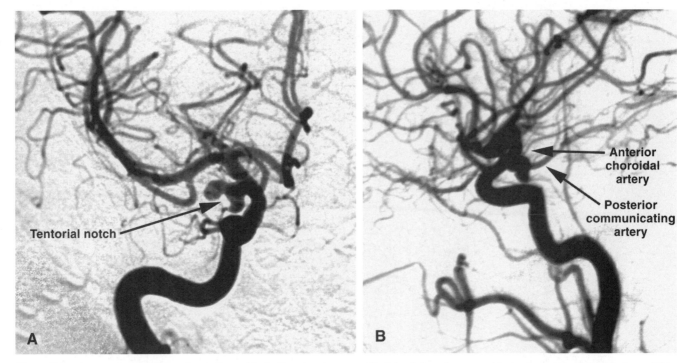

Figure 7.5. *Importance of interpreting angiographic findings in relationship to surrounding structures.*   An unruptured bilobed posterior communicating artery aneurysm is seen on the PA **(A)** and lateral views **(B)** of the right internal carotid artery. Typical of aneurysms in this location, it arises along the distal rim of the ostium of the posterior communicating artery and is distinct from the anterior choroidal artery

on the lateral view. An unusual but extremely important feature of this particular aneurysm is its relationship to the tentorium. The lobule in the supratentorial compartment is very likely to be tightly applied against and adherent to the uncus of the right temporal lobe. Consequently, a surgical approach to this aneurysm must be planned, which does not require uncal retraction.

be predicted when a component of the circle of Willis is less than 2 mm in diameter.

A "typical" circle of Willis, in which all components are robust in diameter and symmetric, is unusual, being present on macroscopic examination in only 21% of autopsy specimens (16). When bilateral small posterior communicating arteries are allowed as part of the normal symmetric configuration, only 30% would be "typical" (17); or if asymmetry of vessel size is allowed with all vessels in the polygon measuring 1 mm or more, the proportion of "normals" is approximately 52% (18). A fetal type posterior communicating artery, i.e. a posterior communicating artery larger than the P1 segment of the posterior cerebral artery or which supplies the bulk of flow to that territory, is seen in 22–26% of cases. A 15% incidence of a more definitive fetal posterior cerebral artery is seen (18), whereas a hypoplastic posterior communicating artery is seen in 32% (3, 19). When there is a fetal type posterior communicating artery present, the P1 segment of the posterior cerebral artery is often longer and more tortuous. In these instances, the course of the fetal posterior communicating artery is more directly posterior off the internal carotid artery or posterolateral compared with the usual posteromedial course of the non-fetal posterior communicating artery. This alters the relationship of the posterior communicating artery to the oculomotor nerve. Instead of running superomedial to the oculomotor nerve,

the fetal posterior communicating artery takes a more superior or superolateral course.

Complete absence of the posterior communicating artery is rare during dissection, 0.6% or less (18), although it is more common during angiographic interpretation not to be able to see any evidence of a hemodynamically significant posterior communicating artery.

Alone or in combination with other variations of the circle, a hypoplastic A1 segment may be seen in 12% of autopsy specimens, a hypoplastic P1 segment in 18%, and a hypoplastic anterior communicating artery in 20% (16).

Other Anomalies

Anomalies other than those related to vessel size fall into three general categories: unusual vessels, duplications of normally present vessels, and origins of normally present vessels from unusual sites.

The anterior communicating artery complex is probably the single most common site in the circle of Willis for anomalous configurations. Duplications or fenestrations of this complex are seen in 9–40% of dissections (7, 18). Alpers et al. (7) found a total incidence of duplications of vessels in the polygon of 19% (Fig. 7.6). A more unusual variant of the anterior communicating artery complex is the *superior anterior communicating artery,* which is occasionally seen more superiorly joining the A2 segments of the distal anterior cerebral arteries.

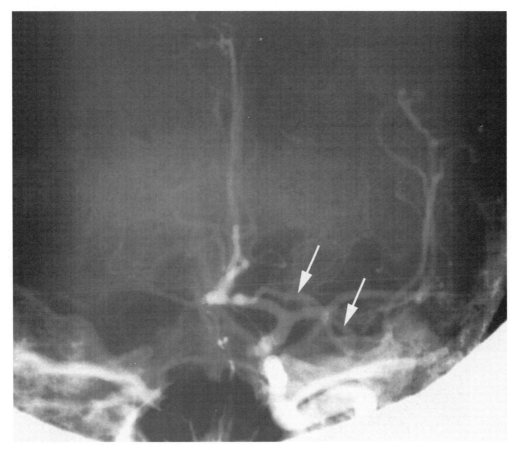

Figure 7.6. *Accessory left middle cerebral artery.* A 35-year-old female with multiple aneurysms demonstrates an accessory left middle cerebral artery (arrows) arising from the distal A1 segment. Such vessels, and the recurrent artery of Heubner on occasion, are sometimes most distinctly seen during the contralateral carotid injection because the remainder of the ipsilateral middle cerebral artery is not then opacified.

Duplication of the anterior choroidal artery is reported in 4% of dissections (3). The anterior choroidal artery, alternatively, may share a common origin with or be a branch of the posterior communicating artery. Up to 24% of anterior choroidal arteries may arise from atypical origins, such as the middle cerebral artery, posterior communicating artery, or posterior cerebral artery with some measure of inter-racial variation (20, 21). A more unusual configuration of the anterior choroidal artery is seen when this vessel retains a portion of its embryologic circulation pattern, continuing to supply much of the posterior cerebral hemisphere. The appearance of this large vessel arising distal to the posterior communicating artery from the internal carotid artery with such a cerebral territory is termed by some authors as a *duplicated posterior cerebral artery or duplicated posterior communicating artery.* This configuration may explain some or most of the reported cases of "duplication" of the posterior communicating artery because true duplication of the posterior communicating artery is not reported in the microanatomical studies of 50 cadaver brains by Saeki and Rhoton (3). Origin of the posterior communicating artery from the ophthalmic artery also during dissection has been described (22).

Other anomalies of the circle of Willis include anomalous relationship of the A1 segments to the optic chiasm or nerve which they usually transcend. Rarely, the A1 segment of one or both sides may loop under the optic structures or may do so in the setting of anomalous origin of the A1 segment from a more proximal point than usual on the supraclinoid internal carotid artery. The latter variant probably represents an unusual persistence of the embryologic origin of the ventral ophthalmic artery from the A2 segment, which normally establishes a connection with the supraclinoid internal carotid artery en route to the orbit. The proximal portion of the primitive ventral ophthalmic artery usually regresses, but if there should be a prenatal occlusion of the proximal A1 segment, the primitive ventral ophthalmic artery may persist as this rare intraoptic anomalous course of the anterior cerebral artery.

Prenatal or developmental occlusions of the internal carotid artery are rare and have differing angiographic manifestations. With an occlusion proximal to the usual site of origin of the ophthalmic artery, flow to the ipsilateral hemisphere will most often be supplied by the contralateral carotid and the vertebrobasilar systems. Congenital absence of the internal carotid artery can occasionally be bilateral (23, 24).

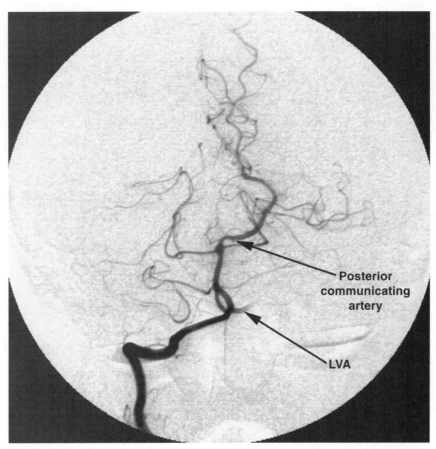

Figure 7.7. *Fenestration of the basilar artery.* An injection of the right vertebral artery demonstrates a fenestration of the proximal basilar artery. The left vertebral artery is briefly opacified (LVA). The right P1 segment is not seen. The left P1 segment is slightly hypoplastic with evidence of widening of the caliber of the posterior cerebral artery distal to the insertion of the posterior communicating artery. In the distal left posterior cerebral artery, there is streaming from posterior communicating artery inflow.

Fenestrations

Fenestrations of the circle of Willis are due to developmental anomalies of vessel fusion, resulting in a segmental separation of the vessel lumen by a pillar or bridge of varying length (Figs. 7.7, 7.8). Bearing in mind that most fenestrations are probably not demonstrated by *in vivo* angiography, the angiographic appearance, when evident, is that of a filling defect separating two channels of flow. The gross, anatomic appearance may range from that of two parallel vessels to a subtle dimple on the adventitial surface. Embryonic fusion of contiguous vessels is most common in the development of the anterior communicating and vertebrobasilar arteries (11), and therefore these are the most common sites of these anomalies. Fenestrations of the vertebro-basilar junction are uncommon during clinical angiography, being seen in less than 1% of studies (25, 26). However, fenestrations can be seen in 5% of postmortem angiographic studies (27) and in 7–16% of autopsy dissections (28, 29). Fenestrations or duplications of the anterior communicating artery complex are seen in up to 40% of dissections (4). Fenestration of the supraclinoid internal carotid artery has been reported in association with aneurysm formation, but is extremely rare (30).

Histologic studies of fenestrations have demonstrated that an apical defect of the media of the vessel wall exists at the proximal and distal ends of the fenestrating bridge, similar to that seen at cerebral artery bifurcations. There is a build-up of subendothelium at the trailing (distal) edge of the bridge, not seen at the proximal (leading) edge (31, 32). Therefore, the leading edge of the fenestration appears to be more vulnerable to the hemodynamic forces of flow in the vessel, and is invariably the site of aneurysm formation in the setting of association of an aneurysm with a fenestration (33, 34). This is particularly the case with aneurysms of the vertebro-basilar junction, approximately one third of which may be associated with fenestrations (33). A large number of reports, particularly from Japan, support the role of fenestrations in the formation of aneurysms (31, 35–37). However, in a review of 38 fenestrations, Sanders et al. (26) concluded that aneurysm formation occurs only in a minority of such anomalies. The accumulation of subendothelium at the distal end of a fenestration is similar to the intimal cushions frequently seen near bifurcation aneurysms elsewhere (28). These cushions are probably an epiphenomenon of the hemodynamic forces at the bifurcation or fenestration, which play a part in the formation of the aneurysm at the site of a medial defect.

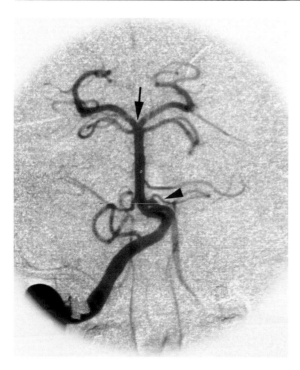

Figure 7.8. *Basilar artery variants.* A fenestration of the vertebro-basilar junction is seen on this right vertebral artery injection. The left posterior inferior cerebellar artery arises from the left limb of the fenestration **(arrowhead)**. The upper basilar artery demonstrates a low bifurcation with sharp angulation of the P1 segments **(arrow)**.

Fenestrations of the other intracranial vessels besides the anterior communicating artery and basilar artery are rare, and their embryological basis is sometimes unclear. Fenestrations of the proximal anterior cerebral artery (29, 38, 39) and middle cerebral artery (40, 41) have been reported, as have rare cases of duplication or fenestration of the internal carotid artery (42–44). Duplication of the cervical internal carotid artery in some instances represents a normal internal carotid artery that is associated with a persistent stapedial artery, which takes a route through the middle ear (45).

Fenestrations or duplications of the extracranial vessels, particularly the vertebral artery, occur by a slightly different phenomenon related to persistence of segmental longitudinal vessels, which normally regress. In a true fenestration of the vertebral artery, which is a rare anomaly, both limbs lie within the vertebral canal. With a duplication of the vertebral artery, one of the limbs lies outside of the canal. In the upper cervical levels, one of the limbs may gain the subarachnoid space at the C1 or C2 level and ascend to the foramen magnum to join its ipsilateral moiety. This subarachnoid location is an alternative expression of the flexibility in ontogeny, whereby a posterior inferior cerebellar artery with origin at C2 may have a similar subarachnoid course (see Chapter 12).

VARIABILITY OF THE TERRITORIES OF THE CEREBRAL ARTERIES

An assumption that the major cerebral arteries have consistent easily identifiable territories of distribution on axial imaging is probably not correct. When considering whether particular ischemic events may be embolic or related to distal hypoperfusion of the watershed zone at the periphery of a territory, an understanding of the territorial boundaries of each of the major vessels is involved. A watershed infarct is one located in the border-zone between two vascular areas, and is related to diminished perfusion of one or both territories (46). If the territories of individual vessels are injected with a marking material, leptomeningeal anastomoses may exaggerate the territory of the injected vessel, an observation known from Heubner (47). Using a technique to inject the three major vessels simultaneously, Van der Zwan et al. (48–50) have demonstrated that there is enormous asymmetry and interindividual variability in the cortical and subcortical territories of the major cerebral arteries (Figs. 7.9, 7.10, 7.11). This variability is directly related to the proximal diameters and peripheral resistance of the major vessels (50). Therefore in considering the possibility of watershed infarcts on axial images or the possible clinical sequelae of a particular single artery occlusion, one must incorporate a degree of latitude into one's understanding of the potential location of the border-zone. For instance, using this technique van der Zwan et al. (49) demonstrated that in approximately 25% of brains the anterior cerebral artery does not perfuse the anterior limb of the internal capsule or lateral segment of the lentiform nucleus, in which cases the middle cerebral artery territory will be correspondingly larger. Also, the superior part of the precentral gyrus concerned with trunk and leg motor function was supplied by the middle cerebral artery in 4% and by the posterior cerebral artery in 2% of cases, implying that lower extremity weakness is not a *sine qua non* of anterior cerebral artery infarction.

With a decrease in perfusion of two neighboring vessels, the location of a distal territory infarct will be different from that caused by a decrease in peripheral perfusion

Maximum

Minimum

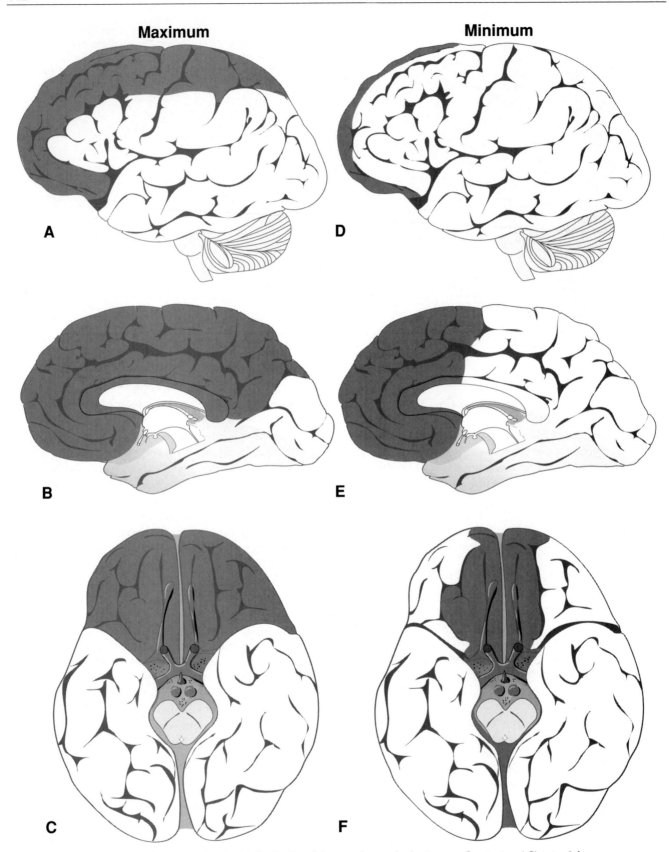

Figure 7.9. *Extremes of territorial distribution of the anterior cerebral artery.* See text and Chapter 9 for discussion. Based on van der Zwan A, Hillen B, Tulleken CAF, et al. Variability of the territories of the major cerebral arteries. J Neurosurg 1992;77 927±940.

Maximum

Minimum

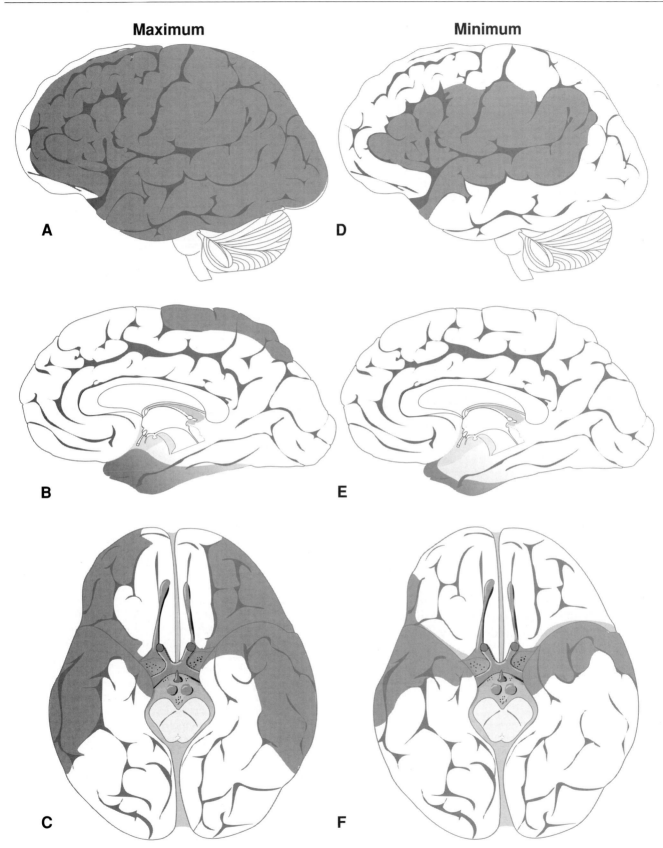

Figure 7.10. *Extremes of territorial distribution of the middle cerebral artery.* See text and Chapter 10 for discussion. Based on van der Zwan A, Hillen B, Tulleken CAF, et al. Variability of the territories of the major cerebral arteries. J Neurosurg 1992;77 927±940.

Maximum   **Minimum**

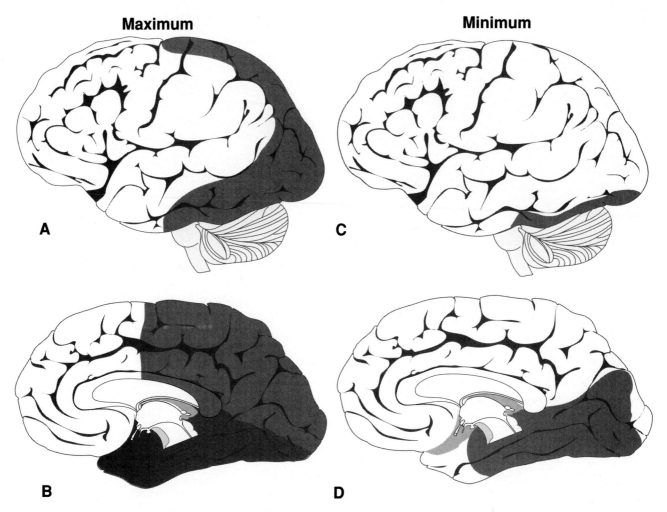

Figure 7.11. *Extremes of territorial distribution of the posterior cerebral artery.*   See text and Chapter 11 for discussion. Based on van der Zwan A, Hillen B, Tulleken CAF, et al. Variability of the territories of the major cerebral arteries. J Neurosurg 1992;77 927±940.

confined to only one of the vessels. The territorial boundaries in life will shift in response to changes in vessel perfusion. They are therefore considered to be dynamic rather than static phenomena.

REFERENCES

1. Willis T. Cerebri anatome; cui accessit nervorum descriptio et usus. London: J. Flesher, 1664.
2. Wildbrand H, Saenger A. Die Neurologie des Auges. 1915. Cited by Berson EC. Arch Ophthalmol 1966;76:52.
3. Saeki N, Rhoton AL. Microsurgical anatomy of the upper basilar artery and the posterior circle of Willis. J Neurosurg 1977; 46:563–578.
4. Alpers BJ, Berry RG. Circle of Willis in cerebral vascular disorders. The anatomical structure. Arch Neurol 1963;8:68–72.
5. Hassler O. Morphological studies on the large cerebral arteries with reference to the aetiology of subarachnoid hemorrhage. Acta Psychiat Neurol Scand 1961;36(Suppl. 154):5–145
6. Rhoton AL. Anatomy of saccular aneurysms. Surg Neurol 1980; 14:59–66.
7. Perlmutter D, Rhoton AL. Microsurgical anatomy of the anterior cerebral-anterior communicating-recurrent artery complex. J Neurosurg 1976;45: 259–272.
8. LeMay M, Gooding CA. The clinical significance of the azygous anterior cerebral artery. Am J Radiol 1966;98:602–610.
9. Nardi PV, Esposito S, Greco R, et al. Aneurysms of azygous anterior cerebral artery. Report of two cases treated surgically. J Neurosurg Sci 1990;34:17–20.
10. Nishio S, Matsushima T, Fukui M, et al. Microsurgical anatomy around the origin of the ophthalmic artery with reference to contralateral pterional surgical approach to the carotid-ophthalmic aneurysm. Acta Neurochir (Wien) 1985;76: 82–89.
11. Padget DH. The development of the cranial arteries in the human embryo. Contrib Embryol 1948;32:205–262.
12. Hillen B. The variability of the circulus arteriosus (Willisii): order or anarchy? Acta Anat 1987;129:74–80.
13. Hillen B, Hoogstraten HW, van Overbeeke JJ, et al. Functional anatomy of the circulus arteriosus cerebri (Willisii). Bulletin de l'Association des Anatomistes 1991;75:123–126.
14. Hillen B, Gassbeek T, Hoogstraten HW. A mathematical model of the flow in the posterior communicating artery. J Biomechanics 1982;15:441–448.
15. Hillen B. The variability of the circle of Willis: univariate and bivariate analysis. Acta Morphol 1986;24:87–101.
16. Riggs, HE, Rupp C. Variation in form of the circle of Willis. The relation of variations to collateral circulation: Anatomic analysis. Arch Neurol 1963;8:24–30.

17. Fisher CM. The circle of Willis: Anatomical variations. Vasc Dis 1965;2: 99–105.

18. Alpers BJ, Berry RG, Paddison RM. Anatomical studies of the circle of Willis in normal brains. Arch Neurol Psychiatr (Chicago) 1959;81:409–418.

19. Wollschlaeger G, Wollschlaeger PB: The circle of Willis. In: Newton TH, Potts DG, eds. Radiology of the Skull and Brain. St. Louis, CV Mosby, 1974;2:1171–1201.

20. Carpenter MB, Noback CR, Moss ML. The anterior choroidal artery. Its origins, course, distribution, and variations. Arch Neurol Psychiatr 1954;71:714–722.

21. Otomo E. The anterior choroidal artery. Arch Neurol 1965;13: 656–658.

22. Bisaria KK. Anomalies of the posterior communicating artery and their potential clinical significance. J Neurosurg 1984;60: 572–576.

23. Moyes PD. Basilar aneurysm associated with agenesis of the left internal carotid artery. J Neurosurg 1969;30:608–611.

24. Tangchai P, Khaoborisut V. Agenesis of the internal carotid artery associated with aneurysm of the contralateral middle cerebral artery. Neurology 1970;20: 809–812.

25. Takahashi M, Tamakawa Y, Kishikawa T, et al. Fenestration of the basilar artery. Report of 3 cases and review of the literature. Radiology 1973;109:79–82.

26. Sanders WP, Sorek PA, Mehta BA. Fenestration of intracranial arteries with special attention to associated aneurysms and other anomalies. Am J Neuroradiol 1993;14:675–680.

27. Wollschlaeger G, Wollschlaeger PB, Lucas FV, et al. Experience and result with postmortem cerebral angiography performed as routine procedure of the autopsy. Am J Radiol 1967;101: 68–87.

28. Hassler O. Morphological studies on the large cerebral arteries with reference to the aetiology of subarachnoid hemorrhage. Acta Psychiatr Neurol Scand 1961;36(Suppl. 154):5–145.

29. Ito J, Washiyama K, Hong Kim C, et al. Fenestrations of the anterior cerebral artery. Neuroradiology 1981;21:277–280.

30. Banach MJ, Flamm ES. Supraclinoid internal carotid artery fenestration with an associated aneurysm. Case report. J Neurosurg 1993;79:438–441.

31. Black SPW, Ansbacher LE. Saccular aneurysm associated with segmental duplication of the basilar artery. A morphological study. J Neurosurg 1984;61:1005–1008.

32. Finlay HM, Canham PB. The layered fabric of cerebral artery fenestrations. Stroke 1994;25:1799–1806.

33. Campos J, Fox AJ, Vinuela F, et al. Saccular aneurysms in basilar artery fenestration. Am J Neuroradiol 1987;8:233–236.

34. Graves VB, Strother CM, Weir B, et al. Vertebrobasilar junction aneurysms associated with fenestration: Treatment with Guglielmi Detachable coils. Am J Neuroradiol 1996;17:35–40.

35. Kowada M, Koichi Y, Takahashi H. Fenestration of the vertebral artery with a review of 23 cases in Japan. Radiology 1972;103: 343–346.

36. Andrews BT, Brant-Zawadzki M, Wilson CB. Variant aneurysms of the fenestrated basilar artery. Neurosurgery 1986;18: 204–207.

37. Miyazaki S, Kamat K, Yamaura A. Multiple aneurysms of the vertebrobasilar system associated with fenestration of the vertebral artery. Surg Neurol 1981;15:192–195.

38. Ito J, Washiyama K, Hong Kim C, et al. Fenestrations of the anterior cerebral artery. Neuroradiology 1981;21:277–280.

39. Baptista AG. Studies on arteries of brain. III Circle of Willis: Morphological features. Acta Neurol Scand 1964;40:398–414.

40. Teal JS, Rumbaugh CL, Bergeron RT, et al. Angiographic demonstration of fenestrations of the intradural intracranial arteries. Radiology 1973;106:123–126.

41. Ito J, Maeda H, Inoue K, et al. Fenestration of the middle cerebral artery. Neuroradiology 1977;13:37–39.

42. Killien FC, Wyler AR, Cromwell LD. Duplication of the interior carotid artery. Neuroradiology 1980;19:101–102.

43. Chess MA, Barsotti JB, Chang JK, et al. Duplication of the extracranial internal carotid artery. Am J Neuroradiol 1995;16: 1545–1547.

44. Hsegawa T, Kashihara K, Ito H, et al. Fenestration of the internal carotid artery. Surg Neurol 1985;23:391–395.

45. Koenigsberg RA, Zito JL, Patel M, et al. Fenestration of the internal carotid artery: a rare mass of the hypotympanum associated with persistence of the stapedial artery. Am J Neuroradiol 1995;16:908–910.

46. Zülch KJ. Über die Entstehung und Lokalisation der Hirninfarkte. Zentralblatt für Neurochirurgie 1961;21:158–180.

47. Heubner O. Die luetischen Erkrankungen der Hirnarterien. Liepzig: FCW Vogel Verlag, 170–214, 1874.

48. van der Zwan A, Hillen B. Review of the variability of the territories of the major cerebral arteries. Stroke 1991;22:1078–1084.

49. van der Zwan A, Hillen B, Tulleken CAF, et al Variability of the territories of the major cerebral arteries. J Neurosurg 1992; 77:927–940.

50. Van der Zwan A, Hillen B, Tulleken CAF, Dujovny M. A quantitative investigation of the variability of the major cerebral arterial territories. Stroke 1993;24:1951–1959.

CHAPTER 8

The Internal Carotid Artery

The common carotid artery usually bifurcates at the C3–C4 level into an external carotid artery trunk and an internal carotid artery. The bifurcation may be lower, occasionally being seen as low as T2–T3, although such extremes are rare (1). Most carotid angiograms are performed on older patients in whom the possibility of atherosclerotic change demands an evaluation of the bifurcation before catheterization of the internal carotid artery (Fig. 8.1). There are other situations in which it is prudent or imperative to perform an angiogram of the common carotid bifurcation before further catheterization or wire-manipulation (Table 8.1). Some of these are obvious and include questions related to the cervical internal carotid artery itself, e.g., dissection, pseudoaneurysm, tumor involvement, etc. Others are less obvious but encompass any situation in which the final interpretation of the angiogram might be seriously compromised by the presence of a minimal amount of cervical carotid spasm induced by the wire, e.g., evaluation of subtle tumor encasement or traumatic injury (Figs. 8.2, 8.3, 8.4, 8.5).

ANATOMY OF THE INTERNAL CAROTID ARTERY

The anatomy of the internal carotid artery is described in segments between the common carotid bifurcation in the neck and the supraclinoid internal carotid bifurcation. In ascending order, these consist broadly of the cervical, petrous, precavernous, cavernous, paraclinoid, and supraclinoid segments (Fig. 8.6). Various numbering and descriptive schemes for the internal carotid artery have been canvassed (2–8). Some schemes number only the intracranial segments of the internal carotid artery, some the entire course. Other schemes number with the direction of flow, more against the direction of flow. Therefore, when one hears, for instance, the "C5 segment" or "C4 branches of the internal carotid artery " mentioned in angiographic discussions, it can be difficult to find an elucidative reference.

The scheme most commonly used in clinical argot in reference to the cavernous internal carotid artery is that of Fischer from 1938 (3), which numbers the segments of the intracranial internal carotid artery from top down, 1 to 5, *against* the direction of blood-flow. This scheme, with its accompanying enumeration of the intracranial cerebral vessels, was devised as a descriptive lexicon primarily for analysis of intracranial mass-effect. Fischer's enumeration schemes (3) of the anterior, middle, and posterior cerebral arteries, which follow *with* the direc-

tion of blood-flow in these vessels, are still commonly used.

To allow for the subtleties of internal carotid artery aneurysm location and surgical techniques, a large number of descriptive anatomic terms has come into use. The names used in these schemes are not necessarily always synonymous, which can make reading on this subject difficult. To encompass the babel of nomenclature and numbers for the segments of the internal carotid artery, Bouthillier et al. (2) described seven segments that will be used as an outline for the following description.

Cervical Segment

This segment spans the common carotid bifurcation to the skull base. At the base of the skull, the internal carotid artery lies anteromedial to the internal jugular vein with which it shares a neurovascular sheath. This sheath also encloses the IXth, Xth, XIth, and XIIth cranial nerves and post-ganglionic sympathetic fibers. The pharyngeal wall lies directly anteromedial to the carotid artery. Instrumentation or biopsy of Rosenmuller's fossa carries a risk of internal carotid injury. Such injuries are also more likely in the setting of unsuspected pharyngeal loops of the internal carotid artery, particularly where these loops have a more medial or directly submucosal course. Parapharyngeal infections may involve the wall of the carotid artery at this level with a risk of pseudoaneurysm formation. At the exocranial ostium of the carotid canal, the carotid sheath splits into two layers. The inner layer becomes the periosteum of the carotid canal, the outer becomes the exocranial periosteum.

The cervical segment usually does not have any branches, except where unusual anatomic variants are encountered (Table 8.2).

Petrous Segment and Laceral Segment

The petrous segment of the internal carotid artery consists of a vertical and a horizontal portion. It enters the skull base at the exocranial opening of the carotid canal, ascends approximately 1 cm, and then turns anteromedially until it enters the intracranial space at the foramen lacerum. The laceral segment is a continuation of the petrous segment ending at the petro-lingual ligament (2, 10). The artery is accompanied along its course by the sympathetic fibers of the stellate ganglion and by a venous plexus (11, 12). Some of the sympathetic fibers part company from

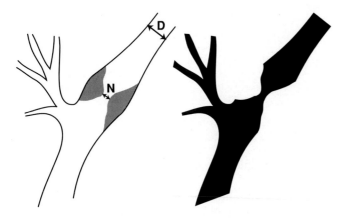

Carotid stenosis % = (1 - $^{N}/_{D}$) x 100

Figure 8.1. *Measurement of carotid artery stenosis.* The formula for calculation of the percentage stenosis of the internal carotid artery is illustrated. In situations of advanced stenosis the distal diameter of ``normal'' vessel, D, is attenuated or underopacified, leading to an underestimation of the percentage stenosis.

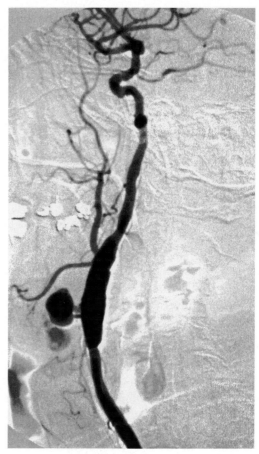

Figure 8.2. *Anastomotic breakdown in a left carotid graft.* A jet of contrast directed anteriorly fills a multilobulated pseudoaneurysm, which presented as a pulsatile mass.

the internal carotid artery at the foramen lacerum and form the deep petrosal nerve. The deep petrosal nerve joins the parasympathetic fibers of the greater superficial petrosal nerve to become the Vidian nerve. This nerve travels anteriorly to the pterygo-palatine fossa via the Vidian (pterygoid) canal. It is unusual in the absence of pathologic conditions to see branches of the petrous segment of the internal carotid artery.

CAROTICOTYMPANIC BRANCH OF THE PETROUS INTERNAL CAROTID ARTERY

This branch of the petrous internal carotid artery is usually too small to see or is obscured by dense petrous bone. It is a vestige of the course of the hyoid artery. Apart from its role as a vestigial remnant in understanding vascular anomalies of the middle ear, the importance of the caroticotympanic artery lies in its potential supply to vascular tumors of the middle ear.

Table 8.1
Clinical Situations in which to Consider a Common Carotid Bifurcation Angiogram Before or Instead of More Selective Injections

Atherosclerotic disease
Dissection (Fig. 8.4)
Pseudoaneurysm (Figs. 8.3, 8.5)
Tumor involvement
Trauma or recent surgery in which external carotid injury is suspected (Fig. 8.5)
Recent carotid angiogram by another radiologist, i.e., avoid catheterizing a vessel in which an undocumented and unsuspected dissection is present
History of endarterectomy

MANDIBULO-VIDIAN BRANCH OF THE PETROUS INTERNAL CAROTID ARTERY

This artery is usually too small to see, but may enlarge quickly in the setting of occlusive disease (see Figs. 3.4, 8.9). It is rare to see this artery in adults. When seen, it is usually in children with a vascular mass of the nasopharynx, e.g., juvenile angiofibroma. It has an origin from the horizontal portion of the petrous carotid artery. The Vidian branch is described as more horizontal and medial than the inferolateral direction of the mandibular branch. The Vidian artery has a straight course along the skull base, anastomosing with branches of the internal maxillary artery anteriorly (13).

Table 8.2
Variant Branches of the Cervical Internal Carotid Artery (9)

Ascending pharyngeal artery or pharyngeal trunk of the ascending pharyngeal artery
Superior thyroidal artery
Occipital artery
Posterior meningeal artery
Persistent hypoglossal artery
Proatlantal intersegmental artery type I
Persistent stapedial artery (Fig. 8.7)

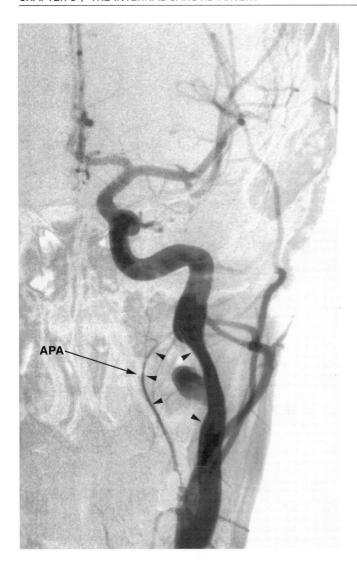

Figure 8.3. *Pseudoaneurysm of the internal carotid artery.* Frontal view of a left common carotid artery injection. A pseudoaneurysm of the left internal carotid artery is associated with surrounding mass-effect (arrowheads) due to unopacified hematoma. The course of the ascending pharyngeal artery is bowed medially (APA) around the aneurysm. In the absence of angiographic evidence of dissection, etiologies to consider include penetrating trauma or parapharyngeal infection.

Cavernous Segment

From the foramen lacerum, the internal carotid artery ascends vertically and medially to the sella where it turns anteriorly within the structures of the cavernous sinus. Anteriorly, the carotid artery makes a 180 turn, pierces the proximal dural ring at the level of the anterior clinoid process, and becomes the clinoidal segment. The level of tortuosity of the carotid artery in this region is variable. Children have a straighter course than adults. In older patients, redundant superimposed loops present problems from the point of view of catheterization, visualization of anatomy of aneurysms, and arterial injury during transphenoidal surgery.

Branches of the juxtasellar internal carotid artery are frequently seen with modern digital technology and may become enlarged in the presence of collateral flow or pathologic conditions (Fig. 8.10). These branches are among the most important for consideration during external carotid artery embolization. They constitute a dangerous system of anastomoses between the external carotid and internal carotid artery systems. Therefore, whether

they are seen on an initial angiogram, embolization is always done with the cautious assumption that they are present.

BRANCHES OF THE CAVERNOUS INTERNAL CAROTID ARTERY

Posterior Bend (Fischer C5) Branches of the Cavernous Internal Carotid Artery

These branches may arise as a common trunk, the meningohypophyseal trunk, or as separate vessels termed the C5 branches (Figs. 8.10, 8.11, 8.12, 8.13). The most consistently present branches from this site are the inferior hypophyseal artery, the marginal and basal tentorial branches, and the dorsal meningeal (lateral clival) branch (14) (Fig. 8.11).

Tentorial Arteries of the Internal Carotid Artery

The marginal artery of the tentorium, regardless of its many possible sites of origin, is sometimes referred to eponymously as the artery of Bernasconi and Cassinari (15)

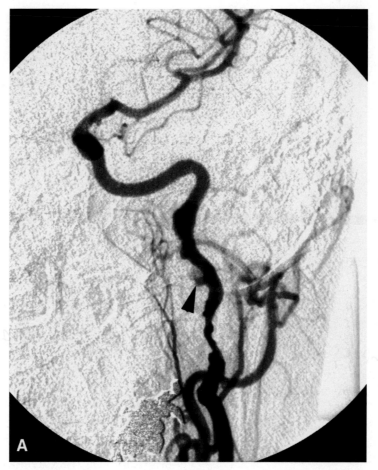

Figure 8.4. *Dissecting pseudoaneurysms of the internal carotid artery.* **(A)** A middle-aged female with angiographic and clinical evidence of deterioration in a left internal carotid artery dissection, even with adequate anticoagulation. A left common carotid artery injection demonstrates irregular attenuation of the artery with pseudoaneurysm or pouch formation at the skull base **(arrowhead)**. Significant other observations on this image include the absence of collateral flow through the circle of Willis. The marginal degree of collateral flow was confirmed on injections of the other cerebral vessels. The patient was advised to undergo a bypass procedure to the left hemisphere, to be followed by endovascular occlusion of the left internal carotid artery.

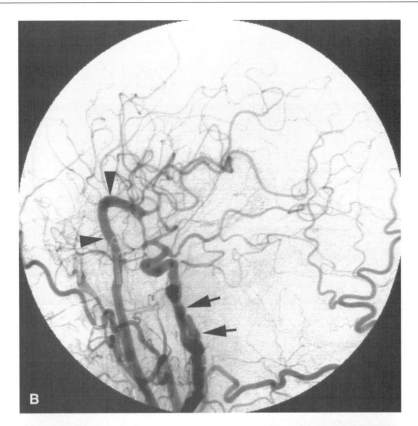

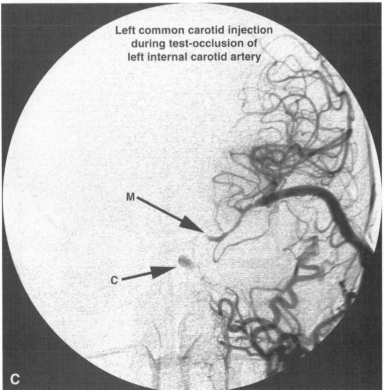

Figure 8.4. *(continued)* **(B)** A left common carotid artery injection, lateral projection, after a venous graft bypass **(arrowheads)** from the left external carotid artery to the left middle cerebral artery. The complex architecture of the pseudoaneurysms can be seen on this oblique projection **(arrows)**. **(C)** A frontal projection of a left common carotid artery injection made proximal to an occluding test-balloon placed proximally in the left internal carotid artery. Reconstitution of the left cavernous internal carotid artery **(C)** via collaterals from the external carotid artery is seen. The M1 segment of the left middle cerebral artery (M) opacifies retrogradely from the anastomotic site.

(Fig. 8.12). The marginal artery of the tentorium runs posteriorly along the free (medial) margin. It therefore ascends and approaches the midline as it progresses posteriorly. It is frequently enlarged in the presence of vascular tumors of the tentorium or other states, such as when involved with a dural arteriovenous malformation. It may occasionally be seen in the normal state.

In contrast, the basal tentorial artery does not ascend in the same manner, but rather diverges laterally along the course of the tentorial insertion on the petrous ridge. Along the petrous ridge and sigmoid sinus it has anastomoses with the middle meningeal artery and dural arteries of the posterior fossa.

Posteroinferior Hypophyseal Artery of the Cavernous Segment

The posteroinferior hypophyseal artery is directed medially from the cavernous segment. It supplies the neurohypophysis and peripheral adenohypophysis of the pituitary gland. It anastomoses with the superior hypophyseal arteries (from the supraclinoid segment), with the capsular arteries of McConnell, and with its contralateral fellow (Figs.

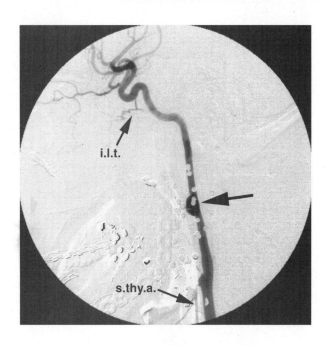

Figure 8.5. *Post-traumatic pseudoaneurysm of the left internal carotid artery.* A young adult underwent emergency embolization of the left external carotid artery following a shotgun blast to the face and neck. The external carotid artery distal to the origin of the superior thyroidal artery (s.thy.a.) is occluded. There is enlargement of the ipsilateral inferolateral trunk (i.l.t.) from the cavernous internal carotid artery, which is participating in collateral flow to the territory of the occluded external carotid artery. On this follow-up angiogram 10 days after the initial embolization, a developing pseudoaneurysm of the cervical internal carotid artery is identified **(arrow)**. In the setting of a lesion such as this, a vital item of surgical interest is the distance from the pseudoaneurysm to the skull-base. This has a large bearing on the difficulty of surgical repair.

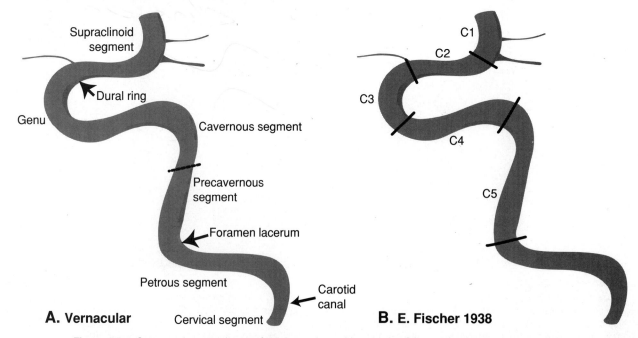

A. Vernacular

B. E. Fischer 1938

Figure 8.6. *Segmental nomenclature of the internal carotid artery.* See text for details. A degree of latitude exists between references on where exactly the internal carotid artery enters the cavernous sinus. The postero-inferior boundaries of the cavernous sinus are variable and difficult to define.

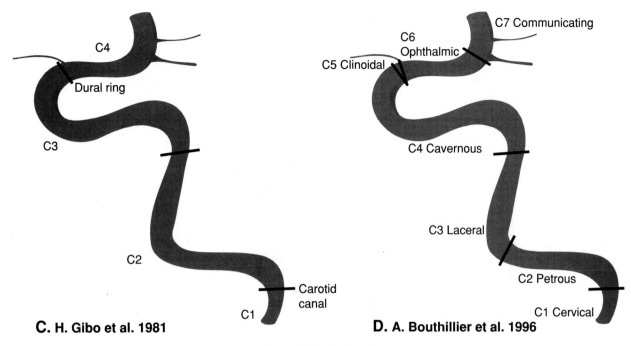

C. H. Gibo et al. 1981

D. A. Bouthillier et al. 1996

Figure 8.6. *(continued)*

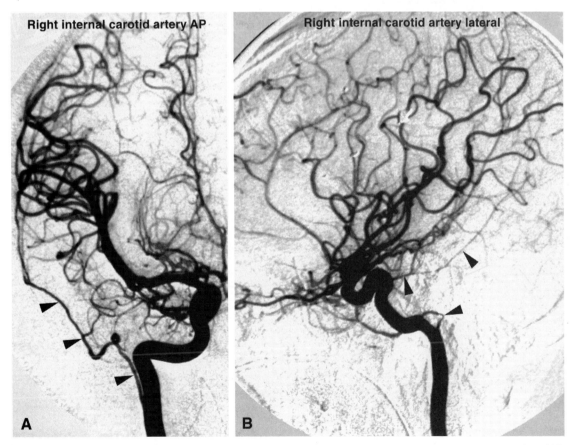

Figure 8.7. *Persistent stapedial artery variant.* An AP and lateral view of the right internal carotid artery in a young adult undergoing angiography because of penetrating injury by metallic fragments after a gun-shot wound. Notice the displacement of the anterior cerebral artery by hematoma on the AP view and artifact from fragments on the lateral view. An unusual vessel **(arrowheads)** arises from the high cervical internal carotid artery and becomes the middle meningeal artery intracranially. The lateral aspect is redolent of the curve evident when the inferior tympanic artery reforms the petrous internal carotid artery in cases of an aberrant internal carotid artery. This particular variant has, therefore, been termed the ``pharyngotympanostapedial'' artery.

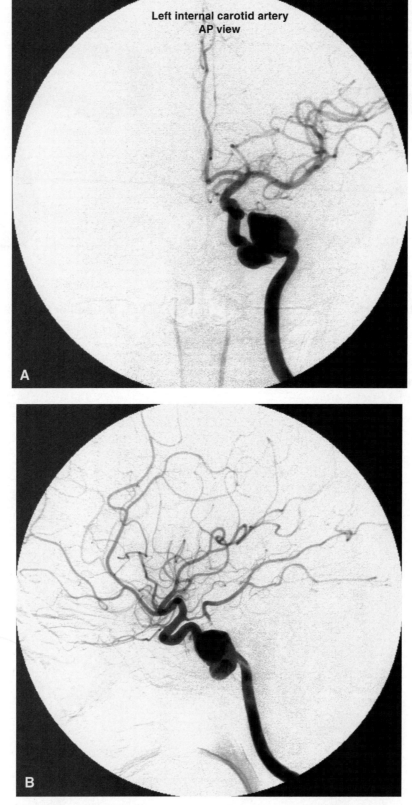

Figure 8.8. *Aneurysms of the petrous internal carotid artery.* **(A, B)** A young adult presented with symptoms of intolerable headache and left V nerve irritation. A lobulated aneurysm of the left petrous internal carotid artery was exercising considerable mass-effect in the left middle cranial fossa. Previous skull trauma or petrous apicitis might be considered as possible etiologies for aneurysms in this location. A small posterior communicating artery is present **(B)**, but the anterior communicating artery was small or absent **(A)**. This demonstrates a need for a surgical bypass procedure before endovascular occlusion of the left internal carotid artery. The complex nature of the aneurysm (better seen on A) presented considerable difficulties during balloon navigation, but the internal carotid artery was finally occluded at the cavernous segment.

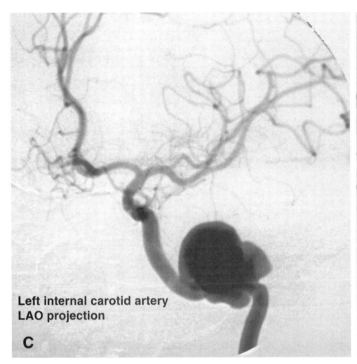

**Left internal carotid artery
LAO projection**

C

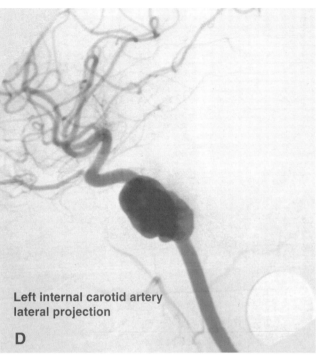

**Left internal carotid artery
lateral projection**

D

Figure 8.8. *(continued)* **(C, D)** A young adult female presented with throbbing headache worsening over months. A complex aneurysm of the left petrous internal carotid artery was discovered. This patient tolerated a test-occlusion of the left internal carotid artery due to the presence of a robust anterior communicating artery. However, balloon navigation of the complex lobulations of the aneurysm proved impossible, and occlusion was performed proximal to the aneurysm.

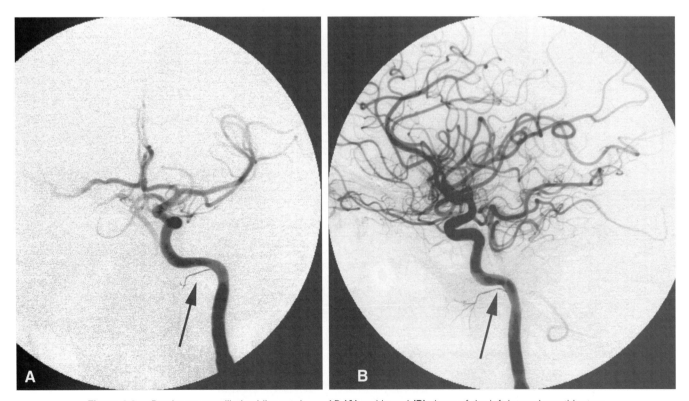

A

B

Figure 8.9. *Persistent mandibulo-vidian trunk.* AP **(A)** and lateral **(B)** views of the left internal carotid artery in a child with a juvenile angiofibroma. An unusual branch of the petrous internal carotid artery (arrows) represents a persistent mandibular or mandibulovidian artery.

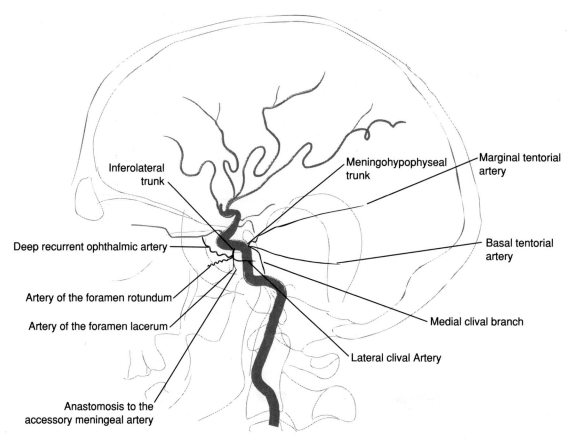

Inferolateral trunk

Meningohypophyseal trunk

Marginal tentorial artery

Deep recurrent ophthalmic artery

Basal tentorial artery

Artery of the foramen rotundum

Artery of the foramen lacerum

Medial clival branch

Lateral clival Artery

Anastomosis to the accessory meningeal artery

Figure 8.10. Angiographically visible branches of the cavernous internal carotid artery.

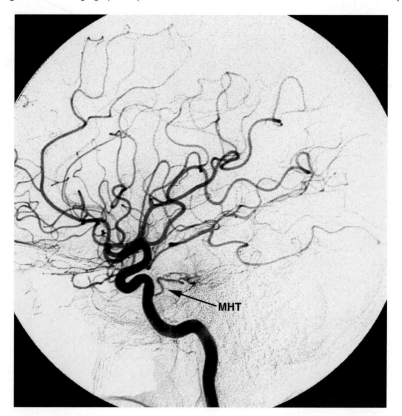

MHT

Figure 8.11. Meningohypophyseal trunk of the internal carotid artery. A lateral projection of the left internal carotid artery in a 60-year-old female with a large meningioma of the tentorium and petrous region. Part of the vascular supply to the tumor derives from the meningohypophyseal trunk (MHT), which supplies the tumor via the lateral clival branch.

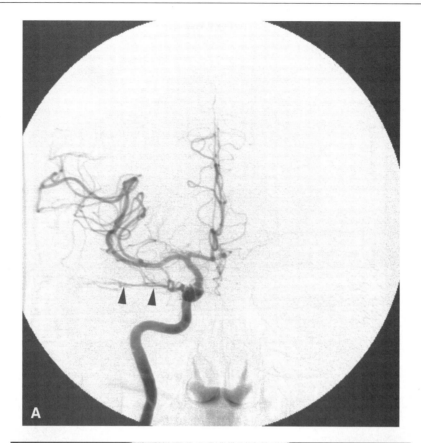

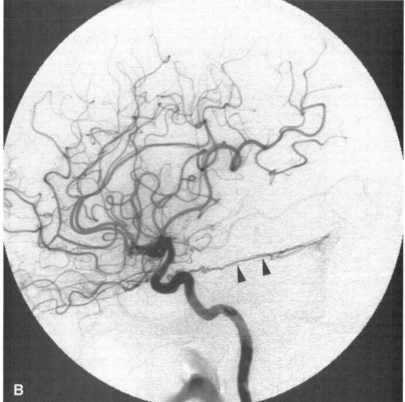

Figure 8.12. *Basal and marginal tentorial arteries.* **(A, B)** Basal tentorial artery. PA view and lateral views of the right internal carotid artery in a patient with a symptomatic dural arteriovenous malformation in the region of the right sigmoid and transverse sinuses. The basal tentorial artery **(arrowheads)** extends laterally and horizontally along the petrous ridge. This could be confirmed by looking at the course of the artery on a non-subtracted image.

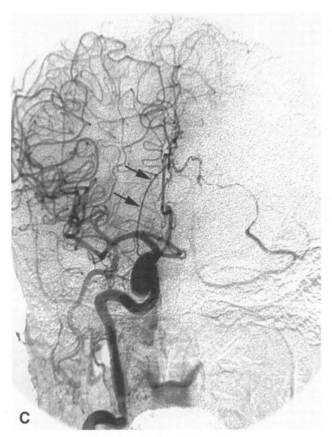

C

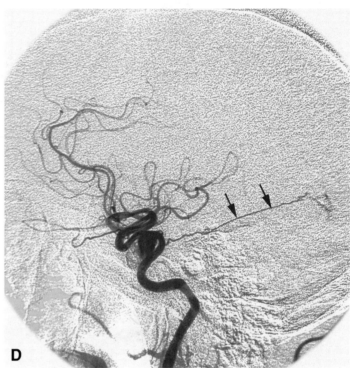

D

Figure 8.12. *(continued)* **(C, D)** Marginal tentorial artery. PA and lateral views of the right internal carotid artery in a different patient being studied for symptoms related to a cavernous internal carotid artery aneurysm. An incidental dural arteriovenous malformation of the tent-orial margin is present. The marginal tentorial artery **(arrows)** follows the tentorial incisura posteriorly and superiorly. Compare with the course of the basal tentorial artery in **A** and **B**.

8.13, 8.14). These branches cause a characteristic early neurohypophyseal blush on carotid angiography. The posteroinferior hypophyseal artery also gives a medial clival branch, which runs near the midline along the clivus to meet the ascending clival branch from the hypoglossal artery (a branch of the neuromeningeal trunk deriving from the ascending pharyngeal artery). This connection explains the occasional visualization of the pituitary blush on ascending pharyngeal artery injections.

Lateral Clival Artery of the Cavernous Segment

The lateral clival artery gives lateral and infero-medial branches along the course of the superior and inferior petrosal sinuses, respectively (Fig. 8.11). The lateral branch of the lateral clival artery thus becomes an anastomosing tributary to the arterial supply of the basal tentorial system. Frequent tributaries in this area with which it may anastomose include the middle meningeal artery and the jugular branch of the ascending pharyngeal artery.

The medial branch of the lateral clival artery, sometimes called the dorsal clival artery (16), passes below Gruber's petroclinoid ligament in Dorello's canal with the VIth nerve. It anastomoses inferiorly with the jugular branch of the neuromeningeal trunk.

Recurrent Artery of the Foramen Lacerum

The recurrent artery of the foramen lacerum may arise from the Fischer C5 branches, but is more commonly associated with the inferolateral trunk. The importance of this vessel lies in its anastomosis in the foramen lacerum with the carotid branch of the superior pharyngeal branch of the ascending pharyngeal artery.

Other C5 Branches of the Internal Carotid Artery

Arterial supply to the trigeminal ganglion from the internal carotid artery may be through specific Fischer C5 branches or through the inferolateral trunk from Fischer C4.

A major vessel seen in less than 1% of the population arising from the Fischer C5 segment of the internal carotid artery is a persistent trigeminal artery. It is most easily recognized on the lateral view, where it is directed posteriorly. The relationship between the site of origin of the meningohypophyseal trunk and the trigeminal artery is disputed. Cases in which the two share a common origin or in which they are distinct have been reported. In the latter instance, the trigeminal artery runs on a plane between that of the meningohypophyseal trunk above and the abducens nerve below (17).

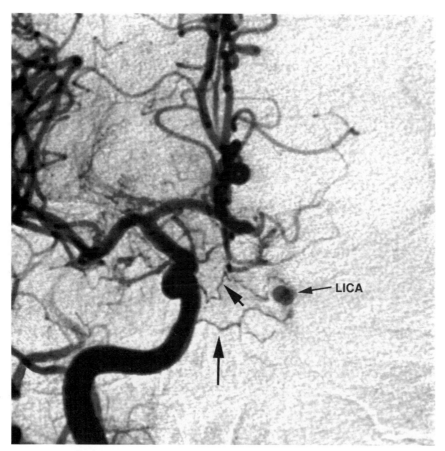

Figure 8.13. *Reconstitution of the left internal carotid artery.* A PA view of a right common carotid artery injection in the setting of occlusive disease of the left internal carotid artery. Early reconstitution of the cavernous left internal carotid artery (lica) is demonstrated. Small collateral vessels (arrows) cross the midline through the sella (inferior hypophyseal arteries) and along the clivus (clival branches from the internal carotid artery and ascending pharyngeal artery).

Horizontal Segment (Fischer C4) Branches of the Cavernous Internal Carotid Artery

Two major groups of arteries are seen in this location. Anteriorly, a number of medially directed microscopic vessels, the capsular arteries of McConnell, supply the periphery of the adenohypophysis and adjacent dura. They can be seen during microsurgical dissection, but are too small to see during angiography.

More posteriorly, a laterally directed group of vessels or a single inferolateral trunk is seen.

CAPSULAR ARTERIES

The anterior group of vessels, McConnell's capsular arteries, from the cavernous segment of the internal carotid artery supplies the inferior and peripheral aspect of the adenohypophysis and adjacent dura of the diaphragm sellae. The bulk of afferent vascular supply to the adenohypophysis is, however, through portal venous channels from the infundibulum and hypothalamus. This accounts for the delayed pituitary blush in the adenohypophysis in the venous phase of an internal carotid artery angiogram. The periphery of the adenohypophysis has vascular supply in addition to that from the portal vessels. These peripheral sources include the capsular arteries, the inferior hypophyseal artery, and the interlobar or middle hypophyseal branches of the superior hypophyseal trunk. These vessels form a capsular arterial rete along the sellar floor (18, 19).

The capsular arteries in the normal state are rarely if ever seen during angiography. However, they may represent one possible site of cavernous internal carotid artery aneurysm formation. Medially directed aneurysms in this location can occupy the sella and are thought to represent a more serious variant of cavernous aneurysms. Their rupture into the sella can penetrate the diaphragm sellae and cause subarachnoid hemorrhage (Fig. 8.15). For this reason, treatment of cavernous aneurysms directed medially into the sella is sometimes recommended even if the patient is asymptomatic. Sella-occupying aneurysms may also cause hypopituitarism as the presenting clinical problem.

INFEROLATERAL TRUNK

The inferolateral trunk (20), sometimes referred to as the artery of the inferior cavernous sinus (14), is the remnant of the embryonic dorsal ophthalmic artery. It is present in more than 80% of microsurgical dissections (21) (Figs. 8.5, 8.10, 8.16). It arises in the mid-portion of the horizon-

Figure 8.14. Agenesis of internal carotid artery with reconstitution via a transsellar anastomosis. Rare cases of unilateral carotid agenesis have been reported. In some of these cases, as illustrated, a large anastomotic bridge between the cavernous carotid arteries has been thought to represent a persistent primitive maxillary artery, the embryologic precursor of the inferior hypophyseal artery.

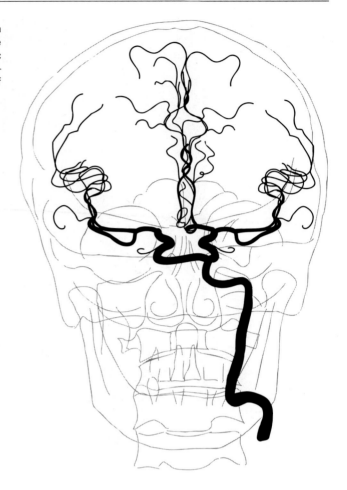

tal cavernous carotid artery, on the lateral aspect of the C4 portion (Fischer Classification), and is directed inferiorly. A branching pattern into three to four divisions is commonly seen.

The most proximal branch is directed posteriorly along the course of the IVth nerve to become part of the vascular supply to the tentorium. The marginal artery of the tentorium may arise from this location.

A branch to the superior orbital fissure is directed anteriorly from the proximal segment of the inferolateral trunk. This branch represents the vestige of the primitive dorsal ophthalmic artery. It meets the deep recurrent ophthalmic branch from the ophthalmic artery, forming an important anastomosis between the ophthalmic artery and the inferolateral trunk.

The inferolateral trunk is then directed laterally over the trochlear nerve and under the ophthalmic division of the trigeminal nerve. It provides an important branch to the foramen rotundum supplying the maxillary division of the trigeminal nerve.

Another branch extends to the region of the foramen ovale to anastomose with the accessory meningeal artery. It contributes to the supply of the gasserian ganglion and the lower two divisions of V (21). When the inferolateral trunk is absent, its territories may be taken over by smaller individual branches of the internal carotid artery,

branches from the meningohypophyseal trunk, or by the accessory meningeal artery.

The recurrent artery of the foramen lacerum is commonly a branch of the inferolateral trunk. It anastomoses through the cartilage of the foramen lacerum with the carotid branch of the superior pharyngeal branch of the ascending pharyngeal artery.

Angiographically the most constantly seen of these branches is the artery of the foramen rotundum directed anteriorly to anastomose with the internal maxillary artery. The artery of the foramen rotundum consistently has a characteristic tortuous and near horizontal appearance, which allows ready recognition on the lateral view. The persistent vestige of the dorsal ophthalmic artery, which enters the orbit via the superior orbital fissure, is sometimes called the deep recurrent ophthalmic artery. It supplies the corresponding segment of the ophthalmic division of V. Very rarely, the dorsal ophthalmic artery may persist beyond embryonic life and be the dominant arterial supply to the orbit (Fig. 8.16). When a dual ophthalmic artery supply to the orbit is present (Fig. 8.17), variations in the pattern of anastomosis between the two arteries may be seen, including the possibility of a complete or partial arterial ring around the optic nerve (22).

Alternatively, the arterial connection through the superior orbital fissure may be enlarged to assume a dominant

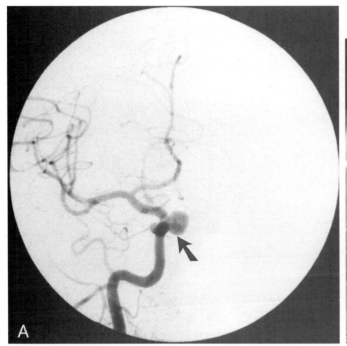

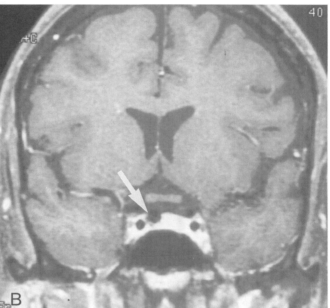

Figure 8.15. *Intrasellar aneurysm from the cavernous internal carotid artery.* A PA angiographic view **(A)** of a right internal carotid artery injection in a middle-aged female with multiple aneurysms. A medially directed aneurysm from the cavernous internal carotid artery is present **(arrow)**. Aneurysms in this location are thought to correspond with the hypophyseal or capsular branches. The intrasellar location was con-firmed on a coronal T1-weighted, gadolinium enhanced MRI study **(B)**. Although this particular aneurysm was asymptomatic, endovascular treatment was recommended. Intrasellar aneurysms that rupture can leak into the subarachnoid space causing significantly greater morbidity than rupture of cavernous aneurysms in other positions.

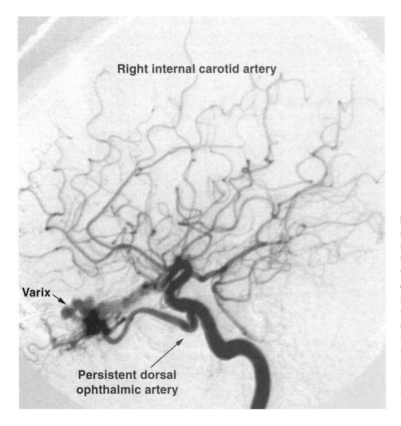

Figure 8.16. *Persistent dorsal ophthalmic artery.* A persistent primitive dorsal ophthalmic artery is present in this middle-aged female who presented with headaches related to a dural arteriovenous malformation of the anterior cranial fossa. The origin of this unusual vessel from the horizontal cavernous internal carotid artery corresponds with that of the inferolateral trunk. Most commonly the dorsal ophthalmic artery regresses to become an anastomotic twig, the deep recurrent ophthalmic artery, between the ophthalmic artery and the inferolateral trunk. Dural arteriovenous malformations of the anterior cranial fossa in this location are typically supplied by ethmoidal branches of the ophthalmic arteries. Because of a propensity for subarachnoid or cortical venous drainage, they are thought to have a high risk of becoming complicated early by subarachnoid hemorrhage.

Figure 8.17. *Dual ophthalmic artery.* Unusual persistence of dual ophthalmic supply from the internal carotid artery to the orbit is seen in association with an aneurysm of the cavernous horizontal segment. The ventral ophthalmic artery (arrowheads) arises from the usual paraclinoidal location; the dorsal ophthalmic artery (arrow) is larger and has a cavernous origin.

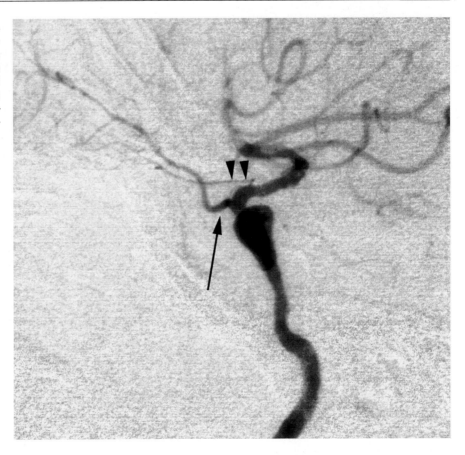

role of supply to the marginal artery of the tentorium, flowing from the ophthalmic artery. The marginal artery of the tentorium may arise from the inferolateral trunk, the middle meningeal artery, the accessory meningeal artery, the internal carotid artery, or the ophthalmic artery.

The arterial system of the inferolateral trunk can be understood as a vascular network in the paracavernous dura. It connects the middle meningeal artery, accessory meningeal artery, internal carotid artery, ophthalmic artery, marginal tentorial artery, and ascending pharyngeal artery. Dominance of one particular vessel can lead to unusual anatomic variants, such as supply of the marginal tentorial artery from the middle meningeal artery. More importantly, the presence of this network is a concern during embolization, lest dangerous anastomoses in this region should open.

Cavernous Carotid Aneurysms

Aneurysms of the cavernous segment of the internal carotid artery account for approximately 5% of intracranial aneurysms and are more likely to be detected in female patients. Idiopathic aneurysms in this location have a strong association with hypertension and advancing age, whereas post-traumatic aneurysms or pseudoaneurysms may be seen in any age-group. Approximately 50% of cavernous aneurysms occur anteriorly adjacent to the carotid genu, and 16% can be giant aneurysms, i.e. 2.5 cm in diameter (23, 24). Most cavernous aneurysms seen during

angiography are incidental, asymptomatic lesions that usually warrant no further evaluation or treatment (25) (Fig. 8.18). Symptoms may develop due to compression of adjacent structures causing cranial nerve deficits, headache, embolic events, or aneurysmal rupture.

Aneurysms close to the genu and the optic nerve frequently present with retro-orbital headache and visual symptoms of blurring or field-deficits. Aneurysms of the horizontal cavernous segment are more likely to affect the VIth, IIIrd, and IVth nerves. There is some debate about whether cranial nerve ischemia, rather than compression by mass-effect, may play a role in the etiology of the cranial neuropathies associated with cavernous aneurysms. However, mass-effect seems to be the most likely explanation.

When cavernous aneurysms rupture, which is an uncommon event, symptoms are related to carotid-cavernous fistula (26), massive epistaxis (27), and subdural (28) or subarachnoid hemorrhage (29, 30). Most spontaneous direct carotid-cavernous fistulas are thought to be related to rupture of a cavernous aneurysm into the surrounding venous structures. The risks of sub-arachnoid hemorrhage are greatest with anterior aneurysms at the genu. Anterior aneurysms may breach the dural ring and expand superiorly into the subarachnoid space. Medially directed aneurysms from the horizontal segment are also thought to represent a risk of subarachnoid hemorrhage if they have an intrasellar location.

Treatment for cavernous aneurysms is indicated for in-

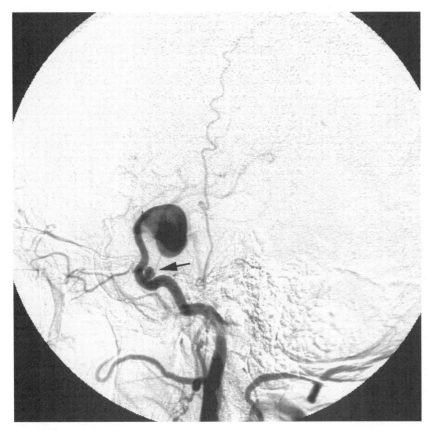

Figure 8.18. *Incidental cavernous aneurysm.* During the course of evaluation of this giant supraclinoid carotid aneurysm, an incidental cavernous aneurysm (arrow) is identified. It lies well below the dural ring and is unlikely to be clinically significant. There is pronounced mass-effect surrounding the larger, supraclinoid aneurysm due to a large quantity of unopacified circumferential thrombus within the periphery of the aneurysm.

tolerable symptoms. They can be approached through surgical or endovascular means, depending on the nature of the presentation and the location of the aneurysm. Endovascular treatment with coil occlusion of the aneurysm can be undertaken if there is a strong indication or preference for preservation of the internal carotid artery. Balloon occlusion of the internal carotid artery with "trapping" of the aneurysm may be undertaken when adequate collateral circulation has been demonstrated. This technique is particularly effective in emergency situations with life-threatening epistaxis from a rent in the internal carotid artery. Endovascular balloon occlusion of a carotid-cavernous fistula can usually preserve the internal carotid artery.

For asymptomatic cavernous aneurysms, treatment is advocated when a risk of subarachnoid bleeding is present, if the aneurysm were to rupture, i.e. aneurysms of the genu encroaching on the dural ring or intrasellar aneurysms (24).

CLINOIDAL SEGMENT

The clinoidal segment of the internal carotid artery is a short wedge-shaped area of the artery between the proximal and distal dural rings. Some authors refer to the lateral aspect of this ring as the clinoidal segment and to the medial aspect as the carotid cave. Aneurysms on the lateral aspect of this segment are extracavernous and, strictly speaking, extradural. However, because of the difficulty in precisely defining the dural margin on angiographic

images, aneurysms in this location are treated with a great deal of caution, as if they were sub-arachnoid. Some authors use the term "carotid cave" for specific reference to subarachnoid aneurysms on the medial aspect of the internal carotid artery in this region. Medial to the carotid genu a redundant fold of dura insinuates itself between the artery laterally and the carotid sulcus of the sphenoid bone medially.

OPHTHALMIC SEGMENT

The ophthalmic segment extends from the distal dural ring to the origin of the posterior communicating artery, thus including the territory referred to as supraclinoidal in some references. There are two major branches of the ophthalmic segment: the ophthalmic artery and the superior hypophyseal artery.

Ophthalmic Artery

EMBRYOLOGY OF THE OPHTHALMIC ARTERY

As described by Padget (13), the ophthalmic artery has two major sources of embryological derivation.

The primitive ventral ophthalmic artery originates from the primitive anterior cerebral artery. By a process of proximal migration, or sequential anastomoses with proximal regression, it assumes a position on the paraclinoid internal carotid artery typically associated with the usual origin of the ophthalmic artery.

The primitive dorsal ophthalmic artery, on the other hand, arises from the primitive internal carotid artery in a location which, in adult life, is typically associated with that of the inferolateral trunk.

Within the orbit, best seen at the 20-mm stage of development, the dorsal and ventral ophthalmic arteries form an embryonic anastomotic ring surrounding the proximal segment of the optic nerve. The dorsal ophthalmic artery usually regresses, and its territory is subsumed by the ventral ophthalmic artery. The anastomotic ring between the ventral ophthalmic artery and dorsal ophthalmic artery undergoes a partial regression, but its form can still be discerned in the intraorbital course of the ophthalmic artery as it spirals around the optic nerve in adults. Rare cases of persistence of a complete vascular ring surrounding the optic nerve are occasionally seen in adulthood.

Typical Course and Configuration of the Ophthalmic Artery

In more than 90% of surgical and anatomic dissections, the ophthalmic artery takes origin from the antero-medial or, less commonly, the superior surface of the internal carotid artery immediately after the latter penetrates the dural ring adjacent to the anterior clinoid process. Thus its proximal stem forms a useful angiographic landmark for the position of the dura. The ophthalmic artery courses antero-laterally from its origin, and again it pierces the dura to enter the optic canal where it occupies a position inferior or inferolateral to the optic nerve. Within the optic canal, the ophthalmic artery lies external to the optic nerve sheath, the latter being an extension of the dural layers. Occasionally, the ophthalmic artery may occupy its own transosseous canal, which may run parallel to or may join the optic canal. Such variant osseous canals may be seen particularly when the ophthalmic artery has a cavernous or extradural origin from the anterior genu of the internal carotid artery. Hayreh and Dass (31) described an 8% incidence of cavernous origin of the ophthalmic artery, a figure supported by other dissection studies but not so frequently observable in angiographic examinations (Figs. 8.16, 8.17, 8.19).

After entering the orbit, the ophthalmic artery approaches that segment representing what was once the embryonic vascular ring surrounding the optic nerve. From the inferior and lateral aspect of the optic nerve, the ophthalmic artery curves around the nerve with an angle that resembles, on the lateral projection, an upturned Civil War bayonet. The central retinal artery is given off at this point and continues anteriorly along the course of the optic nerve. The ophthalmic artery curves from lateral to medial over the optic nerve in approximately 85% of dissections, and under the optic nerve in the remainder (31–33) (Fig. 8.20).

Branches of the Ophthalmic Artery

The named branches of the ophthalmic artery (34) are listed in Table 8.3. They can be simplified into two broad groups, medial and lateral, in addition to the central retinal artery and posterior ciliary arteries (up to five).

Figure 8.19. *Cavernous origin of the ophthalmic artery.* The arrowhead indicates the cavernous origin of this ophthalmic artery. Occasionally a tortuous ophthalmic artery arising from its usual paraclinoidal location may overlap the genu and simulate this appearance.

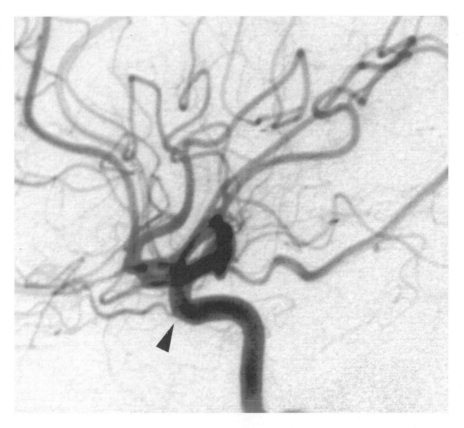

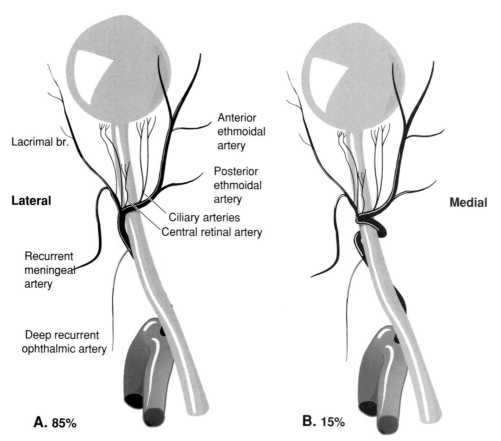

Figure 8.20. *Course of the left ophthalmic artery: superior view.* Seen from above, the ophthalmic artery courses under the optic nerve external to the optic nerve sheath. In 85% of the population, the ophthalmic artery curves around the lateral aspect of the nerve to swing medially over the nerve **(A)**. In 15%, the artery courses under the nerve and curves to the upper aspect of the optic nerve along the medial side **(B)**. Based on Hayreh SS, Dass R. The ophthalmic artery II. Intraorbital course. Br J Ophthalmol 1962;46;165±185.

The central retinal artery is usually the first important intraorbital branch of the ophthalmic artery, given off in close association with the lateral and posterior ciliary arteries. It is directed anteriorly along the optic nerve to the eye (31, 33). As the ophthalmic artery then spirals around the optic nerve, the laterally directed lacrimal branch is most commonly given. However, the order of branching varies and depends in part on the relation between the artery and nerve.

The lacrimal branch (lateral division) of the ophthalmic artery is directed primarily to the lacrimal gland and the related structures. Being lateral in disposition within the orbit, and thus close to the superior orbital fissure, it can be remembered as the branch of the ophthalmic artery that anastomoses most prominently with, or can be supplied preferentially by, the middle meningeal artery (Fig. 8.21). Anteriorly, the lacrimal branch has prominent anastomoses with the zygomatico-orbital branch of the superficial temporal artery.

The larger division of the ophthalmic artery is directed medially towards its termination where it bifurcates into the dorsal nasal artery and supratrochlear artery. Among its most important branches along this route, from an angiographic perspective, are the anterior and posterior ethmoidal branches.

The anterior and posterior ethmoidal arteries supply part of the dura of the anterior cranial fossa by perforating the cribriform plate. They are prominently enlarged in vascular tumors or dural arteriovenous malformations of this region (Fig. 8.22). They also supply the mucosa of the superior nasal septum, and, therefore, can have promi-

Table 8.3
Branches of the Ophthalmic Artery

Ocular group
  Central retinal
  Medial posterior ciliary
  Lateral posterior ciliary
  Anterior ciliary
Orbital group
  Lacrimal
  Muscular
  Periosteal
Extraorbital group
  Anterior ethmoidal, giving the anterior artery of the falx cerebri
  Posterior ethmoidal
  Supraorbital
  Medial palpebral
  Dorsal nasal
  Supratrochlear
  Dural

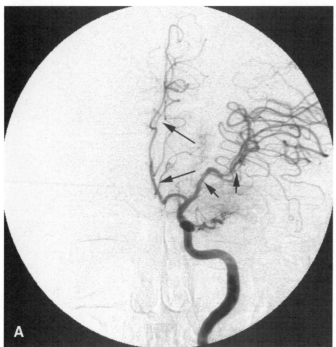

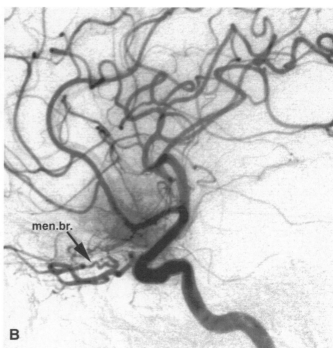

Figure 8.21. *Sphenoid wing meningioma.* A late middle-age female with a symptomatic large left sphenoid wing meningioma. On the PA view **(A)**, there is marked mass-effect on the course of the middle cerebral artery **(small arrows)** and shift of the anterior cerebral artery **(long arrows)**. On the lateral view **(B)**, a characteristic blush of the meningioma is seen on the internal carotid artery injection. The predominant supply to the tumor is via the recurrent meningeal branch of the ophthalmic artery (men.br.) reaching the tumor via the superior orbital fissure.

Figure 8.22. *Ethmoidal and dural branches of the ophthalmic artery.* A large meningioma of the anterior cranial fossa displaces the anterior cerebral arteries posteriorly and superiorly **(small arrows)**. It derives supply from the ethmoidal branches of the ophthalmic artery **(long arrow)** via the cribriform plate. The anterior artery of the falx cerebri is also enlarged **(arrowhead)**.

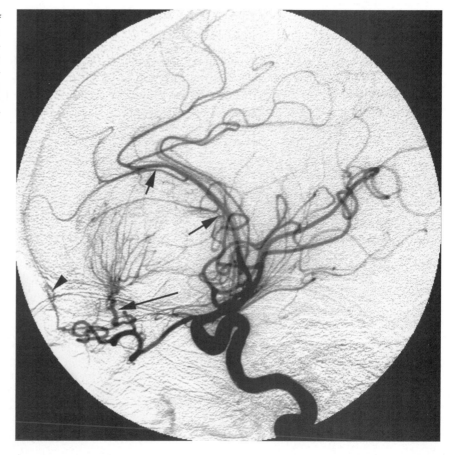

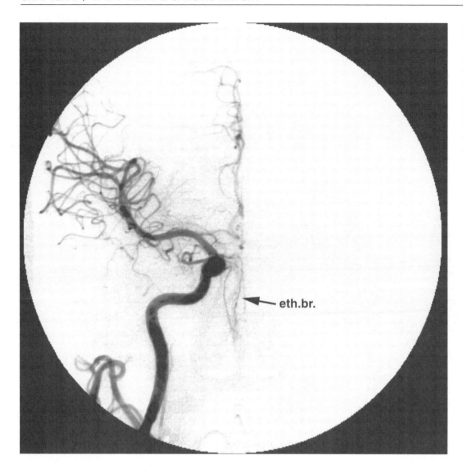

Figure 8.23. *Ethmoidal branches of the ophthalmic artery.* Unusually prominent ethmoidal branches (eth.br.) of the ophthalmic artery are seen on this right internal carotid artery injection. These vessels have large anastomoses along the nasal septum with the long sphenopalatine arteries. Therefore a route of potential hazard to the ophthalmic artery exists through these vessels during embolization of the internal maxillary artery and its branches.

nent anastomoses with the long sphenopalatine branches of the internal maxillary artery (Fig. 8.23). This route along the nasal septum constitutes an anastomotic peril to the ophthalmic artery during embolization of the internal maxillary artery. The anterior ethmoidal artery gives origin to the anterior artery of the falx cerebri, which gains the intracranial space via the foramen cecum. It supplies the anterior portion of the falx cerebri in the midline, in balance with the peripheral territory of the middle meningeal arteries.

Angiographically, many of the remaining named branches of the ophthalmic artery are difficult to identify in the absence of pathologic states. To avoid potential confusion, remember that on the lateral view of an internal carotid artery angiogram, the orbitofrontal branches of the anterior cerebral artery frequently project inferiorly in reference to the distal branches of the ophthalmic artery. This relates to the manner in which the orbital roof bows up into the anterior cranial fossa on each side, while the olfactory sulcus, gyrus rectus, and related medial structures occupy a more caudad position.

Dural Supply from the Ophthalmic Artery

Dural supply from the ophthalmic artery is seen frequently in the setting of meningiomas or other vascular states involving the intracranial space contiguous to the orbit. The ethmoidal branches, the artery of the falx cerebri, the re-

current meningeal artery (to the middle meningeal artery), and deep recurrent ophthalmic artery (to the inferolateral trunk) may be prominently involved by tumors or vascular malformations of the anterior cranial fossa, sphenoid wings, or cavernous sinus. The ophthalmic artery may be one of the sites of origin for the marginal tentorial artery. The proximal ophthalmic artery may therefore be prominent in dural vascular disease of the cerebellar tentorium or of the posterior fossa (Fig. 18.3).

The gravity of inadvertent occlusion of the central retinal artery usually precludes the possibility of direct embolization of these vessels, unless circumstances are extenuating or the eye is already blind.

Choroidal Blush

The choroidal plexus of the eye is supplied by the ciliary branches of the ophthalmic artery. It is evident on lateral projections as a thin, dense crescent. It may remain visible for a few seconds. It is a useful indicator of orbital supply. If it is not seen on an internal carotid artery injection, variant supply from an external carotid source to the orbit can be suspected. Deformity of the choroidal blush may be seen in the presence of intraorbital tumors. Abnormal or absent blush may also be an indirect sign of elevated intraorbital or intraocular pressure. The absence of a choroidal blush on a particular injection, however, does not eliminate the possibility of dangerous anastomoses.

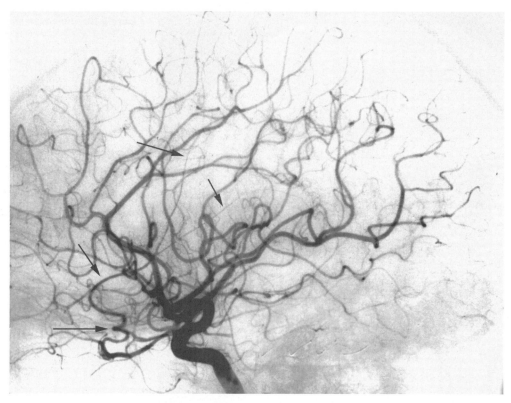

Figure 8.24. Origin of the middle meningeal artery from the ophthalmic artery. It can be easy to overlook this variant due to the multiple overlapping vessels seen on a lateral view. However, the manner in which the relatively straight course of the middle meningeal artery and its branches (arrows) cross the intracranial vessels without joining should catch the eye. This is an example of how vessels that are in different planes cross one another on an angiographic projection without communicating. The course of the middle meningeal artery is buckled at the level of the lowest arrow where it describes a recurrent course through the superior orbital fissure.

Developmental Variations of Orbital Vascular Supply

Anastomotic connections between the ophthalmic artery and the external carotid artery are important for understanding the risks involved in embolization procedures. The central retinal artery is effectively a terminal vessel, inadvertent embolization of which carries little hope for collateralization. Therefore, the utmost care is needed in embolization procedures that involve the collateral relations of the ophthalmic artery to avoid the complication of central retinal artery occlusion and blindness.

Some of the anastomotic relations of the ophthalmic artery are vestiges of embryonic configurations that may occasionally persist into adulthood as anatomic variants.

Middle Meningeal Artery Supply to the Orbit

The middle meningeal artery may have a variable intraorbital territory deriving from the embryologic supraorbital ramus of the hyoid artery. Most commonly, the middle meningeal artery has a small anastomosis, the recurrent meningeal artery, with the lacrimal branch of the ophthalmic artery. This anastomosis enters the orbit via the superior orbital fissure or the foramen of Hyrtl. Occasionally, the lacrimal branch of the ophthalmic artery may be hypo-plastic or absent, and the predominant supply to the territory of the lacrimal artery will be from the middle meningeal artery (see Fig. 5.5A). More rarely, an extensive intraorbital territory is subsumed by the middle meningeal artery that may become the predominant or only source of supply to the ophthalmic territory (see Fig. 5.5B). The degree of this potential state should be evaluated carefully on all external carotid artery angiograms before embolization in the middle meningeal artery territory. The appearance of the choroidal blush on external carotid artery injections is an immediate indicator of the presence of a prominent anastomotic or variant state, but it may not necessarily always be seen.

The converse relationship between the ophthalmic artery and the middle meningeal artery, whereby the ophthalmic artery is the principal source for the middle meningeal artery, may also be seen in approximately 1% of angiograms (35) (see Figs. 5.5E, 8.24).

Origin of the Ophthalmic Artery from the Anterior Cerebral Artery

Rare persistence of the primitive ventral ophthalmic artery is thought to explain the possibility of origin of the ophthalmic artery from the anterior cerebral artery in adulthood (36) (see Fig. 5.5H).

SUPERIOR HYPOPHYSEAL ARTERIES

The superior hypophyseal arteries are the most consistent branches of the supraclinoid segment of the internal carotid artery. They measure 100–500 m in diameter and arise medially or inferomedially between the ophthalmic artery and the posterior communicating artery. They may arise as a single trunk or be up to five in number (4, 21, 37). When present as a single trunk, the artery courses posterosuperiorly towards the pituitary stalk where it divides into several branches. Branches to the upper infundibulum anastomose with branches from the contralateral superior hypophyseal arteries and from the posterior communicating arteries to form a circuminfundibular anastomosis. Some of these branches continue superiorly and supply the hypothalamic structures adjacent to the floor of the third ventricle. Other branches include a recurrent anterior branch along the optic nerve, branches to the inferior part of the optic chiasm, and inferiorly directed branches to the diaphragm sellae and pituitary gland. The branch(es) to the optic nerve may be the dominant vascular supply to the intradural segment of the optic nerve, implying that care must be taken to preserve this artery during resection of sellar and suprasellar tumors.

The optic chiasm, on the other hand, typically has vascular supply from many sources, in addition to that from the superior hypophyseal artery. These include the anterior communicating artery, posterior communicating artery, and basilar artery. A bitemporal visual field-cut seen with superiorly directed pituitary tumors may be due to compromise of the superior hypophyseal artery supply to the lower aspect of the optic chiasm rather than to mechanical compression of the chiasm (38), although this is disputed.

Aneurysms of the supraclinoid internal carotid artery that are directed medially are usually considered to be hemodynamically related to the superior hypophyseal arteries. It is thought that aneurysms in this location are somewhat more likely to bleed at a smaller diameter than subarachnoid aneurysms of a similar size in other locations. Patients with aneurysms in this location may be more prone than other patients to have aneurysms in multiple sites, particularly of the contralateral subarachnoid internal carotid artery, cavernous internal carotid artery, and posterior communicating artery. Superior hypophyseal aneurysms project medially in two patterns. They may extend due medially inferior to the optic chiasm and simulate a suprasellar mass (Fig. 8.25). Alternatively, superior hypophyseal aneurysms may extend inferiorly underneath the anterior clinoid process. In this position, they may be misinterpreted as paraclinoid in location or even as carotico-ophthalmic (39).

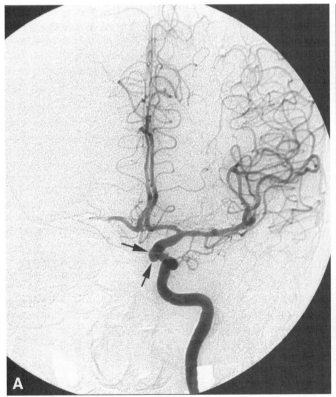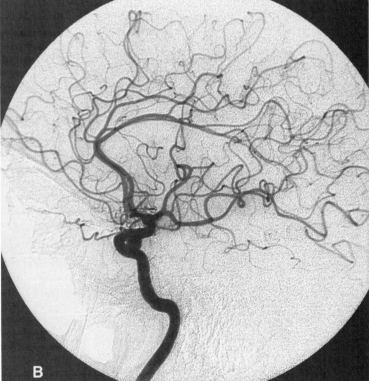

Figure 8.25. *Superior hypophyseal aneurysm.* Aneurysms projecting medially from the supraclinoid internal carotid artery **(A)** distal to the ophthalmic artery and proximal to the posterior communicating artery are most commonly described as being hemodynamically related to the superior hypophyseal arteries. On the lateral view **(B)**, the origin of this particular aneurysm is easy to discern, although the dome overlaps with the horizontal segment of the cavernous internal carotid artery. When such aneurysms enlarge, the precise site of origin can be difficult to clarify. Superior hypophyseal aneurysms may extend proximally and mimic paraclinoidal aneurysms.

Aneurysms of the supraclinoid internal carotid artery at sites other than those related to the origins of identifiable vessels may occur also (40). These are frequently along the anterior (dorsal) or dorsolateral wall of the internal carotid artery, and have been termed "dorsal wall aneurysms" (41).

COMMUNICATING SEGMENT

The communicating segment of the internal carotid artery extends from the posterior communicating artery origin to the internal carotid artery bifurcation. In addition to the posterior communicating artery, it gives rise to the anterior choroidal artery and occasional perforator branches.

PARACLINOID, CAROTID CAVE, AND CAROTID-OPHTHALMIC ANEURYSMS

The high degree of inter-individual variation and complex anatomic relationships under the anterior clinoid process make the region of the carotid genu difficult to evaluate angiographically and surgically. Aneurysms related to the anterior clinoid process account for approximately 1–5% of intracranial aneurysms (42). The principal angiographic question in this region is to discern between intradural and extradural aneurysms. This will direct decisions of management between conservative observation for an asymptomatic cavernous lesion and definitive treatment for a subarachnoid aneurysm. Frequently, a deal of uncertainty over the precise location and risk of a particular aneurysm is unavoidable. When surgical clipping is contemplated, the precise definition of the site of origin of the aneurysm in reference to the anterior clinoidal process is extremely helpful to the surgeon. This helps to plan the extent of bone resection and the approach needed for exposure of the aneurysm.

Anatomy of the Paraclinoid Group of Aneurysms

As the carotid artery makes its 180 posterior turn at the anterior genu of the siphon, it leaves the cavernous space. It makes a short extra-cavernous and extra-dural transition, and then enters the intradural (subarachnoid) space. It immediately gives off the ophthalmic artery from its superomedial (71%) or superior curve (29%) under the optic nerve (43).

The origin of the ophthalmic artery is covered from direct sight laterally by the anterior clinoid process, which lies superolaterally relative to the genu of the internal carotid artery. Dural coverage of this area is extended medially to the tuberculum sellae by a dural shelf from the anterior clinoid process called the *falciform fold*. The optic nerve lies under the falciform fold separating this dural fold above from the vascular structures lying below. As the internal carotid artery curves posteriorly, it cuts a variably

prominent groove in the lateral aspect of the sphenoid body, called the *sulcus caroticus*. The bony rims of the sulcus caroticus can be slight in form or very prominent. When prominent, the posterior tip of the lower rim may be identifiable as the middle clinoid process. Dense fibrous ligaments between the anterior, middle, and posterior clinoid processes are among the difficulties involved in resecting the anterior clinoid process at surgery, while trying to avoid damage to the internal carotid artery or the aneurysm.

Fibrous ligaments between the anterior and posterior clinoid processes may ossify, creating the common interclinoid foramen of Gruber (44). This foramen may be further divided by ossified ligaments connecting the anterior and middle clinoid processes. When the ligaments between the anterior and middle clinoid processes becomes ossified, the internal carotid artery becomes enclosed within an anomalous bony canal, the *clino-carotid foramen* or *anterior interclinoid canal*. The *posterior interclinoid canal* then encircles the venous structures of the cavernous sinus. Variations of these foramina may be present in complete or partial form in up to 40% of skulls (19, 45). These variations can compound the difficulty of surgically exposing aneurysms in this area.

With the anterior clinoid process and related dura removed, the penetration of the dura by the internal carotid artery, known as the *dural ring* is better seen. However, this ring lies on a plane askance that of the artery. The dural ring is more dense and more tightly adherent superolaterally. It slopes inferiorly and medially across the artery so that more of the medial and posterior aspects of internal carotid genu are exposed to the subarachnoid space. In this medial site, the adherence of the dura to the internal carotid artery is less well defined, and a particular fold of redundant dura medial to the artery projects towards the cavernous sinus. Therefore, a subarachnoid space or potential space exists between the medial wall of the carotid artery and the bony wall of the carotid sulcus. This space is termed the *carotid cave* (39, 46). Its importance is that it represents a site of subarachnoid aneurysm formation. Aneurysms in this medial location off the genu may breach the dura to project inferiorly into the cavernous sinus and cause further confusion as to location and origin (see Fig. 16.20). These aneurysms are also difficult to expose and to clip surgically due to the tight bony space and the overlying optic nerve and ophthalmic artery.

The medially located carotid cave is distinguished by some authors from the laterally situated clinoidal space or segment. The latter is a surgical term for the extracavernous, extradural segment of carotid artery exposed by resection of the anterior clinoid process, the lateral rim of the optic canal, and the dural ring. This dissection is limited inferiorly by the cavernous sinus and inferolaterally by the paracavernous cranial nerves.

Aneurysms of the internal carotid artery that arise on the side of the artery opposite to that of the ophthalmic

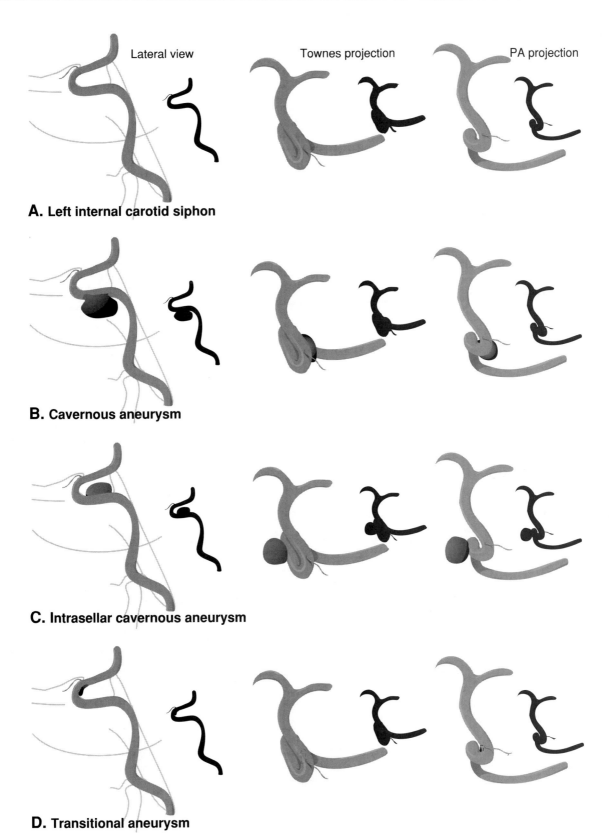

Lateral view   Townes projection   PA projection

A. Left internal carotid siphon

B. Cavernous aneurysm

C. Intrasellar cavernous aneurysm

D. Transitional aneurysm

Figure 8.26. *Paraclinoid internal carotid artery aneurysms.* Aneurysms of the left carotid siphon and paraclinoidal region are illustrated with angiographic silhouettes of each illustration in Townes and PA projection. Where the carotid siphon is markedly tortuous and the an-eurysm large, it can be extremely difficult to define the neck of the aneurysm. This calls for inventiveness in one's projections. Refer to Figures 2.39, 2.41, 2.42.

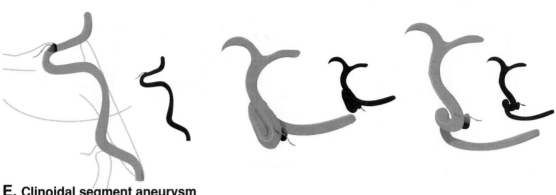

E. Clinoidal segment aneurysm

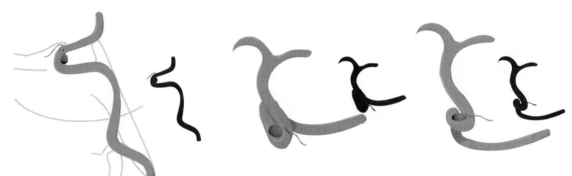

F. Carotid cave aneurysm

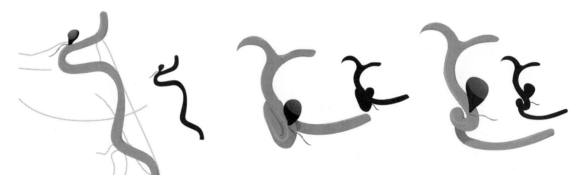

G. Carotid-ophthalmic aneurysm

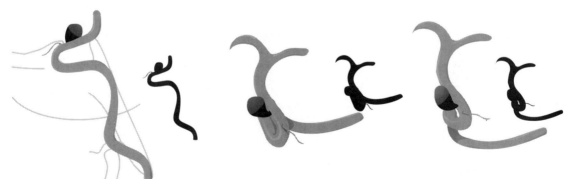

H. Superior hypophyseal aneurysm

Figure 8.26.   *(continued)*

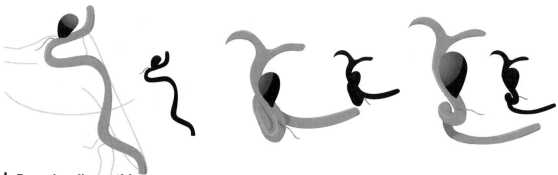

I. Dorsal wall carotid aneurysm

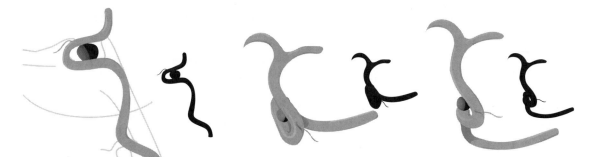

J. Ventral paraclinoid aneurysm

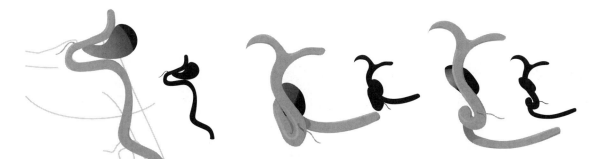

K. Ventral paraclinoid aneurysm

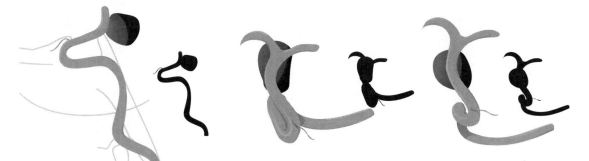

L. Posterior communicating aneurysm

Figure 8.26. *(continued)*

artery have been termed *paraclinoid* or *ventral wall* aneurysms (47). The term "paraclinoid" is frequently used more liberally to refer to a variety of aneurysms close to the anterior clinoid process.

Paraclinoid Aneurysms: Subtypes

Various descriptive terms have been mooted for subarachnoid aneurysms that occur near the anterior clinoid process based on the precise anatomic location of their origin. The general term paraclinoid has been used collectively by some to describe this entire group of aneurysms (48, 49) including those related to the ophthalmic artery (Figs. 8.18, 8.26, 8.27, 8.28, 8.29, 8.30, 8.31). Others reserve this term for ventral paraclinoid aneurysms distal to the ophthalmic artery and not clearly related to the superior hypophyseal artery (47). In proximal to distal order, the nomenclature of subarachnoid aneurysms in this area is as follows:

1. *Transitional aneurysms* (50) are those that arise from the carotid genu outside the dural ring, but which manage to insinuate themselves through the ring and into the subarachnoid space. Occasionally a waist-like constriction due to the stretched dura can be seen on the contour of these aneurysms as they extend superiorly. More than 50% of symptomatic patients with such aneurysms present with subarachnoid hemorrhage, underscoring the need to manage unruptured aneurysms in this location definitively. Other patients present with retro-orbital pain, headache, visual field deficits, and cranial nerve palsies. Contrast en-

hanced coronal MRI images are sometimes useful in evaluating aneurysms of the genu for determining the integrity of the dura.

2. *Carotid cave aneurysms,* sometimes used synonymously with the term *clinoidal segment aneurysms,* are those that arise just as the internal carotid artery enters the dural ring (39, 46, 51, 52). From their origin, these aneurysms tend to extend superiorly. Medial "cave" aneurysms are difficult to access. Laterally projecting clinoidal segment aneurysms may have eroded and become adherent to the clinoid process making bone-resection hazardous (48, 52).

3. *Carotid-ophthalmic aneurysms* (53) arise in close relationship to the ophthalmic artery ostium and usually project superiorly. They displace the optic nerve superiorly and medially against the dural falciform fold. When these aneurysms enlarge beyond 10 mm in diameter, a high incidence (30%) of loss of visual acuity or of visual field defects is seen.

4. *Posterior carotid wall* or *ventral paraclinoid aneurysms* project downward (posteriorly) or a little medially from the artery and tend to splay the genu apart (47, 54). They present significant surgical difficulties as they frequently have a broad atherosclerotic neck that hampers clip-placement. At surgery, they tend to be hidden by the optic nerve, anterior clinoid process, and internal carotid artery. They frequently extend proximally into the cavernous sinus, or are tightly adherent to the dura of the cavernous sinus at surgery (55).

5. *Superior hypophyseal aneurysms* are named for their hemodynamic and anatomic relation to the superior hypophyseal artery origin. They are located along the medial aspect

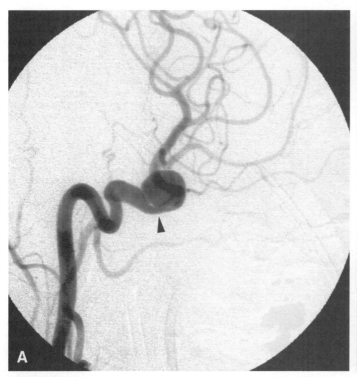
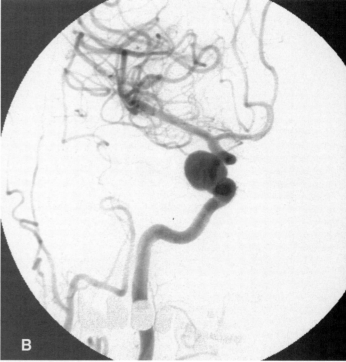

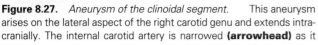

Figure 8.27. *Aneurysm of the clinoidal segment.*   This aneurysm arises on the lateral aspect of the right carotid genu and extends intracranially. The internal carotid artery is narrowed **(arrowhead)** as it approaches the neck of the aneurysm. The importance of varying the window levels at the console to understand the anatomy of an aneurysm such as this is clear.

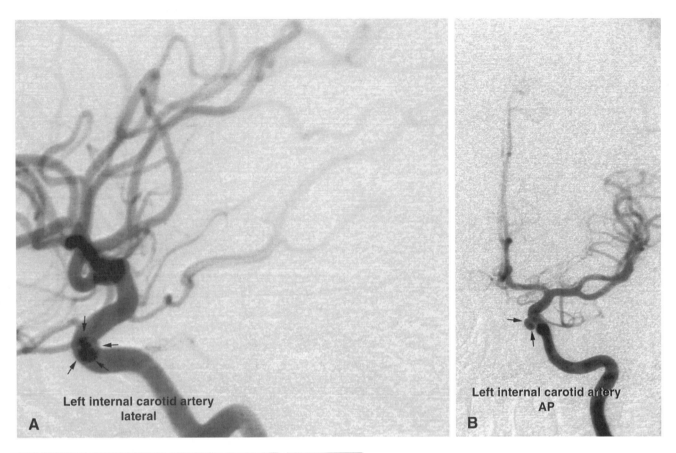

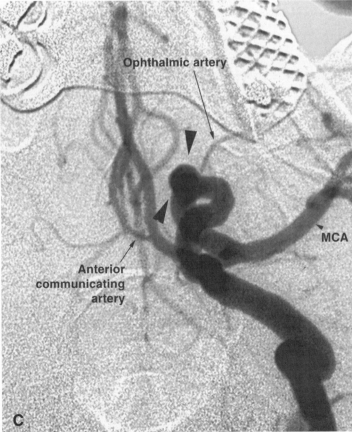

Figure 8.28. *Aneurysms of the carotid "cave."* Lateral **(A)** and PA **(B)** views of a small medially projecting aneurysm **(arrows)** proximal to the origin of the ophthalmic artery. The status of aneurysms in this location can be difficult to ascertain due to the variable anatomy of the dura along the medial aspect of the artery (see text). A base-view of the left internal carotid artery in a different patient **(C)** demonstrates an aneurysm **(arrowheads)** of a similar location.

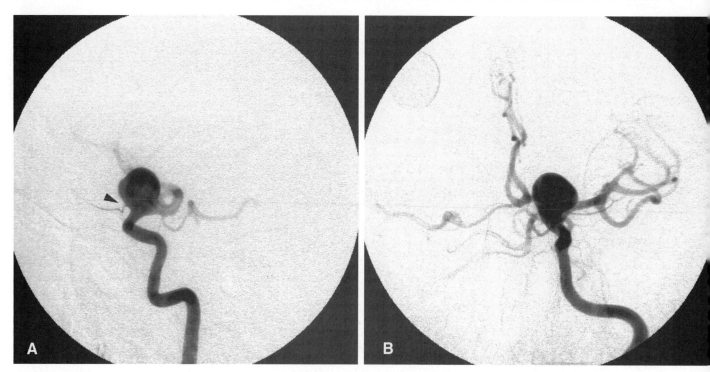

Figure 8.29. *Carotid-ophthalmic aneurysm I.* A wide-necked aneurysm of the supraclinoidal segment of the internal carotid artery from the base of which arises the ophthalmic artery **(arrowhead)**. This aneurysm might be described as carotid-ophthalmic, supraclinoidal, or related to the ophthalmic segment, depending on various literature references.

Figure 8.30. Carotid-ophthalmic aneurysm II. A 7-mm aneurysm (arrowhead) projects superiorly from the area of the ophthalmic artery in a patient with multiple aneurysms. A second aneurysm (arrow) is identified at the junction of the P1 and P2 segments of the posterior cerebral artery. In this particular patient, this was a very useful image, because the patient had a complex multilobulated basilar artery tip aneurysm, which was difficult to discern from the P1-P2 aneurysm on other views of the posterior fossa. This underscores the need to review all runs at the console rather than relying on printed images selected by the technologist. Ancillary information of a critical nature may be available on only one image of a run.

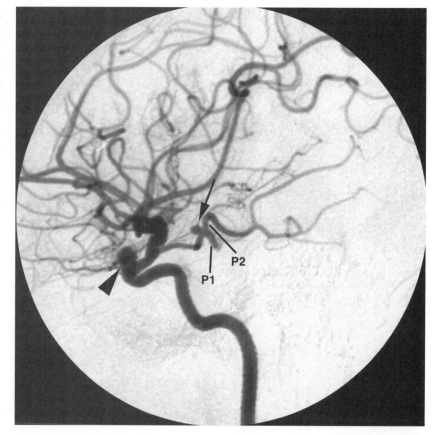

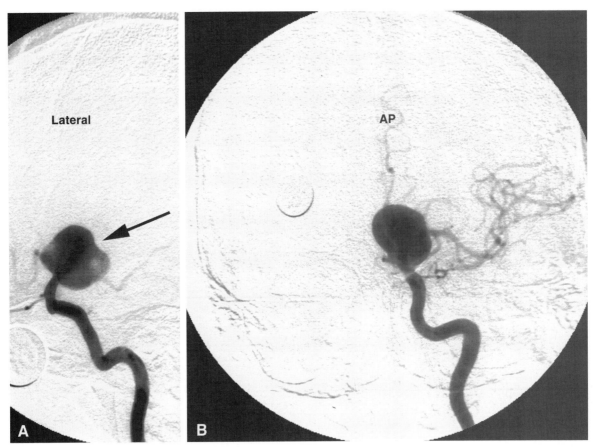

Figure 8.31. *Posterior wall aneurysm.* Aneurysms of the supra-clinoid carotid artery that are not related to the posterior communicating artery and arise from the posterior wall of the artery are termed "posterior wall" or "ventral paraclinoid" aneurysms. On the lateral view **(A)** an indentation **(arrow)** on the posterior surface of the aneurysm probably represents the effect of compression against the optic chiasm. Optic nerve stretching with visual symptoms is common with aneurysms of this size and location.

of the supraclinoid internal carotid artery. They project medially or inferomedially (54) from the vessel which may be displaced superolaterally (Figs. 8.25, 8.32).

Intraoperative Angiography in Paraclinoidal Aneurysms

The technical difficulties involved in surgical clipping of virtually all types of aneurysms in this region are considerable. Intraoperative angiography is extremely useful after clip-placement to evaluate for patency of the internal carotid artery, the ophthalmic artery, and for residual aneurysm. With a giant paraclinoidal aneurysm, surgical reconstruction of the internal carotid artery can be difficult without decompressing the aneurysm first. This can be done by clamping the internal carotid artery proximally and distally, and puncturing the aneurysm (56). Alternatively, suction can be applied in the exposed cervical carotid artery with a needle or by insertion of a double-lumen balloon-catheter (57, 58). However, use of such a device in a nonheparinized patient carries a significant risk of thromboembolic complications.

Clinical Presentation of Paraclinoidal Aneurysms

Aneurysms close to the anterior clinoid process account for approximately 5% of all intracranial aneurysms. Pa-

tients with such aneurysms are likely (45%) to have multiple aneurysms, particularly at sites such as the posterior communicating artery, the contralateral paraclinoid area, and the cavernous segment (39, 49). A female preponderance is consistently reported. Three types of clinical presentation are seen: subarachnoid hemorrhage, visual disturbance, and headache.

Approximately 30% or more of patients with symptomatic aneurysms in this location present with subarachnoid hemorrhage (49, 59). Almost the same proportion present with loss of visual acuity or field-cuts due to the mass-effect of the aneurysm on the optic nerve or chiasm (Fig. 8.31). This is clinically detectable usually only with aneurysms greater than 1 cm in diameter. As the aneurysm expands superiorly, it compresses the optic nerve superiorly and medially against the falciform fold. The maximal impact of compression of the optic nerve is usually on the lateral aspect of the nerve. For this reason, the fibers most commonly affected early may be those for the ipsilateral inferior nasal field (39, 60). Bilateral field defects become more apparent with continued expansion. Numerous patterns of unilateral or bilateral field cuts can be seen (59). The combination of an ipsilateral nasal field cut and a contralateral temporal hemianopsia has been classically

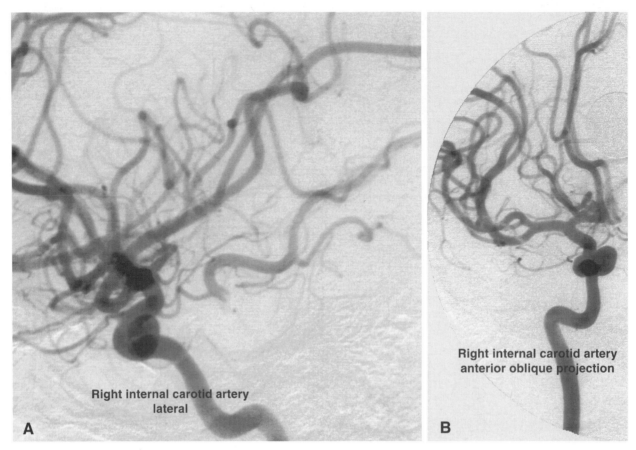

A

**Right internal carotid artery
lateral**

B

**Right internal carotid artery
anterior oblique projection**

Figure 8.32. *Superior hypophyseal aneurysm.*   This aneurysm projects medially and extends proximally. Unless carefully studied, an aneurysm in this location could be misinterpreted as arising from the carotid genu or cavernous segment.

described. It is attributed to compression of the contralateral fibers in the knee of Wildbrand within the posterior part of the ipsilateral optic nerve (39, 61, 62). The taut optic nerve may indent the wall of the expanding aneurysm as it stretches around it (Fig. 8.31). This indentation can be seen occasionally at angiography (48).

Recovery of vision after treatment is unpredictable. A favorable outcome can be hoped for with good decompression of mass-effect on the optic apparatus, preservation of the ophthalmic artery, and a short history. Recovery can continue over a 2-year period (59).

ANATOMIC VARIANTS OF THE INTERNAL CAROTID ARTERY

A number of common vessels with sites of origin usually found elsewhere can be seen occasionally arising from the internal carotid artery (9). More unusual anomalous states include agenesis of the internal carotid artery; persistent stapedial artery; persistent trigeminal artery; proatlantal intersegmental artery type I; otic artery; hypoglossal artery; or primitive maxillary artery.

Agenesis of the Internal Carotid Artery

Rare cases of bilateral or unilateral agenesis of the internal carotid artery have been reported. In this condition, de-

pending on the site of segmental agenesis, the ipsilateral hemispheric circulation may be reconstituted via: the contralateral internal carotid artery through a transsellar anastomosis thought to correspond with the primitive maxillary artery (63, 64) (Fig. 8.14); the ipsilateral inferolateral trunk, predominantly through the accessory meningeal artery, artery of the foramen rotundum, persistent stapedial artery, and other routes (9, 65, 66); the contralateral internal carotid artery via the anterior communicating artery; or the posterior circulation via the posterior communicating artery or via unusual carotid-basilar anastomoses, such as a persistent trigeminal artery (67).

Aberrant Internal Carotid Artery

This unusual but important condition may be an incidental finding or may present with pulsatile tinnitus. An error to avoid is misdiagnosis of this condition as a middle ear mass on axial images with subsequent biopsy, severe bleeding, and pseudoaneurysm formation (68, 69) (Fig. 8.33). This is a rare condition, but because of the surgical risks involved through inadvertent biopsy, it is necessary to be familiar with it. It may occasionally be seen bilaterally (70, 71).

This condition is thought to relate to atresia or regression of the cervical portion of the internal carotid artery.

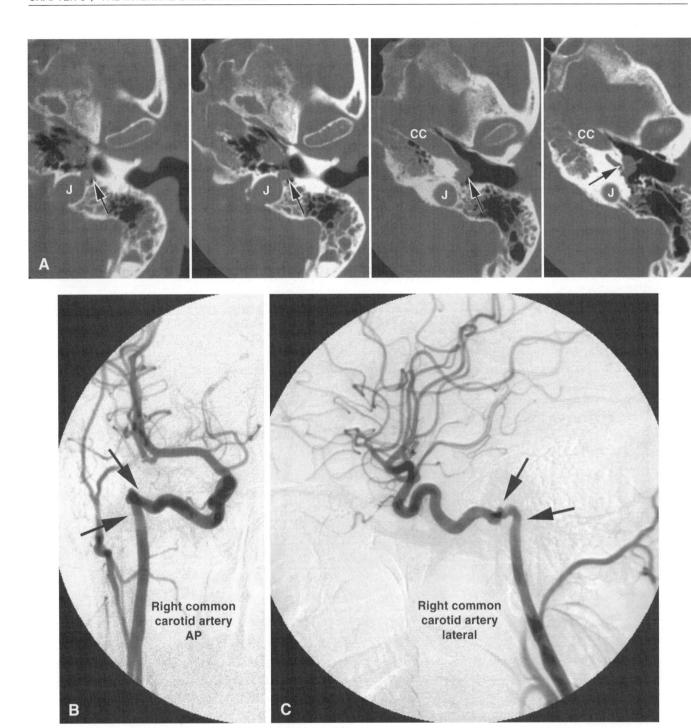

Figure 8.33. *Aberrant internal carotid artery.* An elderly female was studied for evaluation of otosclerosis. A diagnosis of middle ear mass was reached. The ``mass'' was biopsied with a 22 G needle causing profuse bleeding. Axial CT images **(A)** from inferior to superior demonstrate absence of an exocranial ostium of the carotid canal (CC) in the usual location. An unusually large bony canal **(arrow)** is seen adjacent to the jugular bulb (J). Followed from one slice to the next, this canal becomes a tubular soft tissue structure joining the carotid canal (CC). At its apex in the middle ear, the afferent and efferent components of this vessel cannot be perceived on a single image explaining why this entity is sometimes misinterpreted as a mass. Notice how it lies lateral to the semicircular canals of the vestibular apparatus. This is a typical CT appearance of an aberrant internal carotid artery. Right common carotid arteriography demonstrated the typical angiographic appearance of an aberrant internal carotid artery. The artery extends more posteriorly than usual on the lateral view **(C)** with a constrained, knuckled appearance **(arrows)**. On the AP view **(B)**, it projects more laterally than does the usual course of the internal carotid artery. Fortunately for this patient, a pseudoaneurysm at the biopsy-site was not found. Compare the course of the aberrant internal carotid artery with that of the pharyngotympanostapedial artery illustrated in Figure 8.7. In both instances, the inferior tympanic artery of the ascending pharyngeal artery is thought to be identity of the enlarged vessel. The normal inferior tympanic artery is a tiny vessel entering the middle ear via the inferior tympanic canaliculus, the bony canal enlarged in the CT images of **(A)**.

In these cases, what appears to be the internal carotid artery represents an enlarged inferior tympanic branch of the ascending pharyngeal artery. This usually tiny vessel enters the tympanic cavity through the inferior tympanic canaliculus (which it shares with Jacobson's tympanic branch of the IXth nerve). With reconstitution of the petrous internal carotid artery through this route, the vessel has a more lateral and posterior location than the usual carotid canal. This location in association with a pinched contour of the vessel causes a characteristic angiographic appearance. Lapayowker et al. (72) described the vestibular line on the AP view, which is a vertical line dropped from the most lateral aspect of the vestibular apparatus. The petrous internal carotid artery normally lies medial to this line, but swings lateral to it in the setting of an aberrant internal carotid artery.

Persistent Stapedial Artery

A persistent stapedial artery represents a rare anomalous derivative of the hyoid-stapedial artery (see Chapter 5). Usually, this artery regresses at the level of the stapes, becoming the carotico-tympanic branch of the petrous internal carotid artery. A persistent stapedial artery traces a course through the middle ear. Therefore, it represents a surgical hazard during middle ear exploration or biopsy (see Figs. 5.5, 8.7). Most commonly, a persistent stapedial artery retains as its territory the dural branches of the primitive hyoid artery. Therefore, the middle meningeal artery in these cases is supplied by the petrous internal carotid artery, with an accompanying diminution or absence of the foramen spinosum (73). Still rarer cases have been described where the persistent stapedial artery from the internal carotid artery retains the territory of the maxillo-mandibular trunk of the hyoid artery, i.e., that territory usually subsumed by the distal external carotid artery (74).

Persistent Trigeminal Artery

This unusual vessel, seen in approximately 0.3% of cerebral angiograms, extends from the presellar segment of the internal carotid artery to the basilar system (75, 76). It is most commonly seen in two predominant patterns (77). First, it may connect with the upper part of the basilar trunk and supply the posterior cerebral artery and superior cerebellar artery territories (Figs. 8.34, 8.35, 8.36, 8.37). In this instance the inferior part of the posterior circulation below the level of the anterior inferior cerebellar artery is separated from the upper part. Alternatively, there may be one or two fetal type posterior cerebral artery origins present restricting the trigeminal artery supply to the posterior fossa. Other possible variants include origin of a single cerebellar artery from the trigeminal site (78) (Fig. 8.36).

It is important to recognize the trigeminal artery in situations such as Wada testing to avoid embolization or infu-

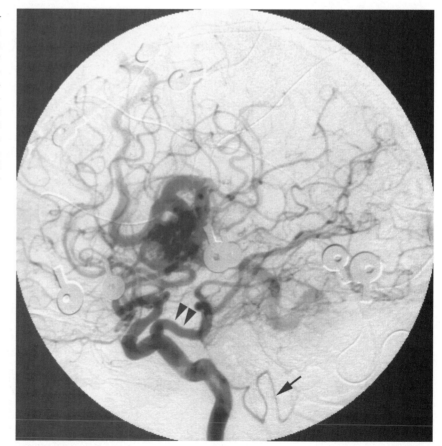

Figure 8.34. *Trigeminal artery in a patient for Wada testing.* A middle-aged female with a left hemispheric AVM referred for preoperative Wada testing. A preliminary internal carotid artery injection demonstrates a persistent trigeminal artery **(arrowheads)** perfusing the posterior circulation as far as the posterior inferior cerebellar artery **(arrow)**. To perform a Wada test safely in this patient, the infusion of amobarbital must be made above the carotid-basilar connection in order to avoid perfusing the posterior circulation. This requires heparinization of the patient and coaxial passage of a microcatheter to the supraclinoid internal carotid artery.

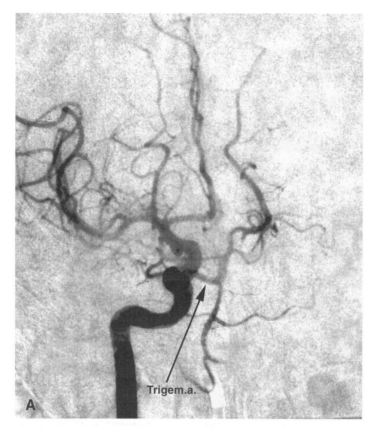

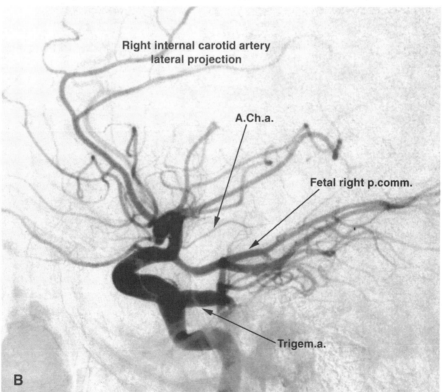

Figure 8.35. *Trigeminal artery.* A variant of the trigeminal artery is demonstrated. An associated ipsilateral fetal posterior communicating artery is present. On the lateral view, confusion over the identity of posteriorly directed vessels from the carotid artery must be avoided by discerning clearly between the posterior communicating artery and anterior choroidal artery (A.Ch.A), which arise from the supraclinoid internal carotid artery, and the persistent trigeminal artery (Trigem.A.), which arises from the cavernous internal carotid artery. As the trigeminal artery enters the basilar artery it frequently makes a loop or turn, well demonstrated in this case. However, in many instances this turn may simulate the appearance of an aneurysm on the lateral view.

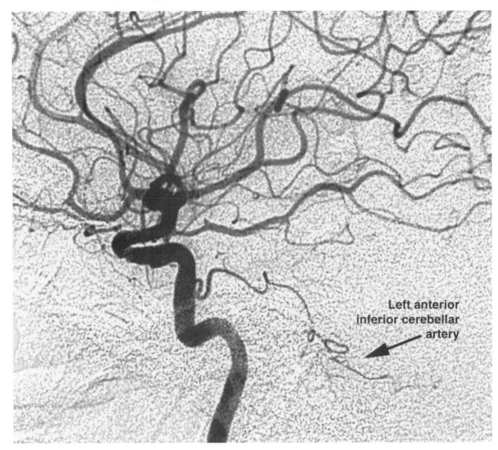

Figure 8.36. *Trigeminal variant to anterior inferior cerebellar artery.*   Incidental finding of a trigeminal variant giving supply to the territory of the ipsilateral anterior inferior cerebellar artery. Cases of posterior inferior cerebellar artery supply in a similar manner have been reported.

Figure 8.37. *Intrasellar course of a persistent trigeminal artery.*   Coronal T1 weighted images demonstrate an intrasellar course of a carotid-basilar anastomotic vessel (white arrowheads). The importance of discerning this entity from intrasellar masses or cysts in which surgery might be considered is self-evident.

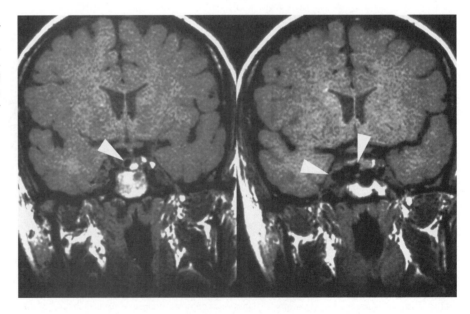

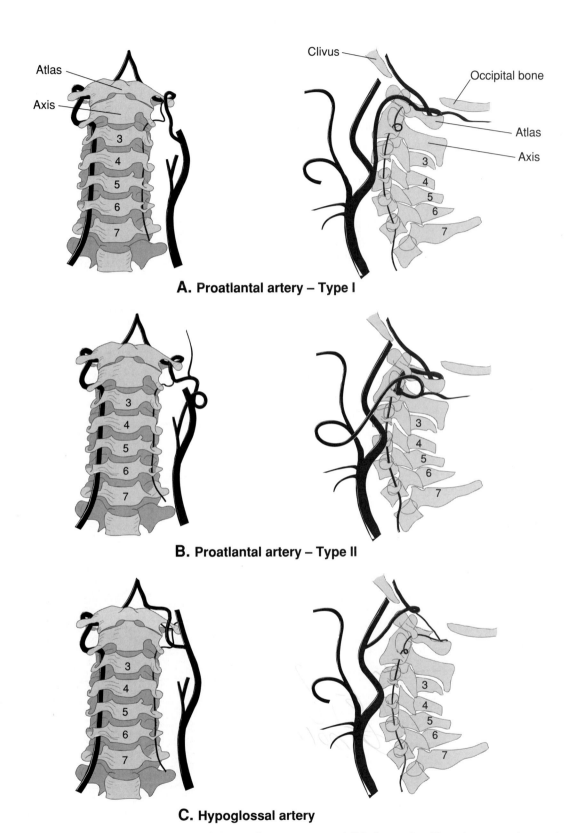

A. Proatlantal artery – Type I

B. Proatlantal artery – Type II

C. Hypoglossal artery

Figure 8.38. *Proatlantal and hypoglossal artery variants.* Proatlantal arteries, types I **(A)** and II **(B)**, and a persistent hypoglossal artery **(C)** are illustrated. For the sake of didactic contrast, hypoplastic ipsilateral vertebral arteries are included, but they are not usually seen in reported clinical examples. Discerning among these variants depends on identifying where they join the normal course of the vertebrobasilar circulation.

sion of barbiturates into the posterior fossa (Figs. 8.34, 8.35, 8.36). The trigeminal artery may also have an intrasellar course and could be mistaken for a pituitary mass or cyst (79) (Fig. 8.37). A persistent trigeminal artery may be a site of aneurysm formation (76, 80). A ruptured aneurysm in this location may leak into the subarachnoid space. Alternatively, leakage into the cavernous sinus presents as a carotid-cavernous fistula. Treatment by endovascular or surgical techniques for fistulas in this location can be undertaken using the same methods as those for carotid-cavernous fistulas in more usual locations (76). However, clarify the vascular anatomy of the posterior fossa before undertaking treatment of a lesion related to a persistent trigeminal artery. In cases in which there is mid-basilar atresia or hypoplasia, it is vitally important to preserve the trigeminal artery as a source of flow to the posterior circulation.

Proatlantal Intersegmental Arteries

The proatlantal intersegmental arteries represent a persistent embryologic connection between the anterior and posterior circulations whereby the vertebrobasilar circulation derives supply either from the internal or external carotid arteries (81). These are extremely rare anomalies of which only a handful have been reported with modern imaging techniques. They are probably associated in embryologic development with the formation of the occipital artery. Therefore, many of the published examples demonstrate a common origin with the occipital artery (82). Kolbinger et al. (83) reported on 39 cases. They observed that the proatlantal artery usually takes origin at the C2-C3 level and is associated with aplasia or hypoplasia of the ipsilateral or both vertebral arteries in about 50% of cases. Cases arising from the external carotid artery are slightly

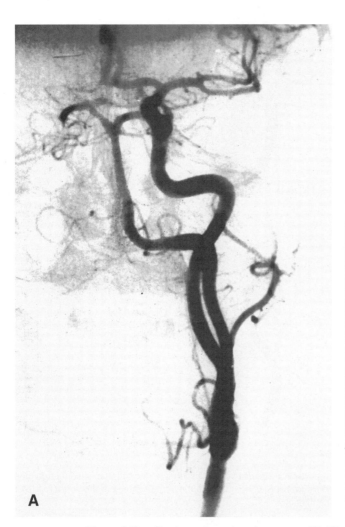

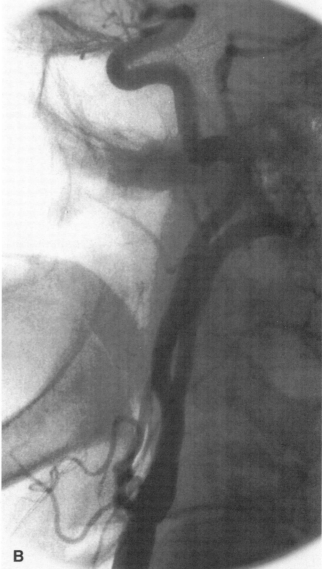

Figure 8.39. *Persistent hypoglossal artery.*   PA **(A)** and lateral **(B)** views of an incidentally discovered hypoglossal artery. Refer to Figure 8.38.

more common than those from the internal carotid artery. The finding of such an anomalous vessel is usually incidental but may warrant specific consideration when associated with ischemic disease or when an endarterectomy or angioplasty is being planned (84, 85).

A persistent proatlantal intersegmental artery type I is usually associated with an origin from the internal carotid artery and is connected to the vertebral artery at the atlanto-occipital space (Fig. 8.38). The type I does not traverse a foramen transversarium. A type II persistent proatlantal intersegmental artery, usually associated with the external carotid artery, joins the normal course of the vertebral artery at the C1-C2 interspace.

Otic and Hypoglossal Arteries

These are extremely rare variants that result in perfusion of the vertebrobasilar system from the internal carotid artery, usually with hypoplasia of the ipsilateral or both vertebral arteries.

The hypoglossal artery has its origin from the internal carotid or common carotid artery between the expected level of the carotid bifurcation and C1-C2 (Figs. 8.38, 8.39). In contrast to the proatlantal intersegmental arteries, which join the extracranial vertebral system gaining access to the intracranial cavity via the foramen magnum, the hypoglossal artery enters the skull via the hypoglossal (anterior condylar) canal (86, 87). The hypoglossal artery has been described on the AP view as having a more medial and direct course in the neck towards the hypoglossal canal, compared with the proatlantal artery, which must join the more laterally disposed course of the cervical vertebral artery (88, 89). On the lateral view, the hypoglossal artery does not have the posterior loop in the atlanto-occipital space seen with both variants of the proatlantal artery (84, 86, 90–93). Rare cases of bilateral primitive hypoglossal arteries or trigeminal arteries have been reported (94, 95).

The otic artery is the most rare of the carotid-vertebral anastomoses (96, 97), and its existence has been disputed by some authors. It is described as a branch of the petrous segment of the internal carotid artery, directed medially, and gaining access to the intracranial cavity via the internal auditory canal (Fig. 8.40). A case of a vessel thought most likely to represent an otic artery remnant in association with a distinct trigeminal artery has been reported by Tomsick et al. (75).

Primitive Maxillary Artery

This is an extremely rare variant of the cavernous segment of the internal carotid artery (C5) that arises at approximately the same level as a persistent trigeminal artery. Unlike the latter which is directed posteriorly, a primitive maxillary artery is directed medially, where it gives branches to the clivus, dorsum sellae, and hypophysis. Inferiorly it anastomoses with the clival branches of the ascending pharyngeal artery, and medially with its contralateral

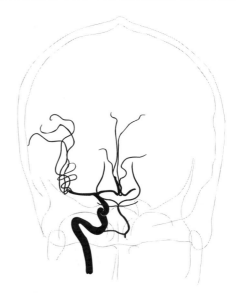

Figure 8.40. *Persistent otic artery.* An illustration of the putative site of origin of the otic artery from the petrous internal carotid artery entering the posterior fossa through the internal acoustic canal.

fellow. It is through the latter route that reconstitution of the contralateral internal carotid artery may take place in cases of prenatal carotid occlusion, giving the appearance of a cavernous origin of the contralateral carotid artery (98) (see Figs. 7.4P, 8.14).

Kissing Carotid Arteries

This variation occurs when redundant loops of the juxtasellar carotid arteries loop medially and touch in the midline. An incidental finding on axial imaging, it is of no consequence except in the setting of transphenoidal surgery, and therefore should be brought to the attention of the surgeon.

ANTERIOR CHOROIDAL ARTERY

Origin of the Anterior Choroidal Artery

The anterior choroidal artery arises from the posterior wall of the internal carotid artery as the most consistently identifiable branch between the posterior communicating artery and the internal carotid bifurcation. It arises most commonly 2–4 mm distal to the origin of the posterior communicating artery. It usually measures about 1 mm in diameter. It is duplicated in approximately 4% of dissection specimens, and its absence is rare (99, 100). Smaller lenticulostriate branches may arise from the carotid artery between the posterior communicating artery and the anterior choroidal artery. Origin of the anterior choroidal artery from the middle cerebral artery or posterior communicating artery has been reported at angiography and at dissection with a frequency of 2–11% (101–103). Rarely, the origin of the anterior choroidal artery may be proximal to that of the posterior communicating artery (104).

The internal carotid artery is ascending in a posterolat-

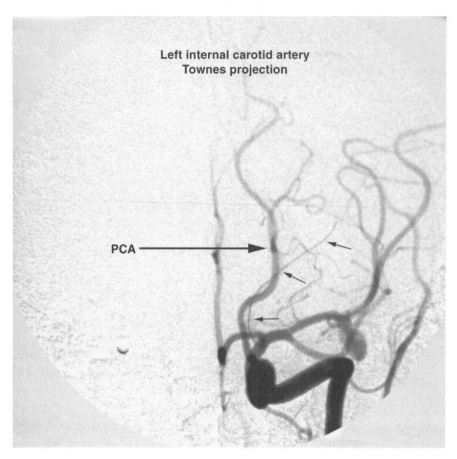

Left internal carotid artery
Townes projection

PCA

Figure 8.41. Origin and course of the anterior choroidal artery in reference to that of the posterior cerebral artery. A Townes projection performed in the evaluation of a left middle cerebral artery aneurysm. There is a fetal posterior communicating artery (PCA) present. The more lateral origin of the anterior choroidal artery **(arrows)**, its initially medially directed course, and its broad curve into the choroidal fissure are well demonstrated.

eral direction in this region. Therefore, the origin and course of the anterior choroidal artery are consistently more laterally disposed than those of the posterior communicating artery (Fig. 8.41). Aneurysms of the posterior communicating artery will therefore most commonly lie inferomedially with reference to the anterior choroidal artery which will be displaced superolaterally. With large posterior communicating artery aneurysms the location of the anterior choroidal artery is of critical importance during surgery. It is extremely useful to the surgeon to gather information, if at all possible, on the disposition of the anterior choroidal artery in reference to the aneurysm.

Course of the Anterior Choroidal Artery

By remembering that the anterior choroidal artery takes its origin more distally and thus more laterally from the internal carotid artery than does the posterior communicating artery, the relationship of the anterior choroidal artery to the adjacent structures can be more easily recalled. In 98% of hemispheres (101), it starts lateral to the optic tract and then crosses under the tract twice, first lateral to medial and then medial to lateral.

After arising from the internal carotid artery, the initial cisternal segment courses posteromedially under the optic tract in a lateral to medial direction. Then it circumvents the cerebral peduncles crossing the optic tract from medial to lateral at the level of the lateral geniculate body

(100). It continues in a posterolateral direction above the uncus to enter the choroidal fissure. After entering the choroidal fissure, the artery is described as becoming the plexal segment with a variable intraventricular and paraventricular supply.

The anterior choroidal artery is considered a crucial vessel in planning neurosurgical and endovascular treatments. The neurally eloquent branches are considered to be the cisternal branches arising proximal to the choroidal point, i.e., the point where it breaches the choroidal fissure. The cisternal segment of the anterior choroidal artery usually measures approximately 24 mm and gives off up to 25 microscopically identifiable branches directed laterally, medially, superiorly and inferiorly, in order of frequency. An average of eight branches are seen at dissection (100). The territories most consistently supplied by the cisternal anterior choroidal artery are the optic tract, cerebral peduncle, temporal lobe, and lateral geniculate body. From the cisternal segment, small perforating branches also ascend into the posterior two-thirds of the optic tract, and from there into the anterior perforated substance to supply the medial parts of the globus pallidus and the internal capsule. Laterally and inferiorly, branches from the anterior choroidal artery supply the piriform cortex, uncus, hippocampus, dentate gyrus, and tail of caudate nucleus. Medial branches enter the middle third of the cerebral peduncle to supply the corticospinal tracts, and penetrate deeply to give a variable supply to the substantia nigra, red nucleus, subthalamus, and ventral nuclei of the thalamus. More posterior branches supply the anterior aspect of the lateral geniculate body in balance with the posterior lateral choroidal artery. These branches also supply the inferior aspects of the posterior limb of the internal capsule, adjacent retrolenticular tracts, and proximal optic radiation fibers.

Anastomoses between the anterior choroidal artery and the middle or posterior cerebral arteries can be a theoretical source of reconstitution of flow in occlusive disease. However, most infarctions involving the anterior choroidal artery usually occur in association with more extensive occlusions; isolated anterior choroidal artery infarcts are extremely rare (105).

The plexal segment usually breaches the choroidal fissure as a single vessel but may divide before entry. Its prominent area of supply involves the choroid plexus of the temporal horn and part of the choroid plexus of the atrium. It anastomoses with the lateral posterior choroidal artery in this area. It may occasionally sweep around the pulvinar to supply the choroid plexus of the body of the lateral ventricle and reach the foramen of Monro.

Angiographic Appearance of the Anterior Choroidal Artery

Analysis of a large series of carotid angiograms by Takahashi (106) demonstrated that approximately two thirds of anterior choroidal arteries have a typical S-shaped curve in the cisternal segment before entering the choroidal fissure. In the AP plane, its course is best studied with a Townes projection. Recognizing the anterior choroidal artery on PA and lateral angiograms can sometimes be hindered by overlapping branches of other vessels. On the lateral projection, the anterior choroidal artery makes an initial downward bend for 1 or 2 mm and turns to form a broad bend convex superiorly, which constitutes the cisternal segment of the anterior choroidal artery (Figs. 8.35B, 8.41, 8.42, 8.43, 8.44, 8.45, 8.46). The choroidal point, where it enters the temporal horn of the lateral ventricle, may be frequently recognized as an abrupt deflection in course 18 to 26 mm posterior to the internal carotid artery (107). There may also be an abrupt discernible change in vessel-caliber at this point.

The appearance of the course of the anterior choroidal artery on the AP view is determined by the degree of

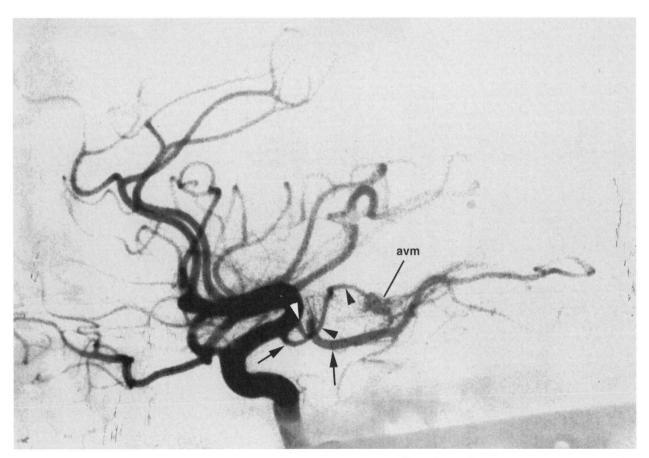

Figure 8.42. *Arteriovenous malformation of the lateral ventricle.* A lateral projection demonstrates overlap of the cisternal segment of the anterior choroidal artery **(arrowheads)** with the junction of the posterior communicating artery and the posterior cerebral artery **(arrows)**. After entering the choroidal fissure, the anterior choroidal artery changes course to a downwards direction and opacifies the arteriovenous malformation. At first glance, the image suggests that the proximal vessel is the anterior choroidal artery and the distal vessel the posterior communicating artery. This inverted arrangement has been seen but is rare; and in this patient, the appearance is an artifact of vessel overlap.

Figure 8.43. Intraventricular AVM supplied by the anterior choroidal artery. After entering the lateral ventricle, the anterior choroidal artery (acha) has a tortuous course before opacifying a small nidus of avm **(arrow)**. An early draining choroidal vein **(arrowhead)** is seen directed anteriorly. An infundibulum of the origin of the posterior communicating artery is present (p).

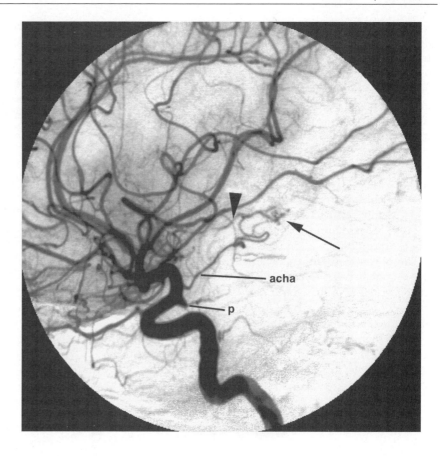

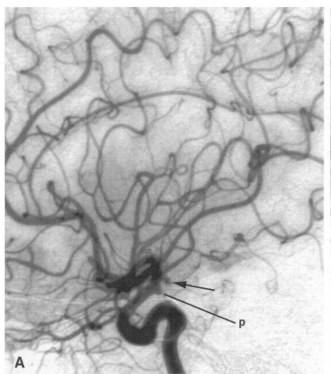

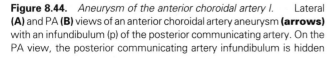

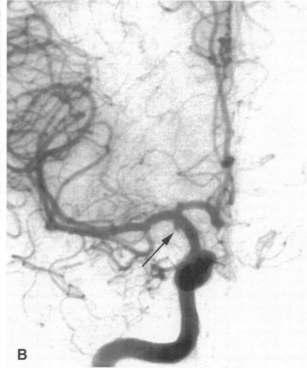

Figure 8.44. *Aneurysm of the anterior choroidal artery I.* Lateral **(A)** and PA **(B)** views of an anterior choroidal artery aneurysm **(arrows)** with an infundibulum (p) of the posterior communicating artery. On the PA view, the posterior communicating artery infundibulum is hidden directly behind the internal carotid artery, whereas the more laterally disposed anterior choroidal artery aneurysm is visible lateral to the contour of the artery.

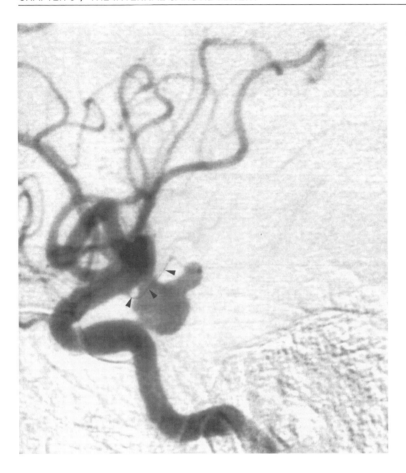

Figure 8.45. *Aneurysm of the anterior choroidal artery II.* This aneurysm was thought at first to be from the posterior communicating artery origin. However, careful windowing demonstrated a tiny thread-like posterior communicating artery arising more proximally **(arrowheads)**. At surgery, the aneurysm was related to the anterior choroidal artery.

cranio-caudad angulation, and it is most easily studied on a steep Townes view (Fig. 8.41). The initial course is usually medially directed under the optic tract. It then takes a lateral course to traverse the crural cistern, and enters the choroidal fissure where it gains the supracornual cleft. The plexal segment of the anterior choroidal artery projects medial to the choroidal blush of the ventricle.

Distortion of the size, course, and contour of the anterior choroidal artery may be seen due to mass-effect involving the adjacent structures with which it has a constrained relationship. It is a sensitive angiographic indicator of central mass-effect. It can be stretched, deflected, or foreshortened depending on the segment and direction involved. Before the advent of axial imaging, changes in the course of the anterior choroidal artery were an important and often the only indicator of central mass-effect (108).

Territory of the Anterior Choroidal Artery

The anterior choroidal artery territory consists in a critical area of the diencephalon and mesencephalon, making it a focus of risk evaluation in planning surgical or interventional treatments. In the embryologic stage, the anterior choroidal artery has a more extensive distribution than is seen in adult angiographic studies. The common pattern of anterior choroidal supply includes the uncus, piriform cortex, much of the tail of the caudate nucleus, hippocampus, amygdala, thalamus, lateral geniculate body, optic

tract, some of the cerebral peduncle, the subthalamic nucleus, and genu and posterior limb of the internal capsule. The importance of the anterior choroidal artery is self-evident, as well as the high risk of severe morbidity related to infarction of this distribution (103). Ischemic infarcts of the anterior choroidal artery are not common, and when they do occur are most likely to involve the posterior two-thirds of the posterior limb and the retrolenticular segment of the internal capsule. An anterior choroidal artery occlusion, accounting for approximately 3% of cerebral ischemic infarcts (109), may cause a clinical syndrome with variable degrees of contralateral hemiplegia, hemianesthesia, and hemianopsia with memory loss and somnolence (110). Hemiplegia is due to involvement of the posterior two-thirds of the posterior limb of the internal capsule; the sensory deficit is due to interruption of thalamocortical fibers; and hemianopsia is due to involvement of the optic tract, the lateral geniculate body, or the geniculocalcarine fibers. This syndrome was not a consistent outcome, however, in all patients who underwent surgical clipping of the anterior choroidal artery in the 1950s for Parkinson's disease, a procedure since abandoned (111). Some patients can have a favorable outcome from a proximal occlusion of the anterior choroidal artery due to distal collateral flow. However, surgical dissection and preservation of the anterior choroidal artery at surgery is considered a priority.

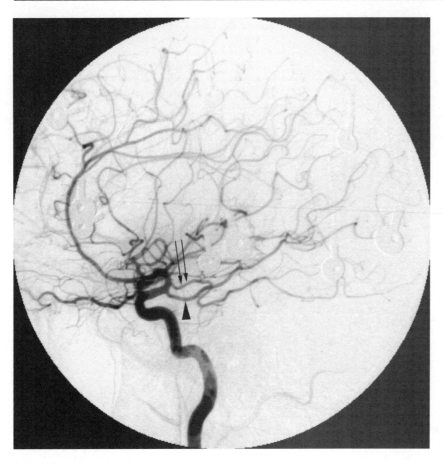

Figure 8.46. *Variant territory of the anterior choroidal artery.* A middle-aged male was referred for Wada testing because of a frontal lobe glioma. Note the artifacts from EEG leads and the taut, displaced appearance of the pericallosal artery. A fetal type posterior communicating artery **(arrowhead)** is present. Another vessel **(double arrow)** with an extensive temporal and occipital territory arises from the internal carotid artery above the posterior communicating artery. This represents a persistence of the embryologic territory of the anterior choroidal artery encompassing much of the temporal and temporo-occipital region. It is sometimes named a ``duplicated posterior communicating artery.''

The anterior choroidal supply exists in balance with a surrounding system of collateral choroidal and parenchymal anastomoses from the anterior, middle, and posterior cerebral arteries. Pathologic lesions or congenital diminution of the adjacent territories account for the variable degree of prominence that the anterior choroidal artery may demonstrate. When the anterior choroidal artery retains a portion of its embryologic territory in the posterior cerebrum, the posterior cerebral artery will be correspondingly smaller (Fig. 8.46). The anterior choroidal artery can have a large posterior and inferior temporal cortical supply, potentially extending to the occipital lobe. This appearance has sometimes been referred to as a *duplicated posterior communicating artery*. Lesser variants of such hyperplastic anterior choroidal arteries were seen in approximately 12% of a large series of angiograms in which the anterior choroidal artery supplied an area usually associated with the posterior cerebral artery (106). These most commonly involved the anterior or posterior temporal regions.

REFERENCES

1. Vitek JJ, Reaves P. Thoracic bifurcation of the common carotid artery. Neuroradiology 1973;5:133–139.
2. Bouthillier A, van Loveren HR, Keller JT. Segments of the internal carotid artery: a new classification. Neurosurgery 1996;38:425–433.
3. Fischer E. Die Lageabweichungen der vorderen Hirnarterie im Gefässbild. Zentralbl Neurochir 1938;3:300–313.
4. Gibo H, Lenkey C, Rhoton AL. Microsurgical anatomy of the supraclinoid portion of the internal carotid artery. J Neurosurg 1981;55:560–574.
5. Lasjaunias P, Berenstein A. Arterial anatomy: introduction. In: Surgical Neuroangiography: Functional anatomy of Craniofacial Arteries. Berlin, Springer-Verlag, 1987;1:1-32.
6. Harris FS, Rhoton AL. Anatomy of the cavernous sinus. A microsurgical study. J Neurosurg 1976;45:169–180.
7. Dolenc VV. A combined epi- and subdural direct approach to carotid-ophthalmic artery aneurysms. J Neurosurg 1985;62:667–672.
8. Debrun G, Lacour P, Vinuela F, et al Treatment of 54 traumatic carotid-cavernous fistulas. J Neurosurg 1981;55:678–692.
9. Teal JS, Rumbaugh CL, Segall HD, et al. Anomalous branches of the internal carotid artery. Radiology 1973;106:567–573.
10. Umansky F, Elidan J, Valarezo A. Dorello's canal: a microanatomical study. J Neurosurg 1991;75:294–298.
11. Overbeeke JJ, Dujovny M, Dragovic L, et al. Anatomy of the sympathetic pathways in the carotid canal. Neurosurgery 1991;29:838–844
12. Paullus WS, Pait TG, Rhoton AL. Microsurgical exposure of the petrous portion of the carotid artery. J Neurosurg 1977;47:713–726.
13. Padget DH. The development of the cranial arteries in the human embryo. Contrib Embryol 1948;32:205–262.
14. Harris FS, Rhoton AL. Anatomy of the cavernous sinus. A microsurgical study. J Neurosurg 1976;45:169–180.

15. Bernasconi V, Cassinari V. Uno sengo carotidografico tipico di meningioma del tentorio. Chirurgia (Pavia)1956;11:586–588.

16. Knosp E, Müller G, Perneczky. The blood supply of the cranial nerves in the lateral wall of the cavernous sinus. In: Dolenc VV (ed). The Cavernous Sinus. New York: Springer-Verlag, 1987;67–80.

17. Parkinson D, Shields CB. Persistent trigeminal artery: its relationship to the normal branches of the cavernous carotid. J Neurosurg 1974;39:244–248

18. Gorczyca W, Hardy J. Arterial supply of the human anterior pituitary gland. Neurosurgery 1987;20:369–378.

19. Inoue T, Rhoton AL, Theele D, et al. Surgical approaches to the cavernous sinus: A microsurgical study. Neurosurgery 1990;26:903–932.

20. Lasjaunias P, Moret J, Mink J. The anatomy of the inferolateral trunk of the internal carotid artery. Neuroradiology 1977;13: 215–220.

21. Krisht AF, Barrow DL, Barnett DW, et al. The microsurgical anatomy of the superior hypophyseal artery. Neurosurgery 1994;35:899–903.

22. Ogawa T, Miyauchi T, Kato T, et al. Internal carotid artery origin of double ophthalmic arteries. Neuroradiology 1990; 32:508–510.

23. Linskey ME, Sekhar LN, Hirsch W, et al. Aneurysms of the intracavernous carotid artery: Clinical presentation, radiographic features, and pathogenesis. Neurosurgery 1990;26: 71–79.

24. Linskey ME, Sekhar LN, Hirsch WL, et al. Aneurysms of the intracavernous carotid artery: Natural history and indications for treatment. Neurosurgery 1990;26:933–938.

25. Kupersmith MJ, Hurst R, Berenstein A, et al. The benign course of cavernous carotid artery aneurysms. J Neurosurg 1992;77:690–693.

26. Obrador S, Gomez-Bueno J, Silvela J. Spontaneous carotid-cavernous fistula produced by ruptured aneurysm the meningohypophyseal branch of the internal carotid artery. Case report. J Neurosurg 1974;40:539–543.

27. Teitelbaum GP, Halbach V, Larsen DW, et al. Treatment of massive posterior epistaxis by detachable coil embolization of a cavernous internal carotid artery aneurysm. Neuroradiology 1995;37:334–336.

28. McLaughlin MR, Jho HD, Kwon Y. Acute subdural hematoma caused by a ruptured giant intracavernous aneurysm. Case report. Neurosurgery 1996;38:388–392.

29. Nishioka T, Kondo A, Aoyama I, et al. Subarachnoid hemorrhage possibly caused by a saccular carotid artery aneurysm within the cavernous sinus. Case report. J Neurosurg 1990;73: 301–304.

30. Lee AG, Mawad ME, Baskin DS. Fatal subarachnoid hemorrhage from the rupture of a totally intracavernous carotid artery aneurysm. Neurosurgery 1996;38:596–699.

31. Hayreh SS, Dass R. The ophthalmic artery. II. Intraorbital course. Br J Ophthalmol 1962;46:165–185.

32. Hayreh SS. Arteries of the orbit in the human being. Br J Surg 1963;938–952.

33. Hayreh SS. The central artery of the retina. Its role in the blood supply of the optic nerve. Br J Ophthalmol 1963;47: 651–659.

34. Hayreh SS. The ophthalmic artery. III. Branches. Br J Ophthalmol 1962;46:212–247.

35. Gabrielle OF, Bell D. Ophthalmic origin of the middle meningeal artery. Radiology 1967;89:841–844.

36. Hassler W, Zentner J, Voigt K. Abnormal origin of the ophthalmic artery from the anterior cerebral artery: Neuroradiological and intraoperative findings. Neuroradiology 1989;21: 85–87.

37. Gibo H, Kobayashi S, Kyoshima K, et al. Microsurgical anatomy of the arteries of the pituitary stalk and gland as viewed from above. Acta Neurochir (Wien) 1988;90:60–66.

38. Bergland R, Ray BS. The arterial supply of the human optic chiasm. J Neurosurg 1969;31:327–333.

39. Day AL. Aneurysms of the ophthalmic segment. A clinical and anatomical analysis. J Neurosurg 1990;72:677–691.

40. Nakagawa F, Kobayashi S, Takemae T, et al. Aneurysms protruding from the dorsal wall of the internal carotid artery. J Neurosurg 1986;65:303–308.

41. Aldrich F. Anterior (dorsal) paraclinoid aneurysm: Case report. Surg Neurol 1991;35:374–376.

42. Knosp E, Müller G, Perneczky A. The paraclinoid carotid artery: Anatomical aspects of a microneurosurgical approach. Neurosurgery 1988;22:896–901.

43. Nishio S, Matsushima T, Fukui M, et al. Microsurgical anatomy around the origin of the ophthalmic artery with reference to contralateral pterional surgical approach to the carotid-ophthalmic aneurysm. Acta Neurochir (Wien) 1985;76: 82–89.

44. Gruber WL. Beiträge zur Anatomie des Keilbeins und Schläfenbeins. St. Petersburg: Eggers und Comp., 1859.

45. Keyes JEL. Observations on four thousand optic foramina in human skulls of known origin. Arch Ophthalmol 1935;13: 538–568.

46. Kobayashi S, Kyoshima K, Gibo H, et al. Carotid cave aneurysms of the internal carotid artery. J Neurosurg 1989;70: 216–221.

47. Fox JL. Microsurgical treatment of ventral (paraclinoid) internal carotid artery aneurysms. Neurosurgery 1988;22:32–39.

48. Heros RC, Nelson PB, Ojemann RC, et al. Large and Giant paraclinoid aneurysm: surgical techniques, complications and results. Neurosurgery 1983;12:153–163.

49. Ogilvy CS. Paraclinoid carotid aneurysms. In: Ojemann RG, Ogilvy CS, Crowell RM, Heros RC, eds. Surgical Management of Neurovascular Disease, 3rd ed. Baltimore, Williams & Wilkins, 1995:185–213.

50. Al-Rodhan NRF, Piepgras DG, Sundt TM. Transitional cavernous aneurysms of the internal carotid artery. Neurosurgery 1993;33:993–998.

51. Yasargil MG, Fox JL. The microsurgical approach to intracranial aneurysms. Surg Neurol 1975;3:7-14.

52. Korosue K, Heros RC. "Subclinoid" carotid aneurysm with erosion of the anterior clinoid process and fatal intraoperative rupture. Neurosurgery 1992;31:356–360.

53. Yasargil MG, Gasser JC, Hodosh RM. Carotid-ophthalmic aneurysms: direct microsurgical approach. Surg Neurol 1977;1: 155–165.

54. Batjer HH, Kopitnik TA, Giller CA, et al. Surgery for paraclinoidal carotid artery aneurysms. J Neurosurg 1994;80: 650–658.

55. Nutik SL. Ventral paraclinoid carotid aneurysms. J Neurosurg 1988;69:340–344.

56. Flamm ES. Suction decompression of aneurysms. Technical note. J Neurosurg 1981;54:275–276.

57. Batjer HH, Samson DS. Retrograde suction decompression of giant paraclinoidal aneurysms. Technical note. J Neurosurg 1990;73:305–306.

58. Mizoi K, Takahashi A, Yoshimoto T, et al. Combined endovascular and neurosurgical approach for paraclinoid internal carotid artery aneurysms. Neurosurgery 1993;33:986–992.

59. Ferguson GG, Drake CG. Carotid-ophthalmic aneurysms: Vis-

ual abnormalities in 32 patients and the results of treatment. Surg Neurol 1981;16:1-8.

60. Berson E, Freeman M, Gay A. Visual field defects in giant suprasellar aneurysms of the internal carotid artery. Arch Ophthalmol 1966;76:52–58.

61. Wildbrand H, Saenger A. Die Neurologie des Auges. 1915. Cited by Berson EC. Arch Ophthalmol 1966;76:52.

62. Jefferson G. Compression of the chiasma, optic nerves and optic tracts by intracranial aneurysms. Brain 1937;60:444–497.

63. Kishore PRS, Kaufman AB, Melichar FA. Intrasellar carotid anastomosis simulating pituitary microadenoma. Radiology 1979;132:381–383.

64. Staples G. Transsellar intracavernous intercarotid collateral artery associated with agenesis of the internal carotid artery. J Neurosurg 1979;50:393–394.

65. Beresini DC, Hieshima GB, Mehringer CM, et al. Bilateral absence of the internal carotid artery with sellar enlargement due to anomalous vascularity. Surg Neurol 1980;16:9-12.

66. Dilenge D, Géraud G. Accessory meningeal artery. Acta Radiol (Suppl) 1975;347:63–69.

67. Lasjaunias P, Santoyo-Vazquez A. Segmental agenesis of the internal carotid artery: angiographic aspects with embryological discussion. Anat Clin 1984;6:133–141.

68. Cole RD, May JS. Aberrant internal carotid artery. South Med J 1994;87:1277–1280.

69. Goldman NC, Singleton GT, Holly EH. Aberrant internal carotid artery. Arch Otolaryngol 1971;94:269–273.

70. Campbell G, Renner G, Estrem SA. Bilateral aberrant internal carotid arteries. Arch Otolaryngol Head Neck Surgery 1992;107:124–128.

71. Glasscock ME, Seshul M, Seshul MB. Bilateral aberrant internal carotid artery case presentation. Arch Otolaryngol Head Neck Surg 1993;119:335–339.

72. Lapayowker MS, Liebman EP, Ronis ML, et al. Presentation of the internal carotid artery as tumor of the middle ear. Radiology 1971;98:292–297.

73. Guinto FC, Garrabrant EC, Radcliffe WB. Radiology of the persistent stapedial artery. Radiology 1972;105:365–369.

74. Rodesch G, Choi IS, Lasjaunias P. Complete persistence of the hyoido-stapedial artery in man. Case report. Intrapetrous origin of the maxillary artery from ICA. Surg Radiol Anat 1991;13:63–65.

75. Tomsick TA, Lukin RR, Chambers AA. Persistent trigeminal artery: unusual associated findings. Neuroradiology 1979;17:253–257.

76. Debrun GM, Davis KR, Nanta JH, et al. Treatment of carotid cavernous fistulas or cavernous aneurysms associated with a persistent trigeminal artery: report of three cases. Am J Neuroradiol 1988;9;749–755.

77. Saltzman GF. Patent primitive trigeminal arteries studied by cerebral angiography. Acta Radiol 1959;51:329–336.

78. Siqueira M, Piske R, Ono M, et al. Cerebellar arteries originating from the internal carotid artery. Am J Neuroradiol 1993;14:1229–1235.

79. Richardson DN, Elster AD, Ball MR. Intrasellar trigeminal artery. Am J Neuroradiol 1989;10:205.

80. McKenzie JD, Dean BL, Flom RA. Trigeminal-Cavernous Fistula; Saltzman anatomy revisited. Am J Neuroradiol 1996;17:280–282.

81. Lasjaunias P, Theron J, Moret J. The occipital artery: anatomy—normal arteriographic aspects—embryologic significance. Neuroradiology 1978;15:31–37.

82. Suzuki S, Nobechi T, Itoh I, et al. Persistent proatlantal intersegmental artery and occipital artery originating from the interior carotid artery. Neuroradiology 1979;17:105–109.

83. Kolbinger R, Heindel W, Pawlik G, et al. Right proatlantal artery type I, right internal artery occlusion, and left internal carotid stenosis: case report and review of the literature. J Neurol Sci 1993;117:232–239.

84. Fantini GA, Reilly LM, Stoney RJ. Persistent hypoglossal artery: Diagnostic and therapeutic considerations concerning carotid thromboendarterectomy. J Vasc Surg 1994;20: 995–999.

85. Ouriel K, Green RM, DeWeese JA. Anomalous carotid-basilar anastomoses in cerebrovascular surgery. J Vasc Surg 1988;7:774–777.

86. Anderson RA, Sondheimer FK. Rare carotid-vertebrobasilar anastomoses with note on the differentiation between proatlantal and hypoglossal arteries. Neuroradiology 1976;11:113–118.

87. Brismar J. Persistent hypoglossal artery, diagnostic criteria. Report of a case. Acta Radiologica Diag 1976;17:160–166.

88. Resche F, Resche-Perrin I, Robert R, et al. L'artère hypoglosse. Rapport d'un nouveau cas. Revue de la littérature. J Neuroradiol 1980;7:27–43.

89. Wardwell GA, Goree JA, Jimenez JP. The hypoglossal artery and hypoglossal canal. Am J Roentgenol 1973;118:528–533.

90. Bahsi YZ, Uysal H, Peker S, et al. Persistent primitive proatlantal intersegmental artery (Proatlantal Artery I) results in "top of the basilar" syndrome. Stroke 1993;24:2114–2117.

91. Lui CC, Liu YH, Wai YY, et al. Persistence of both proatlantal arteries with absence of vertebral arteries. Neuroradiology 1987;29:304–305.

92. Hutchinson NA, Miller JDR. Persistent proatlantal artery. J Neurol Neurosurg Psychiatry 1970;33:524–527.

93. Obayashi T, Furuse M. The proatlantal intersegmental artery. A case report and review of the literature. Arch Neurol 1980;37:387–389.

94. Karasawa J, Kikuchi R, Furuse S, et al. Bilateral persistent carotid-basilar anastomoses. Am J Roentgenol 1976;127:1053–1056.

95. Oertel H. Über die Persistenz embryonaler Verbindungen zwishen der A. Carotid interna und der A. Vertebralis cerebralis. Verhandlungen der Anatomischen Gesellschaft 1922;31:281–295.

96. Reynolds AF, Stovring J, Turner PT. Persistent otic artery. Surg Neurol 1980;13:115–117.

97. Huber G. Die Arteria primitive otica, eine sehr seltene persistierende Primitivarterie. Fortschritte auf dem Gebiete der Röntgenstrahlen und der Nuklear Medizin. 1977;127:350–353.

98. Midkiff RB, Boykin MW, McFarland DR, et al. Agenesis of the internal carotid artery with intercavernous anastomosis. Am J Neuroradiol 1995;16:1356–1359.

99. Rhoton AL, Saeki N, Perlmutter D, et al. Microsurgical anatomy of common aneurysm sites. Clin Neurosurg 1979;26:248–306.

100. Rhoton AL, Fujii K, Fradd B. Microsurgical anatomy of the anterior choroidal artery. Surg Neurol 1979;12:171–187.

101. Carpenter MB, Noback CR, Moss ML. The anterior choroidal artery. Its origins, course, distribution, and variations. Arch Neurol Psychiatr 1954;71:714–722.

102. Morello A, Cooper IS. Arteriographic anatomy of the anterior choroidal artery. Am J Radiol 1955;73:748–751.

103. Herman LH, Fernando OU, Gurdjian ES. The anterior choroidal artery: an anatomical study of its area of distribution. Anat Rec 1966;154:95–102.

104. Moyer DJ, Flamm ES. Anomalous arrangement of the origins of the anterior choroidal and posterior communicating arteries. J Neurosurg 1992;76:1017–1018.

105. Levy R, Duyckaerts C, Hauw JJ. Massive infarcts involving the territory of the anterior choroidal artery and cardioembolism. Stroke 1995;26:609–613.

106. Takahashi S., Suga T., Kawata Y, et al. Anterior Choroidal Artery: Angiographic analysis of variations and anomalies. Am J Neuroradiol 1990;11: 719–729.

107. Théron J, Newton TH. Anterior choroidal artery. I. Anatomic and radiographic study. J Neuroradiol 1976;3:5-30.

108. Théron J, Newton TH. Anterior choroidal artery. II. Pathologic states (tumors). J Neuroradiol 1976;3:31–51.

109. Paroni Sterbini GL, Mossuto Agatiello L, Stocchi A, et al. CT of ischemic infarctions in the territory of the anterior choroidal artery: a review of 28 cases. Am J Neuroradiol 1987;8: 229–232.

110. Foix CH, Chavany H, Hillemand P, et al. Oblitération de l'artère choroidienne antérieure. Ramollissement cérébral, hémiplégie, hémianesthésie et hémianopsie. Société d'Ophthalmologie du 30 mai, 1925; 27:221–223.

111. Cooper IS. Surgical occlusion of the anterior choroidal artery in Parkinsonism. Surg Gynecol Obstet 1954;99:207–219.

CHAPTER 9

The Anterior Cerebral Artery

The anterior cerebral artery and anterior communicating artery, in particular, represent the most common sites of intracranial aneurysms, accounting for approximately 30% in most series (1).

The anterior cerebral artery arises from the medial aspect of the internal carotid bifurcation below the anterior perforated substance. It courses antero-medially towards the interhemispheric fissure. The usual route that it takes is above the optic chiasm or nerve meaning that the optic structures therefore slope through the ring of the circle of Willis. At the level of the interhemispheric fissure, it is joined to the contralateral anterior cerebral artery via the anterior communicating artery in the suprachiasmatic cistern.

SEGMENTAL ANATOMY OF THE ANTERIOR CEREBRAL ARTERY

The A1 segment of the anterior cerebral artery extends from the internal carotid artery bifurcation to the anterior communicating artery; the A2 segment extends from there to the junction of the rostrum and genu of the corpus callosum; the A3 extends around the genu until the artery turns sharply posteriorly. The A4 and A5 segments above the corpus callosum are separated by the plane of the coronal fissure (2–4) (Fig. 9.1).

VARIATIONS OF THE ANTERIOR CEREBRAL ARTERY–COMMUNICATING ARTERY COMPLEX

Variations in the region of the anterior communicating artery are common. The term *anterior cerebral artery–communicating artery complex* is frequently used in clinical parlance. As elsewhere in the circle of Willis, alterations in hemodynamics due to the presence of anomalous vessels are thought to explain the high frequency of such anomalies in patients with aneurysms in this region. The extreme variability of the anatomy in this region, due to redundancy of vessel loops, vessel duplication, and early bifurcation of the A2 segment, can make the anterior communicating artery complex one of the most difficult areas to evaluate angiographically (3) (Fig. 9.2).

Usually the anterior cerebral arteries join the anterior communicating artery superior to the optic chiasm (70%). When the A1 segments are longer or redundant, this union may occur more anteriorly above the optic nerves. Fenestrations or duplications of the A1 portion of the anterior cerebral artery may be seen (Fig. 9.3). More rare anomalies include an interoptic or infraoptic course of the A1 segment (5–7), or even perforation of the optic nerve by the A1 segment (8). Variants involving courses through or below the optic apparatus are rare and are usually discussed as case reports. One possible embryologic explanation for an infra-optic course of the anterior cerebral artery suggests that the A1 segment in these instances represents a persistence of the ventral primitive ophthalmic artery taking origin from the internal carotid artery and flowing retrogradely to the anterior cerebral artery.

Variations in the relative size of the A1 segments and the anterior communicating artery are common. Using a diameter of 1.5 mm or smaller as a definition for hypoplasia, approximately 10% of brains demonstrate hypoplastic A1 segments (3, 9, 10) (Fig. 9.4). The anterior communicating artery varies in length up to 7 mm, may be quite tortuous, and measures up to 3.4 mm in diameter. There is a positive correlation between the diameter of the anterior communicating artery and the degree of asymmetry of the A1 segments. This is to compensate hemodynamically for hypoplasia of the smaller vessel. Asymmetry of the A1 segments has an important impact on the likelihood of aneurysm formation in the anterior communicating artery region. The end-on hemodynamic impact of pulsatile flow in the larger A1 segment directed against the anterior wall of the anterior communicating artery is thought to explain the higher rate of aneurysm formation under these circumstances. Up to 80% of anterior communicating artery aneurysms have significant A1 asymmetry. This hemodynamic force also explains why approximately 70% of such aneurysms here project anteriorly (11, 12) (Figs. 9.5, 9.6). Altered hemodynamics in the anterior communicating artery after therapeutic occlusion of an internal carotid artery are also associated with an increased likelihood of delayed aneurysm formation.

Other common variations in this area include the presence of two or more anterior communicating arteries in 11– 43% of brains (10, 13). This may take the form of a fenestration of the anterior communicating artery or complete duplication or triplication (3, 14) (Fig. 9.2). Another angiographic difficulty in imaging this area occurs when the anterior cerebral arteries are not exactly parallel; the anterior communicating artery must run an oblique course to connect the two. This calls for flexibility in one's positioning for imaging of this region (see Fig. 2.45).

A rare variant of the proximal anterior cerebral artery is a persistent olfactory artery that runs anteriorly from the internal carotid artery bifurcation along the olfactory

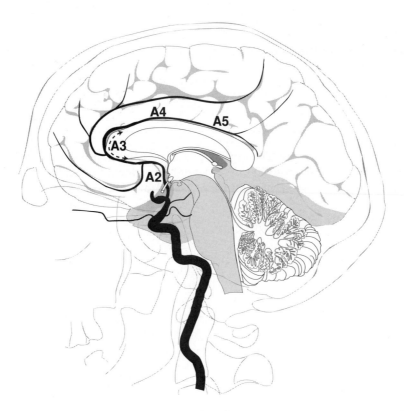

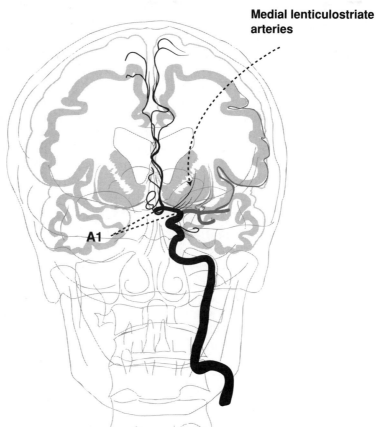

Figure 9.1. Segmental anatomy of the anterior cerebral artery.

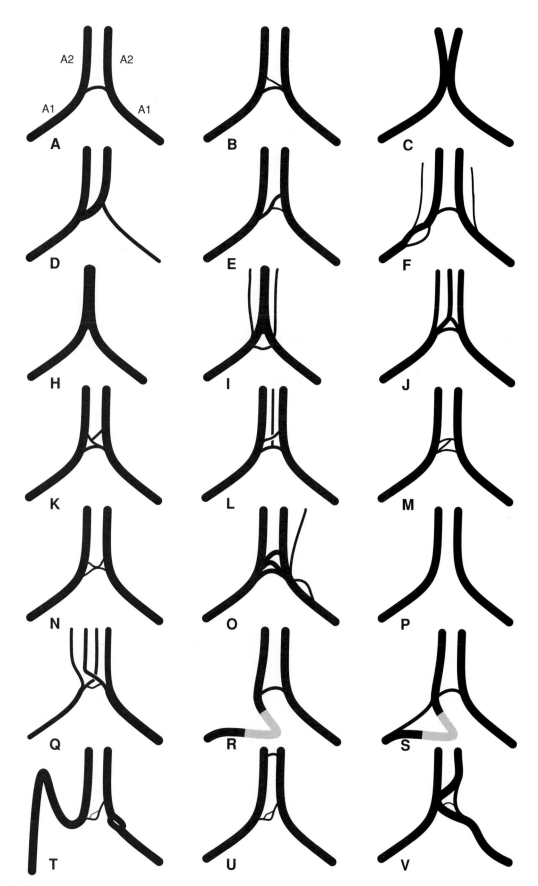

Figure 9.2. A–V Variations in the anterior communicating artery complex. Numerous variants of the junction of the anterior cerebral arteries in the region of the anterior communicating artery make this a difficult area to interrogate angiographically. Schematic illustrations of a range of common and rare variants are represented. Variants R and S represent an infraoptic course of the A1 segment. Variant T represents a persistent primitive olfactory artery.

167

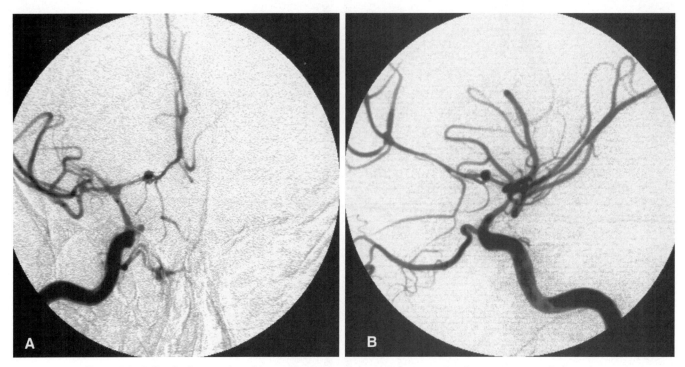

Figure 9.3. A, B *A1 fenestration with associated aneurysm.* A 3-mm ruptured aneurysm extends from the proximal end of a fenestration of the right A1 segment. Evidence of mild intracranial vasospasm is seen in the distal anterior cerebral artery circulation **(B).**

Figure 9.4. *Hypoplastic A1 segment.* Relative hypoplasia of the A1 segment **(arrowhead)** is common, but complete absence is rare.

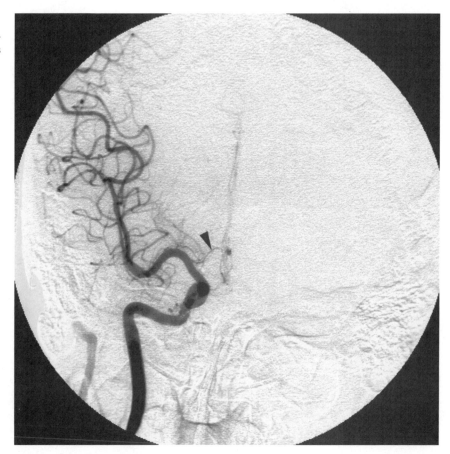

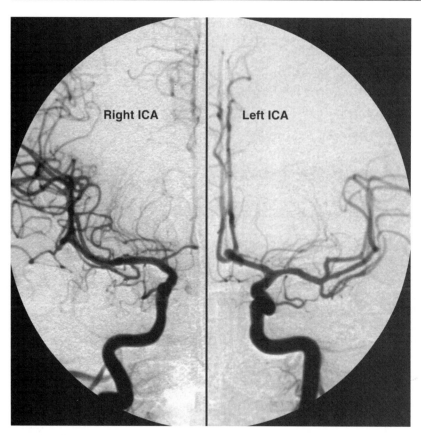

Figure 9.5. A1 asymmetry associated with an aneurysm of the anterior communicating artery complex. Up to 80% of aneurysms in the region of the anterior communicating artery are associated with asymmetry of the A1 segments.

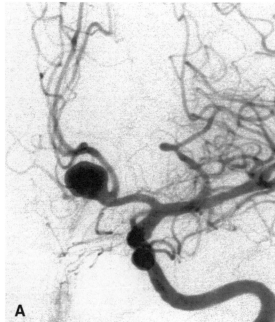
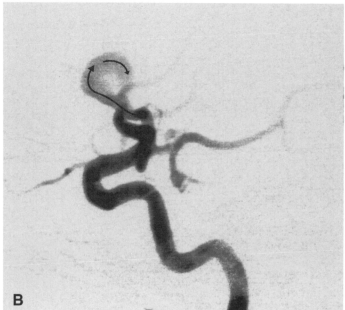
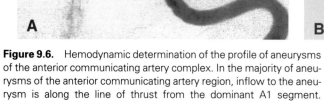

Figure 9.6. Hemodynamic determination of the profile of aneurysms of the anterior communicating artery complex. In the majority of aneurysms of the anterior communicating artery region, inflow to the aneurysm is along the line of thrust from the dominant A1 segment. This, in turn, determines the direction of projection of the aneurysm dome, which in most cases is anterior and towards the opposite side. An early arterial image **(B)** demonstrates the opacified jet as it strikes forward within the aneurysm and is deflected off the dome.

groove. It may supply the territory of the anterior cerebral artery distally (15). Fenestrations of the distal A1 segment, an anomaly that is embryologically difficult to explain in this location, may represent an incomplete fusion of the anterior cerebral artery with the primitive olfactory artery (16) (see Figs. 7.4, 9.2, 9.3).

BRANCHES OF THE PROXIMAL ANTERIOR CEREBRAL ARTERY

Anterior Perforator Vessels

From the A1, proximal A2, and anterior communicating artery, two groups of perforator branches are seen. An inferiorly directed group supplies the optic chiasm and nerve. A superiorly directed group of medial lenticulostriate arteries supplies the anterior hypothalamus, septum pellucidum, the medial part of the anterior commissure, the pillars of the fornix, and the anterior aspect of the striatum (Fig. 9.1). Between 2 and 15 basal arteries arise from the A1 segment, usually from the superior and posterior surfaces, particularly from the lateral half of the A1 segment (3). They enter the anterior perforated substance in the basal forebrain (17). Aneurysms of the A1 segment of the anterior cerebral artery, proximal to the anterior communicating artery, have a high likelihood of being related either to a lenticulostriate origin or cortical branch from this segment of vessel or to a fenestration of the vessel (18).

Anterior communicating artery perforator branches are directed towards the fornix, septal region, anterior cingulum, and corpus callosum (19). Similar to the disposition of the A1 segment, perforators from the anterior communicating artery arise from the postero-superior aspect of the communicating artery. This argues well in terms of surgical risk for aneurysms that project anteroinferiorly rather than those that point posteriorly. Bilobed anterior communicating artery aneurysms, in which one lobe projects posteriorly, warrant specific preoperative consideration due to the difficulty of visualizing the posterior aneurysmal lobe during surgery.

Particular neurologic and psychiatric syndromes have been described when the anterior basal perforators of the anterior cerebral artery-communicating artery complex are compromised by vasospasm or other cause. For example, diminished perfusion of the hypothalamus can result in altered personality, agitation, hypokinesis, and changes in affective state (20, 21).

Recurrent Artery of Heubner

A prominent laterally directed lenticulostriate vessel arising in the region of the anterior communicating artery complex is referred to as the recurrent artery of Heubner (22). It doubles back on the course of its parent vessel. It is directed laterally above the A1 and M1 segments (Figs. 9.7, 9.8). It supplies the anteroinferior portion of the caudate nucleus, anterior limb of the internal capsule, the paraterminal gyrus, and anterior third of putamen (20). It is considered to be an important vessel to identify and preserve during surgery. It arises most often (49–78%) proximally from the A2 segment, or from the anterior communicating artery or A1 segment, or even adjacent cortical branches of the anterior cerebral artery (3, 10, 23). It may occasionally be absent (3%) or duplicated (12%).

Figure 9.7. Inferior frontal AVM supplied by the recurrent artery of Heubner. A tiny AVM nidus along the undersurface of the left anterior perforated substance **(arrowhead)** is opacified by a thin recurrent artery from region of the A1±A2 junction **(arrows).**

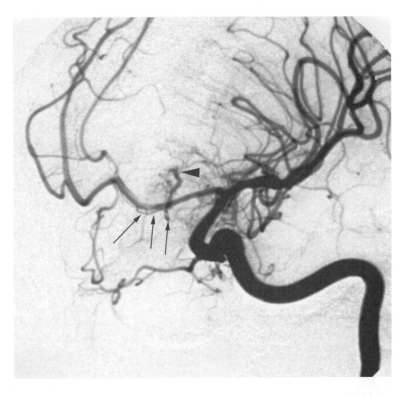

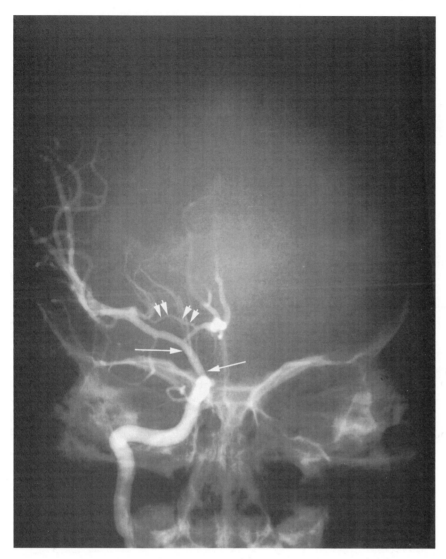

Figure 9.8. Supraclinoid dissection and prominence of the recurrent artery of Heubner. A child recovering from right hemispheric ischemic deficits related to a right supraclinoid carotid dissection. Note the attenuated appearance of the supraclinoid carotid artery and proximal M1 segment **(arrows).** A prominent vessel **(double arrowheads)** from the A1 segment crossing towards the lenticulostriate area probably represents a hyperplastic recurrent artery of Heubner. However, on one view alone, the frontopolar artery of the anterior cerebral artery can simulate such an appearance. The supraclinoid internal carotid artery is a well-recognized site for dissection in children. It may be idiopathic or follow trauma.

Usually it follows a recurrent course along the superior or anterosuperior surface of the A1 segment to which it is attached by arachnoid strands. Less commonly, it may run more posteriorly or within the anterior perforated substance. As it moves laterally, it frequently gives olfactory, frontal, and Sylvian branches and may have a total length along its course of up to 38 mm. It enters the lateral aspect of the anterior perforated substance (i.e., lateral to a sagittal plane described by the olfactory nerve) as a single vessel or with as many as 12 branches. Less commonly, it enters the medial anterior perforated substance. It is thought to represent an important route for preservation of blood flow to the basal ganglia during occlusion of the middle cerebral artery. On the lateral projection, its area of distribution is the anteroinferior portion of the lenticulostriate blush or fan. Because it hugs the course of the A1 segment closely and because of its small size, usually just under 1 mm in diameter, the vessel is not seen as consistently at angiography as it is during surgery. Its preservation is a concern during anterior communicating artery aneurysm clipping. Occlusion of the recurrent artery of Heubner causes a hemiparesis that is most prominent in the upper extremity and face. Despite its proximity, the recurrent artery does not play a significant role in supply of the optic apparatus.

DISTAL ANTERIOR CEREBRAL ARTERY

Aneurysms of the anterior cerebral artery distal to the anterior communicating artery account for approximately 3% of intracranial aneurysms, and most of these occur at the junction of the pericallosal and callosomarginal arteries (24). Post-traumatic pseudoaneurysms of the distal anterior cerebral artery where it crosses the course of the falx cerebri have been described after a shearing motion against the immobile falx (Fig. 9.9).

Early Division of the Distal Anterior Cerebral Artery

Particular angiographic and surgical difficulty may be encountered when an early division of the anterior cerebral artery is present. This results in origin of a duplicated peri-

Figure 9.9. Aneurysms of the distal anterior cerebral artery. A multilobulated aneurysm at the junction of the pericallosal and callosomarginal artery **(arrows in A).** Berry aneurysms of the distal anterior cerebral artery usually occur in this location. When more distal aneurysms are seen **(B),** causes such as trauma or infected emboli should be considered. The aneurysm **(B)** proved fatal in a 43-year-old female with no previous complaints, who collapsed suddenly at work.

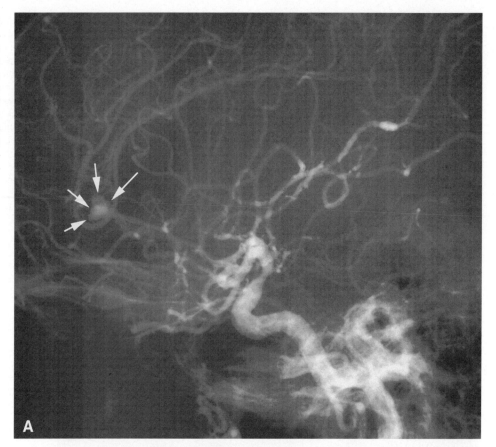

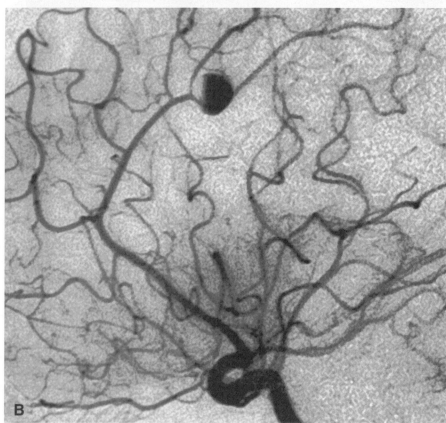

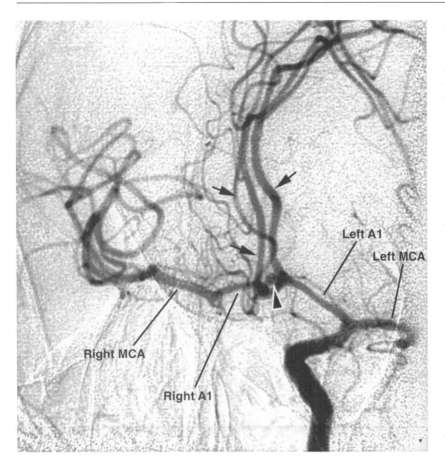

Figure 9.10. *Triplicated A2 configuration.* A left internal carotid artery injection in a 35-year-old male presenting with a Grade II subarachnoid hemorrhage. An aneurysm of the left A1-A2 junction **(arrowhead)** is present. Surgical exploration of the anterior communicating artery complex requires identification of the multiple A2 vessels **(arrows)** emanating from this region.

callosal artery or callosomarginal artery from the immediate region of the anterior cerebral artery-communicating artery complex (Fig. 9.10). This variation is seen in approximately 10% of cases (10). In older publications, an artery of this type was termed the *arteria termatica of Wilder* (25) and was directed along the corpus callosum to the paracentral lobule. A similarly located artery with a distribution more confined to the corpus callosum and lying in the midline is termed the *median artery of the corpus callosum* (26). A large number of variations is possible in terms of which anterior cerebral artery branches may arise proximally. The importance of these vessels is that their presence makes the anatomic and angiographic interrogation of the anterior communicating artery more difficult. It is sometimes impossible to discern between the anterior communicating artery and the pericallosal-callosomarginal junction. The presence of such multiple vessels may also make surgical exploration here extremely difficult.

BRANCHES OF THE DISTAL ANTERIOR CEREBRAL ARTERY

The A2 and more distal segments of the anterior cerebral artery begin at the anterior communicating artery. It extends from the suprachiasmatic cistern to the cistern of the lamina terminalis and curves around the corpus callosum in the sagittal plane. Usually, the anterior cerebral arteries are not side by side here, but rather are staggered in the sag-

ittal plane such that one lies within the concavity of the other. The main trunk of the anterior cerebral artery continues posteriorly as the pericallosal artery in the epicallosal cistern, which gives cortical and callosal branches as it proceeds. Most authors use the term *pericallosal artery* as being synonymous with the anterior cerebral artery distal to the anterior communicating artery. Others prefer to define it as originating at the division of the anterior cerebral artery into pericallosal and calloso-marginal branches. In either event, approximately 18% of hemispheres do not have a definable calloso-marginal branch (4).

The anterior cerebral artery supplies all of the medial aspect of the frontal lobes, most of the anteromedial aspect of the parietal lobes, and a portion of the parasagittal cortex of both lobes, including cortical territories related to motor and sensory functions. Distal anterior cerebral artery occlusion is most prominently associated with contralateral lower extremity weakness or plegia.

BASAL PERFORATING BRANCHES OF THE ANTERIOR CEREBRAL ARTERY

The largest proximal branch of the A2 segment is the recurrent artery of Heubner. Additionally, smaller central perforating branches to the anterior hypothalamus, optic chiasm, lamina terminalis, medial portion of the anterior commissure, and pillars of the fornix may arise distal to the anterior communicating artery. When gathered into a common trunk running in front of the callosal genu, this artery has been termed the *precallosal artery* (4).

Cortical Branches of the Anterior Cerebral Artery

PERICALLOSAL ARTERY

The pericallosal artery ascends under and around the lamina terminalis and genu respectively of the corpus callosum. It passes posteriorly in the cistern of the corpus callosum (Fig. 9.11). Its largest branch is the calloso-marginal artery. The posterior extent of the pericallosal artery holds a balance with the posterior pericallosal branch (artery of the splenium) from the posterior cerebral artery. The course of the pericallosal artery is a useful landmark for the corpus callosum and thus of ventricular size on the lateral view. On the AP view, the positions of all or some segments of the pericallosal artery are indicators of midline shift. The pericallosal sulcus can be seen later in the AP venous phase due to the mustache-like appearance of vessels in the sulcus. The standard descriptions of the pericallosal artery, and its branches categorize them into seven to nine groups.

CALLOSOMARGINAL ARTERY

This is the largest branch of the pericallosal artery. It is defined as a prominent arterial trunk with two or more branches running in the cingulate sulcus. When the callosomarginal artery is not defineable as a distinct trunk, its substituent branches emanate separately from the pericallosal artery. Because it lies higher than the pericallosal artery, the callosomarginal artery crosses the falx cerebri at a more anterior point. The angiographic ramification from this distinction is that the callosomarginal artery is less susceptible to midline shift than the more impressionable pericallosal artery. Moreover, an anterior cerebral artery with bihemispheric supply is most likely to cross the midline via the pericallosal artery than via the calloso-marginal artery. On images precisely aligned in the AP plane, distinguishing between the pericallosal and calloso-marginal arteries can be difficult. Sometimes, the calloso-marginal artery has a more lateral position due to its insinuation into the cingulate sulcus.

ORBITOFRONTAL ARTERY

This is the first cortical branch of the A2 segment and lies close to the midline running anteriorly along the floor of the anterior cranial fossa. It may arise as a common trunk with the frontopolar artery. It may occasionally arise from the A1 segment. The orbitofrontal artery passes down and forward to the level of the planum sphenoidale. In this position, on the lateral angiogram, it can lie on a plane lower than that of the distal ophthalmic artery causing some confusion. It supplies the gyrus rectus, olfactory bulb, and the medial aspect of the orbital surface of the frontal lobe. There may be more than one such vessel present per hemisphere (4).

FRONTOPOLAR ARTERY

This branch usually arises proximal to the origin of the callosomarginal artery, or it may share a common trunk. The frontopolar artery is initially directed anteriorly and superiorly along the medial aspect of the frontal lobe. Then it courses more laterally to supply the medial and lateral aspects of the superior frontal gyrus. The angiographic significance of this vessel is that it is slightly laterally directed. Thus on slightly obliqued AP views, it may be superimposed upon and confused with posterior vessels such as the anterior choroidal or posterior cerebral artery. On more steep ipsilateral anterior oblique views, the frontopolar artery may be superimposed on the contralateral hemisphere and be confused with contralateral branches filled through the anterior communicating artery. On the AP view, its course may appear to parallel the ipsilateral A1 and M1 segments, and it may thus be misinterpreted as Heubner's artery.

INTERNAL FRONTAL BRANCHES

These vessels are named according to which frontal branches are supplying the anterior, middle, or posterior third of the superior frontal gyrus. Their territory extends back as far as the paracentral lobule. They frequently arise as a common trunk. Alternatively, two branches may share a common trunk from the pericallosal artery, and a third may arise from the calloso-marginal artery.

PARACENTRAL ARTERY

This artery may arise in a common trunk with either the posterior internal frontal artery or the superior parietal branch. It is usually seen approximately half-way between the genu and splenium of the corpus callosum arising from either the pericallosal artery or the calloso-marginal artery. It usually courses anterior to the marginal ramus of the cingulate sulcus, and then turns superiorly to supply the paracentral lobule.

INTERNAL PARIETAL ARTERIES

The superior internal parietal artery is the last major branch of the pericallosal artery. Its territory includes virtually all of the precuneus. It anastomoses posteriorly with the parieto-occipital branch of the posterior cerebral artery.

The inferior internal parietal artery is the least consistently present cortical branch of the anterior cerebral artery. It is present in approximately 64% of hemispheres.

CALLOSAL ARTERIES OF THE ANTERIOR CEREBRAL ARTERY

Small perforating branches of the pericallosal artery are directed towards the corpus callosum (27). These usually take the form of ''short callosal arteries.'' Up to 20 such vessels per hemisphere may be present. They traverse the corpus callosum to supply the septum pellucidum, anterior pillars of the fornix, and the anterior commissure.

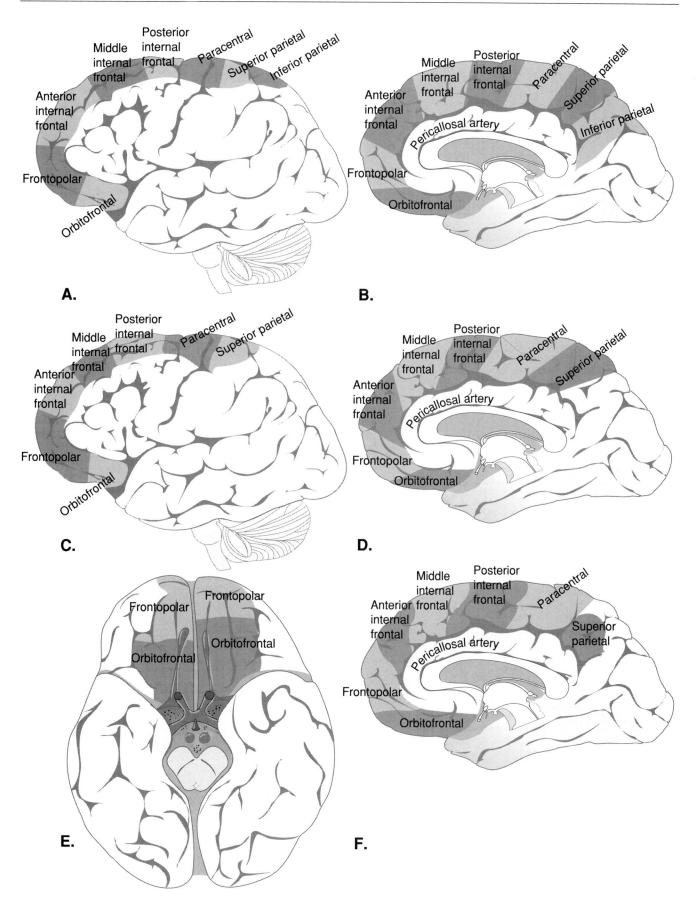

Figure 9.11. Named cortical territories of the anterior cerebral artery. The most typically named branches of the anterior cerebral artery are indicated.

"Long callosal arteries" may be seen which supply the corpus callosum, adjacent cortex, and septal structures. This artery or arteries may sometimes be called the *median artery of the corpus callosum.*

POSTERIOR PERICALLOSAL ARTERY

More posteriorly, the pericallosal artery anastomoses around the splenium of the corpus callosum with the perisplenial branches of the posterior cerebral artery. When this collateral route from anterior to posterior is innately dominant, or becomes so due to pathologic conditions, filling of the medial posterior choroidal area and supply

to the fornix can be seen from the pericallosal artery. Its territory may occasionally extend around the splenium to supply the foramen of Monro. Alternatively, in the setting of anterior occlusive disease, the perisplenial anastomoses become a prominent source of collateral flow to the distal anterior cerebral artery from the posterior cerebral artery.

The anterior cerebral artery may therefore supply the choroidal area in the presence of hypervascular lesions of the third and lateral ventricles. The embryologic basis for this relationship is expressed most vividly in the degree to which prominent anterior cerebral artery supply is frequently seen in vascular malformations of the Vein of

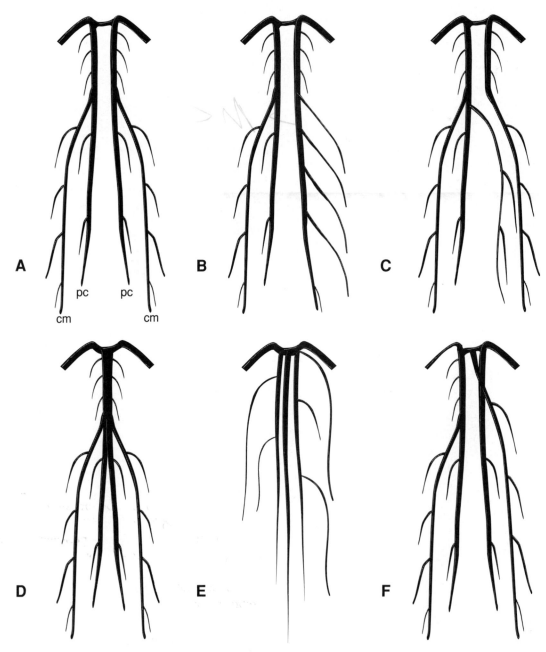

Figure 9.12. *Distal anterior cerebral artery variations.* Schematic illustrations of the range of possible distribution patterns of the distal anterior cerebral arteries are depicted. pc = pericallosal; cm = callosomarginal. Based on Baptista AG. Studies on the arteries of the brain II. The anterior cerebral artery: some anatomic features and their clinical implications. Neurology 1963;13 825±835.

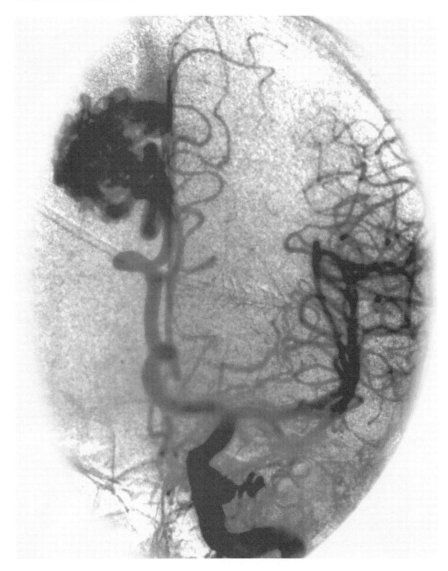

Figure 9.13. Bihemispheric anterior cerebral artery. A left internal carotid artery injection opacifies a right hemispheric AVM. Supply to the AVM is via a right pericallosal branch of the left A2 artery.

Galen (28). In addition to this perisplenial route to the foramen of Monro, anterior cerebral arterial supply may reach this area via perforating hypothalamic branches from the anterior communicating artery and A1 segment.

DURAL BRANCHES OF THE ANTERIOR CEREBRAL ARTERY

Dural supply may be seen from two sources off the anterior cerebral artery. Anteriorly at the cribriform plate, small arteries may cross the dura with the olfactory fibers and anastomose with the ethmoidal arteries. Additionally, the pericallosal artery may give a dural branch to the inferior rim of the falx cerebri, which runs along the course of the inferior sagittal sinus.

VARIATIONS IN THE DISTAL ANTERIOR CEREBRAL ARTERY

Variations of the A2–A4 circulation are common in terms of the degree of bihemispheric supply, which may be pres-

ent from one anterior cerebral artery (Figs. 9.12, 9.13). Using microsurgical techniques, bihemispheric supply can be found in some measure in up to 64% of hemispheres (4), with macroscopically evident bihemispheric supply in 12% (27). An azygous anterior cerebral artery is a rare (0.3%) anomaly, in which only one A2 trunk is present throughout the interhemispheric distribution area (Fig. 9.14). It can be seen in variants of the holoprosencephalic spectrum of congenital disorders. More commonly in situations of bihemispheric supply (29), one anterior cerebral artery will be dominant, and a pericallosal branch of one anterior cerebral artery will have bilateral supply in its distal aspect.

These developmental variants of the distal anterior cerebral artery may be associated with an increased propensity for distal anterior cerebral artery aneurysm formation, particularly at the bifurcation of the pericallosal and callosomarginal arteries. This appears to be especially so for true azygous anterior cerebral artery variants. In a retrospective study of pericallosal aneurysms, which normally

Figure 9.14. Azygous anterior cerebral artery variant.
(A) A left internal carotid artery injection in a patient
with a left middle cerebral artery bifurcation aneurysm
demonstrates prominent cross-flow to the right A1 segment. Only one vessel **(arrowheads)** arises from the
midline to supply both hemispheres. Note the bone
subtraction artifact from having the orbital rims superimposed on the M1 and A1 segments. **(B)** A right internal carotid artery injection in the same patient confirms
the azygous nature of the A2 segment. An internal frontal branch **(double arrow)** arises from the right A1
segment proximal to the midline.

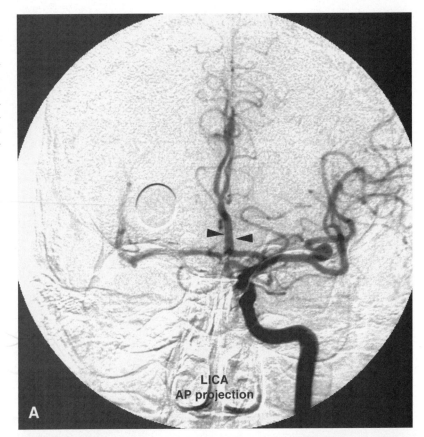

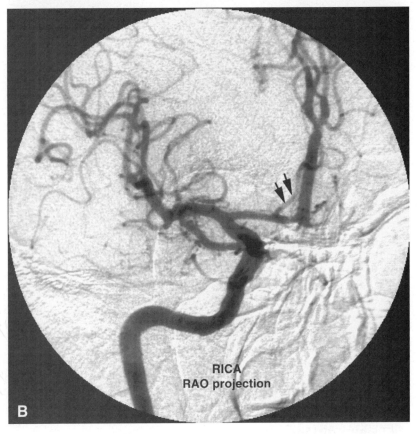

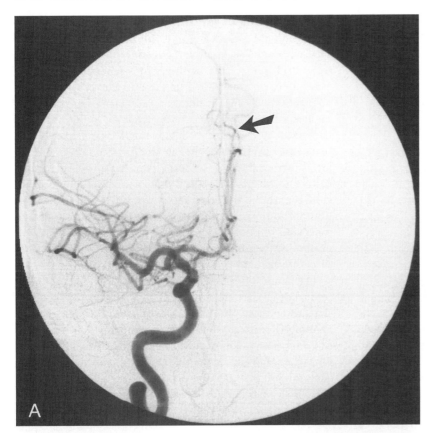

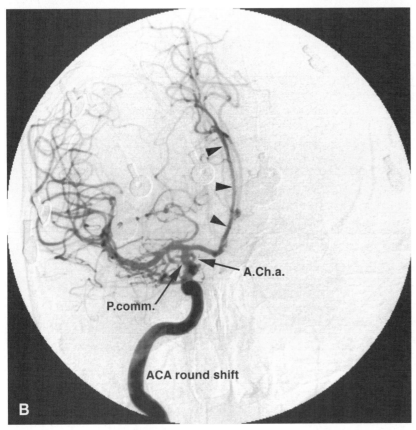

Figure 9.15. *Anterior cerebral artery shift.* **(A)** Midline shift of the anterior cerebral artery to the left is present due to a right hemispheric mass. An abrupt step-like correction (square shift) of the course of the distal anterior cerebral artery is seen at its intersection with the immobile falx cerebri **(arrow). (B)** Round shift of the anterior cerebral artery in a different patient **(arrowheads).** An unusual appearance of vessels is seen behind the internal carotid artery. This is the PA appearance of the variant territory of the anterior choroidal artery (A.Ch.a.) seen in lateral projection on Figure 8.46.

constitute 5% or less of all intracranial berry aneurysms, Huber et al. (30) reported that 25% of such aneurysms occur at the bifurcation of an unpaired pericallosal trunk.

Occasionally, a communication exists between the anterior cerebral arteries near the callosal genu and has been termed the *superior anterior communicating artery* (24, 31).

ANTERIOR CEREBRAL ARTERY SHIFT

The use of cerebral angiography as a primary means for detection of intracranial masses is now of historical interest. However, there are still situations in which a careful analysis of vessel location is of vital interest to surgical planning for a particular patient. An understanding of these phenomena can help prevent misinterpretation of normal variants or obliqued films. Succinctly, angiographic shift of the anterior cerebral artery occurs when mobile median or paramedian structures are displaced. The angiographic signs of shift are analyzed by juxtaposition of the appearance of displaced and fixed structures (Fig. 9.15). The most mobile and, thus, most sensitive paramedian structure is the pericallosal artery. The mobility of the anterior two thirds of this artery relates to the position of the falx cerebri anteriorly. The falx is more remote from the genu of the corpus callosum than it is relative to the splenium posteriorly. Therefore, the pericallosal artery is highly mobile throughout much of its course until it becomes suddenly immobile posteriorly at the point where it crosses the falx. The descriptive categorizations of round, square, or central shift related to the point of maximal impact of mass-effect on the course of the anterior cerebral artery and whether an abrupt step-like deformity of the pericallosal artery could be seen posteriorly at the point of falcine constraint. An understanding of the diffuse effect of such mass-effect should prevent a meandering anterior cerebral artery with relatively smooth turns from being misperceived as displaced. Additionally, a smooth posterior course of the pericallosal artery without a step-like deflection and a normal appearance of the pericallosal venous mustache will help in recognition on oblique films. Gross midline shift will always be accompanied by venous signs of mass-effect.

Interhemispheric masses or collections displace the pericallosal and callosomarginal branches of opposite sides away from one another. The appearance may be asymmetric with a falcine meningioma, which may favor one side. The position of the vessels may also help distinguish between a parasagittal and a falcine meningioma, according to whether the principal displacement is inferiorly (by a parasagittal tumor) or laterally and superiorly (by a falcine mass). With large tumors, the precise location

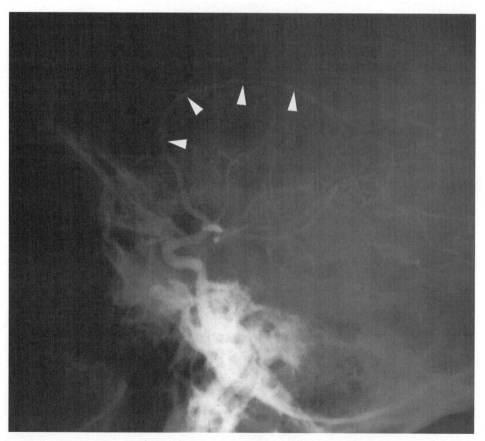

Figure 9.16. *Angiographic appearance of hydrocephalus.*   The pericallosal artery has a taut, stretched appearance **(arrowheads)** due to ventricular dilatation. The patient was a middle-aged female who presented with a tuberculoma of the posterior fossa causing obstructive hydrocephalus.

of critical vessels, which are draped and displaced, should be analyzed before surgery to avoid laceration.

VENTRICULAR DILATATION

The deep venous structures are more sensitive than the arterial to alterations in ventricular volume and early hydrocephalus. With greater degrees of ventricular enlargement, changes in the pericallosal artery become evident. On the lateral projection, the pericallosal artery loses its smooth, undulating appearance and assumes a taut, rounded course displaced superiorly (see Figs. 8.46, 9.16). On the AP projection, branches into the pericallosal sulcus are bowed upwards, and lateral displacement of the lenticulostriate and middle cerebral artery branches is present.

REFERENCES

1. McKissock W, Paine KWE, Walsh LS. An analysis of the results of treatment of ruptured intracranial aneurysms. J Neurosurg 1960;17:762–776.
2. Fischer E. Die Lageabweichungen der vorderen Hirnarterie im Gefässbild. Zentralbl Neurochir 1938;3:300–313.
3. Perlmutter D, Rhoton AL. Microsurgical anatomy of the anterior cerebral-anterior communicating-recurrent artery complex. J Neurosurg 1976;45: 259–272.
4. Perlmutter D, Rhoton AL. Microsurgical anatomy of the distal anterior cerebral artery. J Neurosurg 1978;49:204–228.
5. Friedlander RM, Ogilvy CS. Aneurysmal subarachnoid hemorrhage in a patient with bilateral A1 fenestrations associated with an azygous anterior cerebral artery. Case report and literature review. J Neurosurg 1996;84:681–684.
6. Klein SI, Gahbauer H, Goodrich I. Bilateral anomalous anterior cerebral artery and infraoptic aneurysm. Am J Neuroradiol 1987;8:1142–1143.
7. Fujimoto S, Murakami M. Anomalous branch of the internal carotid artery supplying circulation of the anterior cerebral artery: case report. J Neurosurg 1983;58:941–946.
8. Mäurer J, Mäurer E, Perneczky A. Surgically verified variations in the A1 segment of the anterior cerebral artery. J Neurosurg 1991;75:950–953.
9. Alpers BJ, Berry RG, Paddison RM. Anatomical studies of the circle of Willis in normal brains. Arch Neurol Psychiatr (Chicago) 1959;81:409–418.
10. Nathal E, Yasui N, Sampei T, et al. Intraoperative anatomical studies in patients with aneurysms of the anterior communicating artery complex. J Neurosurg 1992;76:629–634.
11. Wilson G, Riggs HE, Rupp C. The pathologic anatomy of ruptures cerebral aneurysms. J Neurosurg 1954;11:128–134.
12. VanderArk GD, Kempe LC. Classification of anterior communicating aneurysms as a basis for surgical approach. J Neurosurg 1970;32:300–303.
13. Gomes FB, Dujovny M, Umansky F, et al. Microanatomy of the anterior cerebral artery. Surg Neurol 1986;26:65–69.
14. Fisher CM. The circle of Willis: Anatomical variations. Vasc Dis 1965;2: 99–105.
15. Tsuji T, Abe M, Tabuchi K. Aneurysm of a persistent primitive olfactory artery. Case report. J Neurosurg 1995:83:138–140.
16. Minakawa T, Kawamata M, Hayano M, et al. Aneurysms associated with fenestrated anterior cerebral arteries: report of four cases and review of the literature. Surg Neurol 1985;24: 284–288.
17. Rosner SS, Rhoton AL, Ono M, et al. Microsurgical anatomy of the anterior perforating arteries. J Neurosurg 1984;61:468–485.
18. Suzuki M, Onuma T, Sakurai Y, et al. Aneurysms arising from the proximal (A1) segment of the anterior cerebral artery. J Neurosurg 1992;76:455–458.
19. Dunker RO, Harris AB. Surgical Anatomy of the proximal anterior cerebral artery. J Neurosurg 1976;44:359–367.
20. Ostrowski AZ, Webster JE, Gurdjian ES. The proximal anterior cerebral artery; an anatomical study. Arch Neurol 1960;3: 661–664.
21. Webster JE, Gurdjian ES, Lindner DW. Proximal occlusion of the anterior cerebral artery. Arch Neurol 1960;2:19–26.
22. Heubner O. Zur Topographie der Ernahrungsgebrete der eizelnen Hirnarterien. Zentralb Med Wissen 1872;10:816–821.
23. Gomes F, Dujovny M, Umansky F, et al. Microsurgical anatomy of the recurrent artery of Heubner. J Neurosurg 1984;60: 130–139.
24. Yasargil MG, Carter LP. Saccular aneurysms of the distal anterior cerebral artery. J Neurosurg 1974;40:218–223.
25. Critchley M. The anterior cerebral artery and its syndromes. Brain 1930;53:120–165.
26. De Vriese B. Sur la Signification morphologique des artères cérébrales. Archives de Biologie 1905:21:357–455.
27. Baptista AG. Studies on the arteries of the Brain II. The anterior cerebral artery: some anatomic features and their clinical implications. Neurology 1963;13:825–835.
28. Mullan S, Mojtahedi S, Johnson DL, et al. Embryological basis of some aspects of cerebral vascular fistulas and malformations. J Neurosurg 1996;85:1-8.
29. Moniz E. Die Cerebral Arteriographie und Phlebographie. Berlin: Springer-Verlag, 1940:413.
30. Huber P, Braun J, Hirschmann D, et al. Incidence of berry aneurysms of the unpaired pericallosal artery: Angiographic study. Neuroradiology 1980;19:143–147.
31. Laitinen L, Snellman A. Aneurysms of the pericallosal artery. A study of 14 cases verified angiographically and treated mainly by direct surgical attack. J Neurosurg 1960;17:447–458

CHAPTER 10

The Middle Cerebral Artery

The vascular territory of the middle cerebral artery includes some of the most eloquent cortical areas for motor and sensory function. It covers the receptive and expressive components of language, abstract thought, and other faculties of higher cognitive functioning. Additionally, perforating branches of the proximal middle cerebral artery supply the basal ganglia and important descending and corticospinal tracts.

SEGMENTAL ANATOMY OF THE MIDDLE CEREBRAL ARTERY

The M1 (horizontal/sphenoidal) segment of the middle cerebral artery extends from the bifurcation of the internal carotid artery to the limen insulae, where the middle cerebral artery makes a turn or genu superiorly into the insula (Fig. 10.1). The M2 (insular) segment extends from the genu to the circular sulcus of the insula, and the M3 (opercular) extends from the circular sulcus to the opercular turn of the middle cerebral artery branches. The M4 (cortical) segments are those visible on the lateral convexity of the hemisphere (1, 2).

The middle cerebral artery divides in the majority of hemispheres proximal to the genu, and strictly speaking, the M1 segment therefore should have a prebifurcation and a postbifurcation segment. However, clinical use of the term M1 usually implies the segment of the middle cerebral artery proximal to the main division. The *M1-M2 junction* is taken to be synonymous with the main division point.

BRANCHING PATTERNS OF THE MIDDLE CEREBRAL ARTERY

The middle cerebral artery can divide in up to four described patterns: a single trunk with no main division, a bifurcation, a trifurcation, or a quadrifurcation. Of these, the most common is a bifurcation pattern seen in 64–90% of hemispheres (2– 4). Most neurology literature presupposes this pattern (5), and the terminology of "superior" and "inferior" divisions of the middle cerebral artery is in ubiquitous clinical use. A trifurcation pattern may be seen in 12–29% of hemispheres, with other patterns being less common.

Variability within the bifurcation pattern can be evident at microanatomical examination and in the clinical syndromes associated with a division occlusion. It is slightly more common (32%) for the inferior division to be "dominant," covering a more extensive cortical area than the superior division. The superior division is dominant in 28% of hemispheres (Fig. 10.2). Balanced division is seen in approximately 18% of hemispheres (2), in which cases, the superior division spans the orbitofrontal to the posterior parietal areas. When the inferior division is dominant, it covers the temporal and parietal lobes, with the superior division confined to the frontal lobe. When the superior division is dominant its territory may extend as far posteriorly as the angular or temporo-occipital regions. These configurations have clinical relevance. In the dominant hemisphere, the clinical syndrome of a dominant superior division occlusion might include parietal lobe signs such as finger-agnosia, Gerstmann's syndrome of left-right disorientation, acalculia, agraphia, hemineglect, and impairment of discriminative sensation.

PERFORATING BRANCHES

The middle cerebral artery passes laterally from the internal carotid artery bifurcation to the Sylvian fissure. It makes a 90 genu around the falciform curve of the limen insulae as it turns into the insular segment. The trunk of the middle cerebral artery arises under the anterior perforated substance, lateral to the optic chiasm, and behind the division of the olfactory tract. As it proceeds laterally towards the limen insulae, the middle cerebral artery gives off a number of branches that penetrate the base of brain lying immediately above.

The anterior perforated substance is the flat surface at the base of the brain bound medially by the interhemispheric fissure, laterally by the limen insulae, anteriorly by the division of the olfactory tract into the medial and lateral olfactory striae, and posteriorly by the optic tract and temporal lobe (see Fig. 7.3). It is divided along the sagittal plane into medial and lateral components by a line drawn posteriorly from the axis of the olfactory tract (6). This line divides the medial from the lateral anterior perforator or lenticulostriate vessels, which penetrate the perforated substance.

There are between 1 and 21 lenticulostriate branches per hemisphere, with an average of 10 (6–8). Approximately 80% arise usually from the postero-superior aspect of the artery proximal to the middle cerebral artery division. The remainder arise from the proximal branches of the middle cerebral artery, particularly from the superior division. When the recurrent artery of Heubner is large, the number of lenticulostriate branches may be reduced.

The lateral lenticulostriate arteries have a slightly larger

Figure 10.1. *Segmental anatomy of the middle cerebral artery.* The segmental anatomy of the middle cerebral artery is illustrated. Although the M1 segment was originally defined as extending from the carotid bifurcation to the limen insulae, in clinical parlance the term M1 is most frequently applied to the mainstem of the middle cerebral artery extending to the principal division.

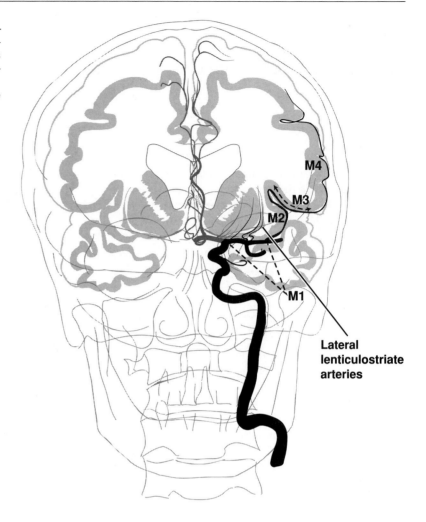

Lateral lenticulostriate arteries

diameter than the medial group. The lateral group in particular describes a recurrent curve before entering the anterior perforated substance. The lateral lenticulostriate arteries arise from the M1 or M2 segments of the middle cerebral artery. On AP projection, they have an S (on the right side) or reverse S (on the left side) shape. From their origin, they follow a sharp posterior and medial turn in the cisternal segment to assume a more lateral curve as they enter the anterior perforated substance. Here they course initially around the lateral aspect of the putamen and fan out to give an important supply to the lateral aspect of the anterior commissure, internal capsule, dorsal aspect of the head of caudate nucleus, putamen, lateral globus pallidus, and substantia innominata. Blood supply to more lateral structures including the claustrum and external capsule derives from insular branches.

More than 70% of all aneurysms of the middle cerebral artery occur at its division. Aneurysms of the M1 trunk of the middle cerebral artery represent 10% of all aneurysms of this artery. They tend to arise either from the superior wall of the artery, in which case they are associated with the lenticulostriate arteries, or from the inferior surface, i.e., associated with the anterior temporal branches (9) (Fig. 10.3).

CORTICAL BRANCHES OF THE MIDDLE CEREBRAL ARTERY

The insula is a fan-shaped area of cortex obscured from lateral view by the frontal, temporal, and parietal opercula. Seen in coronal section it has a laterally convex aspect and is higher posteriorly. At the lowest point of the fan is the limen insulae, from which the sulci and gyri of the insula radiate superiorly and posteriorly. In correspondence with these sulci, the branches of the middle cerebral artery extend until their course is deflected by the circular sulcus or sulcus limitans of Reil. Within the sulcus limitans or circular sulcus, the middle cerebral artery branches change direction 180 and curve around the operculum. They then undergo another 180 turn to start coursing along the surface of the cerebral convexity. The frontal branches of the M2 segments have a shorter insular course than the posterior frontal and parietal branches. The appearance on the lateral projection of the middle cerebral artery branches within the insula turning in the sulcus limitans describes a straight line. This line forms the base of an upturned triangle with the limen insulae at its apex, termed the *Sylvian triangle* (Fig. 10.4). The highest angiographic point posteriorly in this triangle is the Sylvian

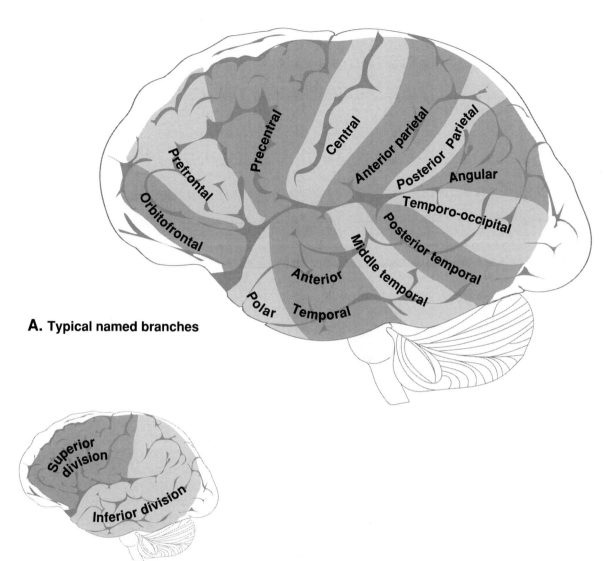

A. Typical named branches

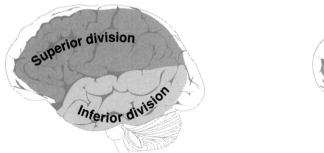

B. Inferior division dominant (32%)

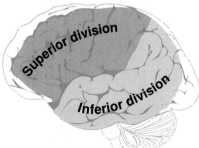

C. Superior division dominant (28%)

D. Equal bifurcation (18%)

Figure 10.2. *Branching pattern of the middle cerebral artery.* The most commonly named branches of the middle cerebral artery and division patterns are illustrated. Compare with lesser and greater extremes of middle cerebral artery territory in Figure 7.10.

Figure 10.3. *Left middle cerebral artery aneurysm.* A PA view **(A)** of a left middle cerebral artery aneurysm demonstrates that its neck appears to be related to a division of the middle cerebral artery **(arrow).** A shallow LAO view **(B)** demonstrates a similar relationship between the aneurysm and this vessel. However, careful windowing shows that the vessel origin is not related to the aneurysm neck **(C).** The middle cerebral artery branch merely projects behind the aneurysm dome. Presurgical analysis of middle cerebral artery aneurysms in particular is important with reference to warning the surgeon whether any vessel arises from the aneurysm.

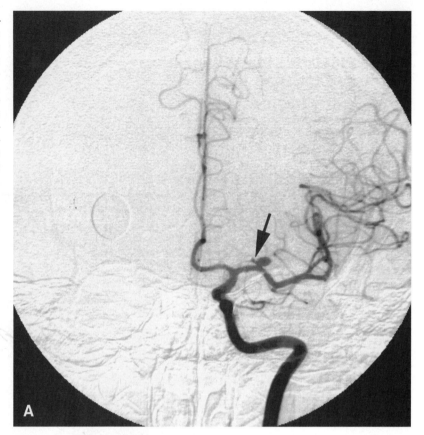

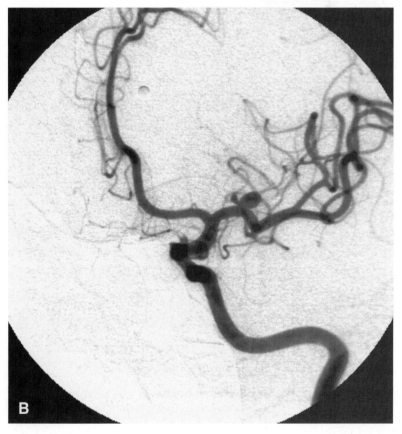

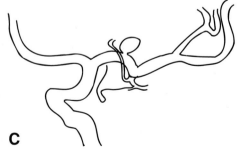

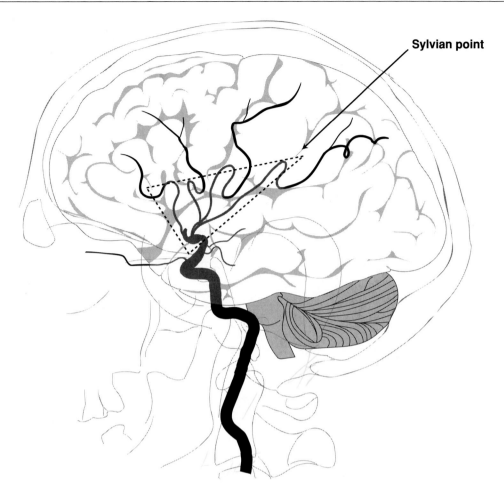

Sylvian point

Figure 10.4. *Sylvian triangle.* The angiographic appearance of the Sylvian triangle is created by deflection of the buried insular branches of the middle cerebral artery by the sulcus limitans to a course that brings them around the opercula to the cerebral convexities. The course of each individual vessel is then made more tortuous by undulation into sulci and over gyri along its course.

point. These angiographic phenomena were used for detection and description of middle cerebral artery shift and mass-effect. An understanding of the route taken by each middle cerebral branch is still valuable, however, in understanding the anatomy of the middle cerebral artery and identifying its individual branches.

The cortical branches of the middle cerebral artery supply most of the lateral convexity of the cerebral hemisphere, the insular and opercular cortex, the lateral part of the orbital surface of the frontal lobe, and the lateral inferior surface of the temporal lobe anteriorly. The border region between the distribution of the middle cerebral artery and the adjacent cerebral arteries is termed the *watershed zone,* meaning that it is at the interface of different circulations. This region is therefore most at risk when conditions of hypoperfusion exist, such as might be due to proximal occlusive disease or systemic hypotension. *Shift of the watershed zone* is an angiographic observation due to adaptive changes in the cerebral circulation when the interface between two territories moves to compensate for a state of hypoperfusion in one territory. It is often most clearly demonstrated

in the presence of chronic adaptation. It may be seen in occlusive disease with proximal thromboembolic or atherosclerotic obstruction of flow. Alternatively, it may be seen in the presence of a high-flow arteriovenous malformation in one territory creating a sump-effect such that the territory of the neighboring vessel becomes extended. This can sometimes generate an angiographic appearance of bizarre-appearing vessels that are tortuous and enlarged. This adaptive response of vessels neighboring an arteriovenous malformation has been termed *angiomatous change.* When interpreting an arteriovenous malformation, it is important to realize that such hemodynamic changes in the adjacent vessels are merely adaptive. These vessels are not part of the arteriovenous malformation nidus. Approximately 10–12 named cortical branches of the middle cerebral artery are described, with much variability (Fig. 10.2). They may arise as common trunks. Particular named branches may not be individually identifiable in every patient. The largest branches, and thus those most useful when an external to internal carotid bypass procedure is performed, are usually the angular (3) or the temporo-occipital branches (2, 10).

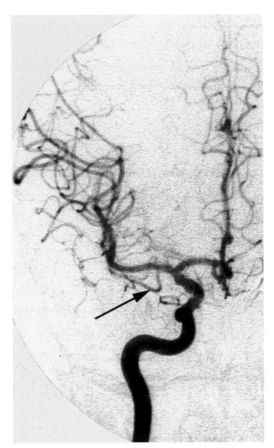

Figure 10.5. *Anterior temporal branch.* A typical appearance of an anterior temporal branch of the middle cerebral artery proximal to the main bifurcation is indicated with the arrow.

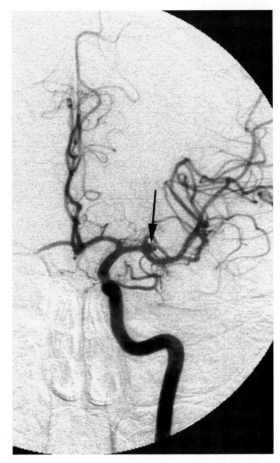

Figure 10.6. *Middle cerebral artery trifurcation pattern.* In contrast to Figure 10.5, the middle cerebral artery in this patient has a short mainstem ending in a trifurcation where an unruptured aneurysm **(arrow)** is identified. More views to establish the profile of the aneurysm in reference to the middle cerebral artery branches would usually be obtained.

Anterior Temporal Branch

This may arise as a separate branch from the horizontal portion of the M1 (Fig. 10.5), share a common trunk with the orbitofrontal branch, or may arise as part of a middle cerebral artery trifurcation (Fig. 10.6). When a middle cerebral artery bifurcation is present, this vessel usually belongs to the inferior division.

The anterior temporal branch is usually a small vessel, approximately 1 mm in diameter. When it arises from the M1 segment proximal to the main division, it can be seen easily on the AP view because it is not as likely to be superimposed on other middle cerebral artery branches. It supplies the anterior portion of the temporal pole with a variable degree of supply to the lateral aspect of the anterior temporal lobe.

Orbitofrontal Artery

This vessel supplies the middle and inferior frontal gyri and part of the pars orbitalis.

The lateral or superficial appearance of the Sylvian fissure is described as having a main sulcal stem and a number of rami or arms. The anterior ascending ramus of the superficial aspect of the Sylvian fissure separates the pars triangularis of the inferior frontal gyrus from the pars

opercularis. The anterior horizontal ramus separates the pars orbitalis from the pars triangularis (see Fig. 7.1).

The orbitofrontal branch of the middle cerebral artery runs most frequently in the anterior horizontal ramus. The bulge of the pars triangularis then pushes the next group of operculofrontal branches, sometimes called the *candelabra group,* back into the anterior ascending ramus.

Prefrontal Artery and Precentral Artery

The appearance of these vessels on the lateral projection has been likened to that of a candelabra. These branches supply a large area of the frontal lobes, including Broca's speech area, the frontal eye fields, and the premotor strip.

The prefrontal artery supplies a large part of the middle frontal gyrus and the opercular part of the inferior frontal gyrus. It also covers the superior part of the pars orbitalis and the pars opercularis.

The precentral artery covers the posterior aspect of the frontal candelabra group. It supplies part of the inferior frontal gyrus, the middle frontal gyrus, and the lower part of the precentral gyrus.

Central or Rolandic Arteries

More than one artery to the area of the central sulcus and motor strip may be present. These arteries have variable supply to the precentral and postcentral gyri.

Anterior and Posterior Parietal Arteries

These are best identified by first defining the Rolandic and angular branches, which are more prominent. The parietal branches lie between the two groups. They can arise from either a superior or inferior division in the context of a middle cerebral artery bifurcation. They supply part of the parietal convexity including the supramarginal gyrus, the anterior parietal lobule, the cortex adjacent to the upper part of the central sulcus, and the inferior parietal lobule.

Angular Artery

This is a large, posteriorly directed branch of the middle cerebral artery running over the posterior aspect of the superior temporal gyrus. Its territory also includes the angular gyrus, supramarginal gyrus, and the occipital convexity. The angular branch is usually one of the most easily

identified on the lateral angiogram. The angular gyrus of the parietal lobe straddles the posterior extent of the superior temporal sulcus. The supramarginal gyrus similarly corresponds to the posterior reach of the Sylvian fissure. Lesions in these loci have specific clinical syndromic correlates. Infarctions of the dominant supramarginal gyrus are associated with ideomotor apraxia. Infarctions of the angular gyrus of the dominant lobe are associated with alexia and agraphia.

Temporal Arteries

These constitute the temporo-occipital, posterior temporal, middle temporal, anterior temporal, and temporopolar arteries. The temporo-occipital artery is frequently large enough to use for bypass procedures. It supplies the posterior aspects of the superior, middle, and inferior temporal gyri, and the lateral occipital gyri.

ANOMALIES OF THE MIDDLE CEREBRAL ARTERY

Anomalies of the middle cerebral artery are more rare than those of the other intracranial vessels. They are seen in approximately 0.6–3% of dissected hemispheres in microanatomical studies (2, 3, 4, 11), but less commonly dur-

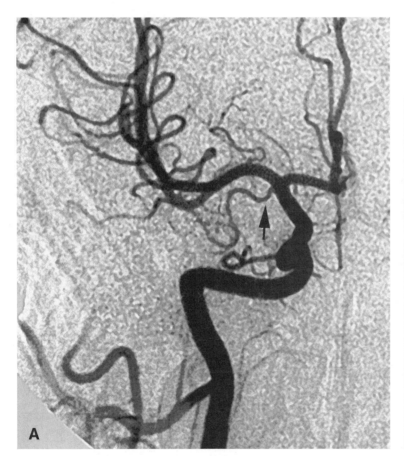

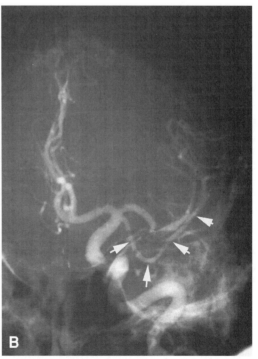

Figure 10.7. *Duplicated middle cerebral arteries.* **(A)** A temporal branch of the right middle cerebral artery territory **(arrow)** has its origin from the supraclinoid internal carotid artery, distinguishing this vessel as a duplicated middle cerebral artery. An incidental finding in this patient, it would, however, be important to clarify such an anomalous finding with the surgeon if treatment of an adjacent aneurysm were contemplated. **(B)** A similar anomaly is seen **(arrows)** from the left internal carotid artery in this different patient.

Figure 10.8. *Accessory middle cerebral artery.* In this patient, an anomalous vessel **(arrows)** to the middle cerebral artery territory arises from the A1-A2 region, qualifying this vessel as an accessory middle cerebral artery. However, some authors would argue this vessel is only a hyperplastic variant of the recurrent artery of Heubner.

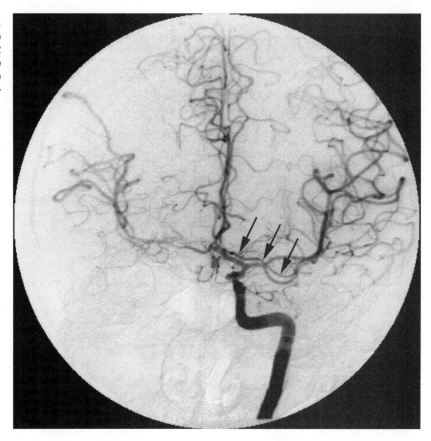

ing angiography (12). Anomalies of the middle cerebral artery usually consist in either:

- A duplicated middle cerebral artery rising from the internal carotid artery
- An accessory middle cerebral artery from the anterior cerebral artery (see Figs. 7.6, 10.7, 10.8).

Many authors consider that these anomalous vessels may be prone to aneurysm formation (13–15). The nature and nomenclature of these anomalous vessels is debated. Although the accessory middle cerebral artery may have lenticulostriate branches, it is distinguished by some authors from a recurrent artery of Heubner by the fact that it has a predominantly cortical distribution. Moreover, it has been seen during dissections to be distinct from or even give provenance to Heubner's artery (4).

Grand (7) suggested that a middle cerebral artery duplication arising from the internal carotid artery probably only represents a very proximal origin of a middle cerebral artery anterior temporal branch in most instances. Van der Zwan et al. (16–18) have demonstrated the enormous variability of the cortical and white matter distribution of the cerebral arteries. This would argue that a territory typically associated with the middle cerebral artery might occasionally be supplied by the anterior cerebral artery. Alternatively, Takahashi et al. (19) have reviewed 14 cases of accessory middle cerebral arteries and consider the vessel to be most clearly understood as a variant of the recurrent artery of Heubner.

REFERENCES

1. Fischer E. Die Lageabweichungen der vorderen Hirnarterie im Gefässbild. Zentralbl Neurochir 1938;3:300–313.
2. Gibo H, Carver CC, Rhoton AL, et al. Microsurgical anatomy of the middle cerebral artery. J Neurosurg 1981;54:151–169.
3. Umansky F, Juarez SM, Dujovy, et al. Microsurgical anatomy of the proximal segments of the middle cerebral artery. J Neurosurg 1984;61:458–467.
4. Jain KK. Some observations on the anatomy of the middle cerebral artery. Can J Surg 1964;7:134–139.
5. Fisher CM. Clinical Syndromes in cerebral thrombosis, hypertensive hemorrhage, and ruptured saccular aneurysms. Clin Neurosurg 1975;22:117–147.
6. Rosner SS, Rhoton AL, Ono M, et al. Microsurgical anatomy of the anterior perforating arteries. J Neurosurg 1984;61:468–485.
7. Grand W. Microsurgical anatomy of the proximal middle cerebral artery and internal carotid artery bifurcation. Neurosurgery 1980;7:215–218.
8. Umansky F, Gomes FB, Dujovny M, et al. The perforating branches of the middle cerebral artery. A microanatomical study. J Neurosurg 1985;62:261–268.
9. Hosoda K, Fujita S, Kawaguchi T, et al. Saccular aneurysms of the proximal (M1) segment of the middle cerebral artery. Neurosurgery 1995;36:441–446.
10. Chater N, Spetzler R, Tonnemacher K, et al. Microvascular bypass surgery. Part I: Anatomical studies. J Neurosurg 1976;44:712–714.
11. Crompton MR, Lond MB. Pathology of ruptured middle cerebral aneurysms with special reference to differences between sexes. Lancet 1962;2:421–425.
12. Teal JS, Rumbaugh CL, Bergeron T, et al. Anomalies of the

middle cerebral artery: Accessory artery, duplication, and early bifurcation. Am J Radiol 1973;118:567–575.

13. Stabler J. Two cases of accessory middle cerebral artery: including one with aneurysm at its origin. Br J Radiol 1970;43:314–318

14. Tacconi L, Johnston FG, Symon L. Accessory middle cerebral artery. J Neurosurg 1995;83:916–918.

15. Takahashi T, Suzuki S, Ohkuma H, et al. Aneurysms of a duplication of the middle cerebral artery. Am J Neuroradiol 1994; 15:1166–1168.

16. van der Zwan A, Hillen B, Tulleken CAF, et al. Variability of the territories of the major cerebral arteries. J Neurosurg 1992; 77:927–940.

17. Van der Zwan A, Hillen B, Tulleken CAF, et al. A quantitative investigation of the variability of the major cerebral arterial territories. Stroke 1993;24:1951–1959.

18. van der Zwan A, Hillen B. Review of the variability of the territories of the major cerebral arteries. Stroke 1991;22:1078–1084.

19. Takahashi S, Hoshino F, Uemura K, et al. Accessory middle cerebral artery: is it a variant form of the recurrent artery of Heubner? Am J Neuroradiol 1989;10:563–568.

CHAPTER 11

The Posterior Cerebral Artery

The embryologic origin of the posterior cerebral artery is from the internal carotid artery, but by the time of full development, the dominant supply to the posterior cerebral artery is usually from the basilar artery (1). A *fetal posterior communicating artery* configuration implies origin of posterior cerebral artery flow from the internal carotid artery. Some authors use this term when the major tributary of posterior cerebral artery flow is from the internal carotid artery; others reserve this term for exclusive origin of posterior cerebral artery flow from the internal carotid artery.

The posterior cerebral artery serves the posterior cerebral hemisphere, thalamus, midbrain, and structures in the walls of the third ventricle and choroidal fissure. Vascular injury to the posterior cerebral artery or its branches causes a range of debilitating deficits, of which the most severe are those related to the realm of vision. These include functions of a higher order for cortical and subcortical integration of visual perception, interhemispheric integration of visual fields, and relay of visual information to the visual association cortex. Ocular functions served by the posterior cerebral artery include many aspects of eye movement, pupillary reflexes, and eye coordination. Other sites of injury to the posterior cerebral artery may result in devastating neurologic syndromes related to thalamic infarction. Other deficits relate to disruption of afferent pathways in the medial lemniscus and of efferent pathways in the corticospinal tracts. Alterations in levels of arousal and consciousness occur with involvement of the midbrain reticular activating system; memory and endocrine disturbances occur with involvement of the hippocampal and hypothalamic vascular supply. Difficulties in surgical access to the proximal posterior cerebral artery and basilar artery tip, combined with the gravity of these syndromic deficits, make the proximal posterior cerebral artery a surgical site approached with some trepidation.

SEGMENTAL NOMENCLATURE

Various short-hand schemes for segmental description of the posterior cerebral artery have been proposed, two of which are most commonly used. A descriptive scheme (2) identifies:

• The *peduncular segment* as that part coursing around the peduncle and bisected by the posterior communicating artery
• The *ambient segment* lying between the midbrain and the hippocampal gyrus
• The *quadrigeminal segment* running in the cistern of that name

More commonly, a symbolic scheme is used (3–5), wherein the P1 segment extends from the basilar tip to the posterior communicating artery insertion, the P2 segment extends from there to the back of the midbrain, and the P3 segment runs through the lateral aspect of the quadrigeminal cistern around the pulvinar and divides into named branches at the anterior end of the calcarine fissure. The patterns of the proximal branches of the posterior cerebral artery vary and cannot always be exclusively assigned to one segment or another.

HERNIATION THROUGH THE TENTORIAL INCISURA

As the posterior cerebral artery and some of its circumflex branches curve around the midbrain, they course parallel and inferior to the basal vein of Rosenthal and to the geniculate bodies. The posterior cerebral artery is separated from the superior cerebellar artery below by the oculomotor nerve medially and the trochlear nerve laterally. Its usual position is superomedial to the tentorium. In the setting of severe asymmetric mass-effect or temporal lobe herniation, the midbrain may become compressed against the tentorium. This causes a classically described indentation in the midbrain contralateral to the mass-effect, Kernohan's notch (6), with an occlusion of the interposed posterior cerebral artery or its branches. Therefore, the clinical phenomenon of a "false localizing sign" occurs with hemiparesis ipsilateral to the side of the tumor or mass-lesion. In addition to occlusion of the contralateral posterior cerebral artery by compression between the midbrain and tentorium, occlusion of the posterior cerebral artery ipsilateral to the side of mass-effect may occur too. This can happen when this vessel or its branches are stretched around the tentorial edge.

Positional variations of the posterior cerebral artery, the superior cerebellar artery, and their branches within the tentorial incisura in relationship to the tentorial edge determine where the impact of tentorial compression or stretching of vessels is most critical (Fig. 11.1) (7, 8). Posterior cerebral arteries with a distal branching pattern experience a compression or stretching of the main division against the tentorium. With a proximal division, herniation or stretching may affect only individual branches. The clinical appearance of these patients is compounded by the shearing effect of herniation on the pons, causing a severing of the pontine and mesencephalic perforating branches. These injuries result in linear median or paramedian brainstem Duret hemorrhages. Midbrain

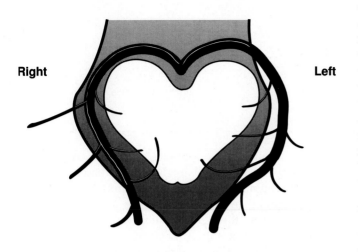

Right   **Left**

Figure 11.1. *Variable course of the posterior cerebral artery in reference to the tentorial edge.* The disposition of the posterior cerebral artery (or superior cerebellar artery in the setting of upward herniation) medial or lateral to the edge of the tentorium determines some of the clinical effects of transtentorial herniation. In this schematic illustration, the main trunk of the right posterior cerebral artery is spared from compression, meaning that mesencephalic and circumflex branches continue to be perfused while parenchymal branches become stretched and occluded. On the left side, the main trunk of the posterior cerebral artery is compressed early in its course by the tentorium. On this side, the mesencephalic branches are also liable to be compressed against the tentorial edge.

compression may also cause hydrocephalus. Dysfunction of the mesencephalic reticular activating system may affect levels of consciousness. Furthermore, the shape of the tentorium and the distances between the midbrain and temporal lobes in the anterior, middle, and posterior incisural spaces are variable. Variability of arterial anatomy implies that very different clinical syndromes may be seen in similar patterns of herniation.

FETAL POSTERIOR CEREBRAL ARTERY CONFIGURATION

Normal physiologic flow in a posterior communicating artery is from anterior to posterior.

A fetal configuration posterior cerebral artery in which the predominant supply is from the internal carotid artery, or where the P1 segment is smaller than the posterior communicating artery, is seen in between 15–40% of hemispheres (5, 9). When the posterior cerebral artery is fetal in

configuration, it is common for the course of the posterior communicating artery to be altered slightly. Usually, in a non-fetal configuration, the posterior communicating artery describes a slightly posteromedial course from the internal carotid artery to the posterior cerebral artery. In this location, the non-fetal posterior communicating artery runs superomedial to the oculomotor nerve. In the setting of a fetal type posterior cerebral artery, the P1 segment is longer and hypoplastic to varying degrees, and the fetal posterior communicating artery has a more posterolateral course lying superior or superolateral to the oculomotor nerve.

POSTERIOR CEREBRAL ARTERY BRANCHES

For purposes of description three broad categories of branches from the posterior cerebral artery are identified (9):

1. Direct or circumflex perforating branches to the brainstem and thalamus
2. Ventricular branches winding around the brainstem to the choroidal fissure
3. Cortical branches

Occasionally, in the setting of a meningioma or a dural arteriovenous malformation of the tentorium or posterior fossa, evidence of dural arteries from the posterior cerebral artery may be seen. Small dural branches from the distal cortical and choroidal branches of the artery, usually too small to image angiographically, can supply the falx cerebri. These vessels were first described by Wollschlaeger and Wollschlaeger in 1965 and were named the artery of Davidoff and Schechter to honor their former mentors (10, 11).

Brainstem and Thalamic Branches of the Posterior Cerebral Artery

These centrally directed branches fall into two patterns (Fig. 11.2).

Direct branches arise from the posterior cerebral artery and enter the brainstem immediately. This pattern includes the posterior thalamoperforator arteries from the P1 segment directed superiorly, the thalamogeniculate arteries from the P2 segment directed superiorly and laterally, and the peduncular perforating branches from the P1 and P2 segments directed centrally into the peduncle and brainstem.

Circumflex branches encircle the brainstem in a course

Figure 11.2. *Lateral view of the posterior cerebral artery.* The principal angiographically identifiable branches of the posterior cerebral artery are illustrated. The curve described by the lateral posterior choroidal artery conforms to the posterior surface of the pulvinar, thus serving as a useful angiographic marker for the anterior margin of the atrium. The curve of the medial posterior choroidal artery depicts the location of the velum interpositum (as does the internal cerebral vein). The calcarine artery demonstrates the position of the calcarine fissure;

the parieto-occipital artery lying in the fissure of that name separates the parietal from the occipital lobes. The posterior curve of the splenium is illustrated angiographically by the perisplenial artery **(B).** These and other relatively fixed angiographic-anatomic relationships can be extremely useful when collating data from angiograms with MRI or CT images where these anatomic structures are identifiable through other techniques.

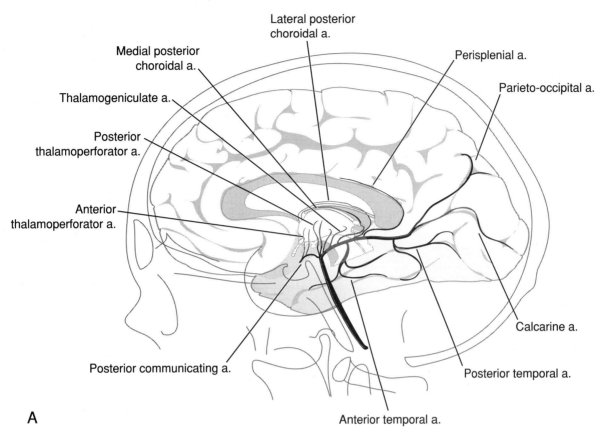

A

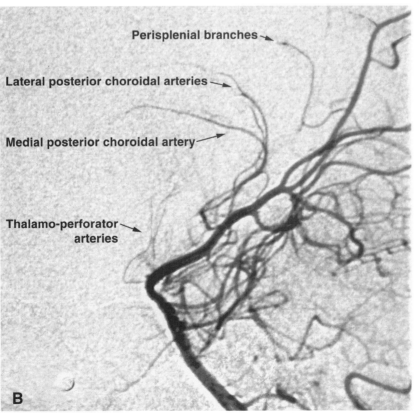

B

parallel to that of the posterior cerebral artery for variable distances before entering the thalamus or mesencephalon.

THALAMOPERFORATOR ARTERIES OF THE POSTERIOR CEREBRAL ARTERY

The anterior thalamoperforator arteries, seven to ten in number, arise from the superolateral aspect of the posterior communicating arteries. A prominently visible artery from among this number directed to the base of the brain between the optic chiasm and the mamillary bodies is sometimes referred to as the premamillary artery or the thalamotuberal artery. The anterior group of thalamoperforator arteries supplies the thalamic nuclei, posterior aspect of the optic chiasm, proximal part of the optic radiations, posterior hypothalamus, and part of the cerebral peduncle. Having traversed the thalamus, they may give a variable supply to the ependyma of the lateral ventricle, and anastomose there with the choroidal vessels.

Up to eight posterior thalamoperforator arteries arise from the posterior or postero-superior aspect of the P1 segment of the posterior cerebral artery. They enter the brain via the posterior perforated substance, the recess of the interpeduncular fossa, and the medial walls of the cerebral peduncles. Together they supply the thalamus, subthalamic nucleus, and the nuclei and tracts of the upper midbrain including the substantia nigra, red nucleus, oculomotor and trochlear nuclei, posterior portion of the internal capsule, and the cisternal segment of the oculomotor nerve (2, 12). Occasionally, posterior thalamoperforating arteries may arise predominantly or exclusively from one side. When a dominant thalamoperforating vessel is seen giving bilateral supply, it is sometimes referred to as *the artery of Percheron* (Fig. 11.3) (13, 14).

An important observation in microsurgical studies is the relative infrequency of thalamoperforating vessels arising directly from the basilar tip in the midline. They arise usually 2–3 mm distally along the P1 segment (5). This has an important bearing on the treatment of basilar tip aneurysms and the need for caution when these aneurysms are off-center in location. Furthermore, the propensity of the perforating vessels from the P1 segments to arise from the posterior or postero-superior aspects of the artery implies that surgical clipping is more favorable when a basilar tip aneurysm projects anteriorly rather than posteriorly.

Surgical or occlusive injury to thalamoperforating branches may result in a number of midbrain or thalamic syndromes due to involvement of the substrates of cranial nerves III and IV, with hemiplegia, hemiballismus, cerebellar ataxia, and choreiform movement disorders. The number and size of thalamoperforating vessels arising from the posterior communicating arteries and P1 segments is fairly constant, even when one or the other is hypoplastic (5, 9). This implies that midbrain and thalamic morbidity is still a consideration and risk if sacrifice or compromise of

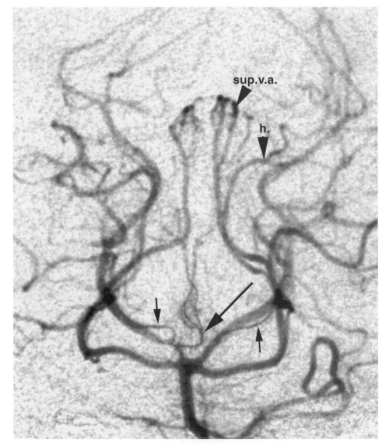

Figure 11.3. *Townes view of basilar artery tip: artery of Percheron.* A hypoplastic right P1 segment is seen, which widens in the P2 segment with dilution (wash-in) indicating that an unseen right posterior communicating artery of substantial size is present. A single midline vessel (Percheron) **(longer arrow)** arises from the right P1 segment and supplies bilateral thalamoperforator vessels. However, even though its course is midline, its origin is off midline, i.e., from the P1 segment rather than from the basilar artery itself. Proximal branches of the P1 segments bilaterally **(shorter arrows),** probably representing medial posterior choroidal arteries or circumflex branches, parallel the course of the posterior cerebral artery.
The superior vermian branches of the superior cerebellar artery (sup.v.a.) describe the peaked surface of the superior vermis. Sloping laterally, the superior surface of the cerebellum is outlined by the medial hemispheric branches (h.) of the superior cerebellar artery.

a hypoplastic P1 segment or a hypoplastic posterior communicating artery is contemplated.

THALAMOGENICULATE BRANCHES OF THE POSTERIOR CEREBRAL ARTERY

Up to 12 thalamogeniculate branches arise from the P2 segment of the posterior cerebral artery or, less commonly, from the P3 segment. They appear either as individual branches or, in approximately a quarter of all hemispheres, as common trunks that subsequently divide (15). They measure up to 580 m in diameter. Like the lateral posterior choroidal artery described below, the thalamogeniculate arteries have a high incidence of recurrent origin from more distal branches of the posterior cerebral artery, particularly from the temporal branches.

The thalamogeniculate arteries perforate the inferior surface of the medial geniculate body, the pulvinar of the thalamus, and lateral geniculate body to supply the posterior half of the lateral thalamus, posterior limb of internal capsule, and part of the optic tract (12, 15). This area may also be supplied by the circumflex branches of the posterior cerebral artery. Infarction in this region of the lateral thalamus and geniculate bodies can cause the classic *lateral thalamic syndrome of Dejerine and Roussy*. This involves contralateral loss of deep or superficial sensation, hemihyperesthesia, contralateral hemiplegia, contralateral hypotonia and incoordination, and homonymous hemianopsia. Isolated components of this syndrome may also be seen with more confined infarcts. Involvement of the posterior limb of the internal capsule or of extrapyramidal pathways accounts for the hemiparetic component of this syndrome. More medial perforators from the posterior cerebral artery may cause involvement of the cerebral peduncle which would have a similar motor effect. Extrapyramidal and cerebellar signs with ataxia may be seen too due to involvement of the dentato-rubro-thalamic pathways with ischemia of the ventrolateral nucleus of thalamus (16, 17).

PEDUNCULAR PERFORATING BRANCHES OF THE POSTERIOR CEREBRAL ARTERY

Up to six branches from the P1 and P2 segments enter the cerebral peduncle directly to supply the corticospinal and corticobulbar tracts, substantia nigra, and red nucleus. They also supply the tegmental and cisternal portions of the oculomotor nerve (5, 18). Close to the midline up to six perforator branches course posteriorly to supply the median portion of midbrain back to the aqueduct. Therefore, occlusion of these medial vessels has a profound impact on the nuclear and fascicular substrates of extraocular movement.

CIRCUMFLEX BRANCHES OF THE POSTERIOR CEREBRAL ARTERY

One or more short circumflex branches arise from the P1 segment or, less commonly, from the P2 segment. They encircle the brainstem, coursing deep to the medial posterior choroidal artery and posterior cerebral artery. En route as far back as the geniculate bodies, they send small twigs to the lateral aspects of the peduncles and the tegmentum.

Up to three long circumflex branches may be seen and are more consistently present (96%) than the short circumflex branches (66%) (Fig. 11.3) (5). They tend to be more distal in origin than the short circumflex arteries. They extend more distally posteriorly and end in the region of the quadrigeminal plate. When a prominent branch to the superior colliculi is present, it may be termed the collicular artery. Supply to the lower aspect of the quadrigeminal plate from the superior cerebellar artery implies that anastomoses between the posterior cerebral artery and superior cerebellar artery can occur at this site.

Ventricular Branches of the Posterior Cerebral Artery

Two groups of branches directed towards the choroid plexus and its adjacent structures arise from the posterior cerebral artery.

MEDIAL POSTERIOR CHOROIDAL ARTERIES

The medial posterior choroidal artery is multiple in up to 40% of hemispheres (9), with 2 or 3 vessels seen per hemisphere (Fig. 11.4). The most common site of origin is from the P2 segment, slightly more proximal on the posterior cerebral artery than the dominant sites of origin of the lateral posterior choroidal arteries. The medial posterior choroidal artery may also arise from the parieto-occipital, calcarine, and splenial branches of the posterior cerebral artery. In these instances, it can sometimes be seen on a lateral angiogram describing a recurrent anterior course to enter the roof of the third ventricle. Anomalous origin of the medial posterior choroidal artery from the basilar artery has been described (Fig. 11.5) (19).

The medial posterior choroidal artery curves around the brainstem deep to the posterior cerebral artery supplying small tegmental branches along its course. The "cisternal segment" of the medial posterior choroidal artery is defined as spanning the origin of the vessel to the point of entry into the velum interpositum. As they course around the ambient cistern, the cisternal branches contribute to the vascular supply of midbrain, tectal plate, pineal gland, posterior thalamus, the habenula, and medial geniculate body. It then curves over the quadrigeminal plate slightly lateral to the pineal gland (19) to enter the roof of the third ventricle where it becomes the "plexal segment." The plexal segment of the medial posterior choroidal artery runs anteriorly within the velum interpositum towards the foramen of Monro supplying the ipsilateral choroid plexus of the third ventricle. The roof of the third ventricle is formed by the inferior tela choroidea suspended from the medial walls of the thalamus close to the stria medullaris (see Fig. 14.8). The medial posterior choroidal arteries may also supply the medial ventricular surfaces of the thalamus, stria medullaris, and fornix.

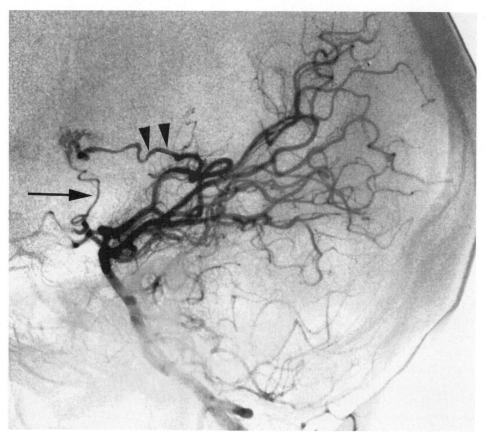

Figure 11.4. *Arteriovenous malformation of the foramen of Monro.* A lateral projection of the posterior fossa demonstrates an enlarged medial posterior choroidal artery **(double arrowhead)** and an anterior thalamoperforator/thalamotuberal artery **(arrow)** directed toward an arteriovenous malformation nidus in the region of the foramen of Monro. The identity of the medial posterior choroidal artery can be confirmed by superimposing the arterial image on the venous. The medial posterior choroidal artery and the internal cerebral vein both course within the cistern of the velum interpositum.

Its terminal branches are directed anteriorly toward the foramen of Monro where they anastomose with the terminal branches of the lateral posterior choroidal artery. The velum interpositum lies slightly below the level of the choroid plexus of the lateral ventricle. Therefore, the course of the medial posterior choroidal artery on a lateral angiogram lies lower than that of the lateral posterior choroidal artery. Recognition is further assisted by the frequent notching of the course of the medial posterior choroidal artery by the quadrigeminal plate, giving it a characteristic "3" pattern.

LATERAL POSTERIOR CHOROIDAL ARTERIES

The lateral posterior choroidal arteries, up to nine per hemisphere, arise typically from the P2 segment of the posterior cerebral artery slightly more distal in origin than the medial posterior choroidal arteries. However, up to 48% can be identified arising from more distal branches of the posterior cerebral artery including the hippocampal, temporal, parieto-occipital, and other arteries (5, 21). Before entering the choroidal fissure lateral to the ambient cistern, the lateral posterior choroidal arteries may give peduncular or tegmental branches. Like the anterior cho-

roidal artery, the posterior choroidal vessels have been described in terms of their cisternal and plexal (intraventricular) segments. As a rule of thumb for all the choroidal arteries, neurologic deficits are more likely to occur with occlusions involving the branches of the cisternal segments than with occlusions confined to the plexal segments. The cisternal segment of the lateral posterior choroidal artery measures approximately 25 mm in length, but can range from 5–70 mm (21). Cisternal branches supply parts of midbrain crus, the pineal body, splenium, posterior commissure, tail of the caudate nucleus, thalamus, and fornix. The thalamic branches supply the dorsomedial nucleus and the pulvinar. Additionally, there may be branches to the anterolateral aspect of the lateral geniculate body important for relaying macular vision to the primary visual cortex.

The lateral posterior choroidal arteries most commonly enter the lateral ventricle posteriorly at the level of the atrium. To gain access from the quadrigeminal region to the choroid plexus of the lateral ventricle, the lateral posterior choroidal artery must swing laterally between the posteroinferior surface of the thalamus and the fimbria or crus of the fornix. The thalamus and forniceal crus, bridged by tela choroidea, define the margins of the cho-

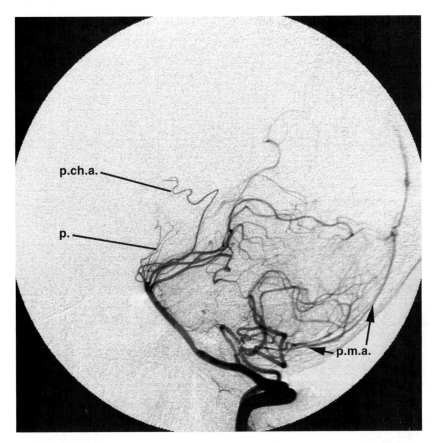

Figure 11.5. *Variant origin of the posterior choroidal arteries.* A posterior fossa injection in a patient with bilateral fetal posterior communicating arteries affords an unobstructed view of the transmesencephalic, thalamoperforator, and circumflex branches of the upper basilar artery (p.), without superimposed posterior cerebral arteries. A medial posterior choroidal artery (p.ch.a.) appears to arise from the basilar artery, a variant that has been described. However, this could also be due to preferential opacification of this vessel via a hypoplastic P1 segment. The course of the posterior meningeal artery (p.m.a.) clinging to the inner table of the skull is well seen.

roidal fissure at this level. In the lateral ventricle, the lateral posterior choroidal artery curves around the pulvinar of the thalamus. It supplies the glomus of the choroid plexus in the atrium and the body of the choroid plexus itself in the lateral ventricle. It then makes its way toward the foramen of Monro. In the temporal horn of the lateral ventricle, its size is in relative counterbalance with that of the intraventricular segment of the anterior choroidal artery. Occasionally the intraventricular choroidal territory may be dominated by the latter. Choroidal vessels are correspondingly enlarged in the setting of intraventricular hypervascular tumors or arteriovenous malformations.

The posterior wall of the pulvinar defines the medial anterior edge of the ventricular atrium, which is therefore accurately described on a lateral angiogram by the curve of the lateral posterior choroidal artery (see Fig. 11.2). This used to be an important marker for thalamic masses and shift, but it can still be useful with modern axial imaging, serving as an easily transposed landmark from one imaging modality to the other. The anastomoses between the lateral posterior choroidal artery and medial posterior choroidal artery anteriorly sometimes serve as a useful angiographic reference point for the foramen of Monro.

Cortical Branches of the Posterior Cerebral Artery

Cortical branches of the posterior cerebral artery are the temporal arteries to the inferior surface of the tem-

poral lobe, parieto-occipital artery, calcarine artery, and splenial artery (Fig. 11.6). During posterior fossa arteriography, they are frequently superimposed on each other and on thalamic, midbrain, and superior cerebellar artery branches. They are therefore most clearly seen on a lateral view of a carotid artery injection in the setting of a fetal posterior cerebral artery origin. When identification of a particular vessel is necessary, it is sometimes useful to trace a line on the lateral view of the arterial phase, representing the straight sinus traced from the venous phase. Branches of the posterior cerebral artery projecting below this line are lateral to the midline and therefore temporal. The artery immediately above the straight sinus and approximately parallel to it will be the calcarine artery, whereas the most prominent branch directed diagonally posteriorly and superiorly will be the parieto-occipital branch. On the AP or Townes view of the vertebral artery injection, the calcarine artery and parieto-occipital artery may be difficult to discern from one another. The calcarine artery can frequently be identified on this view by its position off the midline within the deep calcarine fissure, whereas the parieto-occipital artery lies closer to the falx and midline (Fig. 11.7). Midline vermian branches from the superior cerebellar artery and posterior inferior cerebellar artery may sometimes superimpose on these branches of the posterior cerebral artery on a steep Townes view and be a source of confusion.

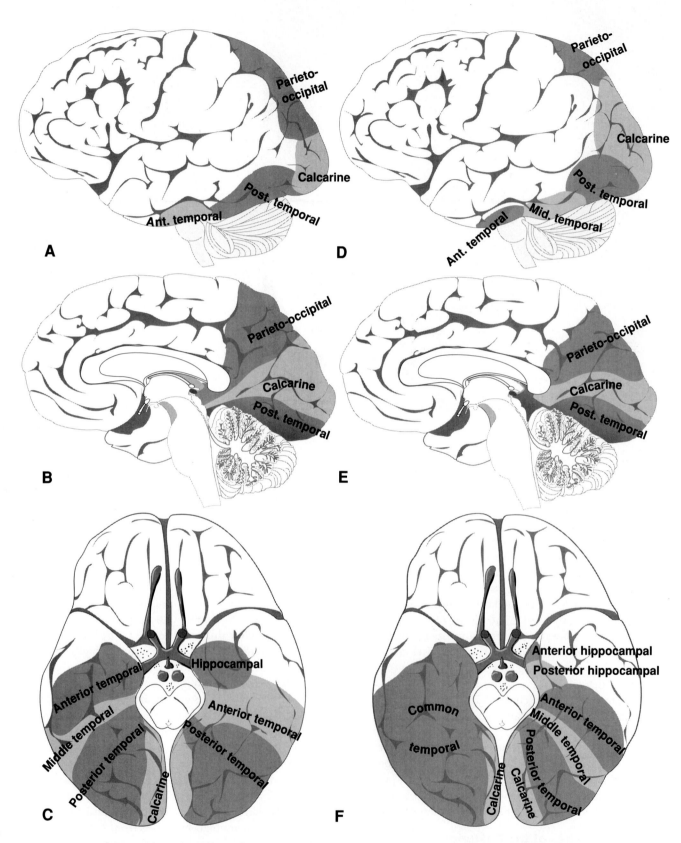

Figure 11.6. *Named cortical branches of the posterior cerebral artery.*   Common division patterns and assigned nomenclature of the cortical branches of the posterior cerebral artery are illustrated.

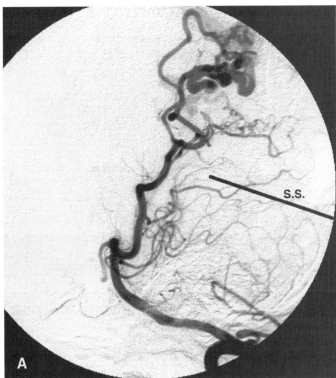 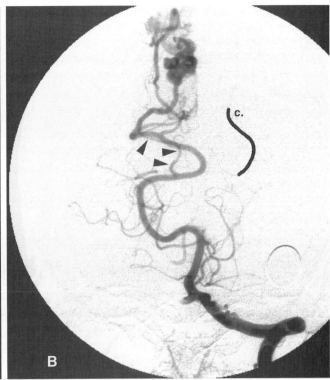

Figure 11.7. *Parieto-occipital arteriovenous malformation.* A right parieto-occipital arteriovenous malformation is opacified in this patient without superimposition on the lateral view **(A)** because of the presence of a left fetal posterior communicating artery. The course of the straight sinus (S.S.) is depicted by the black line **(A)**. On the Townes view **(B),** the arrowheads on the patient's right indicate the course of the calcarine artery as it deviates more laterally than the near midline course of the parieto-occipital artery. This is because the calcarine artery usually lies within the depths of the calcarine fissure; it therefore usually projects more laterally, as illustrated by line c on the patient's left side.

TEMPORAL AND HIPPOCAMPAL BRANCHES OF THE POSTERIOR CEREBRAL ARTERY

The temporal branches of the posterior cerebral artery, sometimes called the inferior temporal branches in distinction from the superior temporal branches of the middle cerebral artery, vary in number (9, 20). Approximately 10% of hemispheres have a full complement of temporal posterior cerebral artery branches including anterior temporal, middle temporal, posterior temporal, and hippocampal branches. These vessels arise from the P2 segment of the posterior cerebral artery either separately or as a common trunk. They can alternatively arise more distally in the quadrigeminal cistern, in which position they may contribute branches to the choroidal fissure.

The hippocampal artery (64% of hemispheres) is the most proximal temporal branch arising from the P2 segment of the posterior cerebral artery. It supplies the medial temporal lobe, specifically the uncus, hippocampal gyrus, and the dentate gyrus. It may send branches anteriorly to the temporal pole, which anastomose with temporal polar branches of the middle cerebral artery.

The anterior temporal artery arises from the P2 segment of the posterior cerebral artery and supplies an area of the inferior and anterior surface of the temporal lobes more lateral to the territory of the hippocampal artery. In more than 50% of hemispheres, its territory may extend around the inferior surface of the temporal lobe and reach the middle temporal gyrus (9).

The middle temporal artery lies more posteriorly and is smaller and less constant than the anterior temporal artery.

The posterior temporal artery is a large branch that runs posteriorly toward the occipital pole and supplies the posterior undersurface of the temporal lobe and the occipital lobe. It supplies the lingual gyrus and gives collateral or accessory vessels to the calcarine fissure in 10–20% of brains. This accessory route of calcarine supply is posed as one explanation for central visual field sparing after a distal posterior cerebral artery occlusion. Collateral supply to the calcarine fissure from this route is more likely to reach the posterior aspect of the sulcus, which is the portion concerned with macular vision.

PARIETO-OCCIPITAL ARTERY

This is the largest and most readily identified terminal branch of the posterior cerebral artery, present in more than 96% of hemispheres, running in the parieto-occipital fissure. It supplies the cuneus, part of precuneus, lateral occipital gyrus, and may occasionally extend to the medial aspects of the precentral gyrus and superior parietal lobule. When the parieto-occipital artery has a proximal origin from the posterior cerebral artery, it frequently serves as a common trunk for distribution of thalamic, choroidal, mesencephalic, thalamogeniculate, splenial, and calcarine branches. More distally, the parieto-occipital artery frequently gives origin to an accessory calcarine artery.

CALCARINE ARTERY

This important vessel to the primary visual cortex buried deep in the calcarine fissure may arise from the posterior cerebral trunk, from the parieto-occipital branch, or from the posterior temporal branch. Accessory calcarine vessels may be present from the posterior temporal or parieto-occipital arteries in 10–20% of hemispheres (9). The calcarine artery supplies the cortex in the reaches of the calcarine fissure and gives branches extending to the surface of the fissure to supply the lingual gyrus and cuneus. Unilateral occlusion of the calcarine artery is associated with homonymous hemianopsia with a variable degree of macular sparing. Bilateral calcarine artery occlusion can cause Anton's Syndrome in which there may be confabulatory denial of blindness.

SPLENIAL ARTERY

This vessel (or vessels) arises most often from the parieto-occipital branch of the posterior cerebral artery, but can arise from the temporal and calcarine branches. It can form a common trunk with the medial posterior choroidal artery, or can arise directly from the main trunk of the posterior cerebral artery. It is sometimes called the posterior pericallosal artery and represents an important source of collateral supply from the posterior to anterior cerebral arteries. It sometimes has a recurrent branch to the fornix which anastomoses with the medial posterior choroidal arteries.

A combination of infarction in the territory of the splenial artery with an infarction of the calcarine artery of the dominant hemisphere can result in the rare syndrome of dyslexia without dysgraphia. This is due to a disconnection of the remaining intact (non-dominant) visual cortex from the (dominant) angular gyrus. This means that the eloquent dominant hemisphere cannot "see" the visual stimulus even though the patient is not blind.

REFERENCES

1. Padget DH. The development of the cranial arteries in the human embryo. Contrib Embryol 1948;32:205–262.

2. Margolis MT, Newton TH, Hoyt WF. Gross and roentgenologic anatomy of the posterior cerebral artery. In: Newton TH, Potts PC (eds): Radiology of the Skull and Brain, Volume II, Book 2, St. Louis; C.V.Mosby, 1974;1551–1576.

3. Fischer E. Die Lageabweichungen der vorderen Hirnarterie im Gefässbild. Zentralbl Neurochir 1938;3:300–313.

4. Krayenbühl HA, Yasargil MG. Cerebral Angiography, ed 2. Philadelphia: J.B. Lippincott, 1968.

5. Saeki N, Rhoton AL. Microsurgical anatomy of the upper basilar artery and the posterior circle of Willis. J Neurosurg 1977; 46:563–578.

6. Kernohan JW, Woltman HW. Incisura of the crus due to contralateral brain tumor. Arch Neurol Psychiatr 1929;21:272–287.

7. Ono M, Ono M, Rhoton AL, Barry M. Microsurgical anatomy of the region of the tentorial incisura. J Neurosurg 1984;60: 365–399.

8. Blinkov SM, Gabibov GA, Tanyashin SV. Variations in location of the arteries coursing between the brainstem and the free edge of the tentorium. J Neurosurg 1992;76:973–978.

9. Zeal AA, Rhoton AL. Microsurgical anatomy of the posterior cerebral artery. J Neurosurg 1978;48:534–559.

10. Wollschlaeger PM, Wollschlaeger G. Eine infratentorielle meningeale arterie. Radiologie 1965;5:451–452.

11. Weinstein M, Stein R, Pollock J, et al. Meningeal branch of the posterior cerebral artery. Neuroradiology 1974;7:129–131.

12. Lazorthes G, Salamon G. The arteries of the thalamus, an anatomical and radiological study. J Neurosurg 1971;34:23–26.

13. Westberg G. Arteries of the basal ganglia. Acta Radiologica (Diagn) 1966;5:581–595.

14. Percheron G. The anatomy of the arterial supply of the human thalamus and its use for the interpretation of the thalamic vascular pathology. Zeitschrift Neurol 1973; 205:1-13.

15. Milisavljevic MM, Marinkovic SV, Gibo H, et al. The thalamogeniculate perforators of the posterior cerebral artery: The microsurgical Anatomy. Neurosurgery 1991;28:523–530.

16. Hayman AL, Berman SA, Hinck VC. Correlation of CT cerebral vascular territories with function: II. Posterior cerebral artery. Am J Radiol 1981;137:13–19.

17. Caplan LR, DeWitt D, Pessin MS, et al. Lateral thalamic infarcts. Arch Neurol 1988;45:959–964.

18. Marinkovic S, Milisavljevic M, Kovacevic M. Interpeduncular perforating branches of the posterior cerebral artery. Microsurgical anatomy of their extracerebral and intracerebral segments. Surg Neurol 1986;26:349–359.

19. Berland LL, Haughton VM. Anomalous origin of posterior choroidal artery from basilar artery. Am J Radiol 1979;132:674–675.

20. Yamamoto I, Kageyama N. Microsurgical anatomy of the pineal region. J Neurosurg 1980;53:205–221.

21. Fujii K, Lenkey C, Rhoton AL. Microsurgical anatomy of the choroidal arteries. Fourth ventricle and cerebellopontine angles. J Neurosurg 1980;52:504–524.

CHAPTER 12

The Extradural Vertebral Arteries

The vertebral arteries derive from eight paired segmental vessels that correspond with the embryologic cervical somites. As the vertebral bodies differentiate, the vessels become intersegmental in location and are so designated thereafter in the embryologic literature, with each numbered to correspond with the vertebral body above. In the embryologic literature, the first segmental artery is therefore displaced from the numbering scheme and is then termed the *proatlantal intersegmental artery* (1). However, in angiographic parlance anastomotic branches of the vertebral artery are numbered according to the corresponding cervical nerve root. For example, the C2 branch of the vertebral artery emerges between the C1 and C2 vertebral bodies (Figs. 12.1, 12.2) (See Chapters 5 and 15).

The plexus, which is formed cranially by the segmental arteries during embryonic life, anastomoses at the level of the hypoglossal nerve with the paired longitudinal neural plexi, which form the basilar artery. The cervical vertebral artery forms from a longitudinal anastomosis between the segmental cervical arteries. A concurrent partial regression of the proximal portions of each of the upper segmental arteries takes place.

It should be theoretically possible for any of the segmental arteries to become the dominant feeder to the forming longitudinal anastomosis, which will become the ipsilateral vertebral artery. Usually the proximal vertebral trunk off the subclavian artery corresponds with the 6th intersegmental artery and enters the foramen transversarium below the C6 vertebral body. When the left vertebral artery arises directly off the aorta proximal to the subclavian artery, the vertebral artery corresponds most commonly with the 4th intersegmental vessel and enters the foramen under the C4 body. Other derivations of the intersegmental arteries are rare. A primitive proatlantal intersegmental artery type I originates from the internal carotid artery. A proatlantal intersegmental artery type II (off the external carotid artery) joins the usual course of the vertebral artery at the C1-C2 interspace (2) (see Fig. 8.38).

The formation of the vertebro-basilar system from the fusion of two sets of vascular embryologic plexi explains the propensity of the vessels in this region to emerge with variable patterns. The vertebral artery itself may retain flow through two parallel channels, giving the appearance of a duplication (Figs. 12.3, 12.4, 12.5). Duplications can be seen at any level of the vertebral artery in 0.7% of studies (3–7). Alternatively ectasia or looping in the high cervical area may result in the vertebral artery assuming an intra-dural course at a level as low as the C2 body. This can be an incidental finding but can also be associated with cord or root compression symptoms (8) and may be seen particularly with somal disorders affecting the cervical area such as Klippel-Feil syndrome (9). An anomalous pattern of regression of elements of the longitudinal neural plexi (in the posterior fossa) and of the cervical plexus can also explain a C1 or C2 origin of the posterior inferior cerebellar artery (Fig. 12.6).

The anatomy of the vertebral artery is sometimes described in four parts (Fig. 12.7).

1. The first segment extends from the subclavian artery to the foramen transversarium of the C6 vertebral body.
2. The second segment ascends vertically within the foramina transversaria from C6 to the atlas.
3. The third segment leaves the transverse foramen of the atlas and extends posteriorly and horizontally on the superior surface of the posterior arch of the atlas.
4. The fourth segment pierces the atlanto-occipital membrane and the dura in turn, and then enters the intracranial cavity via the foramen magnum.

Within the foramina transversaria, the vertebral artery in its usual configuration ascends surrounded by the vertebral venous plexus. It runs immediately adjacent to the uncinate processes medially and the ventral rami of the cervical nerves posteriorly. Above the axis, the artery courses laterally and posteriorly before turning sharply cephalad. It then passes through the foramen transversarium of the atlas, which is located more laterally than those below. It courses posteromedially in a horizontal direction imprinting a groove on the superior surface of the posterior arch of the atlas. In a minority of anatomic specimens, the rims of this groove on the superior atlantal surface become a circumferential bony ring. At the margin of the C1 posterior arch, the vertebral artery turns abruptly antero-medially and pierces the atlanto-occipital membrane to enter the dura where a waist-like impression on the contour of the vessel may be seen angiographically. The vertebral artery then fuses with its counterpart anterior to the medulla to form the basilar artery. This junction is usually at or within a few millimeters of the inferior rim of the clivus.

The distal intradural portion of the vertebral artery may be hypoplastic or absent, implying that the vertebral artery effectively ends with a posterior inferior cerebellar artery as a terminal branch. Although this is uncommon (5%), the consequences of performing a full volume injection

Figure 12.1. *Anastomotic branches of the upper vertebral artery I.* A left vertebral artery injection in a patient with a vascular tumor of the C1 vertebral body. The C1 branches **(large arrowhead)** of the vertebral artery supply the center of the mass directly. The vertebral artery at the C1 level is irregular and narrowed indicating encasement. The C2 branch of the vertebral artery also gives supply to the tumor and has prominent anastomotic connection with the occipital artery (occ.a.). The C3 anastomotic branch of the vertebral artery ascends medially behind the vertebral bodies of C2 and C1 close to the midline and is also involved with supply to the tumor.

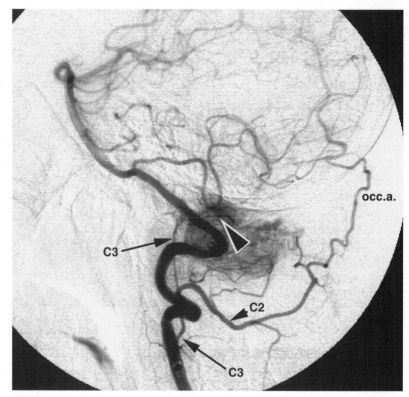

Figure 12.2. *Anastomotic branches of the upper vertebral artery II.* A left vertebral artery injection demonstrates a typical appearance of anastomotic opacification of the ipsilateral occipital artery (occ.a.). The C3 branch of the vertebral artery is prominent in this patient. It gives a characteristic appearance of the arcade of the odontoid process. There is retrograde opacification of the ascending pharyngeal artery and external carotid artery via the neuromeningeal trunk (n.m.t.). The degree of opacification of the external carotid artery and middle cerebral artery (M.C.A.) is a reflection of this patient's ipsilateral occlusive carotid disease.

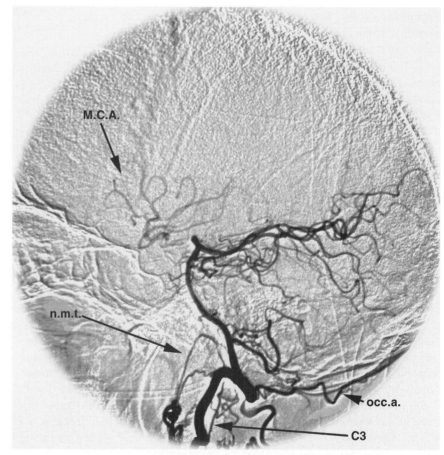

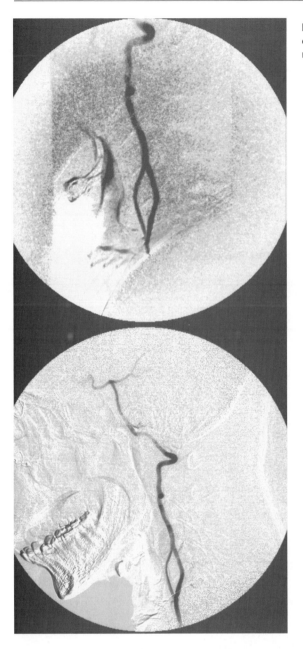

Figure 12.3. *Segmental duplication of the right vertebral artery.* Lateral views of a right vertebral artery demonstrating an incidental finding of a duplicated segment.

into a vertebral artery terminating in a posterior inferior cerebellar artery could be devastating, due to the risk of vessel rupture or infarction. Evaluating the distal runoff from a vertebral artery to exclude this possibility is a routine consideration before performing any vertebral artery injection.

The anterior spinal artery in the cervical area is commonly referred to as the *artery of cervical enlargement*. It is a major focus of concern during embolization of the cervical region, particularly in vessels with anastomotic connections to the C4–C6 level. The artery of cervical enlargement usually arises from the vertebral arteries, often bilaterally. Other origins are frequently seen, particularly from branches of the thyrocervical trunk. During all embolizations or therapeutic vessel-occlusions in the low cervical

area, it is important to identify and preserve the source of the artery of cervical enlargement.

DISSECTION OF THE VERTEBRAL ARTERIES

Like dissection of the internal carotid artery, dissection of the vertebral artery, although clinically less common, is thought to have a similar pathogenesis. With exception of systemic angiopathic syndromes discussed later, most cases of vertebral artery dissection are either of spontaneous origin or are seen following neck trauma. A variety of traumatic etiologies for vertebral artery dissection has been reported, particularly after sport and vehicular accidents (Fig. 12.8). Iatrogenic traumatic etiologies include vessel catheterization, percutaneous needle placement, and chiropractic manipulation. Spontaneous vertebral artery dis-

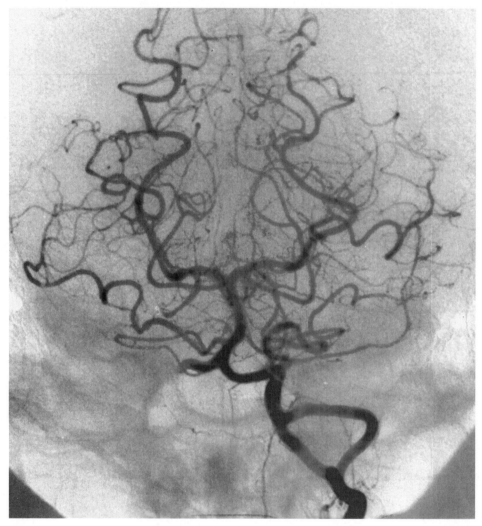

Figure 12.4. *Duplicated upper segment of vertebral artery I.*   A left vertebral artery Townes projection demonstrates an incidentally discovered duplication of the upper segment. The medial limb of such duplications frequently pursues a medial intra-dural course, similar to instances of C1 or C2 origins of a posterior inferior cerebellar artery.

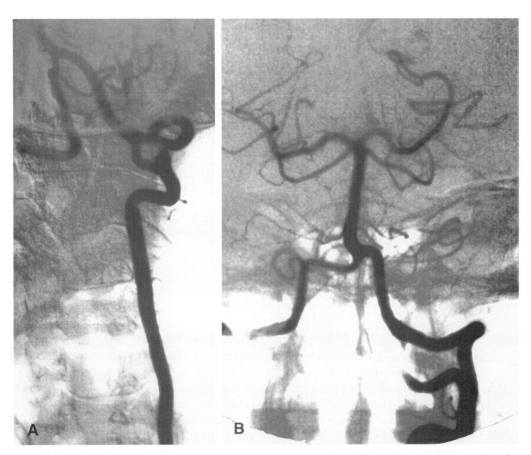

Figure 12.5. *Duplicated upper segment of vertebral artery II.* Oblique **(A)** and Townes **(B)** projections demonstrate a similar anatomic anomaly as in Figure 12.4.

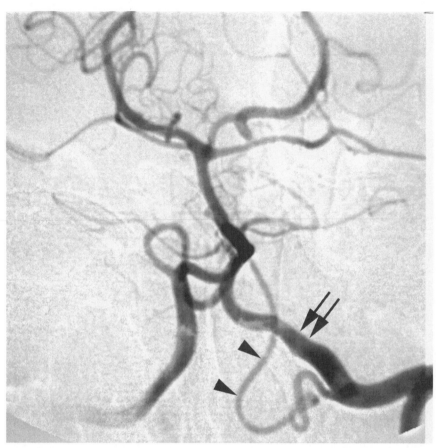

Figure 12.6. *Cervical origin of the left posterior inferior cerebellar artery.* On this Townes projection, the posterior inferior cerebellar artery **(arrowheads)** arises at the C1 level of the left vertebral artery. The dural margin is demonstrated by the cincture **(arrows)** of the vertebral artery above this level.

section occurs most commonly in middle-age females (10). Chiras et al. (11) have emphasized that many cases of ''spontaneous'' vertebral artery dissection in middle-age females may be related to fibromuscular dysplasia or paroxysmal hypertension, with 30% of cases being bilateral (Fig. 12.9).

The incidence of subclinical or mildly symptomatic vertebral artery dissection is unknown. An MRI study of patients who had suffered major cervical nonpenetrating trauma indicated that at least 24% of such patients had sustained an arterial injury to the vertebral arteries, most of which remained asymptomatic (12). An angiographic study of patients with blunt cervical injuries and significant vertebral instability had a 46% rate of major vascular injuries involving the vertebral arteries (occlusion, intimal flap, pseudoaneurysm formation, or dissection), most of which were clinically silent (13). These studies would suggest that many patients who sustain similar or lesser injuries may have arterial dissections or occlusions that do not become clinically relevant.

Moreover the symptoms of vertebral artery dissection can be difficult to discern from musculoskeletal pain. Hinse et al. (10) reported that pain is a prominent symptom in approximately 70% of patients with this disorder.

Pain may be localized to the neck and occiput, or it may give the sensation of a diffuse headache. Therefore, unless the patient develops neurologic symptoms, the possibility of a vertebral artery dissection may be overlooked in many instances.

The neurologic complications of extracranial vertebral artery dissection can be severe or even fatal. Frequently, neurologic symptoms are preceded by pain for a period ranging from hours to weeks. Ischemia of the posterior circulation may be related to embolic events or to complete vessel occlusion in the setting of inadequate collateral circulation. A lateral medullary (Wallenberg) infarct is a typical presenting syndrome (Fig. 12.8).

Angiographic findings of vertebral artery dissection include: long, irregular luminal narrowing; vessel occlusion; a double lumen or intimal flap; and pseudoaneurysm formation. The vertebral artery is most vulnerable to external traumatic injury or to spontaneous dissection, where it is most mobile, i.e., after it leaves the foramen transversarium of C2. Above this level, the normal vertebral artery must conform to physiological rotational maneuvers of the C1-C2 articulation. Narrowing or transient occlusion of flow related to head position or head traction has been reported angiographically at this level and may be symp-

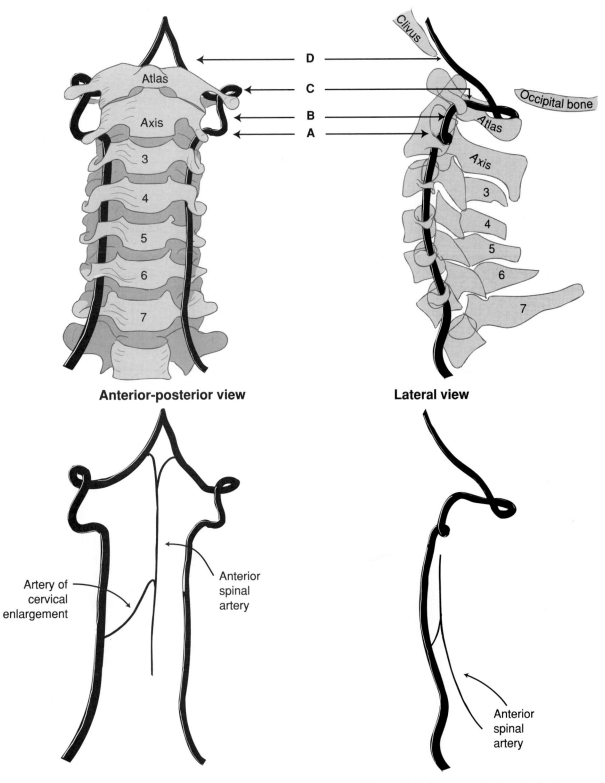

Figure 12.7. *Vertebral arteries.* The course of the vertebral arteries with and without related bony structures is illustrated, as seen on angiographic images. The turns of the vessel at the C1±C2 level are difficult to correlate on direct AP and lateral views without having a mental image of the four turns that the vertebral artery makes in this region. The course of the anterior spinal artery lying anteriorly within the spinal canal is illustrated.

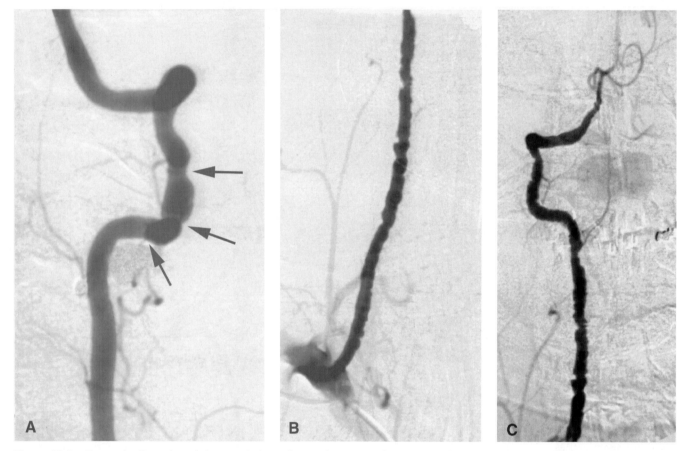

Figure 12.8. *Traumatic dissection of the vertebral arteries.* A young adult female involved in a vehicular accident with severe cervical trauma developed complications from a right internal carotid artery dissection and a right Wallenberg syndrome. MRA demonstrated a normal appearance of the vertebral arteries. During angiographic evaluation of the carotid arteries, injection of the left vertebral artery **(A)** and right vertebral artery **(B, C)** demonstrated multiple areas of intimal irregularity representing dissection and spasm **(arrows).**

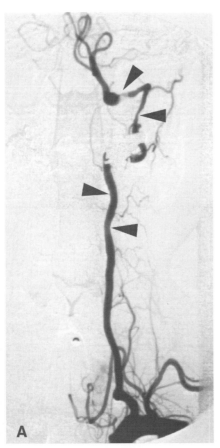 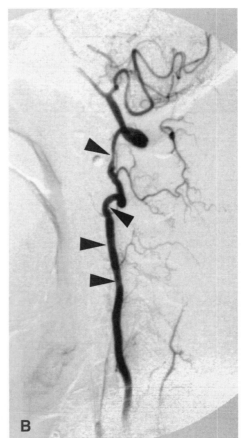

Figure 12.9. *Vertebral artery dissection with presumed fibromuscular dysplasia.* A middle-aged patient with malignant hypertension was found to have renal artery dissections and renal infarcts during angiography. A presumptive diagnosis of fibromuscular dysplasia was established. Subsequent complaints of headache and neck-pain were evaluated by cerebral angiography, which demonstrated carotid (see Fig. 19.2) and vertebral artery irregularities and dissections **(arrowheads)**

Figure 12.10. *Right vertebral artery A-V fistula.* A gunshot to the neck resulted in a high-flow fistula from the right vertebral artery to the adjacent vertebral veins and internal jugular vein. Bullet fragments are seen along the trajectory line. Factors to consider here include the possibility of other vascular injuries, i.e., the ipsilateral external and internal carotid arteries; the evaluation of the ipsilateral ascending cervical and deep cervical arteries; closure of the vertebral artery in an incorrect manner without consideration of the anastomotic connections in this area, which could allow resumption of supply to the fistula from other sources; evaluation of the contralateral vertebral artery to opacify the precise point of the fistula by reflux, and to evaluate the intracranial circulation; identification of the origin of the artery of cervical enlargement before embolization or other treatments.

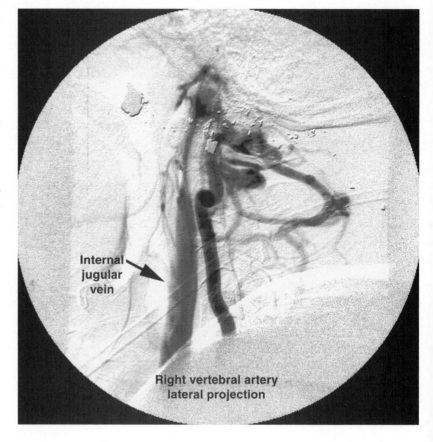

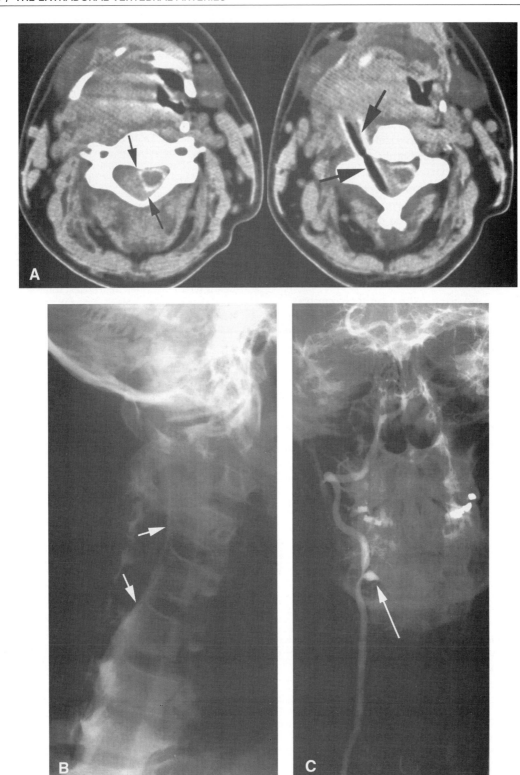

Figure 12.11. *Pseudoaneurysm of the right vertebral artery due to wooden foreign body.* **(A)** CT myelographic images in a middle-aged patient with a history of a fall on deck lumber. A soft tissue mass representing an infected hematoma displaces the airway towards the patient's left. There is soft tissue (hematoma) within the spinal canal displacing the thecal sac **(small arrows).** A linear structure of air-density **(larger arrows)** representing a wooden fragment projects directly through the foramen transversarium of C3, narrowly missing the spine. **(B)** Oblique myelographic image demonstrates displacement of the thecal sac by epidural hematoma **(white arrows). (C)** A PA angiographic image of the right vertebral artery demonstrates a pseudoaneurysm of the right vertebral artery at the site of the wooden missile **(arrow).** The artery was sacrificed using balloon occlusion before surgical evacuation of the hematoma.

tomatic (14–16). This is usually associated with rotational movements of the head, particularly when a combination of extension and rotation is applied. This can be demonstrated on living subjects during angiography or by cadaver studies (17–19). This type of movement or post-traumatic instability at the atlanto-axial level may cause transient *in vivo* vessel occlusion contralateral to the direction of rotation (15). However, the particular vessel compromised by neck movement can be influenced by the particular combination of either flexion or extension with rotation (20). The phenomenon of positional ischemia related to passive or active rotation of the head has been called *bow-hunter's stroke* (21) and may respond well to surgical decompressive procedures (22–24).

A predisposition to positional occlusion may be influenced by the presence of redundancy or loops in the upper cervical vertebral artery. Similar phenomena may also affect the internal carotid artery, which can be compressed against the lateral mass of the atlas in certain positions (25). When a rotational movement is performed suddenly or with force, the vertebral artery may not be able to adapt to the altered position, leaving it vulnerable to mural or intimal injury. Positional occlusion of the vertebral artery ipsilateral to the direction of rotation has been seen angiographically at the C5-C6 level due to compression of the vessel by fascial bands and has responded well in this lower location to surgical release (26).

Traumatic injuries of the vertebral artery that are due to penetrating injuries or catheter manipulations correspond with the site of injury (Figs. 12.10, 12.11). Those related to unsuccessful attempts at percutaneous jugular vein catheterization are typically seen at the C5-C6 level and may be associated with a vertebro-venous fistula.

REFERENCES

1. Padget DH. Designation of the embryonic intersegmental arteries in reference to the vertebral artery and subclavian stem. Anat Rec 1954;119:349–356.
2. Legré J, Tapias PL, Nardin JY, et al. Anastomose intersegmentaire carotide externe—vertébrale d'origine embryonnaire. J Neuroradiol 1980;7:97–104.
3. Takasato Y, Hayashi H, Kobayashi T, et al. Duplicated origin of the right vertebral artery with rudimentary and accessory left vertebral arteries. Neuroradiology 1992;34:287–289.
4. Suzuki S, Kuwabara Y, Hatano R, et al. Duplicate origin of the left vertebral artery. Neuroradiology 1978;15:27–29.
5. Rieger P, Huber G. Fenestration and duplicate origin of the left vertebral artery in angiography: report of 3 cases. Neuroradiology 1983;25:45–50.
6. Hashimoto H, Ohnishi H, Yuasa T, et al. Duplicate origin of the vertebral artery: report of two cases. Neuroradiology 1987;29:301–303.
7. Eisenberg RA, Vines FS, Taylor SB. Bifid origin of the left vertebral artery. Radiology 1986;159:429–430.
8. Sharma RR, Parekh HC, Prabhu S, et al. Compression of the C-2 root by a rare anomalous ectatic vertebral artery. J Neurosurg 1993;78:669–672.
9. Tokuda K, Myasaka K, Abe H, et al. Anomalous atlantoaxial portions of vertebral and posterior inferior cerebellar arteries. Neuroradiology 1985;27:410–413.
10. Hinse P, Thie A, Lachenmayer L. Dissection of the extracranial vertebral artery: report of four cases and review of the literature. J Neurol Neurosurg Psychiatr 1991;54:863–869.
11. Chiras J, Marciano S, Vega Molina J, et al. Spontaneous dissecting aneurysm of the extracranial vertebral artery (20 cases). Neuroradiology 1985;27:327–333.
12. Friedman D, Flanders A, Thomas C, et al. Vertebral artery injury after acute cervical spine trauma: Rate of occurrence as detected by MR angiography and assessment of clinical consequences. Am J Roentgenol 1995;164:443–447.
13. Willis BK, Greiner F, Orrison WW, et al. The incidence of vertebral artery injury after midcervical spine fracture or subluxation. Neurosurgery 1994;34:435–442.
14. Barton JW, Margolis MT. Rotational obstruction of the vertebral artery at the atlantoaxial joint. Neuroradiology 1975;9:117–120.
15. Takahashi I, Kaneko S, Asaoka K, et al. Rotational occlusion of the vertebral artery at the atlantoaxial joint: is it truly physiological. Neuroradiology 1994;36:273–275.
16. Dickinson LD, Tuite GF, Colon GP, et al. Vertebral artery dissection related to basilar impression: case report. Neurosurgery 1995;36:835–838.
17. Brown BSJ, Tatlow WFT. Radiographic studies of the vertebral arteries in cadavers: effects of position and traction on the head. Radiology 1963;81:80–88.
18. Selecki BR. The effects of rotation of the atlas on the axis: experimental work. Med J Aust 1969;1:1012–1015.
19. Toole JF, Tucker SH. Influence of head position upon cerebral circulation: studies on blood flow in cadavers. Arch Neurol 1960;2:616–623.
20. Davis JM, Zimmerman RA. Injury of the carotid and vertebral arteries. Neuroradiology 1983;25:55–69.
21. Sorenson BF. Bow hunter's stroke. Neurosurgery 1978;2:259–261.
22. Fox MW, Piepgras DG, Bartleson JD. Anterolateral decompression of the atlantoaxial vertebral artery for symptomatic positional occlusion of the vertebral artery. J Neurosurg 1995;83:737–740.
23. Hanakita J, Miyake H, Nagayasu S, et al. Angiographic examination and surgical treatment of bow hunter's stroke. Neurosurgery 1988;23:228–232.
24. Vinchon M, Assaker R, Leclerc X, et al. Vertebrobasilar insufficiency resulting from traumatic atlantoaxial instability: case report. Neurosurgery 1995;36:839–841.
25. Bauer R, Sheehan S, Meyer J. Arteriographic study of cerebrovascular disease. II. Cerebral symptoms due to kinking, tortuosity, and compression of the carotid and vertebral arteries in the neck. Arch Neurol 1961;4:119–131.
26. Hardin CA, Poser CM. Positional obstruction of the vertebral artery due to redundancy and extraluminal cervical fascial bands. Ann Surg 1963;158:133–137.

CHAPTER 13

The Arteries of the Posterior Fossa

The basilar artery forms by fusion of the left and right vertebral arteries. It runs from the vertebro-basilar junction at the pontomedullary sulcus to the interpeduncular cistern, where it bifurcates behind the dorsum sellae. The level of the basilar bifurcation in reference to the posterior clinoid processes can have an important bearing on the surgical approach to basilar tip aneurysms (Fig. 13.1). More than 70% of basilar bifurcations lie level with or above the posterior clinoid processes (1).

The vertebro-basilar system gives vascular supply to the posterior cerebral arteries and three pairs of named branches to the cerebellum. Smaller perforating and circumflex branches throughout its length supply the upper spine, medulla, pons, midbrain, and thalamus (Figs. 13.2, 13.3). The posterior circulation is more prone to developmental anomalies than is the anterior circulation.

INTRACRANIAL SEGMENT OF THE VERTEBRAL ARTERY

After traversing the atlantooccipital membrane, the vertebral artery pierces the dura and enters the subarachnoid space usually in the lateral medullary cistern. The point of dural penetration can be seen commonly during angiography as a smooth cincture of the diameter of the artery. In approximately 60% of cases, the left vertebral artery is "dominant" or significantly larger than the right. Hypoplasia of the distal non-dominant vertebral artery can be seen in varying degrees in approximately 5–10% of cases, underscoring the need to check the intracranial run-off before doing a full-volume power-injection in a vertebral artery (Figs. 13.4, 2.28).

From the lateral medullary cistern, the vertebral arteries on their respective sides wind around the medulla oblongata anteriorly into the premedullary cistern. They fuse close to the midline with an angle of incidence between 30 and 90. Their meeting is most commonly at or within a few millimeters of the pontomedullary junction (2, 3). The blood supply of the medulla is therefore predominantly from the intracranial segment of the vertebral arteries proximal to the vertebro-basilar junction, and to a lesser extent from small recurrent basilar artery branches that loop inferiorly.

The branches of the intracranial segment of the vertebral arteries have been classified into medial and lateral branches (3). The medial branches arise from the posterior and posteromedial aspect of the vertebral artery, particularly the distal half, and supply the anterior medulla

and pyramid. The most prominent of these vessels is the anterior spinal artery (Figs. 13.5, 13.6), directed inferiorly along the anterior median sulcus. Other small branches are directed superiorly towards the foramen cecum. The anterior spinal artery is absent unilaterally in approximately 20% of post-mortem angiograms (4). Moreover, the ideal appearance of bilateral symmetric spinal arteries fusing in the anterior median sulcus is frequently replaced by the configuration of a dominant vessel from one side supplying the major portion of flow. A connecting vessel between the left and right anterior spinal arteries can be seen occasionally at dissection and is termed the *anterior spinal communicating artery.*

The foramen cecum, also known as Schwalbe's foramen or the foramen of Vicq d'Azyr, is a median triangle-shaped fossicle on the anterior surface of the medulla at the pontomedullary junction at the superior end of the ventral median sulcus (5). This fossa fills a role analogous to that played by the anterior and posterior perforated substance at the base of the brain, in that it is traversed by a number of small (1 mm) perforator vessels. These vessels penetrate the brainstem to provide vascular supply as far back as the tegmentum and floor of the IVth ventricle. The brainstem-perforators observe a sharp demarcation of the midline and do not give bilateral supply (Fig. 13.7). Compromise of these vessels is responsible for the long tract or nuclear substrate of brain-stem syndromes associated with occlusive infarcts there.

The lateral branches of the intracranial segment of the vertebral artery include the posterior inferior cerebellar artery and circumferential branches to the inferior cerebellar peduncle, lateral medulla, and the olivary structures. The posterior inferior cerebellar artery usually arises from the vertebral artery at the level of the olive, but may be either absent, hypoplastic, or arise from the basilar artery. It may alternatively arise more proximally from the vertebral artery as low as the C2 vertebral body and have an initially extradural course (see Figs. 12.6, 13.8). Rarely the posterior inferior cerebellar artery may arise from an alternative source in the suboccipital region such as the occipital artery, ascending pharyngeal artery, or from the internal carotid artery as a remnant of the trigeminal artery (see Fig. 8.36) (6–8). The medullary segment of the posterior inferior cerebellar artery also gives medullary branches, which anastomose with those arising directly from the vertebral artery.

The lateral spinal artery of the upper cervical cord may

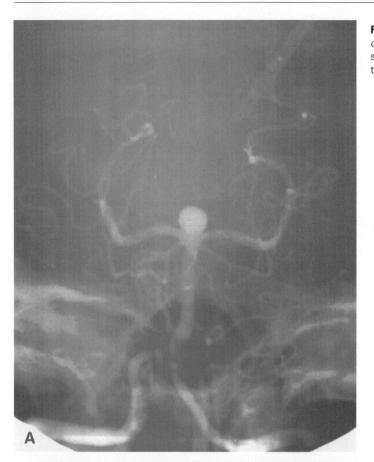

A

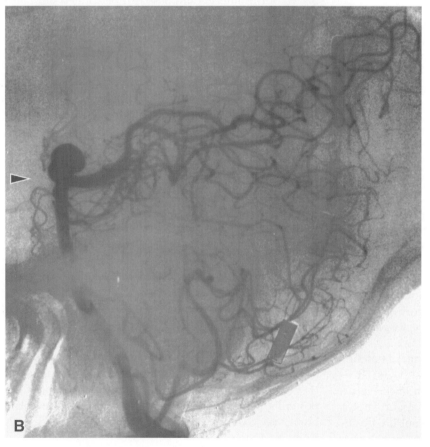

B

Figure 13.1. A–D *Importance of height of the basilar artery bifurcation in surgical planning.* Two basilar aneurysms are demonstrated. In the first patient **(A, B)** the basilar artery has a high bifurcation above the level of the dorsum sella **(arrowhead in B).**

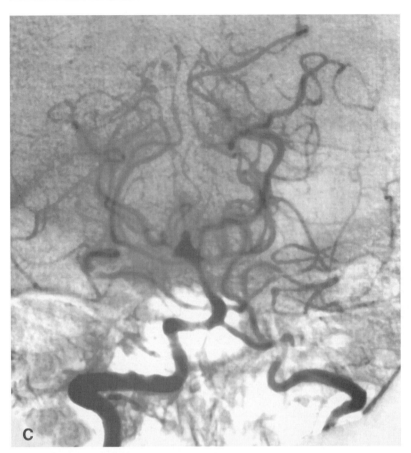

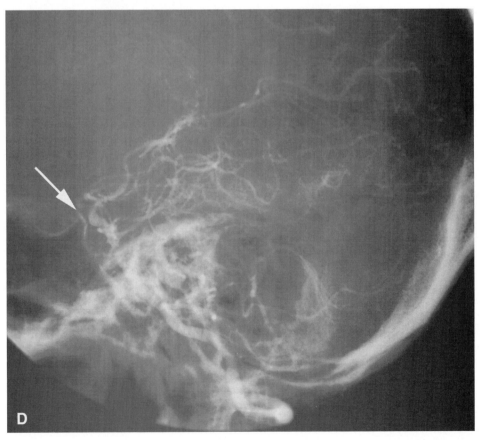

Figure 13.1. *(continued)* In the second patient **(C, D)**, the basilar artery division has a low position with acute angulation of the P1 segments. This aneurysm lies well below the level of the posterior clinoid processes **(white arrow)** on the lateral view **(D).** The aneurysm lies between the superiorly directed P1 segments. This position presents more of a surgical problem for adequate access than the first case.

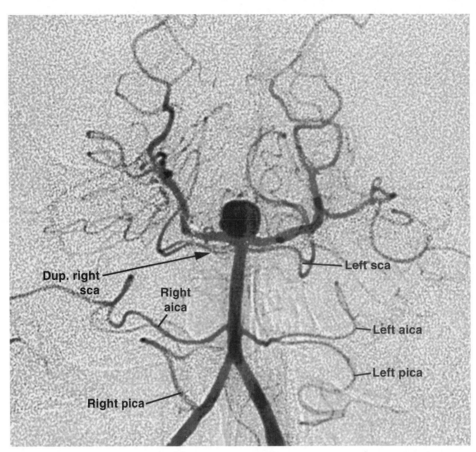

Figure 13.2. *Townes projection of the posterior fossa.*   A young adult male presented with headache and anxiety and was found to have an unruptured basilar artery tip aneurysm. A Townes projection demonstrates common examples of the variability in the configurations of the vessels of the posterior fossa. The left posterior inferior cerebel- lar artery (pica) territory is supplied by the left anterior inferior cerebellar artery (aica). The right anterior inferior cerebellar artery and posterior inferior cerebellar artery have a balanced distribution. The right superior cerebellar artery (sca) has a duplicated origin, the upper branch arising from the posterior cerebral artery.

take origin from the intradural segment of the vertebral artery or from the posterior inferior cerebellar artery posterior to the medulla (8). The lateral spinal artery is usually small and difficult to see during angiography. Augmentation of the vascular territory of the lateral spinal artery can be seen in congenital diminutive variations of the suboccipital vertebral artery and of the posterior inferior cerebellar artery origin. This vessel usually runs caudally posterior to the dentate ligament and anterior to the posterior nerve roots of the upper four cervical levels. Below this point, it joins or is replaced by the posterior spinal artery.

BASILAR ARTERY

From its formation at the pontomedullary junction to its division into the P1 segments of the posterior cerebral arteries, the basilar artery measures approximately 32 mm in length (range: 15–40 mm) with a normal adult diameter of approximately 4 mm (9, 10) (Figs. 13.9, 13.10). The basilar artery is sometimes narrowest at the level of the superior cerebellar arteries, which is a reflection of how this point represents the embryologic junction between the anterior and posterior circulations. The basilar artery frequently has a tortuous course, particularly in older pa-

tients or patients with hypertension and demonstrates a curve away from the side of the dominant vertebral artery inflow. When inflow is balanced from each vertebral artery, the basilar artery can demonstrate slip-streamed laminar flow. This can be seen occasionally during angiography with pusillanimous vertebral artery injection-rates. This phenomenon causes appearances that raise concerns about whether vessel occlusion has occurred. Laminar flow within the basilar artery is most often parallel, meaning that vessels are supplied by inflow from the ipsilateral vertebral artery. In 20% of normal volunteers as demonstrated by Smith and Bellon (11) using selective saturation pulses on MRA, a spiral pattern of flow is seen in the basilar artery.

Therefore during hand injection images, a cerebellar artery or posterior cerebral artery contralateral to the side of the catheter may not fill well because they are being supplied preferentially by unopacified inflow.

Brainstem Branches of the Basilar Artery

An average of 17 perforator branches per brain arise from the basilar artery between the vertebro-basilar junction and the origins of the superior cerebellar arteries (2).

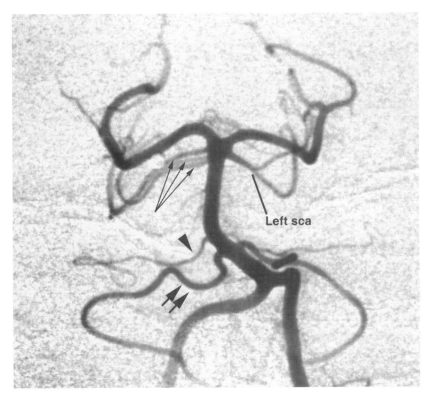

Figure 13.3. *Variability in the posterior circulation.* A Townes projection demonstrates triplication of the right superior cerebellar artery **(triple arrow).** There are bilateral duplications of the anterior inferior cerebellar artery. Alternative nomenclature might denominate the upper branch **(arrowhead)** as an enlarged transverse pontine artery, or the lower branch **(double arrow)** as the origin of the posterior inferior cerebellar artery from the basilar artery. The usual bifurcation pattern of the left superior cerebellar artery (left sca) is well seen in this patient.

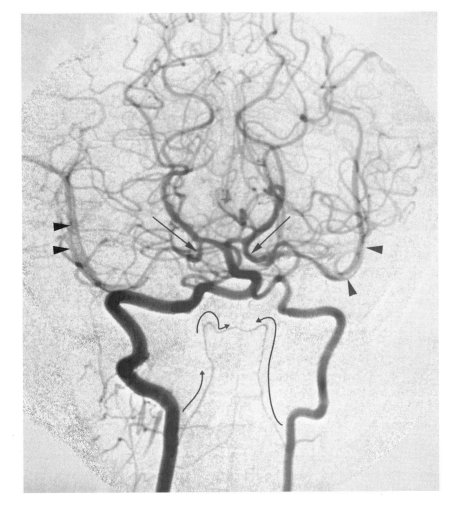

Figure 13.4. *Dominant right vertebral artery.* An injection into the right vertebral artery refluxes the left vertebral artery. To interpret this Townes projection, recall that one is looking at the posterior fossa from above. Therefore, the posterior communicating arteries **(long arrows)** course across the superior cerebellar arteries bilaterally and opacify the middle cerebral arteries **(arrowheads)** bilaterally. The arcade of the odontoid process is well seen in this image filling from the C3 branches of the vertebral arteries bilaterally **(curved arrows).**

Figure 13.5. *Anterior spinal artery and artery of the falx cerebelli.* A lateral projection of the left vertebral artery demonstrates a well-visualized anterior spinal artery (a.sp.a.) directed inferiorly along the anterior surface of the medulla and spine. The left posterior inferior cerebellar artery (pica) has a relatively high origin off the intradural left vertebral artery. The artery of the falx cerebelli (f.cb) arises from the extracranial vertebral artery. It courses diagonally towards the torcular deviating away from the inner table of the skull.

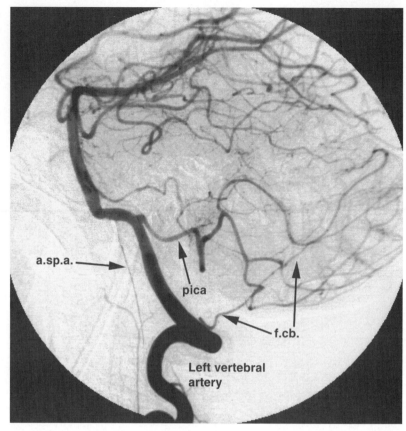

These fall into two patterns. Median branches enter the pons close to the midline in the median sulcus and penetrate to the floor of the IVth ventricle (Fig. 13.7). Short and long circumflex or transverse branches encircle the brainstem and eventually penetrate the surface more laterally (12). Anastomoses may occur within the brainstem between arteries of the same side but do not typically cross the midline. Although these perforator vessels are difficult to see at angiography, they nevertheless play a vital role as they supply the corticospinal and corticobulbar tracts, pontine nuclei, and the lemnisci, fasciculi, and motor nuclei of the midbrain and pons. Diminished perfusion of the reticular activating system is thought to explain the alterations in levels of consciousness seen in cerebral vasospasm, which affects the basilar artery after subarachnoid hemorrhage (13). Because the vertebral arteries and basilar arteries are closely adherent to the brainstem in the posterior fossa, great care is needed to preserve these vessels during aneurysm clipping or other procedures.

BASILAR ARTERY OCCLUSIVE DISEASE

Atherosclerotic narrowing of the intracranial vertebrobasilar vessels is common in later life. In the middle cerebral artery, acute occlusive disease is more likely embolic than thrombotic with a 13 1–16 1 ratio (14, 15). Conversely, in the vertebro-basilar system, most acute occlusions, at least proximally, are thrombotic (16, 17). The complete syndrome of basilar artery occlusion is a devastating and sudden event with loss of consciousness, pupillary abnormalities, bilateral extensor plantar responses, and autonomic dysregulation. Partial thrombosis or occlusion of some of the perforating basilar artery branches may present with lesser degrees of this syndrome. Symptoms of dysarthria, cranial nerve asymmetries, headache, and hemiplegia can be of a fluctuating nature before progressing to full thrombosis. Patients with a fluctuating clinical course are those who respond most favorably to emergency basilar artery thrombolysis, if it can be performed before full thrombosis has become established (see Fig. 21.1).

BASILAR ARTERY BIFURCATION

Approximately 10–18% of intracranial saccular aneurysms occur in the posterior circulation, of which more than half occur at the basilar bifurcation (18). Two major concerns for surgical clipping of aneurysms in this location are access to the aneurysm and the risks of occlusion of perforator vessels at the time of clip placement.

The perforator vessels in the region of the basilar artery bifurcation fall into two categories. The posterior aspect of the upper centimeter of the basilar artery frequently gives horizontally and posteriorly directed branches to the midbrain. These form a complex arterial network or arcade in the interpeduncular fossa mingling with mesencephalic and thalamoperforator branches from the posterior and superior surfaces of the P1 segments (see Figs. 11.5, 13.11, 13.12) (9, 13). The distal centimeter of the basilar

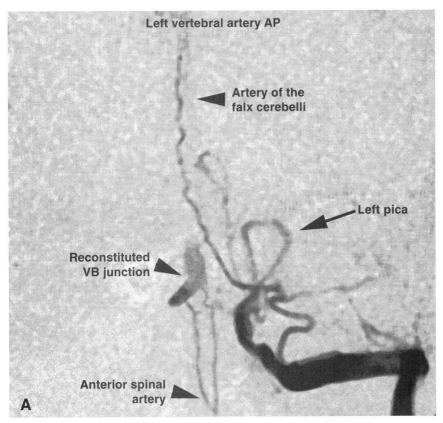

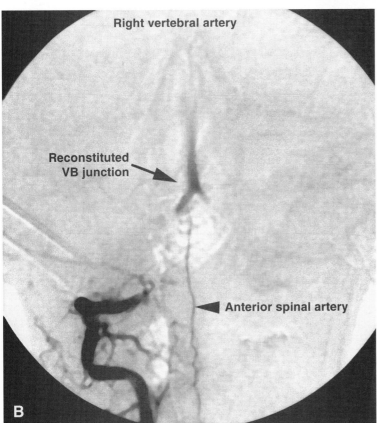

Figure 13.6. *Anterior spinal artery collateral flow to the basilar artery.* PA views of the left vertebral artery **(A)** and right vertebral artery **(B)** in a patient with bilateral distal vertebral artery occlusions and ischemia of the basilar artery territory. The left vertebral artery is occluded distal to the origin of the left posterior inferior cerebellar artery. However, the artery of cervical enlargement lower in the neck opacifies the anterior spinal artery, which has collateralized the vertebrobasilar junction. The midline course of the artery of the falx cerebelli is well seen. The right vertebral artery **(B)** is occluded just proximal to the dural margin. The anterior spinal artery is seen again from this side flowing retrogradely to opacify the intracranial circulation.

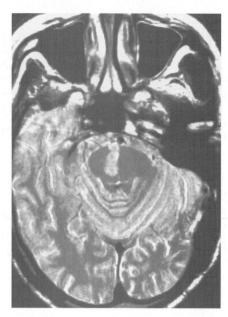

Figure 13.7. *Brainstem perforator infarct.* An axial T2-weighted MRI image in an elderly male demonstrates an infarct of the pons. The pattern of signal hyperintensity conforms to the described pattern of perforator penetration into the brainstem with no transgression of the midline.

artery can have on average about 8 perforating vessels, and the proximal P1 segment an average of 2–4. They measure 200–800 m in diameter (19). The basilar artery tip itself and proximal 2–3 mm of the P1 segments are most often free of vessels, implying that aneurysms in this location can be treated without necessarily threatening an occlusion of the perforator branches. However, the microanatomy of these vessels is extremely complex as some of the perforator vessels often have origin from other posterior cerebral artery branches in this area, such as the medial posterior choroidal artery and collicular artery. Before perforating the peduncular wall or posterior perforated substance, some of the mesencephalic or thalamo-perforator vessels in the interpeduncular fossa give supply to the mammillary bodies and the oculomotor nerves.

The pattern of bifurcation of the basilar artery has bearing on the origins and locations of these important perforator vessels for the midbrain and upper pons. The basilar artery bifurcation angle can vary between 30 and 180, with an average of 109 (1). Most commonly, small perforator vessels are directed posteriorly and vertically from the dorsum of the upper end of the basilar artery when there is a high bifurcation near the diencephalon. This is the most common configuration. When the basilar artery has a proximal (low) bifurcation, midbrain perforator ves-

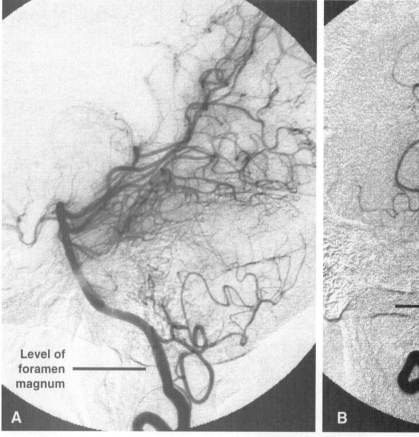

Level of foramen magnum

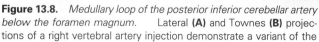

A

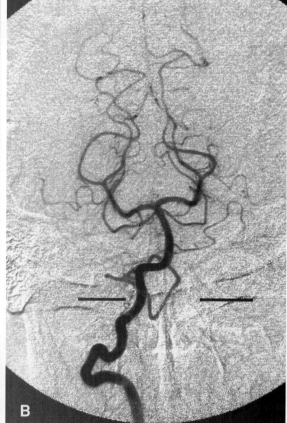

B

Figure 13.8. *Medullary loop of the posterior inferior cerebellar artery below the foramen magnum.* Lateral **(A)** and Townes **(B)** projections of a right vertebral artery injection demonstrate a variant of the right posterior inferior cerebellar artery. The medullary loop of the posterior inferior cerebellar artery sweeps below the level of the foramen magnum to run behind the spine as it reenters the cranium.

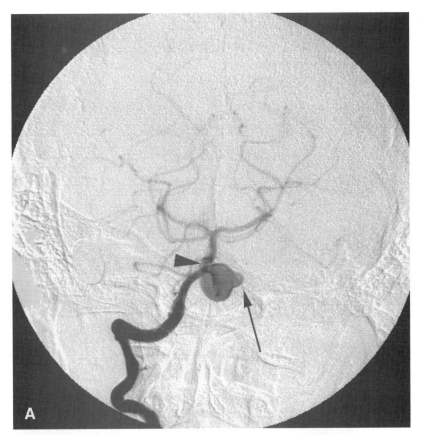

Figure 13.9. *Aneurysm of the vertebrobasilar junction.* Townes and lateral projections of the right vertebral artery injection in a middle-age female presenting with Grade II subarachnoid hemorrhage. A daughter sac of the dome of the aneurysm **(arrow in A)** projects to the left and probably represents the site of hemorrhage. The anterior surface of the aneurysm is flattened against the clivus **(arrowheads in B).** The right vertebral artery appears to deviate away from the aneurysm before joining the basilar artery at the vertebrobasilar junction **(arrowhead in A).** However, the aneurysm also filled readily from the left side. Although it could not be demonstrated clearly in this case, the findings suggest that the aneurysm is related to the presence of a fenestration, and the arrowhead in A points to the right-sided limb of the fenestration.

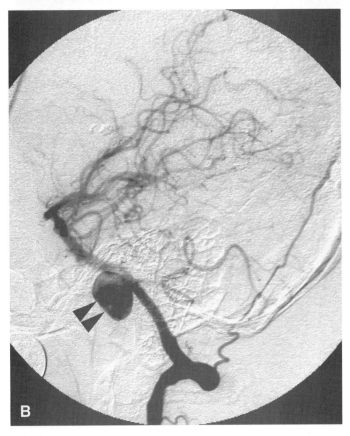

Figure 13.10. *Vertebrobasilar fenestrations.* Vertebrobasilar aneurysms of the proximal basilar artery
related to the presence of a fenestration invariably arise
from the proximal fork of the window (*fenestra* = window, breach). They are frequently multilobulated or
complex in morphology. Their size and shape can make
the underlying fenestration difficult to identify. In **(A
and B),** a slightly obliqued PA view was necessary to
demonstrate a lucency between the two limbs (arrowheads) of the fenestrations.

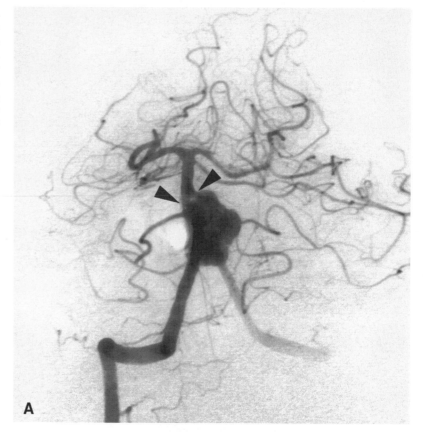

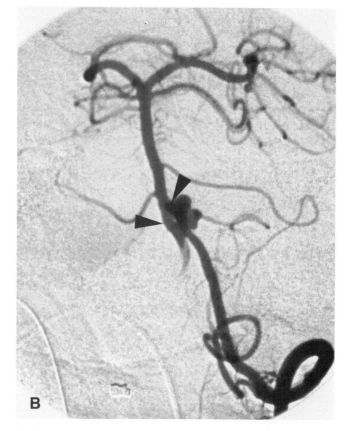

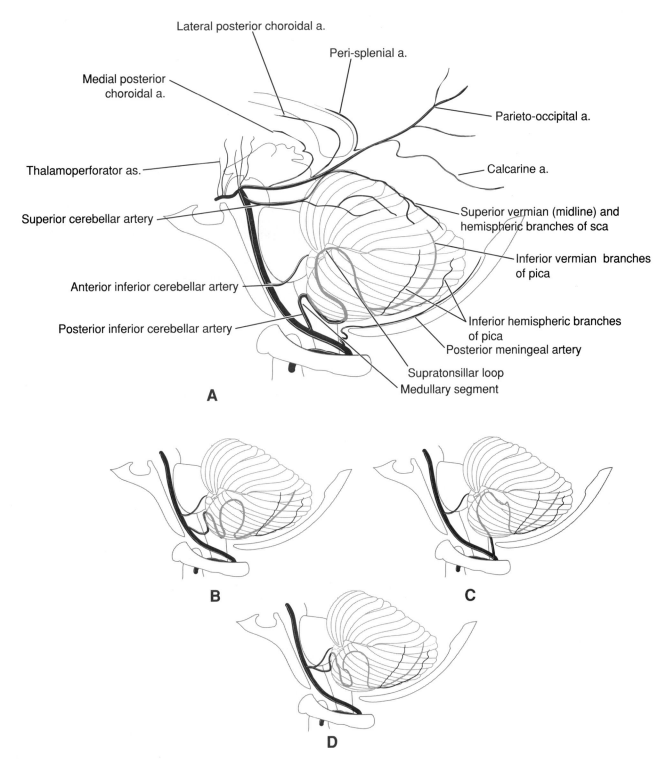

Figure 13.11. *Lateral projection of the posterior circulation:* Variations of the posterior inferior cerebellar artery. The major angiographically identifiable vessels of the posterior fossa are illustrated **(A)**. Variability in the course of the posterior inferior cerebellar artery leads to numerous appearances on the lateral projection **(B, C, D)**. In all configurations, the posterior inferior cerebellar artery circumvents the medulla first, and the cerebellar tonsil second, to finally perfuse the inferior cerebellar hemisphere and inferior vermis.

Figure 13.12. *Basilar artery aneurysm and perforator vessels.* A lateral view of a basilar artery tip aneurysm demonstrates separation of the dome of the aneurysm from the adjacent small vessels with unusual clarity. The reason for this is that the thalamoperforator arteries and circumflex branches **(arrows)** of the posterior cerebral artery are displaced away from the aneurysm by mass-effect from unopacified circumferential thrombus within the aneurysm.

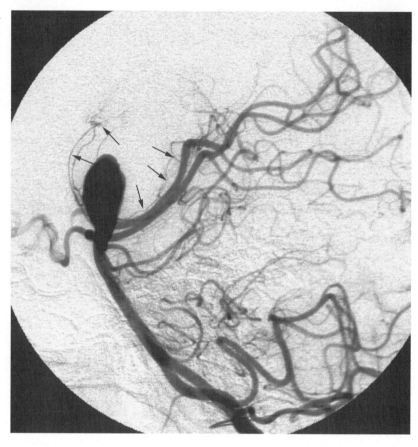

sels arise more commonly from the posterosuperior surfaces of the P1 segments of the posterior cerebral arteries. The direction of projection of the aneurysm, the position of the basilar bifurcation with reference to the posterior clinoids, and the angle of bifurcation of the basilar artery are three major factors to consider in planning a surgical approach (13). With the possible configurations of the perforator vessels in mind, one can understand the more favorable outcome for surgical clipping of an anteriorly directed basilar aneurysm versus one which points posteriorly. In the latter instance, uncomplicated clipping of an aneurysm projecting into the interpeduncular fossa, surrounded by many vital perforator vessels, can be extremely difficult.

ARTERIES OF THE CEREBELLUM

The cerebellum can be described as a three-surfaced organ lying behind the brainstem. The superior or tentorial surface is supplied predominantly by the superior cerebellar artery. The surface facing anteriorly against the anterior wall of the posterior cranial fossa is called the petrosal surface and is dominantly supplied by the anterior inferior cerebellar artery (Fig. 13.11). The inferiorly projecting or suboccipital surface has the most complex topography and is supplied by the posterior inferior cerebellar artery. All of the cerebellar arteries provide important perforating vessels to the brainstem along their early course. They demonstrate a high degree of variability in their origins,

rates of absence or duplication, and in the extent of their territories.

Posterior Inferior Cerebellar Artery

The posterior inferior cerebellar artery is the most complex and variable of the cerebellar arteries. It supplies the lower medulla and the inferior aspects of the fourth ventricle, tonsils, vermis and inferolateral cerebellar hemisphere. An infarction of the entire territory of the posterior inferior cerebellar artery is termed a lateral medullary syndrome or Wallenberg's syndrome (20–22). This includes ipsilateral trigeminal nerve sensory loss, ipsilateral sympathoplegic symptoms, ipsilateral bulbar and pharyngeal paresis, ipsilateral cerebellar symptoms, contralateral hemiplegia, and contralateral numbness to pain and temperature. More distal posterior inferior cerebellar artery infarctions involve only the cerebellar symptoms with sparing of the medullary tracts and nuclei.

The size of the territory of the posterior inferior cerebellar artery is in inverse proportion to that of the ipsilateral anterior inferior cerebellar artery, the larger of the two being referred to as "dominant" in the patois of angiographic interpretation. It is common for a dominant posterior inferior cerebellar artery to arise from the larger of the vertebral arteries with a small ipsilateral and a dominant contralateral anterior inferior cerebellar artery. When a posterior inferior cerebellar artery is absent, its territory is most often taken over by the caudal branch of the ipsilateral anterior inferior cerebellar artery discussed below, in which case, the artery is colloquially termed an *aica-pica complex*. When the anterior inferior cerebellar artery is absent, its territory is taken over by the tonsillo-hemispheric branch of the ipsilateral posterior inferior cerebellar artery. An even more extensive distribution of the posterior inferior cerebellar artery is seen in approximately 14% of brains when the vermian branches of the posterior inferior cerebellar artery cross the midline to establish a bilateral supply, which may include some of the contralateral hemisphere (23). The medullary segments of the posterior inferior cerebellar artery may also give rise to the anterior and lateral spinal arteries.

The posterior inferior cerebellar artery arises from the distal vertebral artery, at or above the level of the foramen magnum in more than 80% of brains, usually at or immediately below the level of the inferior olive. It may arise below that level as far caudally as C2. Rare origins from alternative sources, such as the occipital artery, ascending pharyngeal artery, or the internal carotid artery as a variant remnant of a persistent trigeminal artery can be seen (24–26) (Fig. 13.13). The posterior inferior cerebellar artery may be absent or hypoplastic unilaterally in 4–25%, and absent bilaterally in approximately 2% of cases (23, 27, 28). Rarely, it may be duplicated (29).

After arising from the vertebral artery, it winds around the medulla by looping around or between the rootlets of the XIIth nerve in the preolivary sulcus and those of the IXth, Xth, and XIth nerves in the retro-olivary sulcus. The

posterior inferior cerebellar artery may loop inferiorly or superiorly at this point or may form a complex curve that distorts the course of these rootlets. Even the rootlets of the VIIth and VIIIth nerves more superiorly can be affected. An extremely inferiorly directed loop adjacent to the medulla may sweep below the level of the foramen magnum. The anterior medullary segment of the posterior inferior cerebellar artery is defined as being anterior to the apex of the inferior olive. If the posterior inferior cerebellar artery arises very proximally on the vertebral artery, it will not have an anterior medullary segment. The lateral medullary segment extends from the inferior olive to behind the rootlets of the IXth, Xth, and XIth nerves. The anterior and lateral medullary segments provide direct perforator and circumflex medullary branches similar to the pattern of brainstem branches seen from the basilar artery. The medullary branches of the posterior inferior cerebellar artery may anastomose with those arising directly from the vertebral artery and the basilar artery. A prominent branch of the posterior inferior cerebellar artery running along the lateral aspect of the medulla towards the cervical spine becomes the lateral spinal artery.

COURSE OF THE POSTERIOR INFERIOR CEREBELLAR ARTERY

Much has been written on the course of the posterior inferior cerebellar artery, its segments, routes, and territories of supply. When faced with an angiogram that requires

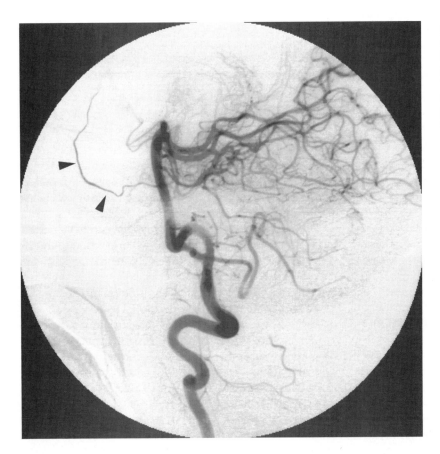

Figure 13.13. *Origin of the middle meningeal artery from the basilar artery.* In addition to origin of various arteries of the posterior fossa from a persistent trigeminal artery off the carotid artery (see Figures 7.4, 8.34, 8.35, 8.36), a variant of the trigeminal route may explain the unusual event of the middle meningeal artery arising from the basilar circulation **(arrowheads)**.

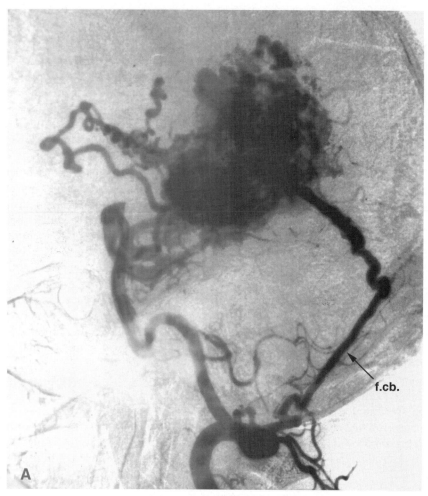

Figure 13.14. Discerning between the inferior vermian vessels, the artery of the falx cerebelli, and the posterior meningeal artery. Angiograms from three patients are presented. A mistake that is occasionally made is misinterpreting an enlarged artery of the falx cerebelli (a dural vessel) as a posterior inferior cerebellar artery or vice versa. The consequences of this can be considerable if it leads to confusion between a vermian and a dural arteriovenous malformation. **(A).** The artery of the falx cerebelli arises from the vertebral artery, posterior inferior cerebellar artery, or less commonly from branches of the external carotid artery. It has a characteristic straight course on the lateral projection (f.cb) as it runs along the edge of the falx towards the Torcular. On a Townes projection it has a midline position (see Figure 13.6). In image A the artery of the falx cerebelli is involved in a large supratentorial arteriovenous malformation which has recruited dural-pial supply.

specific interpretation of the posterior inferior cerebellar artery territory, discerning named loops and segments in the midst of overlapping structures is not done easily (Fig. 13.11). Therefore, to simplify the matter, it is helpful to recall the two major adjacent bodies, the medulla and the cerebellar tonsil, around which the posterior inferior cerebellar artery must insinuate itself. Virtually all posterior inferior cerebellar arteries can be described as having two major destinations, the inferior vermis (median) and the inferior cerebellar hemispheric surface (lateral). Therefore, whether it takes its origin high or low, each posterior inferior cerebellar artery must circumvent its first obstacle, the medulla. On the posterior surface of the medulla, the posterior inferior cerebellar artery is faced with its second obstacle, the tonsillar projection of the cerebellar hemisphere. The course that the posterior inferior cerebellar artery takes to loop over the tonsil, close to the midline, may take many forms and give diverse angiographic ap-

pearances. However, by envisioning the medulla and tonsil superimposed on the lateral angiogram, the location of each idiosyncratic loop of a posterior inferior cerebellar artery will then fall into place.

The course of the posterior inferior cerebellar artery has been described in segments and loops corresponding with the anatomic areas supplied. With particular reference to their relation to the cerebellar tonsil, these are described as an initial caudal loop (lateral medullary) followed by a cranial loop (supratonsillar) (30).

The tonsil is an ovoid or egg-like structure subtended in the paramedian plane by the cerebellar hemisphere to which it is attached at the superolateral tonsillar surface. The remaining free surfaces of the cerebellar tonsil are described in terms of the fissures that separate it from surrounding structures:

The cleft above the superior pole of the tonsil is called the *supratonsillar fissure.*

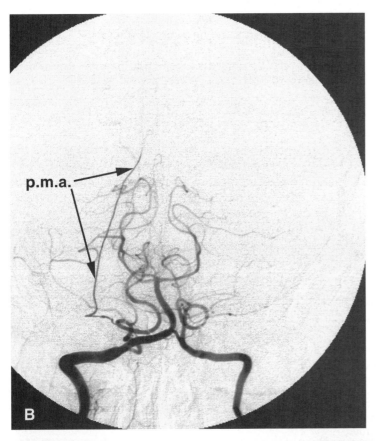

Figure 13.14. *(continued)* **(B).** A Townes projection of the posterior fossa in a different patient demonstrates that neither posterior cerebral artery is opacified, indicating a bilateral fetal posterior communicating artery configuration. The right superior cerebellar artery is duplicated. A curved vessel (p.m.a.) crosses the cerebellar vessels without anastomosing with them; therefore it runs in a different anatomic plane. This off-midline course is typical of the posterior meningeal artery, which curves with the inner table of the skull on the lateral view (see Fig. 13.11). **(C).** Like the artery of the falx cerebelli, the inferior vermian branches (i.v.a.) of the posterior inferior cerebellar artery are elevated away from the inner table. However, the course of the posterior inferior cerebellar artery proximal to the inferior vermian branches should help to avoid any confusion. In this image, the superior vermian branches of the superior cerebellar artery (s.v.a.) are also enlarged in this arteriovenous malformation of the vermis. Notice how the vermian branches of the superior cerebellar artery peak above the more lateral supratentorial branches of the posterior cerebral artery.

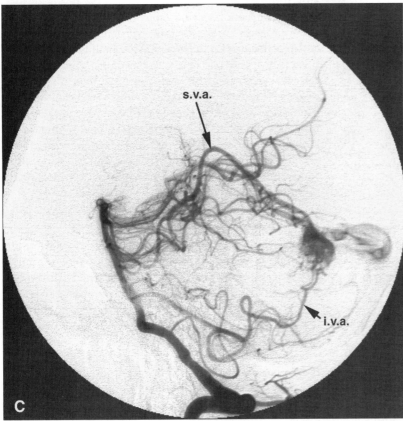

The antero-medial surface of the tonsil is separated from the postero-lateral medulla by the *cerebello-medullary fissure.*

The narrow median cleft between the tonsils posterior to the fourth ventricle is called the *vallecula.*

The roof of the lower half of the fourth ventricle has two components, the inferior medullary velum and the tela choroidea. The inferior medullary velum, a diaphanous neural structure, extends from the fastigium at the apex of the ventricle down to a transverse junction with the lower part of the roof, which is composed of tela choroidea. The transverse junction of these two components is called *the telovelar junction* (29).

Consequently the posterior inferior cerebellar artery, having skirted around the posterolateral aspect of the medulla, encounters the tonsil at approximately mid-equator. To circumvent the tonsil and gain access to the inferior vermis and inferolateral surface of the cerebellar hemisphere, the posterior inferior cerebellar artery must drape itself around the curved surface of the tonsil. It usually takes a superior and medial course over the tonsil forming what is termed the supratonsillar loop in the supratonsillar fissure. The ascending limb of this loop lies immediately behind the roof of the lower half of the fourth ventricle and is called the *telovelotonsillar segment.* These minutiae are relevant in that a surgical and neurointerventional landmark exists at the zenith of the tonsillar segment. Branches to the posterior aspect of the medulla continue to arise from the ascending limb as do a number of branches to the choroid plexus of the fourth ventricle (23). The tip of the supratonsillar arch is known as the "choroidal point," and when occlusion or sacrifice of a posterior inferior cerebellar artery becomes necessary, subsequent morbidity may be significantly less if the occlusion is performed distal to this point. The posterior inferior cerebellar artery does not always take a route through the supratonsillar fissure, however, and may drape itself more laterally along the inferior pole of the tonsil.

At the zenith of the tonsillar loop, the main trunk of the posterior inferior cerebellar artery takes a postero-inferior course to define the posterior border of the upper tonsil as it runs in the retrotonsillar fissure. This course may alternatively have a more transverse aspect to gain the lateral aspect of the dome of the tonsil. Seen from the lateral view, the supratonsillar loop frequently makes an outline of the tonsil along its anterior, superior, and posterior aspects.

DISTAL BRANCHES OF THE POSTERIOR INFERIOR CEREBELLAR ARTERY

At or soon after the zenith of the supratonsillar curve, the posterior inferior cerebellar artery usually bifurcates into two main trunks. The smaller (vermian) stays close to the midline and supplies the median structures along the inferior surface of the vermis (Fig. 13.14). The larger (tonsillohemispheric) trunk serves the posterior aspects of the tonsil and fans over the lateral inferior cerebellar surface. The

median vermian branches and lateral hemispheric branches have prominent anastomoses with the superior cerebellar artery, similar to the anastomoses of pial collateral flow seen in the cerebral hemispheres. These anastomoses can be important in diminishing the extent of ischemia in the event of basilar artery occlusion.

MENINGEAL BRANCHES OF THE POSTERIOR INFERIOR CEREBELLAR ARTERY

The posterior meningeal artery and artery of the falx cerebelli may arise from the vertebral artery, the posterior inferior cerebellar artery, or from another source such as the occipital artery. The artery of the falx cerebelli is distinguished by its near-midline course on the AP angiogram. On the lateral projection its straight course along the falx cerebelli away from the inner table of the skull is like a taut bow-string.

The posterior meningeal artery has a more lateral location. Its curved course conforms in close apposition to the inner table (Figs. 13.11, 13.14).

TOWNES PROJECTION OF THE POSTERIOR INFERIOR CEREBELLAR ARTERY

A Townes projection is the standard initial projection in the AP plane for evaluating the vessels of the posterior fossa because it minimizes foreshortening of the posterior cerebral artery and superior cerebellar artery branches. However, this projection gives a view of the posterior fossa as if one were looking from in front and above. Therefore, the supratonsillar segment and vermian branches appear close to the midline projecting under higher structures, such as the distal basilar artery and thalamoperforator vessels. Discerning on this view alone between inferior vermian and superior vermian branches can be difficult, as can discerning between vermian and supratentorial branches on occasion. The same applies to the venous anatomy of the posterior fossa. For arteriovenous malformations and aneurysms of the posterior fossa, multiple views and obliquities will be necessary to clarify the anatomic relationships.

Anterior Inferior Cerebellar Artery

The anterior inferior cerebellar artery arises from the proximal or middle third of the basilar artery. It courses laterally and inferiorly to embrace the belly of the pons. It runs superior or inferior to the VIth cranial nerve root. In the cerebello-pontine angle it passes above, below, or between the VIIth and VIIIth nerve roots, and divides into two major branches. The lateral (rostral) branch courses around and above the flocculus. It runs in the horizontal fissure between the superior and inferior semilunar lobules which it supplies. The medial (caudal) branch is directed more anteriorly and medially towards the biventral lobule. This branch also gives some supply to the middle cerebellar peduncle, the lateral aspects of the pons, and the choroid plexus in the lateral recess and cerebellopontine angle (23). Other choroidal branches may be seen from the rostral branch or main trunk of the anterior inferior cerebellar artery. The artery of the internal auditory meatus usually arises from the proximal trunk or loop of the anterior inferior cerebellar artery and supplies the nerve roots of the internal auditory canal and the sensory structures of the inner ear. Less frequently, this artery may arise directly from the basilar artery distal to the origin of the anterior inferior cerebellar artery. The anterior inferior cerebellar artery and its branches may become displaced by or involved in supply to tumors of the posterior fossa, such as meningioma or vestibular schwannoma, or tumors that have invaded the posterior fossa, e.g., glomus tumors, craniopharyngioma, chordoma. For this reason, angiographic evaluation of the posterior circulation in certain situations can be very helpful to confirm that intradural extension of a tumor has occurred, as represented by involvement of the anterior inferior cerebellar artery.

Superior Cerebellar Artery

The superior cerebellar artery supplies the lower midbrain, upper pons, upper vermis, and superior aspects of the cerebellar hemispheres. It has a duplicated origin in 14–28% of cases (28, 31–33) (Figs. 13.2, 13.3, 13.14B). With a similar frequency it may share a common ostium with the ipsilateral posterior cerebral artery. Less commonly, it arises from the P1 segment (Fig. 13.15). The

main trunk of the superior cerebellar artery runs in the perimesencephalic cistern above the trigeminal nerve at the pontomesencephalic junction. It is separated from the P1 segment of the posterior cerebral artery above by the oculomotor nerve medially and by the trochlear nerve more laterally. The trigeminal nerve roots come in contact with the superior cerebellar artery in approximately 50% of dissections or with the anterior inferior cerebellar artery in 8% (32). When neurovascular contact of a pronounced degree produces distortion of nerve roots in patients with tic douloureux, some authors have advocated surgical decompression at the site of distortion (34).

When the superior cerebellar artery has a duplicated origin both trunks may arise from the basilar artery. Alternatively, the upper may arise from the P1 segment. The upper trunk of the pair is equivalent to the rostral branch of the non-duplicated superior cerebellar artery, while the more proximal trunk equates with the marginal-hemispheric branch.

The main trunk of the non-duplicated superior cerebellar artery curves around the midbrain in the ambient cistern, which it shares with the trochlear nerve, the posterior cerebral artery and its branches, the basal vein of Rosenthal, and the free edge of the tentorium cerebelli. The course of the superior cerebellar artery in relation to the edge of the tentorium can determine the degree of vascular compromise caused by herniation of the brainstem superiorly through the incisura (see Fig. 11.1) (35, 36).

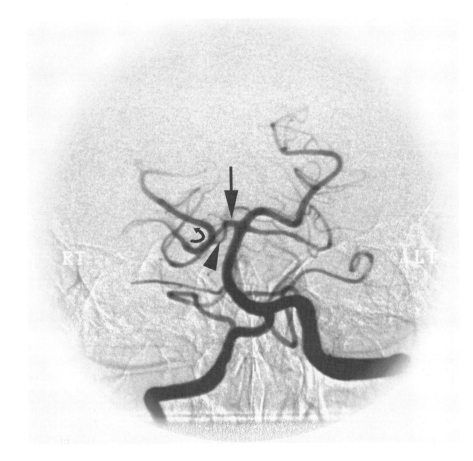

Figure 13.15. *Conjoined variant origin of P1 and superior cerebellar artery.* The P1 segment of the right posterior cerebral artery arises as a branch of the superior cerebellar artery **(arrow)**. The P1 segment is hypoplastic **(arrowhead)** and widens after augmentation by the posterior communicating artery **(curved arrow)**.

Figure 13.16. *Moya-Moya disease of the right hemisphere with a persistent trigeminal variant.* A right internal carotid artery injection opacifies both superior cerebellar arteries (sca) via a persistent trigeminal artery (Trig.). The asymptotic curve of the superior cerebellar surface is adumbrated by the superior vermian and hemispheric branches of the left superior cerebellar artery. A fetal posterior cerebral artery is present on the right side. Anterior and middle cerebral artery flow have been supplanted by a Moya-Moya (``haze'') pattern of lenticulostriate and perforator collateral flow.

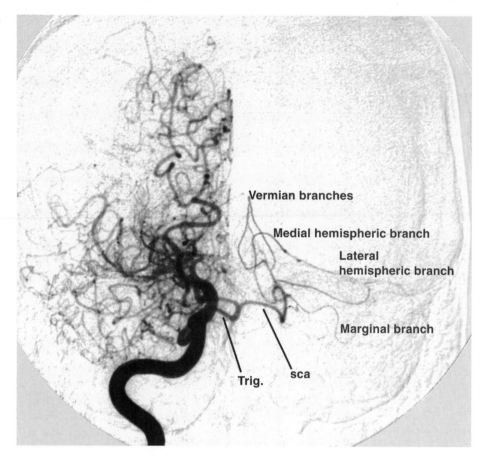

Figure 13.17. *Hemangioblastoma of the right cerebellar hemisphere.* A left vertebral artery injection in a patient with a hemangioblastoma. The vascular tumor-nodule projects in the lateral aspect of the right cerebellar hemisphere. The tumor is supplied by medial hemispheric (M) and lateral hemispheric (L) branches of the right superior cerebellar artery. The presence of a large cystic component of the tumor can be deduced from the marked mass-effect **(arrowheads)** on the surrounding hemispheric and marginal branches (MG) of the superior cerebellar artery.

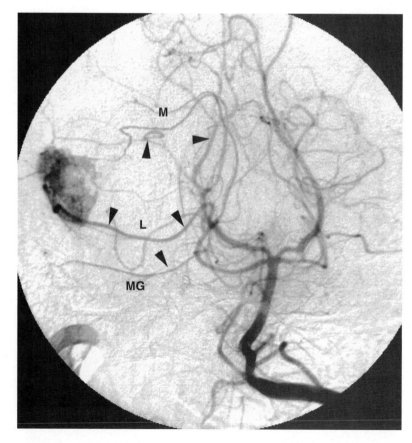

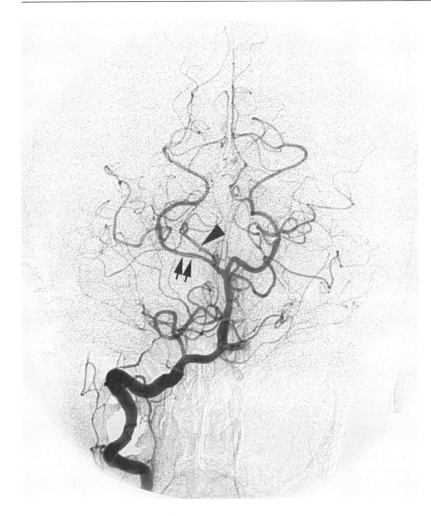

Figure 13.18. *Mass effect on the proximal superior cerebellar artery.* A large sphenoid wing meningioma shows no evidence of opacification on this right vertebral artery injection. However, the proximal course of the right superior cerebellar artery **(single arrowhead)** and, to a lesser extent, that of the proximal right posterior cerebral artery **(small double arrow)** are displaced posteriorly. Because this is a Townes projection, a posterior displacement is represented by a position higher in the field. The mass-effect is more pronounced on the superior cerebellar artery, which therefore is placed higher in the projection than is the posterior cerebral artery.

At a variable distance from its origin, the superior cerebellar artery bifurcates into a rostral and a caudal trunk. The rostral trunk continues a course circumferential to the brainstem to which it gives direct and circumflex perforating branches. It then supplies the superior surface of the vermis and the paramedian aspects of the superior cerebellar hemispheres (Figs. 13.16, 13.17). In the quadrigeminal cistern, the rostral branches of the superior cerebellar arteries may approach one another closely and give small perforating branches to the inferior colliculi, lateral midbrain, and related structures. The collicular branches represent a site of occasional anastomosis with the collicular branches of the posterior cerebral artery.

The cortical cerebellar branches are described as marginal (lateral), hemispheric, and vermian. The marginal branch is usually the first large branch of the superior cerebellar artery. It may have a separate (duplicated) origin from the basilar artery. It extends laterally to the horizontal fissure separating the superior lobe of cerebellum from the inferior (Fig. 13.17). It joins the horizontal fissure at a point more lateral than that supplied by the anterior inferior cerebellar artery. It usually supplies the lateral aspects of the hemisphere including the superior semilunar and quadrangular lobules. It is therefore balanced with

the anterior inferior cerebellar artery with which it shares an inverse relationship of size. The proximal marginal artery also supplies the superior cerebellar peduncle and the superior part of the dentate nucleus (in balance with the posterior inferior cerebellar artery). The dentate nucleus is considered to be an important site of spontaneous hypertensive cerebellar hemorrhage.

Anastomoses between the superior vermian and hemispheric branches of the superior cerebellar artery and the inferior counterparts from the posterior inferior cerebellar artery are commonly seen (Figs. 13.14, 13.17, 13.18). They constitute an important route of flow in situations of midbasilar occlusive disease.

REFERENCES

1. Caruso G, Vincentelli F, Guidicelli G, et al. Perforating branches of the basilar bifurcation. J Neurosurg 1990;73: 259–265.
2. Torche M, Mahmood A, Araujo R, et al. Microsurgical anatomy of the lower basilar artery. Neurol Res 1992;14:259–262.
3. Akar ZC, Dujovny M, Slavin KV, et al. Microsurgical anatomy of the intracranial part of the vertebral artery. Neurol Res 1994; 16:171–180.
4. Wollschlaeger G, Wollschlaeger PB, Lucas FV, et al. Experience and result with postmortem cerebral angiography performed

as routine procedure of the autopsy. Am J Radiol 1967;101: 68–87.

5. Mahmood A, Dujovny M, Torche M, et al. Microvascular anatomy of foramen caecum medullae oblongatae. J Neurosurg 1991;75:299–304.

6. Ito J, Tokiguchi S, Tsuchiya T. Anomalous origin of the posterior inferior cerebellar artery from the external carotid artery. Neuroradiology 1984;26:79–80.

7. Lasjaunias PL. Craniofacial and Upper Cervical Arteries: Functional Clinical and Angiographic Aspects. Baltimore: Williams & Wilkins, 1981.

8. Lasjaunias P, Vallee B, Person H, et al. The lateral spinal artery of the upper cervical spinal cord. J Neurosurg 1985;63:235–241.

9. Saeki N, Rhoton AL. Microsurgical anatomy of the upper basilar artery and the posterior circle of Willis. J Neurosurg 1977; 46:563–578.

10. Shrontz C, Dujovny M, Ausman JI, et al. Surgical anatomy of the arteries of the posterior fossa. J Neurosurg 1986;65:540–544.

11. Smith AS, Bellon JR. Parallel and spiral flow patterns of vertebral artery contributions to the basilar artery. Am J Neuroradiol 1995;16:1587–1591.

12. Hassler O. Arterial pattern of human brainstem. Normal appearance and deformation in expanding supratentorial conditions. Neurology 1967;17:368–375.

13. Pedroza A, Dujovny M, Ausman JI, et al. Microvascular anatomy of the interpeduncular fossa. J Neurosurg 1986;64:484–493.

14. Fisher CM. Clinical syndromes in cerebral thrombosis, hypertensive hemorrhage, and ruptured saccular aneurysms. Clin Neurosurg 1975;22:117–147.

15. Lhermitte F, Gautier JC, Derouesné C. Nature of occlusion of the middle cerebral artery. Neurology 1970;20:82–88.

16. Castaigne P, Lhermitte F, Gautier JC, et al. Arterial occlusions in the vertebro-basilar system. A study of 44 patients with postmortem data. Brain 1973;96:133–154.

17. Adams RD, Victor RD. Cerebrovascular diseases. In: Adams RD, Victor M, eds. Principles of Neurology. New York: McGraw-Hill, 1989; 634–642.

18. Schievink WI, Wijdicks EFM, Piepgras DG, et al. The poor prognosis of ruptured intracranial aneurysms of the posterior circulation. J Neurosurg 1995;82:791–795.

19. Marinkovic S, Milisavljevic M, Kovacevic M. Interpeduncular perforating branches of the posterior cerebral artery. Microsurgical anatomy of their extracerebral and intracerebral segments. Surg Neurol 1986;26:349–359.

20. Senator H. Apoplectische bulbärparalyse mit wechelständiger empfindungslähmung. Arch f. Psychiatr 1881;11:713.

21. Wallenberg A. Acute bulbar affections. Embolie der art. Cerebellar post. inf. sinstra. Arch f. Psychiatr 1895;27:504.

22. Merritt H, Finland M. Vascular lesions of the hind-brain (lateral medullary syndrome). Brain 1930;53:290–305.

23. Fujii K, Lenkey C, Rhoton AL. Microsurgical anatomy of the choroidal arteries. Fourth ventricle and cerebellopontine angles. J Neurosurg 1980;52:504–524.

24. Ito J, Takeda N, Suzuki Y, et al. Anomalous origin of the anterior inferior cerebellar arteries from the interior carotid artery. Neuroradiology 1980;19:105–109.

25. Ahuja A, Graves VB, Crosby DL, et al. Anomalous origin of the posterior inferior cerebellar artery from the internal carotid artery. Am J Neuroradiol 1992;13:1625–1626.

26. Ogawa R, Fujita H, Inugami A, et al. Anomalous origin of the posterior inferior cerebellar artery from the posterior meningeal artery. Am J Neuroradiol 1991;12:186.

27. Margolis MT, Newton TH. The posterior inferior cerebellar artery. In: Newton TH, Potts DG, eds. Radiology of the Skull and Brain: Angiography. St. Louis: CV Mosby, 1974;2:1710–1774.

28. Salamon G, Huang YP. Radiologic Anatomy of the Brain. Berlin: Springer-Verlag, 1976:305–322.

29. Lister JR, Rhoton AL, Matsushima T, et al. Microsurgical anatomy of the posterior inferior cerebellar artery. Neurosurgery 1982;10:170–199

30. Huang YP, Wolf BS. Angiographic features of fourth ventricle tumors with special reference to the posterior inferior cerebellar artery. Am J Radiol 1969;107:543–564.

31. Mani RL, Newton TH, Glickman MG. The superior cerebellar artery: an anatomic-roentgenographic correlation. Radiology 1968;91:1102–1108.

32. Hardy D, Rhoton AL. Microsurgical relationships of the superior cerebellar artery and the trigeminal nerve. J Neurosurg 1978;49:669–678.

33. Hardy DG, Peace DA, Rhoton AL. Microsurgical anatomy of the superior cerebellar artery. Neurosurgery 1980;6:10–28.

34. Jannetta PJ. Arterial compression of the trigeminal nerve at the pons in patients with trigeminal neuralgia. J Neurosurg 1967; 26:159–162.

35. Blinkov SM, Gabibov GA, Tanyashin SV. Variations in location of the arteries coursing between the brainstem and the free edge of the tentorium. J Neurosurg 1992;76:973–978.

36. Ono M, Ono M, Rhoton AL, et al. Microsurgical anatomy of the region of the tentorial incisura. J Neurosurg 1984;60:365–399.

CHAPTER 14

The Venous System

The venous system of the intracranial and extracranial structures of the neck and head is most easily described in separate spaces or compartments. However, it is important to understand the remarkable potential of these layers to communicate. The variable pattern of free communication through certain channels, in combination with selective flow-restriction through others, forms the basis for the pathophysiology of some vascular diseases of the brain and its coverings. A small shunt or fistula in a certain setting can have a catastrophic clinical effect on one patient; another patient with a large shunt in the same location may be asymptomatic and may even be best left untreated. Evaluation of the venous system is important for understanding the pathophysiology of certain disease states. It is particularly important for avoiding the creation of a dangerous restriction on venous flow through incomplete or erroneous interventional procedures.

EXTRACRANIAL VEINS

The scalp and face are highly vascular structures with a rich network of large veins throughout. The superficial temporal vein corresponds with the artery of the same name and runs down anterior to the ear to the posterior aspect of the parotid gland (Figs. 14.1, 14.2). Here it usually joins with the internal maxillary vein to form the retromandibular vein. The retromandibular vein joins the internal jugular vein. The anterior facial vein may also join the retromandibular vein or may empty directly into the internal jugular vein. The angular vein is formed at the junction of the frontal and supraorbital veins and forms an important anastomosis posteriorly with the superior ophthalmic vein. Although it usually drains inferiorly to the facial vein, it can drain into the cavernous sinus if flow is reversed and can become a conduit for propagation of infection or thrombosis. The occipital vein drains inferiorly into the deep cervical or vertebral veins. It may connect with the posterior auricular vein, and then to the external jugular vein.

The intracranial and extracranial venous systems communicate via emissary veins through skull foramina. Important emissary veins connect the superior sagittal sinus and transverse sinus with the suboccipital veins. The pterygoid plexus lies outside the skull base but has a number of important connections with the cavernous sinus via the foramina of the middle cranial fossa, notably the foramen of Vesalius, the foramen ovale, and other foramina innominata (Figs. 14.3, 14.4). The pterygoid plexus usually

drains to the facial vein. It may also connect superiorly into the orbit via the inferior orbital fissure through which it drains part of the inferior ophthalmic vein.

The internal jugular vein runs inferiorly in a position lateral to the internal carotid artery. The internal jugular vein receives input from the inferior petrosal sinus, the facial vein, lingual vein, pharyngeal veins, and thyroidal veins. In the thoracic inlet, it joins with the subclavian vein to form the brachiocephalic vein.

The external jugular vein receives venous outflow from the scalp, occipital region of the neck, and part of the face. It forms in the parotid gland and runs inferiorly superficial to the sternocleidomastoid muscle.

The vertebral vein forms at the level of atlas and runs as a plexus in the foramina transversaria surrounding the vertebral artery. A single outlet vein inferiorly then joins the brachiocephalic vein.

EMISSARY VEINS

These inconstant channels breach the skull and connect the superficial veins with the underlying dural sinuses. Some are more commonly seen.

Parietal emissary veins connect the superior sagittal sinus with the overlying scalp.

Mastoid emissary veins pass through the mastoid foramen and connect the transverse sinus with the occipital or posterior auricular veins.

Anterior condylar veins pass through the anterior condylar canal (hypoglossal canal) and connect the inferior petrosal sinus with the suboccipital veins.

DIPLOIC VEINS

The diploic veins between the two tables of the skull communicate with the overlying scalp veins and with the underlying meningeal veins and dural sinuses. They are not frequently seen at angiography. They do not cross suture lines unless the sutures have been completely obliterated.

MENINGEAL VEINS

Meningeal veins accompany their respective meningeal arteries. The anterior meningeal vein joins the superficial Sylvian vein to form the sphenoparietal sinus. The sphenoparietal sinus then passes below the lesser wing of the sphenoid bone to join the cavernous sinus. Alternatively it may course posteriorly in the middle cranial fossa to join the lateral sinus.

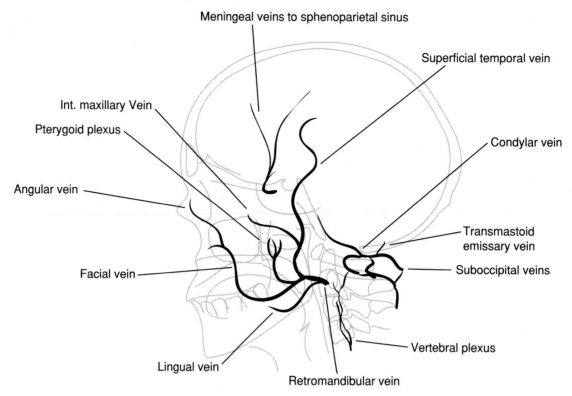

Figure 14.1. Superficial extracranial and middle meningeal veins.

DURAL SINUSES

The dural sinuses are venous channels enclosed between two layers of dura. They do not have valves.

The superior sagittal sinus extends from the foramen cecum posteriorly to the Torcular Herophili (Fig. 14.2). Occasionally, the superior sagittal sinus may bifurcate above the internal occipital protuberance. The superior sagittal sinus drains the superficial cerebral veins from the lateral and medial surfaces of the cerebral hemispheres. The largest such named vein is the vein of Trolard. Venous lacunae along the course of the superior sagittal sinus contain arachnoid granulations which become more prominent with age. They may form filling defects within the sinus itself. Veins entering the superior sagittal sinus may appear constrained at the point of entry giving a false appearance of venous stenosis.

The Torcular Herophili, named for its similarity to the handle of a manually operated wine-press (1), is the confluence of the superior sagittal sinus, the straight sinus, and the occipital sinus. It drains into the two transverse sinuses. The drainage is usually bilateral. If unilateral or asymmetric, the right transverse sinus is usually larger (2).

The inferior sagittal sinus lies along the inferior edge of the falx cerebri. It drains the anterior part of the corpus callosum, the medial portions of the cerebral hemispheres, and the falx. It joins with the internal cerebral vein to form the vein of Galen.

The straight sinus extends posteriorly from the junction between the falx cerebri and the tentorium, where it collects the vein of Galen and related tributaries. It drains to the torcular posteriorly.

The occipital sinus is inconstantly seen (Figs. 14.2B, 14.5). It usually drains upwards to the torcular. It may flow inferiorly and bevel laterally to join the sigmoid sinus, or connect with a sinus around the foramen magnum, termed the *marginal sinus*. The occipital and marginal sinuses are most commonly seen in young children. They diminish in size with age.

The transverse (lateral) sinuses curve laterally in the perimeter of the tentorium until they turn inferiorly to form the sigmoid sinuses. The transverse sinus receives a number of important supratentorial veins from the temporal and occipital lobes, notably the vein of Labbé. Infratentorial veins also drain to the transverse sinus, and it also receives the drainage of the superior petrosal sinus.

The sigmoid sinus represents the anterior, medial, and inferior continuation of the transverse sinus. It becomes the internal jugular vein in the jugular fossa and may receive direct venous channels from the pons and medulla. It communicates with the scalp veins via the mastoid and condylar veins.

The superior petrosal sinus runs from the posterior aspect of the cavernous sinus along the petrosal ridge to the junction of the sigmoid and transverse sinuses within the basal attachment of the tentorium. It receives venous channels from the supratentorial and infratentorial compartments and from the tympanic structures. It may lie either adjacent to or surround the roots of the trigeminal nerve.

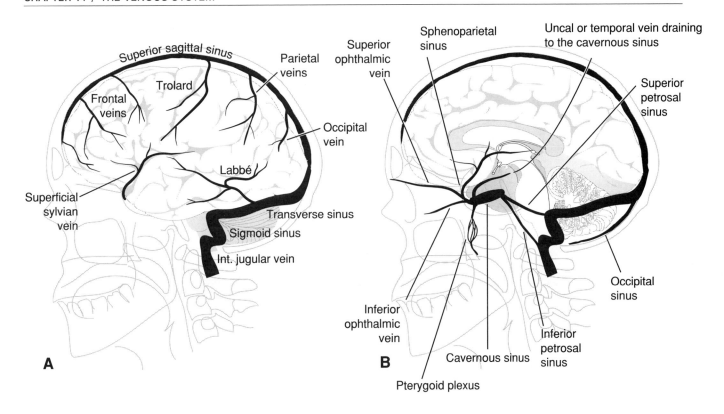

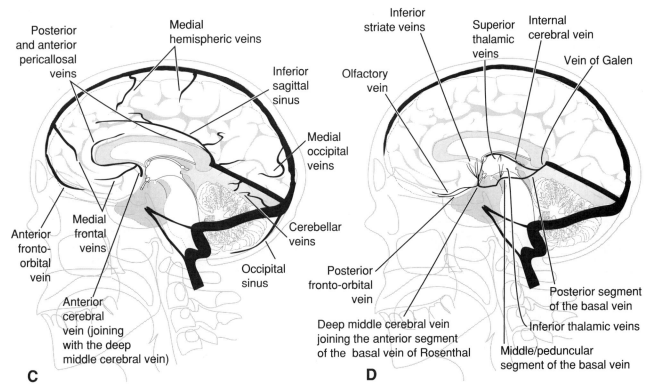

Figure 14.2. *Intracranial dural sinuses and veins.* **(A).** Superficial cortical veins of the left hemisphere are illustrated. A balanced arrangement of the superficial Sylvian vein, vein of Trolard, and vein of Labbé is depicted. **(B).** The left hemisphere has been removed from the illustration. The left superficial Sylvian vein is still in place (from A) to illustrate its relationship to the cavernous sinus. An understanding of the variability of the connections to and from the cavernous sinus is important to explain the clinical and angiographic consequences of arteriovenous shunting in this structure. The most common connection of clini-cal consequence is to the superior ophthalmic vein. A sinister possibility is the presence of connections from the cavernous sinus to the basal vein. Venous hypertension transmitted through this route accounts for the most serious complications of such disorders. **(C).** Superficial veins close to the midline are illustrated. The anterior pericallosal vein becomes the anterior cerebral vein. This vein may communicate across the midline via the anterior communicating vein. The anterior cerebral vein usually joins the anterior segment of the basal vein.

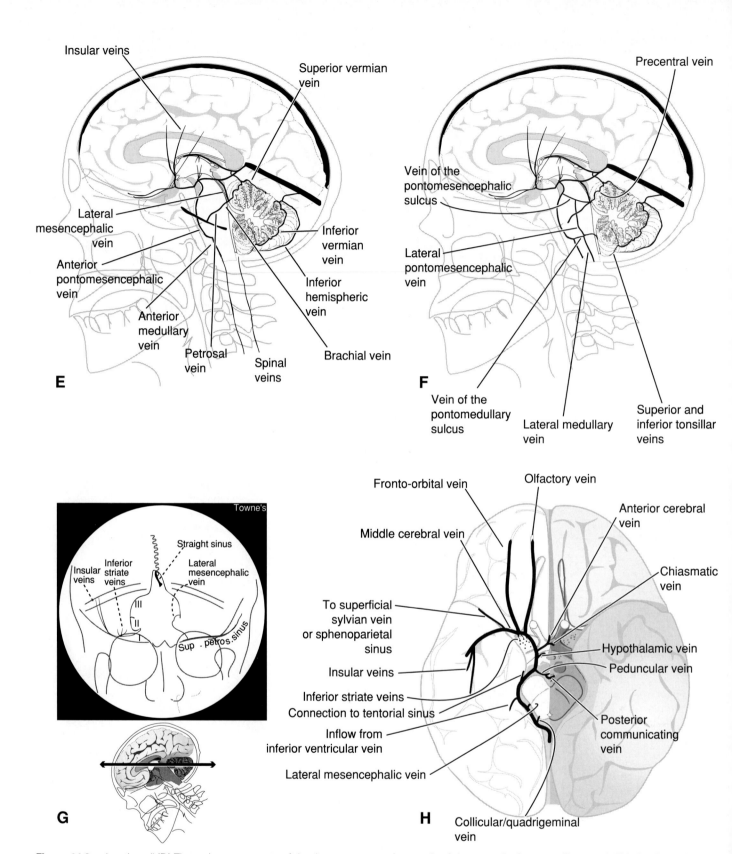

E — Insular veins; Superior vermian vein; Lateral mesencephalic vein; Anterior pontomesencephalic vein; Anterior medullary vein; Petrosal vein; Spinal veins; Brachial vein; Inferior hemispheric vein; Inferior vermian vein

F — Precentral vein; Vein of the pontomesencephalic sulcus; Lateral pontomesencephalic vein; Vein of the pontomedullary sulcus; Lateral medullary vein; Superior and inferior tonsillar veins

G — Towne's; Straight sinus; Insular veins; Inferior striate veins; Lateral mesencephalic vein; III; II; Sup. petros. sinus

H — Fronto-orbital vein; Olfactory vein; Anterior cerebral vein; Middle cerebral vein; Chiasmatic vein; To superficial sylvian vein or sphenoparietal sinus; Insular veins; Hypothalamic vein; Peduncular vein; Inferior striate veins; Connection to tentorial sinus; Inflow from inferior ventricular vein; Lateral mesencephalic vein; Posterior communicating vein; Collicular/quadrigeminal vein

Figure 14.2. *(continued)* **(D).** The major components of the deep venous system are illustrated. The insular veins, which are defining tributaries of the middle cerebral vein, usually superimpose on the inferior striate veins and are illustrated in **(E)** and **(H)**. The internal cerebral vein runs in the velum interpositum; it should therefore be superimposed on the course of the medial posterior choroidal artery from the arterial phase of the posterior circulation. **(E, F).** The insular veins are demonstrated without the underlying inferior striate veins. The major anasto-motic vessels of the posterior fossa are illustrated. **(G).** A schematic illustration of the shape of the basal vein and middle cerebral vein as seen on a Townes projection. The segments of the basal vein are numbered I, II, and III. The lateral mesencephalic vein slopes medially along the surface of the midbrain. Therefore, it usually has a character-istically medial course relative to the basal vein, demonstrated on the anatomic left side here. It drains to the superior petrosal sinus via the petrosal vein.

238

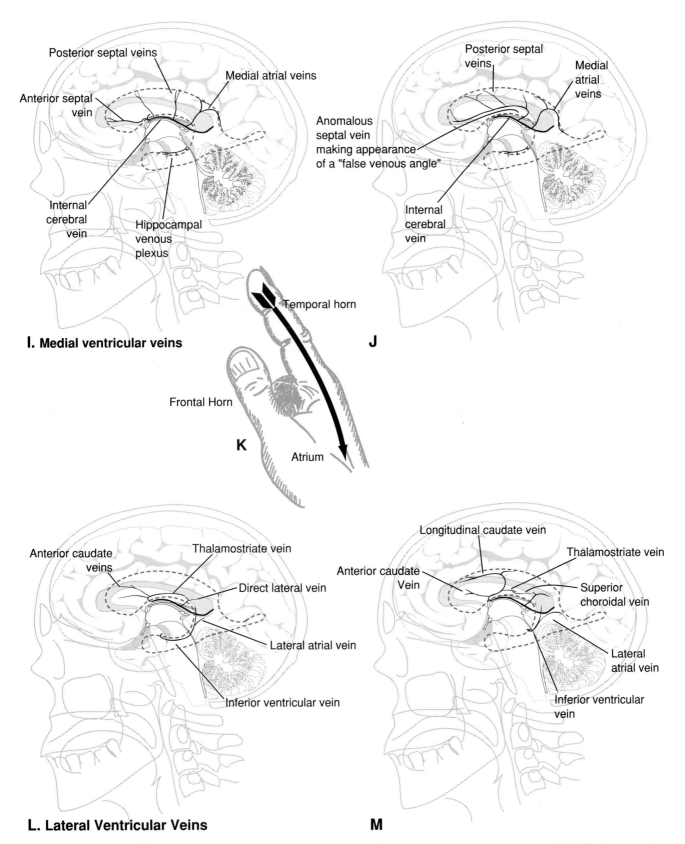

I. Medial ventricular veins

Posterior septal veins

Medial atrial veins

Anterior septal vein

Internal cerebral vein

Hippocampal venous plexus

Posterior septal veins

Medial atrial veins

Anomalous septal vein making appearance of a "false venous angle"

Internal cerebral vein

Temporal horn

J

Frontal Horn

K

Atrium

L. Lateral Ventricular Veins

Anterior caudate veins

Thalamostriate vein

Direct lateral vein

Lateral atrial vein

Inferior ventricular vein

Longitudinal caudate vein

Thalamostriate vein

Anterior caudate Vein

Superior choroidal vein

Lateral atrial vein

Inferior ventricular vein

M

Figure 14.2. *(continued)* **(H).** A base view of the brain demonstrates the complete territory of the basal vein. In reality, it is common for the basal vein to be a fragmented structure with preferential drainage through alternative pathways other than the vein of Galen. **(I, J).** The outline of the lateral ventricle is depicted by the dotted line. The medial ventricular veins are demonstrated in lateral appearance. It is rare to identify the hippocampal veins unless there is a high flow state such as might be related to the presence of an AVM. **(K).** A mnemonic to recall the relationship of the inferior ventricular vein to the lateral group of deep veins can be constructed by viewing the forefinger as the temporal horn of the lateral ventricle. The inferior ventricular vein runs in the roof of the temporal horn and connects with the veins on the lateral wall of the atrium. **(L, M).** The lateral ventricular veins of the deep system are illustrated in lateral projection.

Figure 14.3. *Intercavernous venous connections in a dural arteriovenous malformation of the left cavernous sinus.* A left common carotid artery injection opacifies a multitude of venous structures in the region of the left cavernous sinus through involved branches of the external carotid artery. Prominent intercavernous connections through the sella and along the clivus connect across the midline **(arrowheads)** to opacify the right cavernous sinus. Within the latter, a lucency is preserved by the course of the unopacified right internal carotid artery (RICA). Prompt drainage to the right inferior petrosal sinus (i.p.s.) is seen. On the left side, the superior ophthalmic vein (s.o.v.) is massively distended. It projects foreshortened along the plane of viewing.

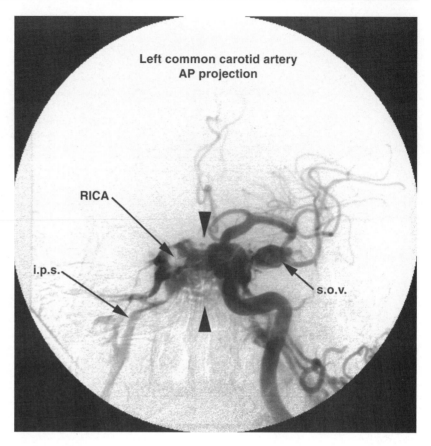

Figure 14.4. *Venous hypertension due to restricted outflow from the cavernous sinus.* Unlike the patient in 14.3, this patient with the same diagnosis, dural arteriovenous malformation of the cavernous sinus, does not have ready outflow from the cavernous sinus to the contralateral side or to the superior ophthalmic vein. At least this is the case for the involved compartment of the cavernous sinus. This injection is made into the ascending pharyngeal artery in the lateral projection. There is early opacification of the cavernous sinus via the carotid branch of the pharyngeal trunk **(double arrowhead)** and clival branches **(triple arrowhead)** from the neuromeningeal trunk. The superior ophthalmic vein (SOV) is small. The cavernous sinus decompresses itself via the basal vein (BV) with connections to the Sylvian veins (SSV), the vein of Galen (VOG) and straight sinus (SS). There is prominent opacification of cerebellar veins (CbV) in the posterior fossa. This is because of drainage from the cavernous sinus via the superior petrosal sinus **(double arrow)**. The patients symptoms were related to venous hypertension of the posterior fossa.

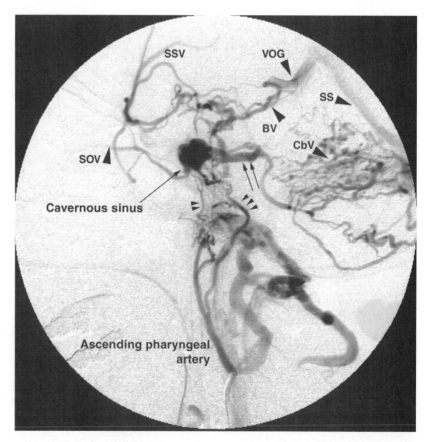

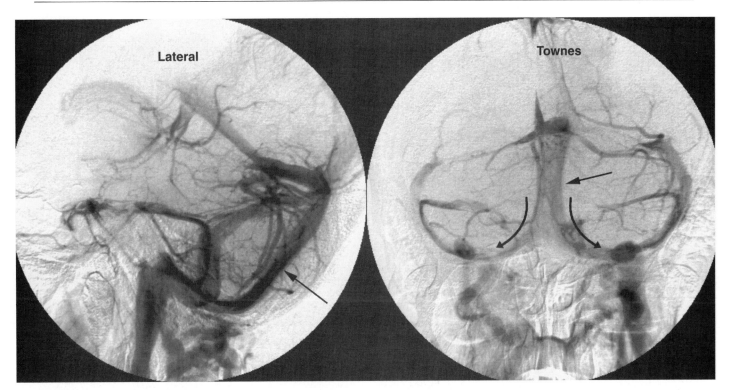

Figure 14.5. *Prominent occipital sinus.* An incidental observation of a large occipital sinus in an adult patient. The occipital sinus **(arrows)** descends along the falx cerebelli and divides into the marginal sinus around the foramen magnum joining the jugular foramen on each side. The transverse sinuses are correspondingly hypoplastic.

The inferior petrosal sinus runs inferiorly and laterally from the posterior part of the cavernous sinus to join the jugular vein in the pars nervosa which it shares with the glossopharyngeal nerve. The inferior petrosal sinus may receive channels from the medulla, cerebellum, and internal auditory veins.

The sphenoparietal sinus drains the superficial Sylvian vein into the cavernous sinus along the lesser wing of sphenoid behind the orbit. It receives variable contributions from meningeal, orbital, medial anterior temporal (uncal), and inferior frontal veins. Less commonly, this venous system may not reach the cavernous sinus. Alternatively, it can turn posteriorly in a sinus, most commonly referred to as the sphenopetrosal sinus (3), running along the floor of the middle cranial fossa to drain along the tentorium and into the superior petrosal sinus (see Fig. 17.3). An alternative variant drains into the pterygoid plexus and bypasses the cavernous sinus.

The cavernous sinus represents the most important site of confluence of intracranial and extracranial venous structures. Variations in the configuration of the outlets from the cavernous sinus are of little significance in the normal state. However, in the setting of pathologically increased blood flow through the sinus, the varied nature of the resulting clinical conditions is determined by the restrictions on venous outflow from the cavernous sinus.

Orbital venous drainage is via the superior and inferior ophthalmic veins, normally in an anterior to posterior direction. There are important variable anastomoses anteriorly with angular branches of the facial vein and frontal veins. The superior ophthalmic vein communicates posteriorly with the cavernous sinus and occasionally with the sphenoparietal sinus. The inferior ophthalmic vein also connects anteriorly with the facial vein and drains posteriorly to the cavernous sinus separate from or after joining the superior ophthalmic vein. It also connects inferiorly via the inferior orbital fissure with the pterygoid plexus.

The cavernous sinuses are multicompartmental extradural spaces that lie on either side of the sella on the surfaces of the greater wing of the sphenoid bone. They are interconnected by the anterior and posterior coronary (intercavernous) sinuses under the diaphragm sellae and by variable sinuses on the clivus (Fig. 14.3). Anteriorly, they accept venous drainage from the ophthalmic veins and the sphenoparietal sinus. Posteriorly they can accept parenchymal draining channels from the temporal lobe, particularly the uncal vein or middle cerebral vein. They also receive flow from the hypophyseal veins.

Outflow from the cavernous sinuses is mainly posteriorly to the petrosal sinuses. There are also draining connections to the pterygoid plexi through the foramina of the middle cranial fossa. The superior petrosal sinus and inferior ophthalmic vein may be either afferent to or efferent from the cavernous sinus.

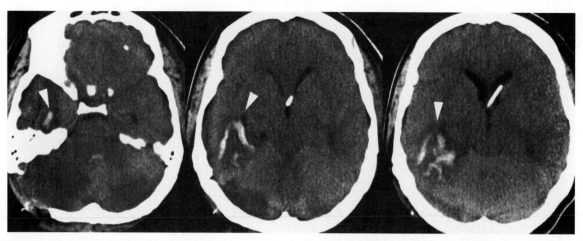

Figure 14.6. *Venous infarction after surgery.* An infratentorial surgical approach to a ruptured aneurysm in the posterior fossa was complicated by presumed occlusion of the right transverse sinus. Hypodensity of the infratentorial tissues may represent effects of retraction during surgery. However, a supratentorial hemorrhagic infarct is seen with a serpentine density representing a thrombosed vein and/or hemorrhage **(white arrowheads).** The findings probably relate to compromise of the right vein of Labbé.

SUPRATENTORIAL INTRADURAL VENOUS SYSTEM

The venous drainage pattern of the supratentorial structures is described as having a superficial system and a deep system. This is a useful division, but there are some superficial areas of cortex that drain via veins of the deep system. In the setting of anomalous or pathologic venous flow, the distinction between the two systems becomes blurred. Nevertheless, where surgery is planned, it is important to be able to recognize the major veins and sinuses present and to describe their direction of flow. Sacrificing major cortical veins or subdural bridging veins carries some risk of venous infarction and is therefore kept to a minimum during surgery (Fig. 14.6).

Superficial Supratentorial Cortical Veins

The superficial veins lie on the surface of the cerebral cortex. On the basal surface of the brain, many of the surface veins drain to the basal vein of Rosenthal and are considered part of the deep drainage system (Fig. 14.2). The superficial veins of the cerebral convexities drain to four major destinations or groups of bridging veins (4):

1. Superior sagittal sinus
2. Sphenoparietal sinus and cavernous sinus
3. Inferior sagittal sinus and vein of Galen
4. Tributaries of the sinuses related to the tentorium cerebelli

The superficial surface veins of the cerebral hemispheres drain the outer 1–2 cm of cortex and white matter. They have no muscle layers or valves. As they approach their sinus of destination, they assume a fibrous layer. When seen from a particular angle, they may give an appearance of constriction or pseudo-stenosis at the point of piercing the dura. Bridging veins of varying length may assume a tortuous course in the subdural space. They frequently fuse with meningeal veins to form common conduits before joining a major sinus.

Medial Hemispheric Superficial Veins

Anteriorly and superiorly in the frontal and parietal areas, superficial veins named for their respective sulci are directed superiorly and anteriorly towards the superior sagittal sinus. The superficial medial veins curve around the superior rim of the hemispheres and join with the superficial veins from the convexities to form common subarachnoid veins, which then pierce the dura (5). Collecting veins may run for variable distances in the subdural space. They may run within the falx itself, particularly posteriorly.

Not all the venous drainage from the medial aspect of the hemispheres enters the superficial system. Veins from the anterior cingulate gyrus and paraterminal gyrus are collected towards the anterior pericallosal vein, the paraterminal vein, and the anterior cerebral vein, which become tributaries of the basal vein. More posteriorly, veins from the central frontal and parietal lobes drain to the inferior sagittal sinus and posterior pericallosal vein, both of which join the vein of Galen. In the occipital lobe, peripherally disposed veins drain centrifugally towards the superior sagittal sinus, while more central veins drain to the straight sinus, to the vein of Galen, or to lesser tentorial sinuses.

Convexity Hemispheric Veins

Veins of the lateral hemispheric convexities drain via three major routes.

1. Veins adjacent to the Sylvian fissure collect into a common channel, the superficial Sylvian vein, which usually drains along the lesser sphenoid wing as the sphenoparietal sinus. The sphenoparietal sinus most often drains to the anterior part of the cavernous sinus.
2. Superiorly directed veins, up to 14 in number per hemisphere (6), empty into the superior sagittal sinus. The largest of these veins usually has an anastomosis with the Sylvian system and is called the *anastomotic vein of Trolard* (Fig. 14.7).

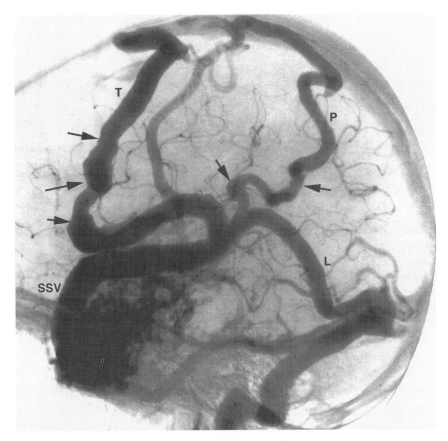

Figure 14.7. Superficial anastomotic veins. A brain arteriovenous malformation of the left temporal lobe drains predominantly through superficial convexity veins. The superficial Sylvian vein (SSV) drains retrogradely from the arteriovenous malformation to the superiorly directed Vein of Trolard (T), a lesser parietal convexity vein (P), and an anastomotic Vein of Labbé (L). The observation that venous outflow from this arteriovenous malformation is through a single channel (SSV) is concerning because this has some correlation with the risk of hemorrhage. Furthermore, the vein of Trolard (T) and parietal vein (P) demonstrate signs of early stenotic change or venous aneurysm formation **(arrows).**

3. Inferiorly disposed veins are directed toward the transverse sinus and other smaller dural sinuses of the middle cranial fossa. The largest of these, again with anastomosis to the Sylvian system, is termed the *anastomotic vein of Labbé.*

Of the three major anastomotic veins—the vein of Labbé, the vein of Trolard, and the superficial Sylvian vein—usually only one or two are present to a substantial degree. The vein of Labbé is most frequently prominent in the dominant hemisphere and the vein of Trolard is so in the non-dominant hemisphere (7). The superficial Sylvian vein is relatively constant in its location lying along the length of the superficial aspect of the Sylvian fissure. The vein of Trolard, by definition the largest anastomotic channel connecting the superficial Sylvian vein with the superior sagittal sinus, most commonly corresponds with the level of the post-central sulcus. It can be represented as far forward as the anterior frontal convexity veins, or as far posteriorly as the anterior parietal veins. It may be duplicated. The vein of Labbé is defined as the largest channel crossing the temporal lobe convexity from the superficial Sylvian vein to the transverse sinus. It usually crosses the middle third of the temporal lobe, but can be inconstant in location or duplicated.

The superficial hemispheric veins of the convexities are frequently described as making an acute angle against the direction of flow as they address the sinus. This appearance is most prevalent posteriorly and is thought by Padget (2) to be a mechanical stretching of the superficial veins away

from their site of dural drainage by expansion of the cerebral hemisphere during forebrain development. Piffer et al. (5) have described how the pattern of insertion into the superior sagittal sinus by the veins changes from anterior to posterior. Anterior veins have a superolateral insertion site; posterior veins approach the superior sagittal sinus from inferiorly along or within the falx cerebri.

BASAL HEMISPHERIC SUPERFICIAL VEINS

Veins from the basal or inferior surface of the frontal lobes may drain in two directions, which can be especially obvious with the patterns of venous drainage from anterior cranial fossa dural arteriovenous malformations. Anterior orbitofrontal branches drain into the superior sagittal sinus. Posteriorly directed veins, i.e., the posterior orbitofrontal and olfactory veins, join the confluence of veins under the anterior perforated substance, and so become tributaries of the middle cerebral veins (Fig. 14.2H). The veins in this area may also drain to the cavernous sinus or sphenoparietal sinus.

Veins from the basal surface of the temporal lobes are divided into medial and lateral according to their direction. Laterally directed veins drain to the tentorial sinuses. Medially directed veins may drain to the superior petrosal sinus or to the basal vein of Rosenthal. With the typical configuration of the basal vein, this implies that the medial temporal lobe structures are drained usually to the vein of Galen. However, the basal vein of Rosenthal varies in its configuration, and the anterior territory of this vein may drain to the cavernous sinus. Therefore in the setting of a high flow state through the cavernous sinus, such as a carotid cavernous fistula or dural arteriovenous malformation, venous hypertension of the temporal lobes may be an alarming complication of the disease with onset of seizures or venous infarction.

The inferior surface of the occipital lobe is drained by occipitobasal veins, which can be directed either to the transverse sinus or toward the basal vein.

Deep Supratentorial Veins

The deep venous system consists of the internal cerebral vein, the basal vein of Rosenthal, and their tributaries (8). The tributary branches of these veins are either ventricular or cisternal in location. The deep veins are concerned with the venous drainage of the central structures of the hemispheres, basal ganglia, corpus callosum, pineal region, midbrain, parts of the limbic system, and thalamus.

The intraventricular veins initially have a subependymal location. They used to be the most reliable angiographic indicators of central or deep mass lesions. In modern times, their relative importance for detection of mass-effect has decreased. They remain a strong consideration in analysis of the drainage patterns of arteriovenous malformations and for surgical planning. They are also used as landmarks for endoscopic navigation of the ventricles, particularly when other landmarks have been obliterated by the effects of hydrocephalus.

The earliest venous pattern seen embryologically is almost exclusively centrifugal to the pial veins. With enlargement of the brain, the deep, centripetal venous structures develop and become prominent, but being late in development are prone to anomalous configurations.

The deep white matter of the hemispheres is drained by medullary veins, which are characteristically straight in appearance. This appearance is thought to be related to the centrifugal pattern of migration of cells from the germinal matrix. The medullary veins collect in subependymal veins, which run along the surface of the lateral ventricles. For purposes of description the deep ventricular veins are divided into lateral and medial groups. The ventricular

veins drain towards the choroidal fissure and eventually join either the internal cerebral vein in the roof of the third ventricle or the basal vein of Rosenthal (Fig. 14.8). The medial group of ventricular veins passes through the outer or forniceal edge of the choroidal fissure; the lateral ventricular group passes through the thalamic or inner edge of the fissure (9). The thalamic veins contribute to both groups. An embryologic torsion of the lateral ventricle in the formation of the temporal horn results in a correspondence of the roof of the temporal horn with the lateral wall of the atrium, while the floor of the temporal horn corresponds with the medial wall of the atrium. Therefore, veins of the roof of the temporal horn (specifically the inferior ventricular veins) are classified with the lateral group of subependymal veins.

The medial group of ventricular veins drains the inner surface of the corpus callosum, septum pellucidum, the fornix, and the hippocampus. The lateral group drains the body, floor, and lateral wall of the lateral ventricle and roof of the temporal and occipital horns.

Medial Group of Deep Veins

The anterior septal vein drains the deep structures of the frontal lobe. It gathers three to five medullary tributaries into a single channel, which runs along the septum pellucidum, making a detour around the fornix. It forms "the venous angle" with the thalamostriate vein (from the lateral group) at the anterior end of the internal cerebral vein thus demarcating the location of the foramen of Monro (Fig. 14.9). Anomalous insertion of the anterior septal vein more posteriorly into the internal cerebral vein is common. In these instances, the vein pursues a course within the lateral ventricle as far back as the splenium. It then enters between the two halves of the fornix into the velum interpositum to join the internal cerebral vein. This more posterior junction with the internal cerebral vein gives an appearance of a "false venous angle" on the lateral view.

Posterior septal or direct medial veins drain the posterior aspect of the frontal lobe and the parietal lobe into subependymal veins in the superior aspect of the lateral ventricle. These two to five veins turn inferiorly along the

---

Figure 14.8. *Deep ventricular veins and the choroidal fissure.* **(A).** A coronal illustration of the cistern of the velum interpositum at the level of the thalami demonstrates the internal cerebral vein and choroidal arteries, which run within this space or potential space. The velum interpositum is defined on each side by the medial walls of the thalami and superiorly by the fornices. The cleavage between the fornix and thalamus on each side represents the uppermost extension of the choroidal fissure. The fissure is bridged by tela choroidea from which is suspended the choroid plexus of the ventricles. The floor of the velum interpositum is composed of a layer of tela choroidea extending between the stria medullaris on each side. The choroid plexus of the third ventricle below is suspended from this layer of tela choroidea. The dotted line in A runs through the choroidal fissure separating the medial from the lateral ventricular veins. The medial veins run close

to the fornix, the lateral group close to the thalamic side of the fissure. Notice the shape of the epicallosal cistern or sulcus between the cingulate gyrus and the corpus callosum. Venous opacification in this space causes the "mustache" appearance on a direct PA view. Asymmetric hydrocephalus or midline shift causes a tilting of the venous mustache. **(B).** An illustration in the coronal plane of the choroidal fissure at the level of the perimesencephalic cistern. Because of embryologic torsion in the formation of the choroidal fissure, the lateral ventricular veins correspond with those in the roof of the temporal horn, i.e., the inferior ventricular vein. The hippocampal plexus of veins drains on the other side of the choroidal fissure via the fimbrio-dentate sulcus to the hippocampal vein in the hippocampal sulcus. Notice how the lateral mesencephalic vein bevels medially from the basal vein, corresponding with its appearance in Townes projection in Figure 14.2G.

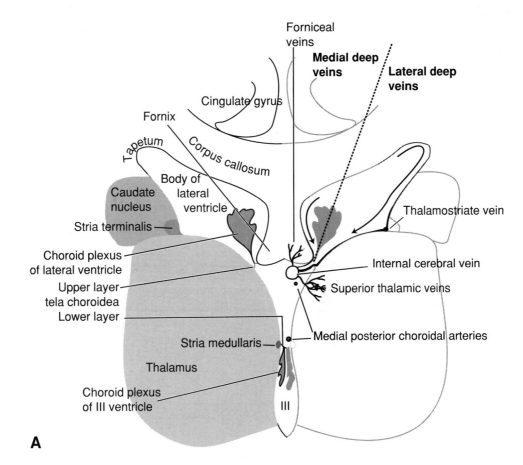

A

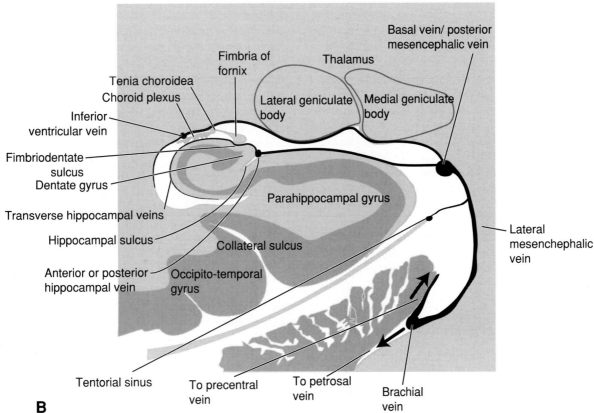

B

Figure 14.9. *Venous angle.* The venous angle **(arrowhead)** is formed by the junction of the thalamostriate vein and anterior septal vein. This junction occurs within a few millimeters of the posterior rim of the foramen of Monro. It serves as a useful landmark.

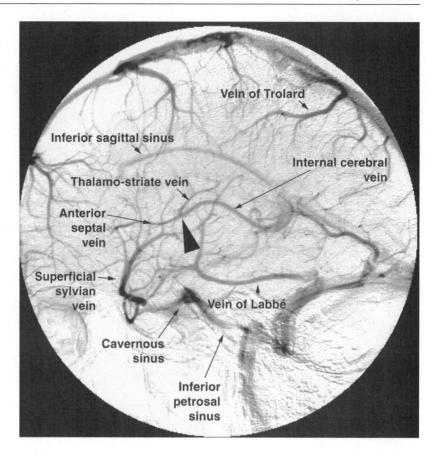

medial ependymal surface. Similar to, or after joining with the previously described course of an anomalous anterior septal vein, they enter the cistern of the velum interpositum between the two halves of the fornix to join the internal cerebral vein.

The medial atrial veins of the lateral ventricle represent the collections of the medullary veins of the posterior parietal and occipital lobes. When a single vein is prominent, it may be termed the *vein of the posterior horn.* The medial atrial veins perforate the fornix and unite in an extraventricular location behind the pulvinar. This common medial atrial vein may receive lateral atrial contributions, and thus, be termed the *common atrial vein.* This vein enters the posterior aspect of the internal cerebral vein or the vein of Galen.

The medial ventricular veins of the temporal horn lie atop the hippocampal structures, which they drain. This collection of transverse veins, the hippocampal venous formation, unites and exits from the ventricle on the dentate gyrus. It enters the basal vein of Rosenthal.

Lateral Group of Deep Veins

Veins that drain the caudate nucleus are named the anterior caudate vein, longitudinal caudate vein, or anteroinferior caudate vein. The anterior caudate vein is the standard described variant, which represents a collection of a number of tributaries from the medial surface of the caudate nucleus. It drains into the thalamostriate vein. The

longitudinal caudate vein has a higher more posterior curve above the caudate nucleus. It curves inferomedially into the thalamostriate vein. The anteroinferior caudate vein variant is significant only for its course and appearance being in the same plane as the anterior septal vein as seen on the lateral view. In the body of the lateral ventricle, the posterior aspect of the caudate nucleus may be drained by the transverse caudate veins, which also drain to the thalamostriate vein.

The thalamostriate vein is usually a prominent tributary of the internal cerebral vein. It drains the posterior frontal and anterior parietal lobes, caudate nucleus, and the internal capsule. However, it does not give significant direct drainage to the thalamus. It begins posteriorly near the atrium, but may arise as far posteriorly as the temporal horn. It runs anteriorly in thalamo-caudate groove. It defines the junction between the diencephalon and telencephalon in adults. At the anterior aspect of the thalamus it turns inferiorly and medially and passes behind and within a few millimeters of the foramen of Monro at the angiographic venous angle. It collects the caudate veins, anterior septal vein, anterior thalamic veins, and superior choroid vein. When the thalamostriate vein is hypoplastic, its territory may be drained by a transverse direct lateral vein, which enters the internal cerebral vein posterior to the foramen of Monro. Alternatively with hypoplasia of the thalamostriate vein, its territory may be drained by the inferior ventricular vein into the temporal horn by virtue

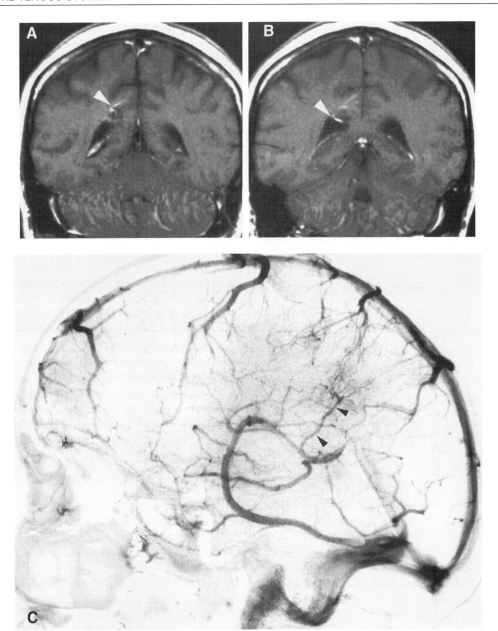

Figure 14.10. *Anomaly of venous drainage to an atrial vein.* An anomaly of venous drainage is seen as an incidental finding in the roof of the occipital horn of the lateral ventricle above the calcar avis (arrowhead). On the coronal gadolinium-enhanced images **(A, B)**, the subependymal collector of this anomaly is easily seen. On a cerebral angiogram **(C)**, the subsequent course of this vein **(arrowheads)** is evident on the late venous phase as it joins the internal cerebral vein.

of a persistent embryologic anastomosis between the thalamostriate vein and the inferior ventricular vein.

The lateral atrial vein lies along the lateral wall of the atrium and receives drainage from the posterior temporal and parietal lobes (Fig. 14.10). It runs anteroinferiorly along the lateral atrial wall and can join the basal vein through the choroidal fissure. Alternatively, it can turn medially along the anterior atrial wall, exit through a higher site in the choroidal fissure, and join the medial atrial veins to form the common atrial vein.

The lateral group is represented in the temporal lobe by the inferior ventricular vein, which lies in the roof of the ventricle. This vein receives drainage from the supero-

lateral areas of the temporal lobe. It runs anteriorly along the course of the tail of the caudate nucleus. After receiving the inferior choroid vein, it exits from the temporal horn through the choroidal fissure and becomes a tributary of the basal vein.

CHOROIDAL VEINS OF THE DEEP VENOUS SYSTEM

There are two named choroidal veins that receive drainage only from the choroid plexus.

The superior choroid vein runs from posterior to anterior in the floor of the body of the lateral ventricle in a course medial to the thalamostriate vein and lateral to the fornix. It drains to the thalamostriate vein or directly to the internal cerebral vein.

The inferior choroid vein drains the choroid plexus of the temporal horn. It also runs from posterior to anterior and joins the inferior ventricular vein or runs directly to the basal vein.

THALAMIC VEINS

The superior thalamic vein is a centrally directed structure that emerges from the thalamus above the pineal gland. It enters the most posterior aspect of the internal cerebral vein or the vein of Galen.

The anterior thalamic vein lies medially and anteriorly and becomes a tributary of the thalamostriate vein, septal vein, or internal cerebral vein.

The inferior thalamic veins are very fine vessels that exit inferiorly through the posterior perforated substance to the posterior mesencephalic vein. They drain the infero-medial portion of the thalamus.

The posterior thalamic veins drain the posterolateral portion of the thalamus to the posterior mesencephalic vein or basal vein of Rosenthal. Superficial thalamic veins drain along the ventricular surface of the thalamus or on the surface contiguous with the cistern of the velum interpositum. They join the tributaries of the internal cerebral vein anteriorly or may join atrial veins posteriorly.

INTERNAL CEREBRAL VEINS

The paired internal cerebral veins run from anterior to posterior in the roof of the third ventricle enclosed between two layers of tela choroidea. This potential space between the two layers is called the cistern of the velum interpositum. As this space emerges into the supra-pineal area, the veins diverge from one another to run around the pineal gland and then reconverge. Underneath the tip of the splenium, they unite into the great cerebral vein of Galen.

GREAT CEREBRAL VEIN OF GALEN

This is a midline, unpaired, subarachnoid structure. Its length is from 5–20 mm. It forms below the tip of the splenium around which it then curves posteriorly. In addition to the internal cerebral veins, it receives tributaries from the basal vein of Rosenthal, the inferior sagittal sinus, the posterior pericallosal vein, the internal occipital veins, and veins from the posterior fossa.

BASAL CEREBRAL VEIN OF ROSENTHAL

The standard configuration of the basal vein forms under the anterior perforated substance, and runs posteriorly on the undersurface of the brain to its termination with the vein of Galen or the internal cerebral vein. It is the collector of venous output from an extensive distribution of tissue encompassing the orbital surface of the frontal lobe, insula and medial temporal lobe, hypothalamus, striatum,

thalamus, and midbrain. It has important anastomoses with the superficial Sylvian vein, the veins of the posterior fossa, and the petrosal and cavernous sinuses.

The formation of the basal vein is defined as the junction of the inferior striate veins with the middle cerebral vein under the anterior perforated substance (Fig. 14.11). The venous system of the brain is characterized by a closer adherence of venous channels to the adjacent brain structures than is seen with the arterial counterparts, thus making the veins a more precise adumbration of anatomic landmarks. Unlike the lateral lenticulostriate arteries, which weave medially in the subarachnoid space before entering the anterior perforated substance, the inferior striate veins have a shorter subarachnoid stem and immediately enter the basal vein. The basal vein is described in three segments. The first (anterior or striate) segment runs from the anterior perforated substance to the anterior margin of the cerebral peduncle. The second (peduncular) extends from there to the lateral mesencephalic sulcus on the lateral aspect of the midbrain. The third (posterior mesencephalic) segment continues to the junction with the great vein of Galen. By evaluating each of these segments, the adjacent anatomy outlined by the basal vein and its tributaries can be more easily inferred. Furthermore, in variant configurations of the basal vein, where the venous collecting system is not united into a single channel, these segments form the basis for alternative collectors and their respective outflow channels.

Anterior Segment of the Basal Vein

The anterior segment of the basal vein is formed by the junction of the inferior striate veins with the middle cerebral vein. After formation under the anterior perforated substance, the anterior segment runs posteriorly and medially. The point at the anterior margin of the cerebral peduncle is the most medial in the course of the basal vein as seen on PA views and the most inferior on lateral views.

The striate veins are described as superior, draining to the internal cerebral venous system, or inferior, draining with a fan-shaped aspect as seen on lateral views. The middle cerebral vein is formed at the limen insulae by the confluence of the insular veins. The insular veins, like the arterial counterparts, have a straight radiating appearance and can be named according to their relation with the sulci of the insula—anterior, precentral, central, or posterior. These vessels are longer and more widely spaced than the fan of the inferior striate veins which may be superimposed on the lateral view. As it curves medially, the middle cerebral vein is also concave posteriorly.

The basal vein is also joined in this anterior segment by veins from the frontal lobe, the olfactory vein and the posterior orbito-frontal veins, medially and laterally respectively. The olfactory vein originates near the olfactory bulb. On the lateral view it initially runs superiorly into the olfactory groove, then descends forming a curve concave superiorly. The posterior orbito-frontal vein(s) lies more laterally and inferiorly. The anterior pericallosal vein is

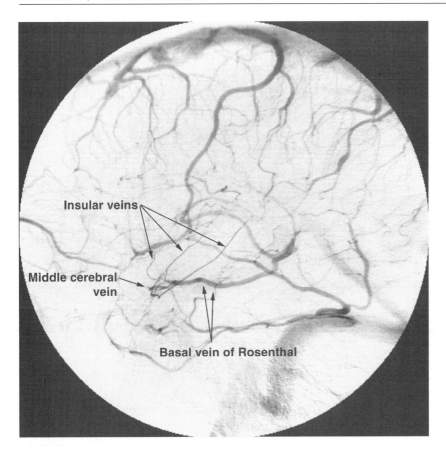

Figure 14.11. *Basal vein of Rosenthal, insular veins, and middle cerebral vein.* In this example, the superficial Sylvian vein is not well seen. This affords an unobstructed view of the insular veins. The insular veins course along the sulci of the insular triangle, forming the middle cerebral vein at their confluence around the limen insulae. The middle cerebral vein collects the inferior striate veins **(see Figs. 14.2D, G, H)** along the anterior perforated substance to form the anterior segment of the basal vein of Rosenthal. A deflection in the course of the basal vein is frequently seen **(between the arrows)** as it circumvents the cerebral peduncle.

the small venous counterpart of the pericallosal artery. It is likely to have anastomoses or channels to the inferior sagittal sinus more posteriorly. It may be connected to the contralateral anterior pericallosal vein by the anterior communicating vein, below which the vessel is then named the anterior cerebral vein. It joins the basal vein at the anterior perforated substance.

Middle Segment of the Basal Vein

The middle segment of the basal vein is closely applied to the upper surface of the peduncle where it lies medial to the uncus and is closely related in course to the optic tract. Within the interpeduncular cistern, a peduncular vein functions as a collector for venous vessels from the midbrain and from the thalamus superiorly. The inferior thalamic veins exit via the posterior perforated substance in the depth of the interpeduncular cistern and enter the peduncular vein. A communication with the contralateral peduncular vein may be prominent, named the posterior communicating vein (Fig. 14.12). Large or dominant connections to the anterior pontomesencephalic vein in the midline may also be present draining into or from the posterior fossa. On its lateral side the basal vein gathers the hippocampal veins. From the temporal horn of the lateral ventricle, it gathers the inferior ventricular vein, the inferior choroidal vein, and occasionally the lateral atrial vein. These veins exit through the choroidal fissure to reach the basal vein.

Posterior Segment of the Basal Vein

From the level of the lateral mesencephalic sulcus, the third segment of the basal vein curves around the pulvinar in a medial and superior direction, enters the quadrigeminal cistern, and then joins the vein of Galen. It is joined on its inferior surface by the lateral mesencephalic vein. The lateral mesencephalic vein lies along the lateral mesencephalic sulcus parallel to the main axis of the brainstem (Fig. 14.13). It is an important collector of the venous system of the posterior fossa. It is also an important potential connection between the supratentorial and infratentorial venous systems, and between both of these systems and the superior petrosal sinus. It may drain into or from the basal vein. Another vessel, the posterior mesencephalic vein having a course similar to the described course of the third segment of the basal vein, may be connected to the lateral mesencephalic vein in this area. The basal vein and the posterior mesencephalic vein may be synonymous.

It is common for the third segment of the basal vein to collect venous output from the posterior fossa by receiving the precentral and superior vermian veins. Other venous tributaries in the supratentorial area include the posterior thalamic veins, the thalamogeniculate veins, the splenial vein, the medial atrial or common atrial vein, and small occipital and temporal cortical veins.

Anatomic Variants in the Basal Vein

Variations are common in the configuration of the basal vein and relate to the degree to which the various segments

Figure 14.12. *Venous drainage of a posterior fossa arteriovenous malformation.* A Townes view of an arteriovenous malformation in the region of the left middle cerebellar peduncle. The route of venous drainage is superiorly through the lateral mesencephalic vein **(see Fig. 14.2G),** which is considerably distended in this patient. When it reaches the posterior mesencephalic vein (synonymous with the basal vein), flow is directed posteriorly to the Galenic system. Flow is also directed anteriorly around the peduncle and opacifies the contralateral posterior mesencephalic vein via the posterior communicating vein. The right side also decompresses via the petrosal vein to the right superior petrosal sinus.

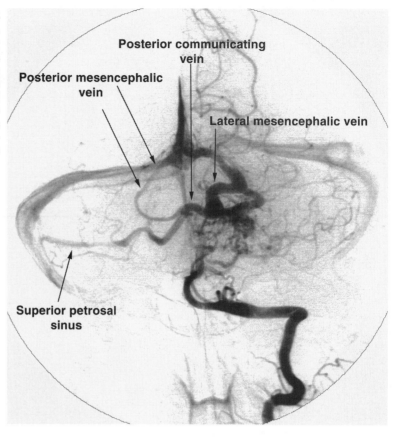

Figure 14.13. *Venous drainage of collicular arteriovenous malformation.* A lateral projection of a left vertebral artery injection in a patient with an arteriovenous malformation of the region of the quadrigeminal plate. Restriction of venous flow is present with no evidence of a straight sinus. Instead, venous flow is directed into alternative routes, principally the lateral mesencephalic vein. The latter drains to the sigmoid sinus via the superior petrosal sinus.

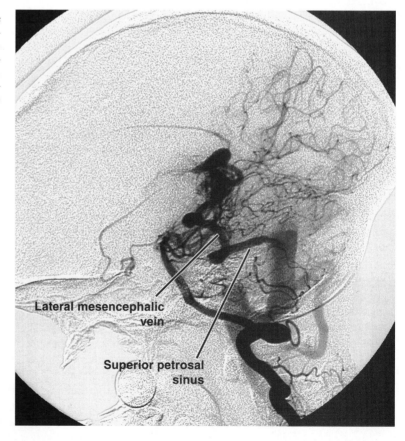

of the basal vein fail to unite, and to alternative outflow routes draining parts or all of this venous system (10).

When there is failure of communication between the anterior and middle segments, venous outflow from the anterior segment is preserved through routes usually directed anteriorly to the cavernous sinus. Union of the middle cerebral vein and the inferior striate veins forms the uncal vein with other tributaries from the frontal and temporal lobes. This vein most commonly drains directly to the cavernous sinus or may do so indirectly by draining laterally to the superficial Sylvian vein and the sphenoparietal sinus. More posteriorly, alternative outflow routes include drainage via the lateral mesencephalic vein to the superior petrosal sinus (via the petrosal vein). The basal system may drain alternatively via tentorial sinuses to the transverse and superior petrosal sinuses. Hypoplasia of the basal vein may occur, in which case a posteriorly directed vein lying more lateral than is usually associated with the position of the basal vein, may be seen. This laterally disposed vein represents an enlarged hippocampal vein.

SEQUENCE OF DEEP VENOUS FILLING

After a carotid injection, the earliest deep venous structures to fill are the thalamostriate and internal cerebral veins, at the same time as the posterior frontal veins. The septal vein fills last, at the same time as the dural sinuses, vein of Trolard, and the occipital veins. The basal vein normally has an intermediate timing. On vertebral artery injections, the transit time for the thalamic circulation is shortest, which means that thalamic veins will be seen during the time that the cerebellum and posterior hemispheres are still in the capillary phase (11, 12).

INFRATENTORIAL VENOUS SYSTEM

The elegance of angiographic depiction of the veins of the posterior fossa lies in the close relationship between the more constant members of this group and their associated anatomic landmarks. More importantly, the functional significance of the configuration of these veins derives from the multitude of possible connections to and from the venous system of the supratentorial space and that of the spinal cord. Therefore, more germane than the enumeration of tiny, obscure veins encountered in this enclosed space is a knowledge of these connections. This prompts an evaluation of the effects of vascular lesions of this area on local and remote venous fields. Conversely, an evaluation of the effects of vascular lesions elsewhere may include examination of effects on the venous system of the posterior fossa (see Fig. 16.5). For instance, a carotid-cavernous fistula or dural arteriovenous malformation of the cavernous sinus can present only with symptoms of posterior fossa venous hypertension. An arteriovenous malformation of the posterior fossa may mimic a spinal dural arteriovenous fistula and present with symptoms of conal myelopathy (see Fig. 18.15).

The veins of the posterior fossa collect to three principal destinations (13–15): the petrosal sinuses, the Vein of Galen and related tributaries, and the dural sinuses bordering on or between the leaves of the tentorium cerebelli.

No single configuration is typical, but certain members of these veins are more commonly and clearly visualized, and certain connections between these three groups will be seen in typical locations (Figs. 14.2, 14.3, 14.12, 14.13).

Anatomic variations can be seen in the drainage of the basal vein of Rosenthal to the dural sinuses, and these will affect the pattern of drainage seen in the posterior fossa. Persistence of embryonic venous sinuses may be seen through which the basal vein may drain to the lateral mesencephalic vein or tentorial sinuses (16).

VEINS RELATED TO THE SURFACE OF THE BRAINSTEM

The major veins related to and named correspondingly with the structures of the brainstem are easily identified on normal angiograms. They frequently act as collectors for smaller cerebellar veins. They are named according to their relationship to the mesencephalon, pons, or medulla, and according to whether they lie in a transverse or longitudinal disposition.

At the interpeduncular fossa, the inferior thalamic veins exit the posterior perforated substance and join with mesencephalic veins to form the peduncular vein. This vein skirts anteriorly around the peduncle from medial to lateral to enter either the basal vein or posterior mesencephalic vein in the ambient cistern.

On the lateral aspect of the midbrain, the lateral mesencephalic vein runs in a cephalad-caudad direction in the lateral mesencephalic sulcus, draining superiorly to the posterior mesencephalic vein or basal vein (16).

The anterior pontomesencephalic vein runs from the peduncular vein in the interpeduncular cistern in a longitudinal direction in approximately the midline along the anterior rim of the pons. It frequently connects with its inferior midline counterpart, the anterior medullary vein, which in turn connects inferiorly with the anterior spinal vein. The anterior pontomesencephalic vein may preferentially connect laterally at the level of the mid-pons through a transverse pontine vein with the petrosal vein. The petrosal vein is a final collector for many cerebellar and brainstem veins draining into the midpoint of the superior petrosal sinus. The single median pontomesencephalic vein may be paralleled along some of its course by bilateral lateral pontomesencephalic veins to which it is connected by transversely oriented pontine veins. The lateral pontomesencephalic veins connect with the posterior mesencephalic vein above and with the petrosal vein below. The longitudinal vein on the lateral surface of the medulla, the lateral anterior medullary vein, is the medullary counterpart of the lateral pontomesencephalic vein; it is sometimes called the preolivary vein. The lateral medullary vein, counterpart of the lateral mesencephalic vein, is sometimes called the retro-olivary vein.

CEREBELLAR VEINS

The complex anatomy of the cerebellum can be simplified into a description that allows three surfaces (17).

The superiorly directed tentorial surface facing the tentorium is the least complex and features a central peak sloping laterally with a smooth transition between the superior vermis (culmen and declive) medially and the cerebellar hemispheres laterally.

The rounded suboccipital surface of the cerebellum faces inferiorly and features two large cerebellar hemispheres separated by a depression or incisura, which straddles the falx cerebelli. The midline surface of this median depression, the posterior cerebellar incisura, is formed by the vermis superiorly and by the intertonsillar fissure or vallecula inferiorly.

The anterior surface of the cerebellum faces the brainstem medially and the petrosal bones laterally. The petrosal surface is bisected transversely into a superior and inferior part by the horizontal fissure of the cerebellum.

The cerebellomesencephalic fissure lies above the cerebellar peduncles and separates the quadrangular lobule of the cerebellar hemisphere from the brainstem. Inferiorly, the cerebellomedullary fissure separates the tonsils from the posterolateral surface of the medulla.

Within the cerebellomesencephalic fissure, the superior and inferior cerebellar peduncles are distinguishable on their surfaces by a shallow interpeduncular sulcus (not to be confused with the midline interpeduncular fossa of the midbrain). The interpeduncular sulcus is contiguous anteriorly with the transversely oriented pontomesencephalic sulcus, separating the midbrain from the pons, and superiorly with the longitudinally directed lateral mesencephalic sulcus on the posterolateral aspect of the midbrain. These confluent sulci frequently contain large correspondingly named veins through which normal and abnormal venous flow can be routed in a variety of directions. Superiorly directed flow through the lateral mesencephalic vein drains to the posterior mesencephalic vein or basal vein of Rosenthal. Anterior drainage from this point via a vein sometimes named the brachial vein (because of its relation to the brachium pontis and brachium conjunctivum) connects to the petrosal vein and thus to the superior petrosal sinus. Matsushima et al. (17) refer to this vein more anteriorly as the ponto-trigeminal vein. Posteriorly the cerebello-mesencephalic fissure extends behind the brainstem to the midline where it continues as the fissure in front of the central lobule of the vermis. The vein in this fissure was called the precentral cerebellar vein by Huang and Wolf (14) and was a useful angiographic guide to the presence of midline mass-effect in the posterior fossa. Matsushima et al. (17) refer to this vein as a continuation of the vein of the cerebello-mesencephalic fissure. It usually drains superiorly and posteriorly to enter the galenic vein after receiving superior hemispheric and superior vermian tributaries. In situations of reversed venous flow, this route back into the cerebello-

mesencephalic fissure allows drainage of these regions into the confluence on the superior aspect of the cerebellar peduncles and thus towards the petrosal vein or other veins.

The vein of the cerebellomedullary fissure drains the inferior vermis, the structures related to the lower part of the fourth ventricle, the inferior cerebellar peduncle, and some of the tonsillar veins. The vein of the cerebellomedullary fissure was termed the *vein of the lateral recess* by Huang and Wolf (18).

The tentorial surface of the cerebellum is drained by the superior hemispheric and the superior vermian veins. The more peripheral superior hemispheric veins drain centrifugally to the transverse sinus and torcular. Centrally, the superior hemispheric veins may drain anteriorly to the superior petrosal sinus, or centripetally to join the superior vermian vein or the veins in the cerebello-mesencephalic fissure, and ultimately the galenic system. The superior vermian veins drain anteriorly to the galenic system or posteriorly to the torcular or straight sinus.

The suboccipital surface of the cerebellum is drained by the inferior hemispheric veins and the inferior vermian veins. The latter also drain the superior and inferior tonsillar veins. The inferior hemispheric veins may drain to the adjacent transverse or tentorial sinuses. Alternatively they may be collected by tributaries to the vein of the cerebellomedullary fissure and ultimately become part of the petrosal drainage system.

REFERENCES

1. Scatliff JH, Clark JK. How the brain got its names and numbers. Am J Neuroradiol 1992;13:241–248.
2. Padget D. The development of the cranial venous system in man, from the viewpoint of comparative anatomy. Contrib Embryol 1957;37:80–140.
3. Wolf BS, Huang YP, Newman CM. Superficial Sylvian venous drainage system. American J Roentgenol 1963;89:398–410.
4. Oka K, Rhoton AL, Barry M, et al. Microsurgical anatomy of the superficial veins of the cerebrum. Neurosurgery 1985;17:711–748.
5. Piffer CR, Horn Y, Hureau J, et al. Étude anatomique des veines cérébrales supérieures. Anat Anz 1985;160:271–283.
6. Andrews BT, Dujovny M, Mirchandani HG, et al. Microsurgical anatomy of the venous drainage into the superior sagittal sinus. Neurosurgery 1989;24:514–520.
7. DiChiro G. Angiographic patterns of cerebral convexity veins and superficial dural sinuses. Am J Roentgenol 1962;87:306–321.
8. Wolf BS, Huang YP. The subependymal veins of the lateral ventricles. Am J Roentgenol 1964;91:406–426.
9. Ono M, Rhoton AL, Peace D, et al. Microsurgical anatomy of the deep venous system of the brain. Neurosurgery 1984;15:621–657.
10. Babin E, Megret M. Variations in the drainage of the basal vein. Neuroradiology 1973;6:154–161.
11. Bub B, Ferris EJ, Levy PS, et al. The cerebral venogram: A statistical analysis of the sequence of venous filling in cerebral angiograms. Radiology 1968;91:1112–1118.
12. El-Banhawy A, Walter W. Incidence and significance of early filling of veins in normal carotid angiography. J Neurosurg 1961;19:717–729.

13. Huang YP, Wolf BS. Veins of posterior fossa—superior or galenic draining group. American J Roentgenol 1965;95:808–821

14. Huang YP, Wolf BS. Precentral cerebellar vein in angiography. Acta Radiol (Diagn) 1966;5:250–262.

15. Huang YP, Wolf BS. Antin SP, et al. The veins of the posterior fossa—anterior or petrosal draining group. Am J Roentgenol 1968;104:36–56.

16. Wolf BS, Huang YP, Newman CM. The lateral anastomotic mes-encephalic vein and other variations in drainage of the basal cerebral vein. Am J Roentgenol 1963;89:411–422.

17. Matsushima T, Rhoton AL, De Oliveira E, et al. Microsurgical anatomy of the veins of the posterior fossa. J Neurosurg 1983; 59:63–105.

18. Huang YP, Wolf BS. The vein of the lateral recess of the fourth ventricle and its tributaries. Roentgen appearance and anatomic relationships. Am J Roentgenol 1967;101:1–21.

CHAPTER 15

The External Carotid Artery and Extracranial Circulation

The branches of the external carotid system are named according to their respective territories without regard to the site of origin of the vessel or pattern of division of the external carotid artery. Certain patterns of branching can be seen as characteristic and, when present, will help in identification of named vessels. Pre-embolization angiography of the external carotid artery is analogous to an attempt to discern the main routes of a great city in the patterns of night-time traffic seen from a high altitude. The main thoroughfares and secondary roads are easily seen in the darkness by the moving headlights. The pattern will remain relatively stable over the period of observation and will give little indication of the multitude of alternative routes and byways available to the traffic in the event of a major restriction or diversion. The capacity of the external carotid artery to compensate for a restriction on flow in one branch by collateral flow through a number of other pathways becomes a major consideration in interventional procedures. The pre-occlusion angiogram does not necessarily indicate which anastomoses are lying dormant waiting to assume a greater hemodynamic role. In a vascular field being embolized, potential anastomoses with dangerous collateral pathways to the internal carotid artery or ophthalmic artery may not fill during the initial part of the procedure. However, as the outflow from the field becomes restricted by progressive embolization, previously unseen pathways emerge, turning what may have initially seemed a safe embolization procedure into a dangerous one.

Therefore in learning the anatomy of the external carotid system, flexibility must be incorporated into one's conception of the arborization of the vessel. The territory of destination is the factor that determines the nomenclature of a vessel; its relationship to bony structures and tissue planes help to confirm its identity. A vessel's location and identity guide the interpreter towards an awareness of the potentially dangerous anastomoses that may be relevant. One's thinking should also take reckoning of nonvisualization of supply to a particular area. An assumption that the supply is coming from an alternative source must be entertained.

The external carotid artery is usually described as having eight to nine major branches, and this description serves as a useful starting point towards a more precise identification of particular smaller vessels. Particular emphasis on the possibility of dangerous anastomoses must be placed in the regions of the orbit, cavernous sinus, middle ear, upper cervical area, and foramen magnum.

On the AP view of the external carotid artery, most of the proximal vessels are superimposed on the lateral aspect of the face in an area that is prone to technical overexposure. For these reasons, and because most of the branches of the external carotid artery run in an AP plane, most images of the proximal external carotid artery branches are depicted in the lateral plane. An important component for understanding the angiographic anatomy of the external carotid artery is the tissue plane in which a particular vessel lies. Vessels that cross one another on the angiographic image without anastomosing lie in different anatomic planes. Vessels that appear to cross a bony barrier, such as the skull base, without a deflection in their course, must lie in a more superficial tissue plane.

BRANCHES OF THE EXTERNAL CAROTID ARTERY

Superior Thyroidal Artery

In approximately 75% of patients, the external carotid system arises as a common trunk in an anteromedial relationship to the internal carotid artery between C3 and C5. It usually divides quickly, giving an inferiorly directed superior thyroidal artery as the first branch (Figs. 15.1, 15.2). In the normal state, this is a small, tapered vessel projecting anteriorly and medially with a number of branches to the larynx and related structures, thyroid gland, and parathyroid glands. If injected directly, the normal thyroid gland will give a discernible dense blush. The superior thyroidal artery may arise as a common trunk with other branches of the external carotid artery or from the common carotid artery. There are rich anastomoses within and around the thyroid gland between the superior and inferior thyroidal arteries. The inferior thyroidal artery is a branch of the thyrocervical trunk or, less commonly, of the vertebral artery, subclavian artery, or common carotid artery. The thyroid ima artery arises from the aortic arch.

Ascending Pharyngeal Artery

The ascending pharyngeal artery is usually a long, needle-thin vessel arising from the posterior aspect of the proximal external carotid trunk. Variant sites of origin include a common trunk with the occipital artery or origin from the internal carotid artery.

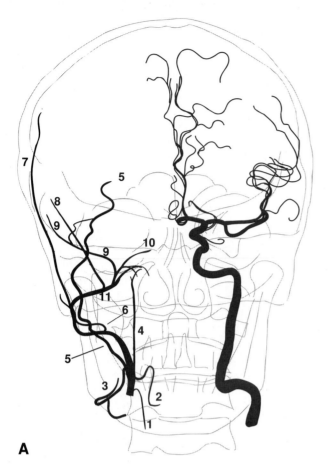

A

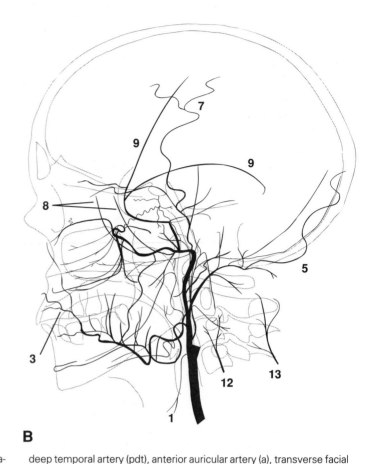

B

Figure 15.1. *External carotid artery.* **(A, B)** PA and lateral illustrations of the external carotid artery circulation, while the internal carotid artery is illustrated on the anatomic left side for reference. 1. Superior thyroidal artery; 2. Lingual artery; 3. Facial artery; 4. Ascending pharyngeal artery; 5. Occipital artery; 6. Posterior auricular artery; 7. Superficial temporal artery; 8. Deep temporal artery; 9. Middle meningeal artery; 10. Accessory meningeal artery; 11. Internal maxillary artery; 12. Ascending Cervical artery (from thyrocervical trunk); 13. Deep cervical artery (from costocervical trunk). **(B)** Template for subsequent illustrations of individual arteries. **(C)** The superior thyroidal artery (s) and occipital artery (o) are highlighted. The C1 and C2 branches of the occipital artery are indicated, as are the stylomastoid (st) and transmastoid (tm) branches of the occipital artery. The stylomastoid and transmastoid branches may arise from other external carotid branches. The occipital artery may also give rise frequently to the neuromeningeal trunk, which is illustrated in Figure 15.1H in its more common form as a branch of the ascending pharyngeal artery. The occipital artery is illustrated giving rise to the artery of the falx cerebelli (fc). This dural artery more commonly arises from the vertebral artery or posterior inferior cerebellar artery. **(D)** The facial artery and posterior auricular artery (pa) are highlighted. The branches of the facial artery are labeled: a., angular branch; ap., ascending palatine artery; il., inferior labial artery; j., jugal branches; m., masseteric branches; mt., mental branch; sl., superior labial artery. The shepherd's hook appearance of the ascending palatine artery illustrated here is characteristic of this vessel. It is often this curve that catches one's attention when this territory is filled via collateral flow. In **(A)**, notice the superficial course of the posterior auricular artery relative to the occipital artery. They may occasionally arise together as a common trunk. The curve of the posterior auricular artery in **(A)** is characteristic of the vessel. It can be difficult to cannulate if the external carotid artery proximal to that point is tortuous. **(E)** The lingual artery is highlighted. The dorsal artery of the tongue with its ranine branches (r) is a characteristic feature. Its circulation at the floor of the mouth and around the submandibular gland is in variable balance with the adjacent branches of the facial artery. **(F)** The middle meningeal artery is highlighted. It is illustrated here with a common exocranial trunk shared by the accessory meningeal artery (a). However the accessory meningeal artery may have a separate origin from the internal maxillary artery. The branches of the middle meningeal artery are indicated: p., petrous branch (a dangerous vessel during embolization as it can supply the vasa nervorum of the VIIth nerve in the middle ear); o., lacrimal branch to the orbit (variable); f., frontal branch; s., squamous branch. **(G)** The superficial temporal artery and related arteries are highlighted. These include the posterior

deep temporal artery (pdt), anterior auricular artery (a), transverse facial artery (tf), and masseteric branches of the latter (m). The arrow indicates the characteristic intersection of the transverse facial artery and the underlying buccal artery. The zygomatico-orbital branch of the superficial temporal artery (zo) is indicated because this is an important branch for superficial temporal artery to ophthalmic artery reconstitution. When the zygomatic branch is prominent, the transverse facial artery is not well seen, and vice versa. **(H)** The lateral appearance of the ascending pharyngeal artery is illustrated. The main branches of the ascending pharyngeal artery are labeled (see text for discussion): ip., inferior pharyngeal branch of the pharyngeal trunk; mp., middle pharyngeal branch; sp., superior pharyngeal branch; c., carotid branch of the superior pharyngeal branch anastomosing to the inferolateral trunk; it., inferior tympanic branch; nmt., neuromeningeal trunk; cl., clival anastomoses from the neuromeningeal trunk extending towards the medial and lateral clival branches of the internal carotid artery (see Fig. 8.10); pma., posterior meningeal artery, a variant branch of the hypoglossal branch of the neuromeningeal trunk; od., odontoid arcade connecting the hypoglossal branch of the neuromeningeal trunk to the C3 branch of the vertebral artery; spm., spinomuscular branch anastomosing with the C3 and C4 branches of the ipsilateral vertebral and cervical arteries. **(I)** Various branches and anastomotic relations of the internal maxillary artery are highlighted: adt., anterior deep temporal; mdt., middle deep temporal; fr., artery of the foramen rotundum connecting to the inferolateral trunk (ilt); ldp., lesser descending palatine artery supplying the soft palate; gdp., greater descending palatine artery; sp., sphenopalatine arteries; io., infraorbital artery.The deep temporal arteries are sometimes described as having a ``pseudomeningeal appearance,'' which refers to their smooth straight course. However, they do not deflect at the skull base as is the case of the middle meningeal artery. Furthermore, they have a very straight superficial course on the PA view **(see A).** The tortuous appearance of the artery of the foramen rotundum is very characteristic as it directs itself towards the floor of the sella. This is one of the most important anastomoses in internal maxillary artery embolization.The infraorbital artery is easy to recognize. It has the shape of an upturned boat-hull, giving a small orbital branch directed superiorly as indicated. The lateral (short) sphenopalatine arteries conform to the curves of the turbinate bones. **(J)** More branches of the internal maxillary artery are labeled: pv., ptergyo-vaginal artery; ia., inferior alveolar (dental) shown here arising from a common trunk with the middle deep temporal artery, a common variant; ant., antral branch arising as a common alveolo-antral trunk with the superior alveolar artery (sa); b., buccal artery connecting the facial and internal maxillary arteries.

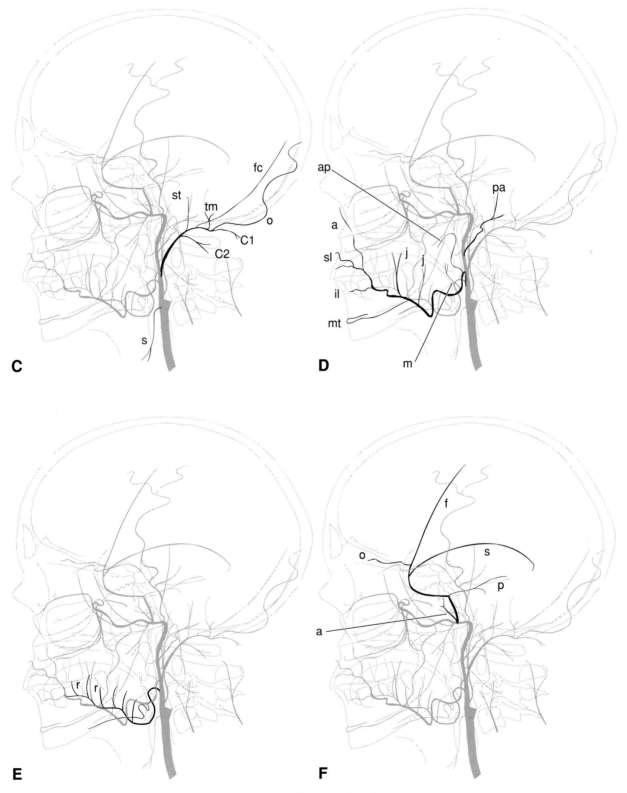

Figure 15.1. *(continued)*

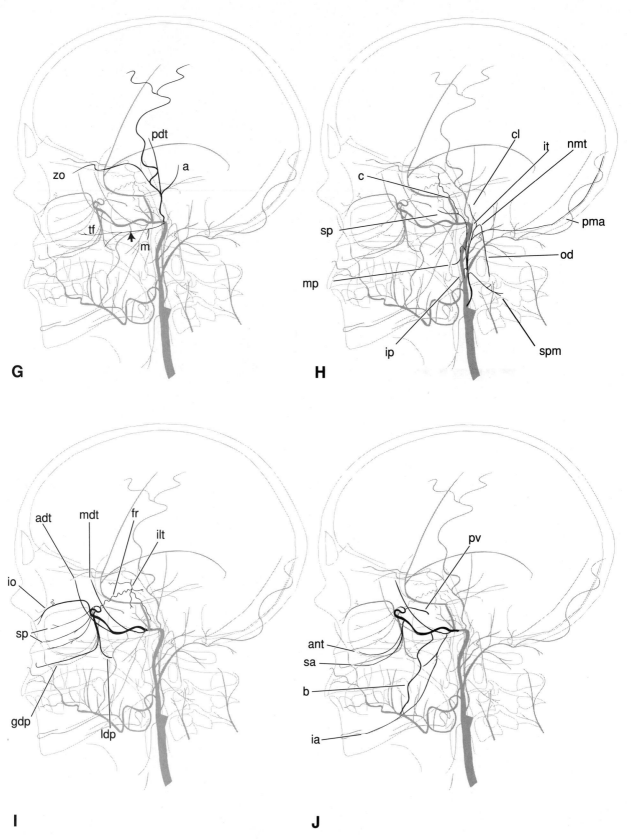

Figure 15.1. *(continued)*

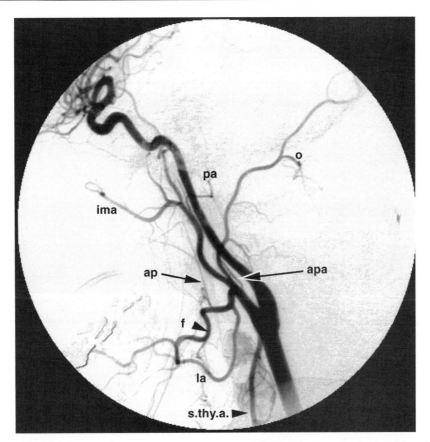

Figure 15.2. *Superior thyroidal artery.* A common carotid injection in a patient with a thyroid adenoma. A hypervascular blush is seen from an enlarged superior thyroidal artery (s.thy.a.). Labels: ap., ascending palatine artery; apa., ascending pharyngeal artery; o., occipital artery; ima., internal maxillary artery; pa., posterior auricular artery; f., facial artery; la., lingual artery.

The ascending pharyngeal artery is directed superiorly in a straight course toward the posterior nasopharynx, appearing to lie in front of or on the vertebral column on the lateral view, and in a position medial to the main external carotid trunk on the AP view. It is an important supply route to the pharynx, dura, and lower cranial nerve foramina of the skull base, and to the middle ear. The ascending pharyngeal artery usually divides into a number of identifiable branches or trunks:

1. Pharyngeal trunk
   Superior pharyngeal branch
   Middle pharyngeal branch
   Inferior pharyngeal branch
2. Neuromeningeal trunk
   Hypoglossal branch
   Jugular branch
3. Inferior tympanic artery
4. Musculospinal artery

The configuration is prone to variability. The pharyngeal trunk may not have all three branches present in an identifiable form. The inferior tympanic artery may be a branch of one of the other trunks. Some components or all of the neuromeningeal trunk may be a branch of the occipital artery.

The pharyngeal branches of the ascending pharyngeal artery can be most easily seen on the lateral view anterior to the ascending pharyngeal artery itself and are described and frequently seen as three in number: superior, middle, and inferior (Fig. 15.3). These can be thought of as corresponding with the nasopharynx (Eustachian tube region), oropharynx (and soft palate), and hypopharynx respectively.

The superior pharyngeal branch gives an important intracranial anastomosis through the foramen lacerum, the carotid branch, which anastomoses with the recurrent laceral branch of the inferolateral trunk of the internal carotid artery. In the posterior nasopharynx, the superior pharyngeal branch anastomoses with the internal maxillary artery system via the pterygo-vaginal artery. This is a small vessel running in an AP direction close to the midline in a similarly named bony canal in the nasal roof. It usually has a particular curve, like an upturned saucer, which makes for easy recognition. The superior pharyngeal branch also makes variable anastomoses with pharyngeal branches of the accessory meningeal artery and with the mandibular artery, when present.

The neuromeningeal trunk is also a long straight artery diverging posteriorly from the pharyngeal trunk, ascending to overlap the foramen magnum on the lateral view. Its major posteriorly directed branches are the hypoglossal artery and the jugular artery, which access the endocranial space through the respectively named foramina. The hy-

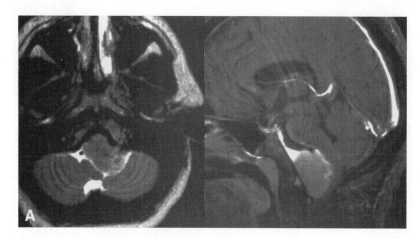

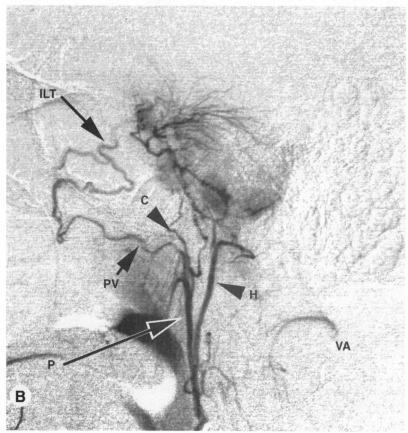

Figure 15.3. *Ascending pharyngeal artery.* **(A).** Axial T2-weighted and sagittal T1-weighted (fat-saturation post-gadolinium) MRI images demonstrate a typical appearance of a near midline clival meningioma. There is pronounced deformity of the structures of the posterior fossa. A dural tail of enhancement extends up to the dorsum sellae. **(B).** A microcatheter injection of the right ascending pharyngeal artery, lateral projection, demonstrates a pronounced tumor blush corresponding with the sagittal appearance of the tumor. The pharyngeal trunk (P) and hypoglossal branch (H) of the neuromeningeal trunk are well seen. The superior pharyngeal branch of the pharyngeal trunk anastomoses to the territory of the internal maxillary artery via the pterygovaginal artery (PV). This results in opacification of the inferolateral trunk (ILT) via the artery of the foramen rotundum. The superior pharyngeal artery may also connect with the middle cranial fossa via the foramen lacerum through its carotid branch (C). The vertebral artery (VA) is transiently opacified on this injection.

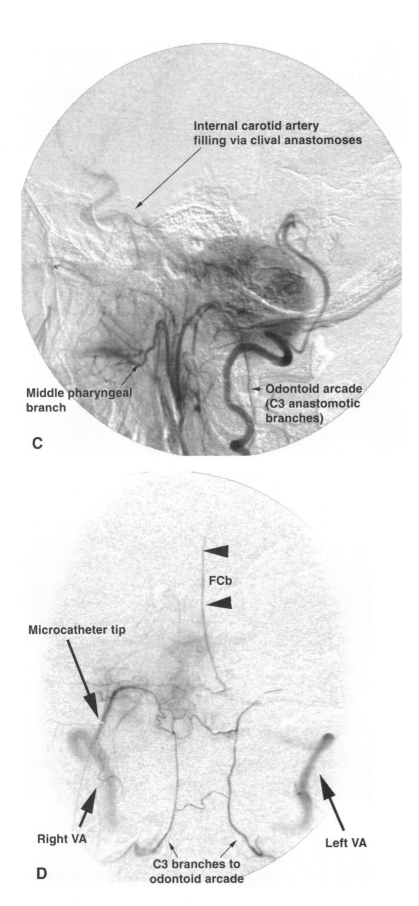

Internal carotid artery filling via clival anastomoses

Middle pharyngeal branch

Odontoid arcade (C3 anastomotic branches)

C

FCb

Microcatheter tip

Right VA

C3 branches to odontoid arcade

Left VA

D

Figure 15.3. *(continued)* **(C).** A lateral projection of the left ascending pharyngeal artery injection demonstrates a tumor blush with a tail extending to the dorsum sellae. Faint opacification of the internal carotid artery is seen, probably through clival anastomoses. The left vertebral artery is compressed by the tumor and shows slow run-off. It is opacified by the odontoid arcade from the neuromeningeal trunk. **(D, E)** A selective PA injection **(D)** and lateral view **(E)** of an injection in the neuromeningeal trunk of the right ascending pharyngeal artery demonstrates the odontoid arcade and its anastomoses across the midline. Both vertebral arteries are opacified by this injection through the C3 branches. A midline artery extends high above the sella on this view; therefore, it represents the artery of the falx cerebelli (Fcb). (Case courtesy of F. Huang-Hellinger, MD, PhD, Boston, MA.)

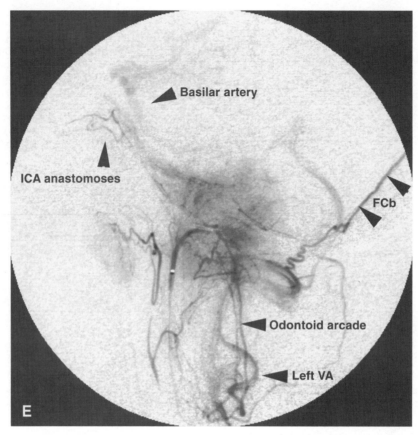

Figure 15.3. *(continued)*

poglossal artery is the more medial of the two branches on the AP view.

The hypoglossal branch of the neuromeningeal trunk is an extremely important vessel. Its normal function is to supply the neural structures of the hypoglossal canal and a variable dural territory in the posterior fossa. It may give rise to the artery of the falx cerebelli, the posterior meningeal artery, or, rarely, the posterior inferior cerebellar artery. Its important anastomotic branches can be divided into those that ascend along the back of the clivus, and those that descend through the foramen magnum and along the back of the body of the C2 vertebral body.

Clival branches of the hypoglossal branch of the neuromeningeal trunk ascend the dorsum of the clivus to meet with medial clival branches from the meningohypophyseal trunk or equivalent internal carotid artery hypophyseal branches (Fig. 15.3). Thus, opacification of the posterior aspect of the pituitary gland can be seen occasionally during superselective injections of the ascending pharyngeal artery. More importantly, this route of collateral flow from the ascending pharyngeal artery to the internal carotid artery can form the basis for dangerous anastomoses during embolization. Alternatively, flow through this route may be visible on the lateral angiogram allowing reconstitution of the cavernous internal carotid artery. In this manner, clival branches of the neuromeningeal trunk may simulate the "string-sign" for persistent internal carotid

artery flow in the setting of internal carotid artery occlusive disease.

A descending anastomosis from the hypoglossal branch of the neuromeningeal trunk exits the foramen magnum and extends inferiorly behind the body of C2 giving branches across the midline to its contralateral fellow. At the C2-C3 interspace, this descending branch becomes the C3 branch of the ipsilateral vertebral artery. This bilateral connection between the vertebral artery and the ascending pharyngeal artery behind the body of C2 is called the arcade of the odontoid process.

The jugular branch of the neuromeningeal trunk supplies the neural structures and adjacent dura of the jugular foramen. It is prominently seen in the setting of vascular tumors, such as glomus jugulare, in the region of the jugular foramen. In the normal state, it may also send branches anteromedially towards Dorelo's canal containing cranial nerve VI. It anastomoses in this region with lateral clival branches of the internal carotid artery. Dural branches of the jugular branch of the neuromeningeal trunk directed towards the sigmoid sinus may have prominent anastomoses with dural branches of the middle meningeal artery and transosseous dural branches of other sources from the external carotid artery.

The inferior tympanic artery is usually a tiny vessel and steers a middle course between the neuromeningeal and pharyngeal trunks on the lateral view. It may arise from either. It gains access to the middle ear via the inferior tympanic canaliculus, which it shares with Jacobson's branch of the glossopharyngeal nerve. It is therefore prominently involved in glomus tympanicum tumors. Within the middle ear the inferior tympanic artery anastomoses with: the stylomastoid branch of the occipital artery, which enters the middle ear via the canal of that name, running with the VIIth nerve; the petrosal branch of the middle meningeal artery; and the carotico-tympanic branch of the internal carotid artery.

The musculo-spinal branch of the ascending pharyngeal artery is directed posteriorly and inferiorly on the lateral view at the level of the third cervical space. It supplies the cervical musculature, cranial nerve XI, and the superior sympathetic ganglion. It has important anastomoses to the ascending and deep cervical arteries and with the vertebral artery.

Lingual Artery

The lingual artery supplies the tongue, floor of mouth, and suprahyoid area. The largest branch is the terminal dorsal artery of the tongue, which is most easily identified on the lateral view. It extends towards the tip of the tongue and gives characteristic parallel ranine branches to the musculature of the tongue (Fig. 15.1E). In the floor of the mouth, the lingual artery has rich anastomoses with the facial artery. The facial artery territory in the region of the mandible, floor of mouth and lower face may be supplanted completely by the lingual artery. The lingual artery contributes in varying degrees to the supply of the submandibular and sublingual salivary glands. The lingual artery and facial artery may arise as a common linguofacial trunk. These two arteries are hemodynamically balanced; hypoplasia of one is compensated by dominance of the other.

Facial Artery

The facial artery arises more distally than the lingual artery, or they may share a common origin from the external carotid artery (Fig. 15.4). The usual musculocutaneous distribution of the facial artery is extensive, and its many branches have rich anastomoses to territories supplied by other external carotid artery branches. Therefore, when these other branches are prominent or "dominant," the facial artery will be correspondingly smaller or hypoplastic. Two general courses of the facial artery are described as it crosses the face diagonally from inferolateral to superomedial. A posterolateral course over the cheek is termed *jugal,* whereas a course more anterior and medial, closer to the mouth, is termed *labial.* The facial artery usually arises medial to the angle of the mandible. Therefore to gain access to the facial structures outside the plane of the mandible, the facial artery must make an inferiorly and laterally directed loop to course around the body of the mandible. This point corresponds with the anterior edge of the masseter muscle insertion (Fig. 15.1D). To make

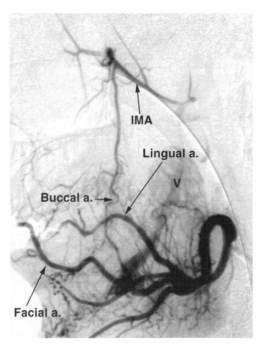

Figure 15.4. *Linguo-facial trunk and buccal artery.* A lateral projection of an injection in the left linguo-facial trunk of a teenager with an arteriovenous malformation of the floor of the mouth. Early venous opacification is seen directed to a large varix (V). A prominent buccal artery allows opacification of the internal maxillary artery (IMA) from the facial artery.

this loop on the lateral projection, it must dip below the level of the lingual artery, creating potential confusion between the two vessels at this point.

The ascending palatine artery arises from the proximal deep segment of the facial artery or adjacent external carotid artery. It ascends towards the soft palate along the levator palati muscle. It anastomoses with the other arteries to the soft palate, particularly: the middle branch of the pharyngeal trunk of the ascending pharyngeal artery; the descending palatine artery from the internal maxillary artery; and the pharyngeal branch of the accessory meningeal artery.

The facial artery supplies the superficial facial structures giving named branches to the submandibular gland, the submental foramen, the mandible (mental branch), the superior and inferior labial area, the cheek (jugal branches), and the ala of the nose (alar branch). It terminates as a naso-angular branch tapering along the lateral aspect of the bridge of the nose, or alternatively as a naso-orbital branch when directed towards the inner canthus of the eye.

Branches to the submandibular gland are given as the main trunk of the facial artery makes its way from medial to lateral under the body of the mandible. During superselective injections, these can cause a pronounced parenchymal blush, which should not be interpreted as pathologic when evaluating tumors or bleeding sites. Bleeding in this area requires evaluation of the ipsilateral lingual artery and the superior thyroidal artery too, as there are common anastomoses between these vessels medial to the angle of the mandible.

Musculocutaneous and periosteal structures of the angle and body of the mandible are supplied by the submental branch posteriorly and the middle mental branch more anteriorly. The latter vessel anastomoses with the terminal branches of the inferior alveolar artery as they emerge anteriorly from the mental foramen.

The jugal vessels may arise as a common trunk or as separate anterior, middle, and posterior branches from the facial artery. The jugal branches are directed superiorly towards the muscles of the cheek and masseter muscle. A prominent buccal branch may be seen connecting this system to the internal maxillary artery superiorly (Figs. 15.1J, 21.18, 21.19). Identification of the buccal artery can be assisted sometimes by identifying how it crosses deep to the transverse facial artery without intersecting with it at the level of the pterygoid plates. The buccal artery and posterior jugal artery may be the site of origin of lower masseteric branches from the facial artery.

The labial vessels are termed superior and inferior, and they have rich anastomoses with adjacent territories. The superior labial arteries may have a considerable circulation to the nasal septum in the midline, raising the possibility of anastomoses with the ethmoidal branches of the ophthalmic artery and with the long sphenopalatine arteries.

In the setting of a proximal ligation or congenital hypoplasia of the facial artery, the surrounding vascular territories will be enlarged to assume supply to the facial distribution. These territories particularly include the following:

Infraorbital artery, which can assume supply equivalent to the anterior jugal branches of the facial artery
Buccal branch of the internal maxillary artery
Transverse facial branch of the superficial temporal artery
Lingual artery
Palatine arteries
Masseteric branches of the external carotid trunk

Discerning between the proximal portions of the lingual and facial arteries can be confusing. A few helpful characteristics can be sought. On the lateral view, the lingual artery, if separate from the facial artery, will arise proximally from the external trunk. The loops of both vessels may be difficult to disentangle from one another under fluoroscopy, but on the AP view, the facial artery is compelled to clear the mandible by looping under its body to access the lateral plane. The lingual artery has a more direct route toward the midline and the tip of the tongue. The facial artery will also have a distribution that ascends above the upper limit of the tongue profile. On the lateral view, the overlapping loops of the facial and lingual artery form an illustration of an important tenet of vessel identification in angiography, i.e., vessels that overlap on a particular projection without connecting with one another must lie in different tissue planes. Although this may appear self-evident in this location, this rule-of-thumb is very useful in

other circumstances in which vessels may be seen through anastomotic connections for only a frame or two.

Occipital Artery

The occipital artery is a posteriorly directed branch of the external carotid artery, which has an extensive musculocutaneous, meningeal, and scalp distribution at the craniocervical junction and above. It runs medial to the sternocleidomastoid muscle, where it cuts a prominent groove in the undersurface of the temporal bone, medial to that cut by the posterior belly of digastric muscle. Like its more anterior counterpart, the superficial temporal artery, the occipital artery may have a sinuous appearance. The occipital artery is embryologically related to the first segmental artery of the cervical vasculature and, therefore, it may arise from the internal carotid artery as a form fruste of a proatlantal intersegmental artery. In the setting of rare cases of a persistent proatlantal intersegmental artery, the occipital artery usually arises from this variant vessel. The occipital artery, in the normal state, has important anastomotic relationships with the C1, C2, C3, and C4 anastomotic systems. In the C1 and C2 spaces, it anastomoses freely with the equivalent branches of the ipsilateral vertebral artery. At the C3 and C4 level, the occipital artery frequently anastomoses with the distal field of the deep cervical artery. It may also anastomose in the third space with the musculospinal branch of the ascending pharyngeal artery (Fig. 15.1C, 15.1H).

It gives two named endocranial branches: the stylomastoid artery and the transmastoid branch. The stylomastoid artery is a superiorly directed straight vessel along the anterior aspect of the mastoid process in the stylomastoid canal thus identifying the course of the distal canal of the VIIth nerve. The stylomastoid artery is an important supply route to the middle ear and a potential site of VIIth nerve morbidity during embolization. More posteriorly the artery of the mastoid foramen (transmastoid branch) describes a transosseous route to gain access to the dura of the posterior fossa. It is an important route of supply to vascular lesions of the dura in this region, including tumors and dural vascular malformations. The mastoid branch is one of the most frequently involved vessels seen in high flow vascular lesions or tumors in the posterior fossa floor. In this capacity, the possibility of anastomoses with the subarcuate branch of the ipsilateral anterior inferior cerebellar artery should be considered. These two named endocranial branches of the occipital artery may have alternative sites of origin, e.g., from the ascending pharyngeal artery or from the posterior auricular artery, and therefore are not dependent on the occipital artery for their nomenclature. Alternatively, other endocranial vessels usually associated with other sites of origin may arise from the occipital artery, e.g., the posterior meningeal artery and artery of the falx cerebelli.

Posterior Auricular Artery

The posterior auricular artery may arise separately from the external carotid artery, or it may share a common auriculo-occipital trunk with the occipital artery (Fig. 15.1D). In either event, it can be thought of as a scalp vessel existing in hemodynamic balance with the occipital artery posteriorly and with the superficial temporal artery anteriorly. It usually supplies the superficial structures of the outer ear. It runs behind the ear where it can sometimes be palpated under the skin against the mastoid bone. It may be the source of origin for the artery of the stylomastoid canal.

The denomination of "posterior" obviously connotes the presence of an "anterior" auricular artery. The latter is a branch of the superficial temporal artery, which anastomoses with the posterior auricular artery above the ear forming an arcade of vessels in the scalp. A more superficial arcade in the earlobe may be seen in superselective magnification views.

Superficial Temporal Artery

The superficial temporal artery, as its name describes, runs on the outer surface of the temporalis muscle for much of its course giving named terminal branches to the frontal and parietal areas of the scalp (Fig. 15.1G). More proximally, it makes a turn around the zygomatic arch where it gives posteriorly directed branches. The anterior auricular branch was described earlier. The posterior deep temporal artery runs deep to the temporalis muscle along the surface of the skull. Anteriorly directed named branches from the superficial temporal artery at the level of the zygomatic arch include the zygomatico-orbital branch superiorly towards the lateral rim of the orbit, and the more inferior alternative, the transverse facial artery (Figs. 15.5, 15.6). The zygomatico-orbital artery may be most prominently seen when the frontal branch of the more distal superficial temporal artery is diminutive or weak. Being directed to the lateral aspect of the orbit, it has important anastomoses with the palpebral and lacrimal arteries.

The transverse facial artery lies slightly lower along the lower rim of the zygomatic arch or along the parotid duct. The transverse facial artery supplies the superficial area of the temple bridging the transition between face and scalp. It carries particular supply to the upper masseteric muscles. Being in this transitional position, it can be thought of as a vessel that will be prominently seen when one or more of the vessels in the adjoining areas is weak, i.e., zygomatico-orbital above or distal facial artery or internal maxillary artery below. When seen, it has a characteristic relationship with the buccal artery, which it crosses at a near 90 angle.

Internal Maxillary Artery

The internal maxillary artery and its branches constitute a distribution of vessels emanating from or best understood in relationship to the sphenopalatine fossa. The sphenopalatine fossa is a slit-like cavity defined by the curve of back wall of the maxillary sinus anteriorly and the pterygoid plates of the greater wing of the sphenoid bone posteriorly. In addition to serving as a focal point for arterial anatomy of the central face and skull base, it also functions as a distribution point for the neural branches of the maxillary division of the Vth nerve and parasympathetic fibers of the superior salivatory nucleus, which synapse in the spheno-palatine ganglion.

The named arterial branches of the internal maxillary artery number between 14 and 16. Their nomenclature follows that of the surrounding osseous structures and bony foramina (Figs. 15.7, 15.8). See Table 15.1.

Middle Meningeal Artery

The middle meningeal artery arises from the internal maxillary artery on the lateral angiogram soon after the origin of the superficial temporal artery. However, this appearance is deceptive and it is frequently necessary to demonstrate the origin of the middle meningeal artery on an AP view for catheterization (Figs. 15.1A, F). On this view, the middle meningeal artery is medial to and at some distance from the superficial temporal artery. The middle meningeal artery enters the cranium via the foramen spinosum. This foramen is hypoplastic or absent in variants where the middle meningeal artery has origin from an alternative source, such as a persistent stapedial artery (Fig. 5.5). The middle meningeal artery is easily recognized by the sharp turn it makes along the floor of the middle cranial fossa after entering via the foramen spinosum (Fig. 15.9). Furthermore its course along the inner aspect of the skull is characterized, for the most part, by smooth curves, in contrast to the sinuous course of the overlapping superficial temporal artery.

The middle meningeal artery supplies named dural branches to the frontal area, temporal squamous region, petrous area, parietal dural convexity, and to the region of the sigmoid and transverse sinuses. The latter branches may also give supply to hypervascular lesions of the tentorium cerebelli and posterior fossa. The middle meningeal artery also supplies the dura in the area of the middle cranial fossa adjacent to the cavernous sinus where it can give rise to prominent orbital branches as described elsewhere. The middle meningeal artery may also give origin to the marginal tentorial artery. At the level of the superior sagittal sinus, the middle meningeal artery anastomoses with the artery of the falx cerebri and together they supply the dural layers of the falx and associated lesions.

Accessory Meningeal Artery

The accessory meningeal artery arises from a common trunk with the middle meningeal artery, or it may arise distal to the middle meningeal artery from the internal maxillary artery (Figs. 15.1A, F). On the lateral view, it has a more oblique, anterior slant in contrast to the straight course of the exocranial trunk of the middle meningeal artery. On the AP view, the accessory meningeal artery is slanted medially towards the cavernous sinus and specifically towards the point of arborization of the inferolateral trunk (Fig. 15.10).

Figure 15.5. *Transverse facial artery.*   A lateral, slightly skewed, projection of the distal external carotid artery in a patient being studied for intractable epistaxis. There is pronounced blush (B) of nasal mucosa in the territory of the distal internal maxillary artery (I). A characteristic 90 turn of the middle meningeal artery (M) is seen as it enters the foramen spinosum. The accessory meningeal artery **(single arrow)** is seen as a proximal branch of the middle meningeal artery; its branches in the nasopharynx can be seen extending forwards to meet the pterygovaginal branch (PV) of the internal maxillary artery. A prominent vessel running anteriorly crosses the course of the internal maxillary artery. This is the transverse facial artery **(arrowheads).**

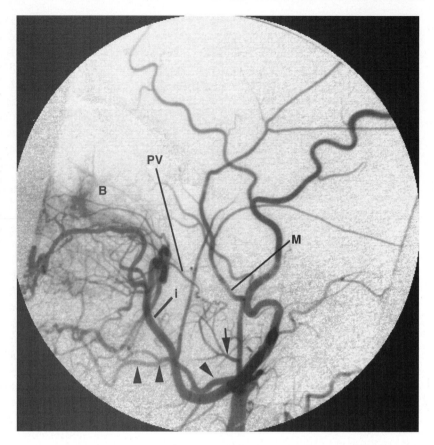

Figure 15.6. *Superficial temporal artery to ophthalmic artery anastomoses.*   A lateral projection of a common carotid artery injection in the setting of occlusive internal carotid artery disease. It demonstrates that a frontozygomatic (f.z.) branch of the superficial temporal artery contributes significantly to retrograde opacification of the ophthalmic artery **(double arrow).** A lesser degree of input is seen from the orbital branch **(arrowhead)** of the infraorbital artery (i.o.). Notice that the timing of external carotid artery opacification is ahead of that of the internal carotid artery, an indication of incipient hemodynamic failure of the internal carotid artery.

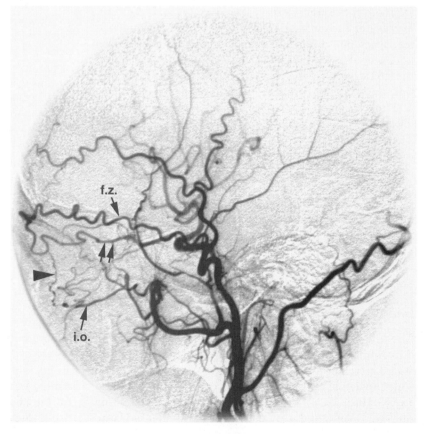

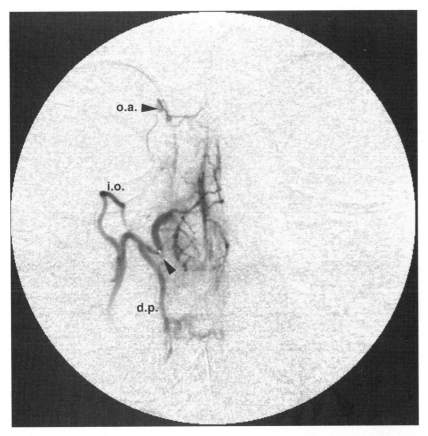

Figure 15.7. *Ethmoidal branches of the sphenopalatine arteries.* An AP view of a microcatheter **(arrowhead)** injection in the distal internal maxillary artery. In this projection the infraorbital artery (i.o.) is in the plane of projection and foreshortened. The descending palatine artery (d.p.) in the greater palatine canal turns at the palate into the plane of imaging. Beading and irregularity of the sphenopalatine vessels is a typical finding in patients with posterior epistaxis. On this injection ethmoidal anastomoses from the long sphenopalatine arteries to the ophthalmic artery result in opacification of the ophthalmic artery (o.a.), prompting caution during embolization.

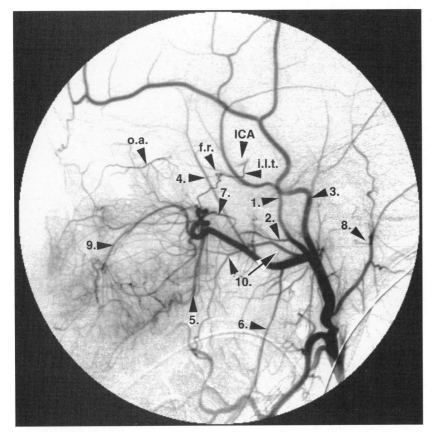

Figure 15.8. *Anatomy of the distal external carotid artery.* A lateral projection of the distal external carotid artery anatomy presents a typical angiographic appearance. However, the image must be inspected closely to reveal dangerous anastomoses to the ophthalmic artery (o.a.) and the internal carotid artery (ICA) via artery of the foramen rotundum (f.r.), and the inferolateral trunk (ilt). 1. Middle meningeal artery; 2. Accessory meningeal artery; 3. Superficial temporal artery; 4. Middle deep temporal artery; 5. Greater descending palatine artery; 6. Inferior alveolar artery; 7. Pterygo-vaginal artery; 8. Posterior auricular artery; 9. Infraorbital artery; 10. Transverse facial artery.

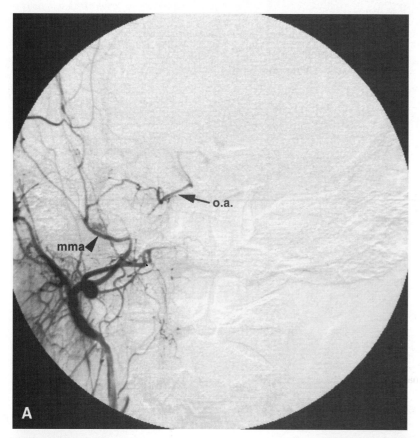

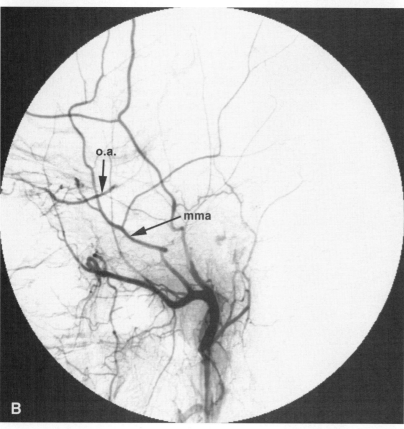

Figure 15.9. *Orbital anastomoses of the middle meningeal artery.* Every embolization of the middle meningeal artery (MMA) must be preceded by a selective microcatheter injection to evaluate for possible anastomoses to the ophthalmic artery (o.a.) via the superior orbital fissure or foramen of Hyrtl (see Chapter 5). On this PA **(A)** and lateral view **(B),** there is prompt opacification of the ophthalmic artery. Because this critical information might be available from only one or two images in a complete run, all images must be reviewed carefully before proceeding.

Figure 15.10. *Dangers to the inferolateral trunk during external carotid artery embolization.* **(A)** A pre-embolization right internal carotid artery injection in a patient with a large meningioma behind the orbit demonstrates some deformity of the course of siphon but no evidence of internal carotid artery supply to the tumor. Notice the draped appearance of the posterior communicating artery **(arrows)**. However, a tortuous little vessel is seen **(arrowhead)** near the genu. The precise identity of this vessel became evident later in the case. **(B)** A pre-embolization injection of the distal external carotid artery demonstrates a complex network of vessels in the paracavernous area supplying the tumor. M., middle meningeal artery; A., accessory meningeal artery; FR., artery of the foramen rotundum. The characteristic appearance of the inferolateral trunk is not specifically identified, but its presence must be suspected. **(C)** A lateral projection of a microcatheter injection in the internal maxillary artery to check on the interim effects of careful embolization. It demonstrates a change in the hemodynamics of the vascular network feeding the tumor. A tortuous vessel **(double arrowheads)** is now seen in the upper anterior aspect of the network opacifying the ophthalmic artery (O), which immediately washes out the opacification. Therefore, the tortuous vessel seen on the internal carotid artery injection **(arrowhead in A)** represents the deep recurrent ophthalmic artery which anastomoses the ophthalmic artery to the inferolateral trunk. Therefore, the margin for error in this situation is extremely narrow. The chances of damaging the ophthalmic artery by forceful injection of emboli are considerable.

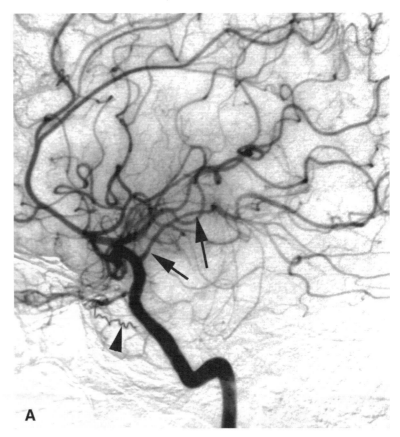

A

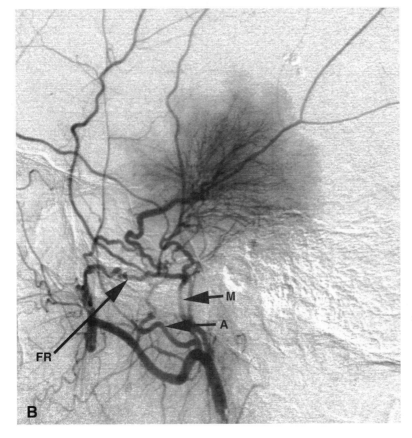

B

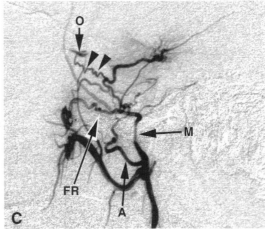

C

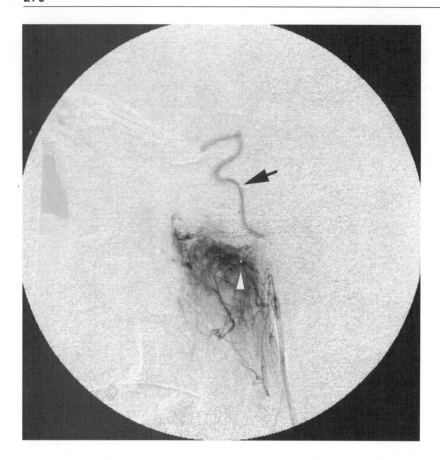

Figure 15.11. *Intratumoral anastomoses.* A lateral projection of a microcatheter injection **(white arrowhead)** into the accessory meningeal artery of a young male with a juvenile angiofibroma of the nasopharynx demonstrates extensive tumoral blush. Transient opacification of the internal carotid artery **(arrow)** from the petrous section is seen due to presumed intratumoral anastomoses with a mandibulo-vidian artery seen on the internal carotid artery injection (same patient in Fig. 8.9).

The dominant territory of supply of the accessory meningeal artery is exocranial. Ascending and descending branches supply the tensor veli palatini, pterygoid muscles, distal Eustachian tube, and soft palate. Therefore, this artery is considered in vascular lesions of the nasopharynx and palatal region. Its principal exocranial anastomoses are with the superior and middle pharyngeal branches of the ascending pharyngeal artery; the ascending and descending palatine arteries; the mandibulo-vidian artery; and the pterygovaginal branch of the internal maxillary artery.

The mandibulo-vidian artery arises from the petrous internal carotid artery (Fig. 15.11). It may anastomose with the accessory meningeal artery, particularly in the setting of juvenile angiofibroma or other hypervascular lesions in children.

A small fraction of the flow of the accessory meningeal artery reaches the endocranial circulation via the foramen ovale or, less commonly, via the foramen of Vesalius. In this location, it anastomoses with the internal carotid artery via the inferolateral trunk. It is frequently involved in paracavernous tumors and dural arteriovenous malformations (Fig. 15.12).

Sphenopalatine Arteries

The long sphenopalatine and short sphenopalatine arteries are directed medially through the sphenopalatine foramen into the nasal cavities, where they supply the septal and lateral surfaces of the ipsilateral nasal airway. On the lateral view, the arteries on the lateral wall, i.e., the short sphenopalatine arteries, describe a curve parallel to that of the turbinates (Fig. 15.1I). Medially, branches of the sphenopalatine arteries near the roof of the nasal cavity may be directed superiorly along the ethmoidal air-cells and anastomose with inferiorly directed ethmoidal branches from the ophthalmic artery. Anteriorly, the long sphenopalatine arteries contribute to Kiesselbach's plexus on the septum. This is the site of idiopathic venous epistaxis in younger patients. Along the nasal septum, the long sphenopalatine vessels anastomose with distal branches of the descending (greater) palatine artery, which have reentered the nasal cavity from the oral cavity via the incisive canal of the hard palate.

The sphenopalatine arteries are the primary target for embolization in the setting of idiopathic arterial (posterior) epistaxis. This is a condition of arterial bleeding thought to be centered around the sphenopalatine foramina or more posteriorly in the nasopharynx. It is therefore distinct from the venous bleeding of more anteriorly centered epistaxis. Collateral supply to the distal sphenopalatine arteries via the superior labial branches of the facial artery is usually embolized too during treatment of idiopathic epistaxis.

Descending (Greater) Palatine Artery

The descending palatine artery is easy to recognize on the lateral arteriogram as it conforms closely to the osseous

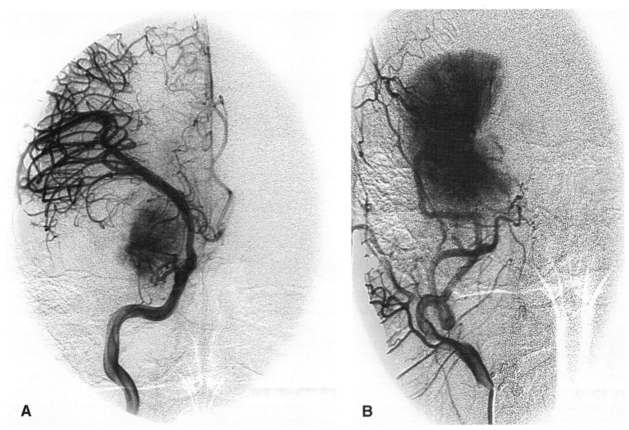

A   **B**

Figure 15.12. *Tumor compartments.* A right sphenoid wing meningioma in a middle-age male presenting with severe right-sided proptosis demonstrates the angiographic appearance of tumor compartmentalization. The right internal carotid artery injection **(A)** opacifies the superior-medial quadrant of the tumor via the recurrent meningeal branch of the ophthalmic artery. There is pronounced mass-effect on the course of the middle cerebral artery. The anterior cerebral artery is displaced to the left. The external carotid artery injection **(B)** opacifies the remainder of the tumor via the middle meningeal artery. The images are complementary.

anatomy of the greater palatine canal and hard palate (Fig. 15.1I). From the sphenopalatine fossa, it descends directly inferiorly and enters the oral cavity at the greater palatine foramen posterolaterally. It makes a 90 turn anteriorly, seen from the lateral view, and from there runs in the roof of the mouth directly anteromedially to the incisive foramen. At the incisive foramen, it makes a direct 90 turn superiorly to re-enter the nasal cavity close to the midline. In the nasal cavity, its distal branches along the septum anastomose with those of the long sphenopalatine arteries and ethmoidal arteries.

Lesser Descending Palatine Artery

The lesser palatine artery in the lesser palatine canal parallels the initial course of the greater palatine artery. At the lesser palatine foramen on the oral surface of the hard palate, it turns directly posteriorly (Fig. 15.1I). Here, it supplies the soft palate and upper faucial area and has potentially significant anastomoses with the other vessels which supply this area, particularly the middle pharyngeal branch of the ascending pharyngeal artery, the accessory meningeal artery, and ascending palatine artery.

Infraorbital Artery

The infraorbital artery enters the orbit through the inferior orbital fissure and describes a characteristic curve like an upturned boat-hull on the lateral view (Fig. 15.1I). In the anterior third of the orbit, it temporarily enters the infraorbital canal curving inferiorly onto the anterior aspect of the maxillary bone. Anterolaterally its zygomatic branches anastomose with the adjacent branches of transverse facial and facial arteries. Medially, palpebral and nasoorbital branches anastomose with terminal branches of the ophthalmic artery. Although it is in the orbit itself for much of its early course, its importance as a source of collateral reconstitution of the ophthalmic artery is less important than other collateral vessels.

Deep Temporal Arteries

The deep temporal arteries are usually three in number. They lie along the outer skull surface deep to the temporalis muscle. The anterior and middle deep temporal arteries arise from the internal maxillary artery while the posterior deep temporal artery arises from the proximal superficial temporal artery (Figs. 15.1G, I). The deep temporal arteries share with the middle meningeal artery a quality of having smooth unbroken curves, referred to as a "pseudo-meningeal" appearance, best perceived in contrast to the tortuosity of the surrounding extracranial and intracranial vessels. Unlike the meningeal vessels, the deep temporal arteries do not change course as they cross the skull base, i.e., they lie outside the skull. The anterior deep temporal artery is of most practical importance because it contributes an important branch to the lateral aspect of the orbit. A branch of the anterior deep temporal artery reaches the orbit via the inferior orbital fissure or by penetrating the malar bone along the lateral aspect of the orbit where a large anastomosis to the lacrimal vascular territory may be seen. This is a frequent route for retrograde collateral flow into the ophthalmic artery in the setting of carotid occlusive disease.

Masseteric Branches

Masseteric arteries fall into four groups: superior, middle, inferior, and deep. The superior arises from the transverse facial artery, the middle from the distal external carotid artery or internal maxillary artery, the inferior from the facial artery, and the deep from the internal maxillary artery. These vessels follow the course of the masseter muscle and therefore on the AP view project lateral to the ramus of the mandible.

Inferior Alveolar (Dental) Artery

The inferior alveolar artery arises proximally from the internal maxillary artery either alone or in a common trunk with other vessels, particularly the middle deep temporal artery. On the medial surface of the mandible it enters the mandibular canal. As it runs forward to anastomose with the mental branches of the facial artery via the submental foramen, it supplies the roots of the lower teeth.

Superior Alveolar (Dental) Artery

The superior alveolar artery supplies the roots of the upper teeth. This branch arises from the internal maxillary artery and gives an antral branch to the floor of the maxillary sinus (Fig. 15.1J). The superior alveolar artery may arise in a common trunk with other branches of the internal maxillary artery (Fig. 15.1I).

Buccal Artery

The buccal artery is frequently seen as an almost straight vessel connecting the facial artery with the internal maxillary artery. It is characterized by a 90 overlap with the transverse facial artery (Figs. 15.1G, J, 15.4). It is an important route of reconstitution of the facial artery after a proximal ligation.

Pterygovaginal Artery

The pterygovaginal artery projects posteriorly from the distal internal maxillary artery on the lateral view within the pterygovaginal canal to the region of the eustachian tube (Figs. 15.1J, 15.5). Here it exists in balance and anastomoses with the pharyngeal branches of the accessory meningeal artery, the ascending pharyngeal artery, and the mandibular artery when present.

Mandibular-Vidian Artery

The mandibular-vidian artery lies within the Vidian canal connecting the anterior wall of the foramen lacerum and the sphenopalatine fossa (see Figs. 3.4, 8.9). It may be opacified via an injection of the internal maxillary artery or through the petrous internal carotid artery. The artery of the vidian canal derives from the embryologic mandibular artery.

This vessel can have anastomoses with pharyngeal branches of the ascending pharyngeal artery and with the ascending and descending palatine arteries, particularly in the setting of hypervascular masses. Such anastomoses form the basis of intratumoral anastomotic connection between branches of the external carotid artery and the petrous internal carotid artery (Fig. 15.11). Therefore, during embolization of the soft palate and nasopharynx care must be directed toward this possibility, in addition to the dangers to the inferolateral trunk and the ophthalmic artery.

Table 15.1.
Pterygopalatine Fossa

Wall	Foramina	Arterial Contents	Neural Contents
Posterior	Foramen rotundum	Artery of the foramen rotundum	Maxillary division (V_b) of Vth nerve
	Pterygo-vaginal canal	Pterygovaginal artery	Pharyngeal branch of V_b
	Vidian Canal	Vidian artery	Parasympathetic fibers from superior salivatory nucleus, i.e., greater superficial petrosal nerve from VII.
			Deep petrosal nerve (sympathetic fibers) leaving the carotid sheath.
Superior	Inferior orbital fissure	Infraorbital artery	Infraorbital nerve
Medial	Lesser sphenopalatine foramen	Lesser (short, lateral) sphenopalatine arteries	Short sphenopalatine nerves
	Greater sphenopalatine foramen	Greater (long, medial) sphenopalatine arteries	Long sphenopalatine nerves
Lateral	Pterygo-maxillary fissure	Internal maxillary artery and branches	
Inferior	Greater palatine canal	Descending (greater) palatine artery	Greater palatine nerve
	Lesser palatine canal	Lesser palatine artery	Middle and posterior palatine nerves

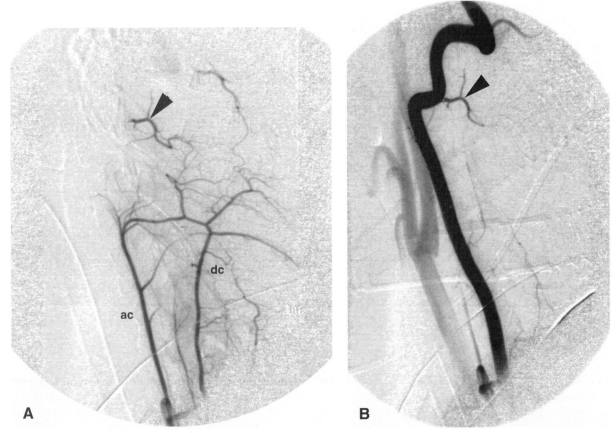

Figure 15.13. *Ascending and deep cervical arteries.* A lateral projection **(A)** of an injection in the right costocervical trunk demonstrates an anastomotic arcade between the deep cervical artery (dc) and the ascending cervical artery (ac). The vertebral artery is not seen directly. However careful comparison with the injection of the right vertebral artery **(B)** demonstrates that the entire C2 branch **(arrowhead)** of the vertebral artery is visible on the cervical injection. Important anastomoses are often recognized in this fashion by comparing the curves, positions, and branching patterns of vessels seen on different runs.

Artery of the Foramen Rotundum

The artery of the foramen rotundum is a posteriorly directed branch of the internal maxillary artery. It forms one of the most dangerous collateral pathways directly to the inferolateral trunk. It is recognized by its tortuous course directed at the base of the sella (see Figs. 8.10, 15.1I, 15.8).

VASCULAR SUPPLY OF THE MIDDLE EAR

Familiarity with the arterial supply of the middle ear is necessary for evaluation of the surgical and endovascular risks involved in treating vascular tumors, particularly glomus tumors, which involve this area. Furthermore, the vessels involved in this region are likely to be closely related to feeding vessels of other vascular lesions such as tumors and dural vascular malformations. They are liable to be exposed to collateral embolization. Moreover, because the vessels in this region have evolved from important embryonic precursors, the middle ear is a site of important aberrant vasculature. Specifically, the risks involved with the latter include inadvertent surgical biopsy of an aberrant internal carotid artery or persistent stapedial artery in the middle ear.

The arterial supply to the middle ear involves six possible routes of supply, which require evaluation:

1. The *inferior tympanic artery* of the ascending pharyngeal artery enters the middle ear through the inferior tympanic canaliculus. It shares this foramen with the tympanic branch of IX (Jacobson's nerve). This foramen is an early site of growth of glomus tympanicum tumors causing early erosion of the bony margins of the canal. In the normal state, the inferior tympanic artery is very small and difficult to see on digital images because of the density of surrounding bone. In the middle ear, its branches in part follow those of Jacobson's nerve towards the cochlear promontory. Its branches follow the respective nerve fibers destined for the greater and lesser superficial petrosal nerves.

2. Along the greater superficial petrosal nerve, the inferior tympanic branches anastomose with the superior tympanic artery, a branch of the petrosal branch of the middle meningeal artery.

3. The inferior tympanic artery also anastomoses posteriorly with the *artery of the stylomastoid canal*. This is a branch usually of the occipital artery or posterior auricular artery; it ascends vertically in the stylomastoid canal along the course of the VIIth nerve. On superselective injections, the petrous and mastoid course of the facial nerve can

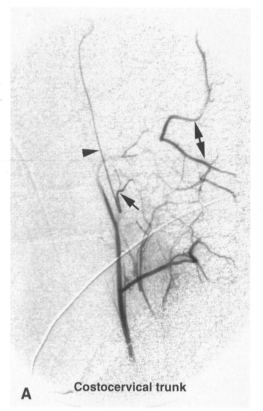

A Costocervical trunk

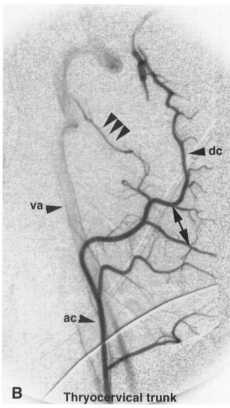

B Thryocervical trunk

Figure 15.14. *Cervical anastomoses.*   Lateral projections of the left costo-cervical trunk **(A)**, left thyrocervical trunk **(B)**, and left vertebral artery **(C)**, performed in that order, are presented. Only by collating all three runs can the potential anastomotic vessels be identified. In B, the ascending cervical artery (ac) has taken over the distal deep cervical (dc) territory. In A, the ascending cervical artery (ac) was opacified therefore by reflux or by muscular anastomoses off-screen. The anastomotic branch that opacifies the vertebral artery in A **(arrow)** is seen again in C. The apparent caliber of the vertebral artery in A is due to slip-streaming of flow along the posterior wall of the vertebral artery.

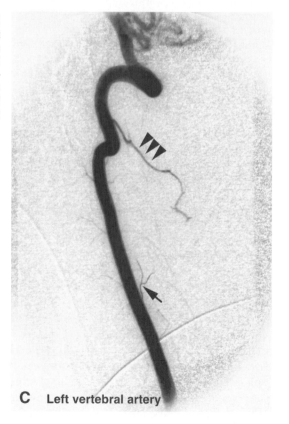

C Left vertebral artery

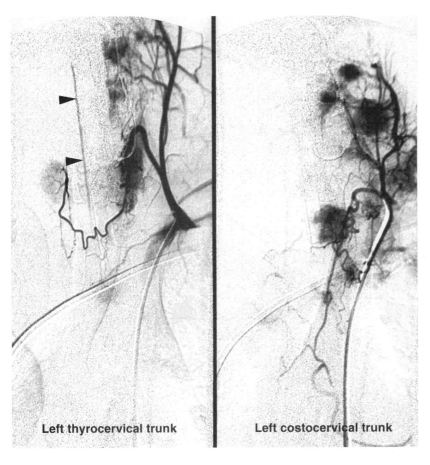

Figure 15.15. *Dangers of cervical embolization.* AP projections of the left thyrocervical trunk and left costocervical trunk in a young adult with metastatic paraganglioma. Hypervascular metastases were evident on virtually every injection of this spinal embolization being performed preoperatively to reduce vascularity in a T3 spine compression. Nevertheless, dangerous vessels must be identified and avoided. The artery of cervical enlargement arose from the left thyrocervical trunk and was only faintly evident in the midline **(arrowheads).**

Left thyrocervical trunk

Left costocervical trunk

be outlined by the opacified vessels from the petrosal branch of the middle meningeal artery and the stylomastoid artery.

4. The *anterior tympanic artery* is a branch of the internal maxillary artery or of the anterior auricular artery and gains access to the middle ear through the petrotympanic (Glasserian) fissure, which it shares with the chorda tympani. On the lateral projection, it runs obliquely posteriorly and superiorly just anterior to the external auditory meatus to anastomose with the stylomastoid artery.

5. The *carotico-tympanic branch* arises at the junction of the vertical and horizontal petrous segments of the internal carotid artery and is directed towards the tympanic cavity. It is usually very small and is rarely, if ever, seen angiographically due to the density of overlying bone.

6. The final artery to consider in evaluating middle ear lesions is the *artery of the internal auditory canal.* This supplies the internal canal and is not thought to have prominent anastomoses with the external and internal carotid branches supplying the middle ear. Nevertheless, it warrants consideration, particularly in larger lesions, which extend beyond the middle ear. The artery of the inner auditory canal may arise directly from the basilar artery or from the anterior inferior cerebellar artery. The latter artery may also supply dural branches to a glomus or other vascular tumor that has involved the dura of the cerebello-pontine angle. This is an important feature to evaluate in pre-surgical patients.

Therefore, consideration to the middle ear anastomoses must be given in embolization of the middle meningeal artery, the ascending pharyngeal artery, and the occipital artery. Aggressive particle embolization or use of sclerosing agents affecting the vasa nervorum may result in permanent lower motor neuron damage to the motor fibers of VII and of the chorda tympani. With highly vascular tumors, the possibility of intratumoral anastomoses with retrograde embolization of the internal carotid artery may need to be considered.

CERVICAL ARTERIES

In addition to the branches of the external carotid artery, when considering angiographic evaluation of the upper neck and skull base, it is necessary to include the ascending cervical artery, usually from the thyrocervical trunk of the subclavian artery, and the deep cervical artery, usually from the costocervical trunk (Fig. 15.1B). These trunks will be also of vital interest in evaluation of cervical spinal lesions.

In the upper cervical levels, there is a system of anastomotic connections between the ascending and deep cervical arteries, the occipital artery, the vertebral artery, and the ascending pharyngeal artery. Because of this propensity for anastomotic collateral flow, the area is an important route for vessel reconstitution in the setting of occlusive

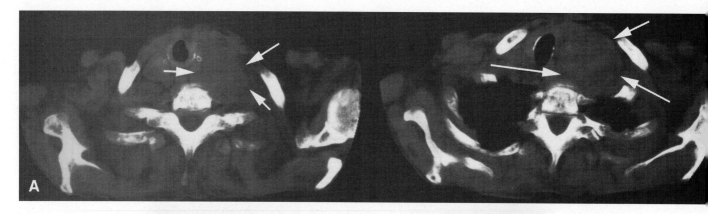

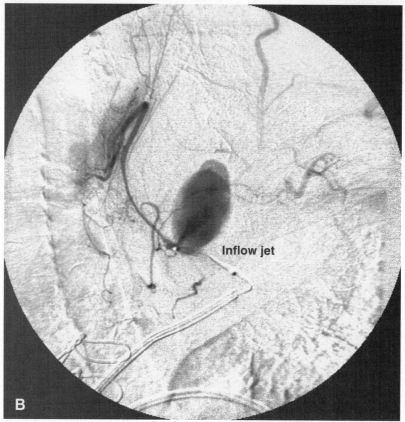

Figure 15.16. *Importance of the jet effect in localizing the precise point of inflow to an aneurysm.* An elderly female developed a pulsatile mass and a thrill in the left supraclavicular fossa following attempted placement of a central line. A CT demonstrated a centrally enhancing mass, and indicated a large amount of circumferential thrombus **(white arrows in A).** An arch aortogram demonstrated what appeared to be a left subclavian artery pseudoaneurysm. Because of extremely tortuous great vessels selective injections were not performed. She was referred for embolization treatment. The case was extremely difficult. Although the aneurysm could be seen, its entrance was elusive despite a multitude of angled views of the left subclavian artery. Finally, a jet of contrast from a single image **(B)** in the filling phase demonstrated that the aneurysm was from the inferior thyroidal artery. Notice the mass-effect on the thyro-cervical trunk by the uno-pacified component of the pseudoaneurysm. The position and direction of the jet during filling can sometimes yield important information about the parent vessel of the aneurysm or pseudoaneurysm.

disease. It is also an area of critical concern during neuro-interventional procedures. The dangers of inadvertent embolization to the posterior circulation are real. Embolization with sclerosing agents in the upper cervical level may also threaten the vasa nervorum of the lower cranial nerves (Fig. 15.13).

On the lateral projection, the ascending cervical artery is a straight vessel that lies at about the level of the vertebral bodies (Figs. 15.14, 15.15, 15.16). The deep cervical artery lies more posteriorly close to a level with the spinous processes. Frequently, one or the other will be absent higher in the neck and the distal territory will be assumed by the other. In such instances, the principal vessel will make a swing on the lateral projection towards the territory of the deficient vessel.

The branch vessels in this region are named according

to the cervical space or neural foramen with which they correspond, i.e., a vessel lying between the bodies of vertebrae C4 and C5 will be the C5 branch. The vertebral artery has segmental branches at each level corresponding with the neural foramina. The C1 and C2 branches of the vertebral artery have a particular propensity to anastomose with the occipital artery. The deep cervical artery is also likely to be involved in the C2, C3, and C4 anastomoses posteriorly. At levels C3 and C4, the anastomoses are also likely to involve respective branches of the vertebral artery with the ascending cervical artery and the ascending pharyngeal artery.

Due to the possibility of the artery of cervical enlargement taking origin from the cervical trunks, embolization in these vessels proximally should be done with extreme caution.

The involvement of the ascending pharyngeal artery in the upper cervical vascular system is twofold:

1. The C3 anastomotic branch of the vertebral artery ascends within extradural space of the spinal canal behind the odontoid process to anastomose with the descending branch of the hypoglossal branch of the neuromeningeal trunk.
2. More laterally the musculospinal branch of the ascending pharyngeal artery anastomoses with the C3 branches of the vertebral artery.

SINUS PERICRANII

Sinus pericranii is a vascular anomaly usually seen in the pediatric age group, characterized by anomalous communication between the intracranial and extracranial venous systems. It occurs close to the midline, usually in the frontal or parietal areas. It can be associated with an underlying anomaly of venous drainage affecting the frontal lobes.

Being composed of predominantly venous structures adherent to the outer surface of the skull, the palpable mass associated with this disorder is usually compressible and increases in size with Valsalva maneuvers. Hemangiomatous variants that are not fully compressible are also described.

SUGGESTED READINGS

Djindjian R, Merland JJ. Superselective arteriography of the external carotid artery. Berlin: Springer-Verlag, 1978.

Lasjaunias P, Berenstein A. Surgical Neuroangiography: Functional Anatomy of Craniofacial Arteries. Berlin, Springer-Verlag, 1987, Vol. 1.

Lasjaunias P, Guibert-Tranier F, Braun JP. The pharyngo-cerebellar artery or ascending pharyngeal artery origin of the posterior inferior cerebellar artery. J Neuroradiol 1981;8 317–325.

Lasjaunias P, Moret J, Mink J. The anatomy of the inferolateral trunk of the internal carotid artery. Neuroradiology 1977; 13 215–220.

Lasjaunias P, Moret J. The ascending pharyngeal artery: normal and pathological radioanatomy. Neuroradiology 1976;11 77–82.

Lasjaunias P, Theron J, Moret J. The occipital artery: anatomy—normal arteriographic aspects—embryologic significance. Neuroradiology 1978;15 31–37.

Lasjaunias P, Vignaud J, Hasso AN. Maxillary artery blood supply to the orbit: Normal and pathological aspects. Neuroradiology 1975; 9 87–97.

Lasjaunias PL. Craniofacial and upper cervical arteries: Functional clinical and angiographic aspects. Baltimore: Williams & Wilkins, 1981.

Osborn AG. The vidian artery: normal and pathologic anatomy. Radiology 1980;136 373–378.

Poppel MH, Roach JF, Hamlin H. Cavernous hemangioma of the frontal bone with report of a case of sinus pericranii. Am J Roentgenol 1948;59 505–510.

PART III / VASCULAR DISEASES

CHAPTER 16

Aneurysms, Subarachnoid Hemorrhage, and Dissections

The term "aneurysm" usually refers to a persistent patho-logic dilatation of an arterial wall. In certain diseases, par-ticularly arteriovenous malformations, the possibility of an-eurysms affecting venous structures must be considered also. Arterial aneurysms may be described according to configuration as fusiform, when the whole vessel circum-ference is involved (Figs. 16.1, 16.2, 16.3), or saccular, when the lesion is eccentric. Mild dilatation of a segment of vessel is called ectasia. The point at which diffuse ectasia becomes an extended fusiform aneurysm is often difficult to define objectively.

EXTRADURAL ANEURYSMS AND PSEUDOANEURYSMS

Extradural aneurysms are unlikely to cause subarachnoid hemorrhage, unless they rupture with particular force against the dura. They are therefore usually considered to be less immediately life-threatening than subarachnoid aneurysms. The commonest location for true aneurysms of the extradural carotid artery is in the cavernous segment.

Aneurysms of the Petrous and Cervical Segments of the Internal Carotid Artery

Aneurysms of the petrous and cervical segments are un-common. They are sometimes seen in patients with con-nective tissue diseases. However, pseudoaneurysms in these areas are encountered more frequently. They can be related to complications of post-traumatic or idiopathic dissection, parapharyngeal infection, infection of the pe-trous air-cells, skull fracture, surgical or traumatic lacera-tion, or tumor invasion. When complications of bleeding or embolic phenomena in the internal carotid artery terri-tory occur, these lesions can constitute a serious risk to life. Bleeding from a petrous aneurysm may occur when erosion of the adjacent supporting bone permits rupture of the aneurysm into the middle ear or sphenoid sinus. These aneurysms or pseudoaneurysms may also present with mass-effect as they bulge into adjacent structures, par-ticularly the floor of the middle cranial fossa where they may compress branches of the trigeminal nerve (see Figs. 8.3, 8.8).

Aneurysms of the Cavernous Segment of the Internal Carotid Artery

Aneurysms in this location are relatively common and are seen particularly in older patients. They may be fusiform or have a relatively defined neck. Frequently there are vari-able degrees of intraluminal thrombus and atherosclerotic mural changes. They are often giant in size (25 mm), in which case they are likely to present with mass-effect and neuropathy of the paracavernous cranial nerves. They may rupture into the cavernous sinus and establish a carotid-cavernous fistula. It is uncommon for them to rupture into the subarachnoid or subdural spaces, but it can happen.

Cavernous aneurysms projecting medially into the sella turcica are thought to carry a particular risk of subarach-noid hemorrhage if they rupture (see Fig. 8.15). Addi-tional care is advised for large cavernous aneurysms when the support of the sphenoid sinus wall has become eroded. Rupture of an aneurysm in this direction is life-threatening due to exsanguinating epistaxis. Therefore, evaluation of the CT bone-windows for this finding is an important com-ponent of treatment decision-making (see Fig. 18.9).

Most small cavernous aneurysms are incidental observa-tions on angiographic or axial examinations. Asymptom-atic cavernous aneurysms are usually not treated unless there is compelling evidence of imminent complications.

FALSE ANEURYSMS OF THE INTRACRANIAL CIRCULATION

Cerebral aneurysms can be classified according to loca-tion, size, etiology, or configuration. When classified by the integrity or otherwise of their mural components, they can be separated into true aneurysms (intima and adventi-tia intact) or pseudoaneurysms. A pseudoaneurysm is one in which the wall of the artery has been perforated. The apparent lumen of the opacified aneurysm is contained by an organized extraluminal hematoma. Pseudoaneurysms occur when the wall of a vessel has been compromised by trauma, dissection, surgical injury, biopsy, or adjacent infection.

Post-surgical Pseudoaneurysms

False aneurysms of the proximal or distal intracranial ves-sels after surgery are rare. They have been seen following vessel injury in the course of open or endoscopic sinus surgery (1–4), transsphenoidal pituitary procedures (5, 6), stereotactic biopsy (7), or craniotomy for a variety of rea-sons (8).

Traumatic Intracranial Aneurysms

Pseudoaneurysms of the intracranial circulation may be seen as a result of penetrating or non-penetrating head-

Figure 16.1. *Fusiform aneurysm.* A fusiform aneurysm **(arrows)** of the right middle cerebral artery involves the entire circumference of an extended segment of vessel.

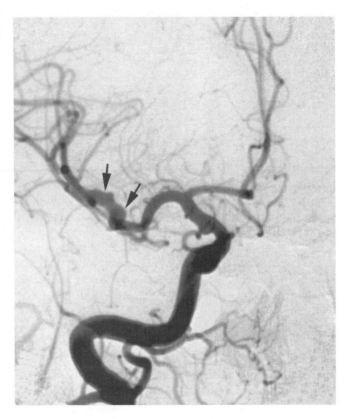

Figure 16.2. *Mild dysplasia.* The communicating segment of the supraclinoid right internal carotid artery in this patient demonstrates mild ectasia **(arrowheads)** and an alteration in caliber, in contrast to the more proximal internal carotid artery. Infundibular widening **(arrow)** of the origin of the posterior communicating artery extends posteriorly from this segment.

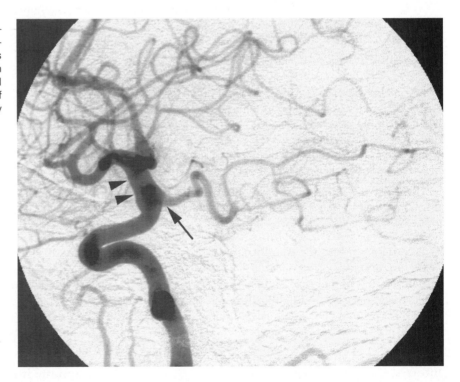

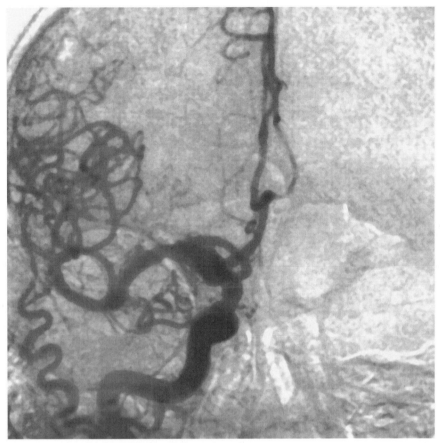

Figure 16.3. *Dysplasia progressing to fusiform aneurysm.* A PA view of the right internal carotid artery demonstrates irregular dysplasia of the supraclinoid internal carotid artery and proximal middle cerebral artery. The point at which such changes become categorized as aneurysmal is often subjective.

injuries (9), impaction on the vessel by bone fragments (10), or following surgical injury (11, 12). They are typically seen in young males after severe injury to the head (Fig. 16.4), but more than 30% are identified in children (13, 14). Post-traumatic lacerations of intracranial major vessels are usually fatal, and it is unusual for a patient so injured to reach medical attention. Some authors maintain that when the adventitia of the vessel is preserved as the retaining layer, then some of these aneurysms may be classified as "true aneurysms."

A consistent theme in the literature dealing with post-traumatic pseudoaneurysms is that their discovery depends entirely on the index of suspicion of the managing physician. Without angiography, they frequently elude early detection. They can present with subacute or delayed rebleeding or other complications, typically after a period of one or two weeks, but possibly as long as months (9, 15).

These injuries can be seen in the anterior or posterior circulation (16), and most frequently have a contiguous or related bone injury. Their discovery is usually associated with penetrating injuries in which the missile impact has scattered numerous fragments of bone or metal in diverging trajectories, particularly when fragments are seen close to the skull base (17).

Pseudoaneurysms in the setting of closed head injury have also been seen where no violation of the dura or skull

is present (18). Pseudoaneurysms may be seen with closed head-injury, particularly in children, when fronto-lateral shear injuries cause significant impaction of the pericallosal (see Fig. 9.9B) and callosomarginal branches against the falx cerebri, or of the middle cerebral artery against the sphenoid ridge (19). Traumatic aneurysms may account for 14–39% of intracranial aneurysms in the pediatric population (20). Nakstad et al. (19) have commented that with the replacement of angiography by CT for evaluation of head injuries, a number of traumatic aneurysms may be overlooked compared with the 1960s.

Military experience suggests that traumatic intracranial pseudoaneurysms are not as rare as was once supposed. Identification of such injuries was rare during the Vietnam and Korean Wars (21, 22), but was seen in 3.6–8% of head-injury patients undergoing angiography after the Iran-Iraq War (9, 17, 23). Intracranial pseudoaneurysms were also found to be a familiar injury during the Civil War in Lebanon by Haddad (24) who worked there as a neurosurgeon throughout the war.

Pseudoaneurysms reaching medical attention may be more likely to be seen in a patient with a low-velocity injury such as a stabbing, rather than a more devastating high-velocity injury from which the victim is less likely to survive. One paper reports an incidence of 10% for pseudoaneurysms after low-velocity, penetrating stabbing injuries to the head (25). The same paper from South Africa by Kieck

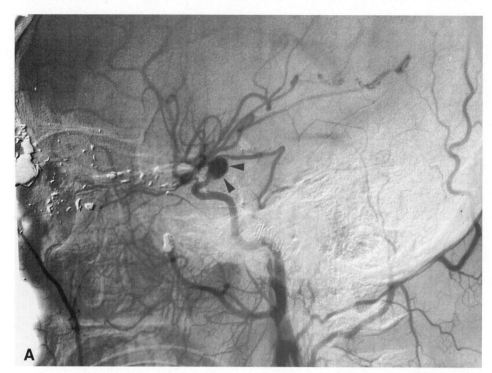

Figure 16.4. *Traumatic intracranial pseudoaneurysm.* **(A)** A young adult was shot accidentally behind the left mastoid bone. The bullet traversed the intracranial space and lodged in the left orbit which it enucleated. A left common carotid arteriogram demonstrates bullet fragments extending from the middle cranial fossa to the orbit. The supraclinoid left internal carotid artery is attenuated and fills a pseudoaneurysm in the expected region of the posterior communicating artery (arrows).

and de Villiers (25) reported a 30% overall incidence of vascular abnormalities on angiograms after such injuries, including arterio-venous fistulas, transections, occlusions, spasm, and pseudoaneurysms (Figs. 16.4, 16.5, 16.6). Pseudoaneurysms may be delayed in formation and be detected only by sequential angiography. They may spontaneously thrombose (26), possibly in as many as 20% of cases on serial angiography (17). However, these patients do better with active surgical intervention (18, 27).

Complications specifically related to false aneurysms include delayed rupture, mass-effect on adjacent brain or cranial nerves, or an associated intraparenchymal, subarachnoid, or subdural hematoma. Delayed presentation months or years after the initial injury may be seen (28). A carotid-cavernous fistula may result when the cavernous carotid artery is torn in association with a sphenoid fracture (Fig. 16.5). Alternatively, massive epistaxis may follow a similar injury when there is free communication of the bleeding site with the paranasal sinuses.

Post-traumatic aneurysms represent a difficult management problem as there is a significant risk of profuse bleeding at surgery when the dura is opened. Trapping of the pseudoaneurysm or occlusion of the parent-vessel proximal to the laceration by surgical or endovascular means may represent the best therapeutic option in certain circumstances (29, 30).

Immediate angiography for patients with penetrating head injuries has been advised by du Trevou and van Dellen (31) who compared angiographic findings in groups of patients studied immediately after admission versus those studied after a delay of over a week. The timing of angiography did not affect the sensitivity of the test to the presence of pseudoaneurysms, the incidence of which was 12% in both groups. Follow-up angiography may be necessary for patients in whom spasm or other vascular abnormalities preclude adequate evaluation.

FUSIFORM INTRADURAL ANEURYSMS

Fusiform aneurysms are frequently associated with vessel tortuosity, hypertension, atherosclerosis, and advancing age. They typically affect the cavernous or supraclinoid internal carotid artery and the basilar trunk. They often present with symptoms related to mass-effect (Fig. 16.7). With large aneurysms stagnation of blood can lead to thrombus formation, and patients may present with embolic stroke (32, 33). Rupture is not common when the condition is mild (34). Surgical management of a ruptured fusiform segment of vessel can be difficult (35). Techniques, including wrapping, proximal occlusion, or bypassing, must make allowance for preserving important perforator vessels, which might take origin from the dysplastic segment (36).

When ectasia of the basilar artery reaches bizarre proportions, the terms "megadolichobasilar anomaly" or "giant fusiform aneurysm" are used (Fig. 16.8A, B) (33, 37). They represent less than 1% of intracranial aneurysms. Although they are classically described as affecting the vertebrobasilar circulation, giant fusiform or serpen-

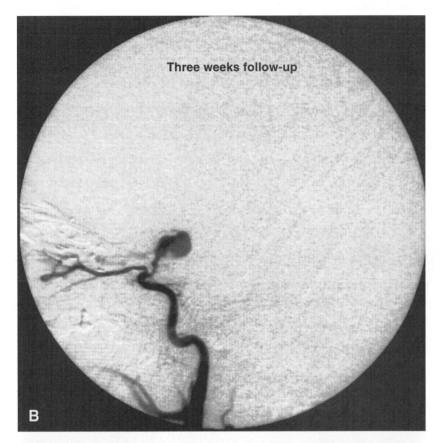

Three weeks follow-up

Figure 16.4. *(continued)* **(B)** Endovascular treatment was planned but delayed because of prolonged sepsis. A left common carotid arteriogram performed three weeks after the first study demonstrates change in the contour of the pseudoaneurysm and less filling of the ipsilateral hemispheric circulation. **(C)** The left internal carotid artery was therapeutically occluded using detachable balloons proximal to the pseudoaneurysm. A right internal carotid artery injection following left internal carotid artery occlusion shows no evidence of filling of the aneurysm. The patient recovered with moderate right sided paretic and language deficits. (Courtesy of Frank R. Huang-Hellinger, MD, PhD, Boston, MA.)

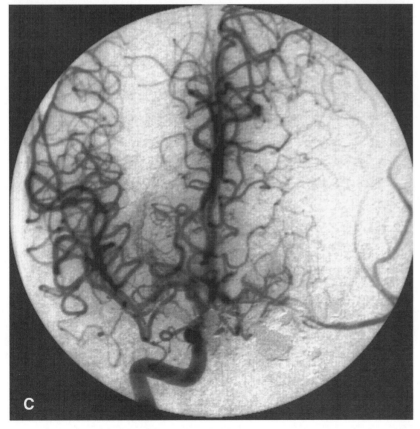

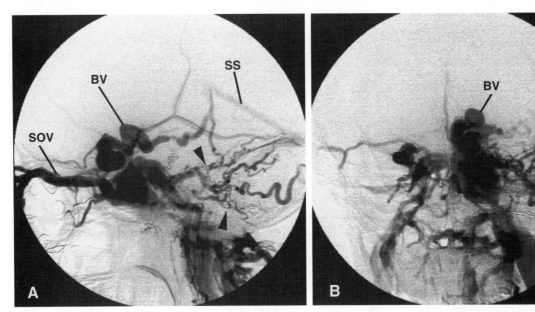

Figure 16.5. *Carotid cavernous fistula following trauma.* Lateral **(A)** and PA **(B)** views of the left internal carotid artery injection in a young adult following severe head trauma. There is immediate and profuse opacification of venous structures due to fistulous flow from the cavernous internal carotid artery. Intercavernous connections fill the contralateral cavernous sinus. Although his symptoms were rela-

tively mild, the angiographic appearance of varicose distention of the anterior segment of the basal vein (BV), and opacification of parenchymal veins of the posterior fossa **(arrowheads)** suggest that complications of venous hypertension may be imminent. SOV = superior ophthalmic vein; SS = straight sinus.

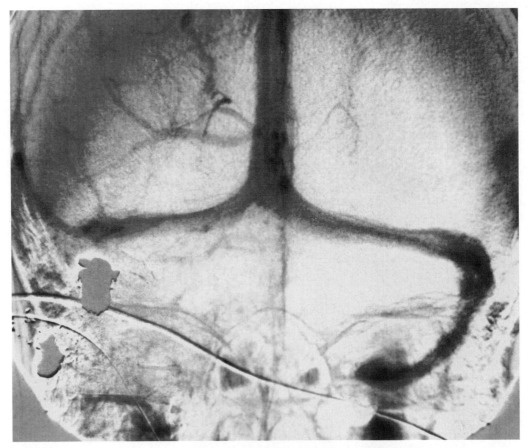

Figure 16.6. *Remember to examine the venous structures when evaluating penetrating missile injuries.* Venous injury may follow penetrating injuries. In this patient, the right transverse sinus has been occluded by bullet fragments lodged in the right mastoid bone.

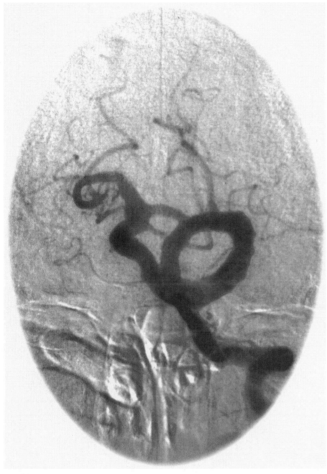

Figure 16.7. *Fusiform dysplasia/aneurysm of the basilar artery.* Changes of this degree are frequently associated with a history of long-standing hypertension. Vessel changes may be more extreme than indicated on an angiogram. Circumferential thrombus augments the degree of mass-effect on surrounding structures.

tine aneurysms are also seen in the anterior circulation (36) (Fig. 16.8C, D). This group of usually elderly patients typically presents with mass-effect, brainstem compression, cranial nerve deficits, obstructive hydrocephalus, subarachnoid hemorrhage, and embolic strokes due to stagnation of blood. Mizutani (38) has presented MRI evidence that many of these aneurysmal vessels demonstrate intimal flaps and a pseudolumen on axial imaging, indicating that dissection plays a role in the growth of these lesions. Furthermore, long-term clinical follow-up of this group of patients indicates a poor prognosis due to recurrent subarachnoid hemorrhage or progressive mass-effect.

INFLAMMATORY AND MYCOTIC ANEURYSMS

Mycotic aneurysms are classically described as occurring distally in the cerebral circulation and as being not necessarily related to vessel bifurcation points. They may be subtle in appearance and are frequently best seen in the parenchymal phase of the injection when the arteries are already washing out.

Intracranial aneurysms of inflammatory origin may be of several types: bacterial, syphilitic (Heubner's arteritis), related to angiocentric organisms such as mucor, aspergillus, or other fungi, or associated with systemic arteritides such as giant cell arteritis and polyarteritis nodosa.

In the modern era, an increased incidence of aneurysms related to the HIV virus or its associated infections has been described. This may be primarily due to a necrotizing vasculitis related to the virus itself, particularly in congenital infections, or due to acquired diseases such as tuberculosis or syphilis (39–41).

Aneurysms associated with infectious diseases are collectively referred to as "mycotic," although some authors reserve this term for those related only to fungal infections.

Presentation and Incidence of Mycotic Aneurysms

Mycotic intracranial aneurysms present most commonly with acute subarachnoid hemorrhage or intraparenchymal hematoma developing as a complication of already established septic disease. Occasionally, young patients may present with an embolic neurologic deficit, such as hemiplegia, as the presenting event of bacterial endocarditis (Figs. 16.9, 16.10)(42, 43). Other common presentations include seizure or focal neurologic signs due to vasculitis, or vegetative emboli in an area of the brain distal to a silent aneurysm. Direct vessel invasion from adjacent infected paranasal sinuses may also be seen (Fig. 16.11). CSF spread of infection has been implicated in a series of mycotic intracranial aneurysms related to *Aspergillus* meningitis, probably due to contaminated equipment during spinal anesthesia (44).

Although mycotic aneurysms are typically described as being found in unusual, peripheral locations, multiple in number, and not necessarily related to vessel bifurcations, this archetype is not always valid. In a series of patients with bacterial endocarditis and related intracranial aneurysms, Corr et al. (45) found that approximately 70% of patients had single aneurysms, and approximately a third of the aneurysms were centrally located. Mycotic aneurysms can be seen in the cavernous carotid artery when a systemic illness is complicated by cavernous thrombophlebitis (46). When an aneurysm is seen in an unusual peripheral location, the possibility of an infectious embolic etiology should be considered, but not all mycotic aneurysms are atypical in appearance or location.

Bacterial aneurysms were typically associated with bacterial endocarditis when this disease was more common, but can be seen with any septicemic state particularly with respiratory infections. Older studies suggest that the incidence of intracranial aneurysms in patients with endocarditis varies between 4 and 15%, or perhaps higher considering that many of these aneurysms remain asymptomatic (47–49).

Mycotic aneurysms are related to impaction of a septic embolus in the intima of a peripheral cerebral artery with

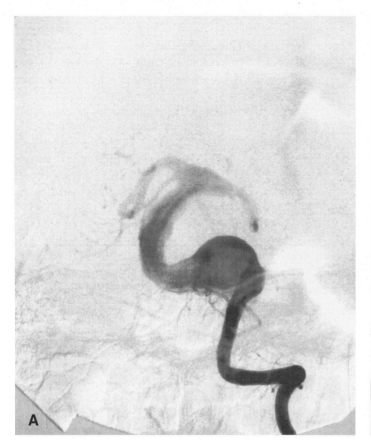

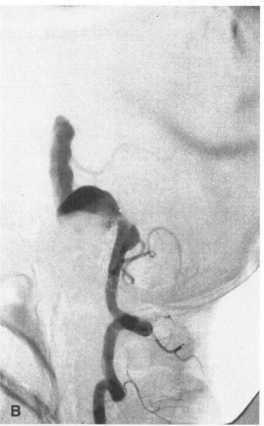

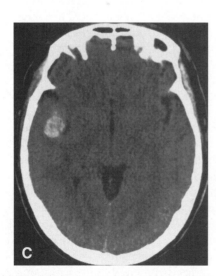

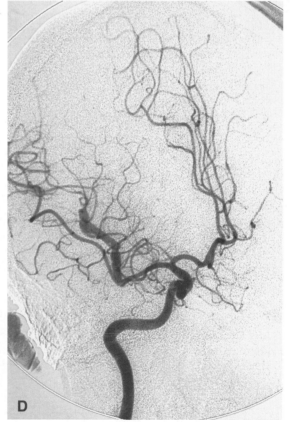

Figure 16.8. *Megadolichobasilar anomaly and serpentine aneurysm.* Townes **(A)** and lateral **(B)** projections of a megadolichoectatic basilar artery in an elderly hypertensive patient. A CT scan of the head **(C)** in a young adult presenting with sudden headache demonstrates a focal collection of blood in the right Sylvian fissure. An oblique RAO view **(D)** of the right internal carotid artery injection demonstrates an elongated fusiform or ``serpentine'' aneurysm of the parietal branch of the right middle cerebral artery. (Case courtesy of T. Gudas MD, Boston, MA)

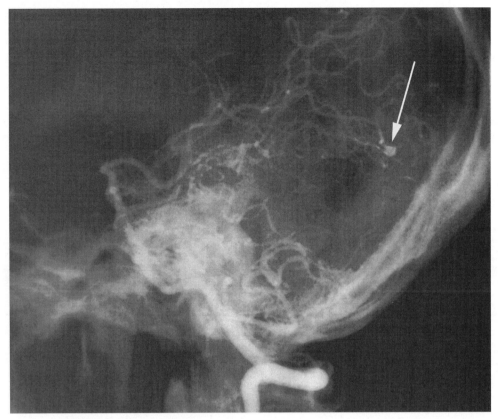

Figure 16.9. *Mycotic aneurysm of the calcarine artery.* A young adult patient with sepsis and a history of intravenous drug abuse demonstrated a small aneurysm **(arrow)** of the distal right calcarine artery on this left vertebral artery injection. Two weeks later after antibiotic treatment, the aneurysm was no longer evident.

development of a resulting arteritis, focal mural necrosis, and aneurysm formation. This explains the friable nature of the wall of these lesions and their propensity to bleed spontaneously or during surgery.

Role of Angiography in Management of Mycotic Aneurysms

Some inflammatory aneurysms tend to regress with treatment of the primary infection (46, 50, 51). Bohmfalk (46) identified complete resolution of mycotic aneurysms without surgical intervention in approximately 12% of patients, while Corr et al. (45) found that 33% of patients with intracranial mycotic aneurysms responded completely during antibiotic therapy. Better results were seen in patients with single, unruptured aneurysms. They also commented that surgical treatment of persistent aneurysms was made easier by antibiotic therapy, the wall of the aneurysm being less friable and less prone to rupture after antibiotic treatment. Early surgical intervention for a mass lesion associated with a mycotic aneurysm appears prudent because the mass could represent an intracerebral abscess. Similarly, early surgical intervention for single, accessible aneurysms has been recommended. However, in situations with multiple aneurysms, delayed surgery after antibiotic therapy may be the safer route.

Bohmfalk et al. (46) advocated that endocarditis pa-

tients without neurologic signs should be considered for cerebral angiography as a screening measure, with the caveat that an initial angiogram was not always positive. Repeated angiography can demonstrate development of mycotic aneurysms in this group of patients. Their recommendation of screening cerebral angiography was based on the mortality rate of up to 80% in endocarditis patients after aneurysmal rupture, contrasted with the low risk of cerebral angiography and a 30% mortality in endocarditis patients with unruptured aneurysms (43). Bingham (50) also stressed the importance of obtaining a baseline angiogram following the treatment of mycotic intracranial aneurysms. Sequential angiography every 2 to 3 weeks during and after antibiotic therapy allows detection of alterations in size or number of intracranial aneurysms (Fig. 16.11). Any growth in size of an aneurysm during therapy or persistence after therapy (4–6 weeks) should be an indicator for surgical treatment (46, 50). Some mycotic aneurysms in peripheral vessels have been successfully treated by endovascular occlusion or sclerosis of the vessel (52, 53)

ONCOTIC INTRACRANIAL ANEURYSMS

Invasion of the intracranial vessel wall with destruction of the internal elastic lamina, and cavitation with aneurysm or pseudoaneurysm formation is a rare but well recognized

Figure 16.10. *Mycotic aneurysm of the right middle cerebral artery.* This peripheral aneurysm **(arrows)** in a patient with infective endocarditis is demonstrated on a skewed lateral view **(A)**. The aneurysm has a fusiform, tapered appearance extending into adjacent branches. Small peripheral mycotic aneurysms are frequently best seen on a late arterial phase when the main arterial structures have begun to lose density **(B)**.

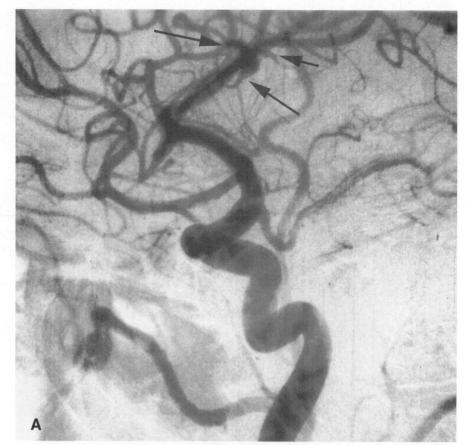

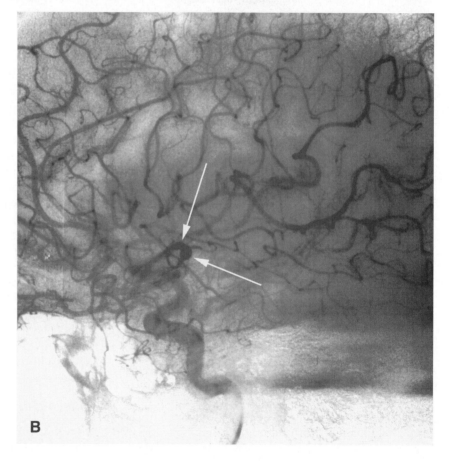

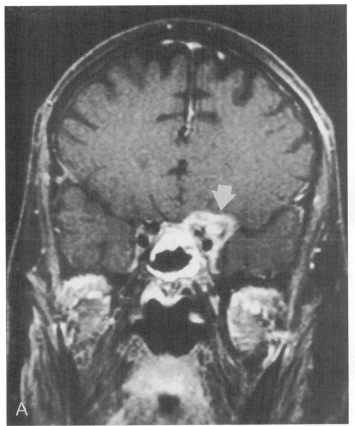

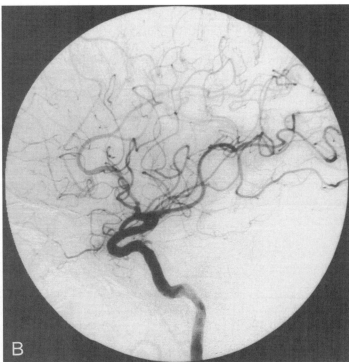

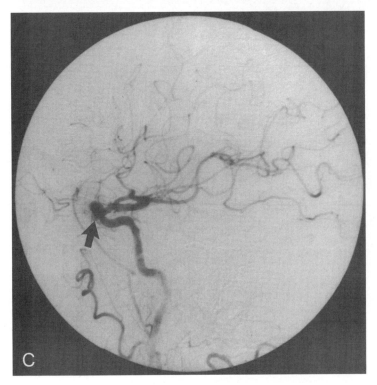

Figure 16.11. *Carotid pseudoaneurysm with aspergillus infection.* An elderly patient with intractable Aspergillus infection of the left orbital apex extending to the left cavernous sinus, seen on the gadolinium-enhanced MRI image **(arrow in A).** An angiogram **(B)** was performed to evaluate for possible pseudoaneurysm formation but was negative. Two weeks later, with a suspicious flow-void evident on a follow-up MRI, a rapidly developing pseudoaneurysm was demonstrated on a second angiogram **(arrow in C).**

event from metastatic deposits of atrial myxoma, chorio-carcinoma (54, 55), renal cell carcinoma, or bronchogenic carcinoma (56–58). Invasion of arteriolar walls by gliomatous tumors may explain the very rare association of false aneurysms with primary brain tumors (59). Features shared by oncotic aneurysms are that they may be delayed in onset (i.e., they may not be seen on an initial angiogram), may be multiple, may grow rapidly, or thrombose spontaneously. They may resolve with chemotherapy for the primary lesion (60).

Left atrial myxoma may be complicated by or present with neurological symptoms related to arterial obstruction by myxomatous emboli, or intracranial aneurysmal rupture with subarachnoid or intraparenchymal hemorrhage (Fig. 16.12) (61–65). Subintimal invasion by myxomatous cells has been verified histologically in such lesions (66). Although this is a rare clinical presentation, it is a treatable disease that can be seen in otherwise healthy young patients. Systemic emboli from myxoma have been reported in up to 45% of patients, half of these going to the cerebral circulation (61, 62, 67). The diagnosis may be delayed due to the initially small size of the cardiac tumor (68). Angiographic features described in these patients include intraluminal filling defects, fusiform or saccular peripheral an-

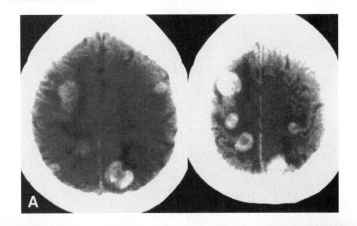

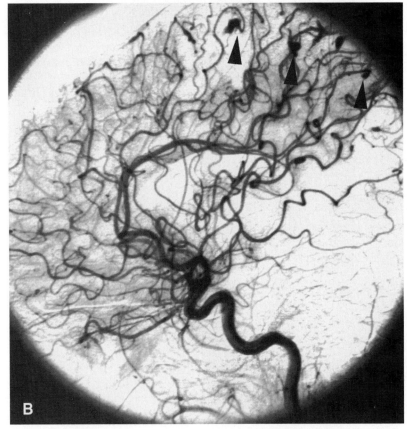

Figure 16.12. *Myxomatous emboli and aneurysms.* A non-enhanced CT **(A)** examination in a young adult patient with a known cardiac myxoma demonstrates multiple intraparenchymal hemorrhagic foci. Lateral **(B)** and PA **(C)** views of the left internal carotid arteriogram demonstrated multiple peripheral areas of pseudoaneurysm formation **(arrowheads)**. (Case courtesy of T. Ptak, MD, PhD, Boston, MA.)

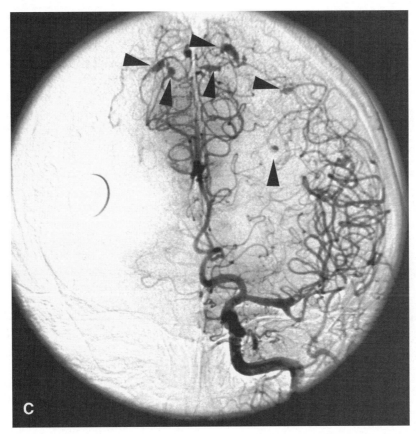

Figure 16.12. *(continued)*

eurysms, vessel occlusions, and delayed passage of contrast. Some peripheral aneurysms may be extremely subtle and could be missed if not looked for carefully on the late arterial or parenchymal angiographic phase. Magnification views can be helpful (69).

DISSECTIONS AND DISSECTING ANEURYSMS

Extracranial Dissections and Dissecting Aneurysms

Dissections of the intracranial and extracranial arteries occur due to disruption of the vessel intima and insinuation of flowing blood between the mural layers of the vessel. Dissection of the extracranial carotid and vertebral arteries is a potentially serious disease due to occlusive or embolic cerebrovascular complications, particularly in young or middle-age adults. Patients with internal carotid dissections present with hemispheric occlusive symptoms, amaurosis fugax, or sympathoplegic signs related to compression of the sympathetic plexus around the internal carotid artery, i.e. an ipsilateral Horner's syndrome. Head pain and tenderness around the orbit or forehead, neck pain along the course of the sternocleidomastoid muscle, or carotid tenderness may also be seen. Patients with vertebral artery dissections present with neck pain, transient ischemic attacks or strokes of the posterior circulation, often with a Wallenberg syndrome due to occlusion of the ipsilateral posterior inferior cerebellar artery.

Dissections of the internal carotid artery or vertebral artery may be idiopathic, post-traumatic (Fig. 16.13), iatrogenic following manipulation of the cervical spine, associated with the effects of fibromuscular dysplasia, or related to minor physical strains in an unusual position, e.g., starting a lawn-mower. Patients with a familial history of arterial dissections are more prone to recurrent dissection (70).

A delayed neurologic event in a patient with history of trauma is a typical clinical presentation for arterial dissection. Injury to the carotid artery in children who fall while running with a pencil or other object in their mouth is a well-recognized danger. Compared with spontaneous dissections, traumatic dissections of the internal carotid artery have a more severe angiographic appearance, a greater likelihood for complete luminal occlusion, a greater likelihood of pseudoaneurysm formation, and less probability of spontaneous complete recovery (71, 72).

Dissections of the internal carotid artery have a predilection for two particular locations. They occur just distal to the common carotid bifurcation and between C2 and the skull base. In the higher location, medial defects in the arterial wall related to changes in the configuration of the mural layers may contribute to a propensity for injury. The intramural hematoma may dissect subintimally and cause narrowing or occlusion of the vessel lumen. It may dissect into the subadventitia forming a protruding pouch. Luminal pouches in a dissection are histologically distin-

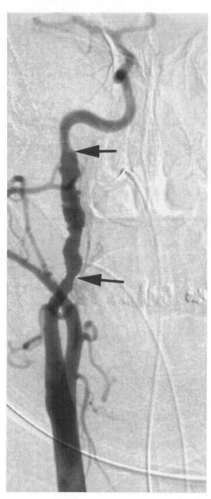

Figure 16.13. *Post-traumatic dissection of the right internal carotid artery.* A non-occluding dissection of the right internal carotid artery extends from the mid-cervical level to the skull-base **(arrows)**. The patient had multiple arterial injuries after a vehicular accident.

guished from a pseudoaneurysm by the presence of a retaining adventitial layer. Dissection-pouches may be the source of emboli to the cerebral circulation or may rupture into the extravascular space forming a pseudoaneurysm. A dissection may occasionally propagate into the petrous carotid artery, but usually stops at the skull base.

Vertebral artery dissections usually start at the point of maximal cervical mobility around C1–C2 (see Chapter 12). The dissection site may be focal or may propagate intradurally and occlude intracranial vessels. Alternatively, emboli may emanate from a dissection-pouch in the neck. Massive bleeding in the neck and hematoma formation may occur from rupture of a dissected extracranial artery, but this is very rare. Occlusion of the dissected vessel may be partial or complete, or flow may be preserved through a false lumen.

A variety of angiographic signs can be seen during evaluation of internal carotid artery dissection, depending on the severity and duration of the disease. In the acute phase, the vessel may be completely occluded with a gradually tapered appearance. A non-occlusive dissection frequently

shows a narrowed irregular lumen with resumption of a normal contour in the petrous segment. Pouching of the carotid lumen, intimal flaps or, less commonly, a double lumen can be seen. In a series of 18 patients with traumatic internal carotid artery dissections, mostly young adults after vehicular accidents, Mokri et al. (72) described the angiographic signs of traumatic dissection in order of frequency: dissecting aneurysm, luminal stenosis, occlusion, intimal flap, distal branch occlusion, and slow flow to the middle cerebral artery.

During angiography of a patient with a spontaneous dissection, most authors advise caution in evaluation of the contralateral internal carotid artery or vertebral arteries lest the catheter should induce another dissection in a patient with a predilection for intimal disease. Nevertheless, an evaluation of the remaining vessels is necessary as bilateral dissections can be seen. In particular an evaluation of the collateral circulation of the circle of Willis is prudent for consideration of treatment possibilities should the patient fail anticoagulant therapy or develop a persistent pseudoaneurysm. Thrombus emanating from the dissection site may be seen on an angiogram as irregular filling defects. Occlusions of the intracranial vessels due to emboli may also be seen. Where such complications are present, in spite of anticoagulation, treatment of the dissection or the pseudoaneurysm by surgical or endovascular techniques often becomes necessary. Where intervention is necessary, the most favorable and least invasive methods usually involve endovascular use of balloons or coils to trap the diseased segment or occlude the parent vessel proximally (73). In particular cases, preservation of the parent vessel by packing the pseudoaneurysm with coils may be possible. In patients with embolic events during anticoagulant treatment for dissection, bypass surgery of the internal carotid artery or vertebral artery has been successfully performed with favorable results (74). This option might be a particular consideration where bilateral dissections are present.

Intracranial Dissections and Dissecting Aneurysms

Dissection of intracranial vessels, once considered an extremely rare disease (75), is now a more recognized entity representing as many as 3–7 % of patients presenting with non-traumatic subarachnoid hemorrhage (76–78). Intracranial dissections are usually clinically idiopathic but have been reported after head trauma, electrocution, with syphilitic and other arteritides of the intracranial vessels, and with conditions such as polyarteritis nodosa, fibromuscular dysplasia, and migraine (Figs. 16.14, 16.15, 16.16). Before 1950 more than half of recognized cases were associated with the meningovascular phase of syphilis (Heubner's endarteritis), a disease now seen more frequently as a result of the AIDS epidemic.

Intracranial dissections are more common in the posterior than in the anterior circulation (78), and patients typically present with suboccipital headache, and with focal

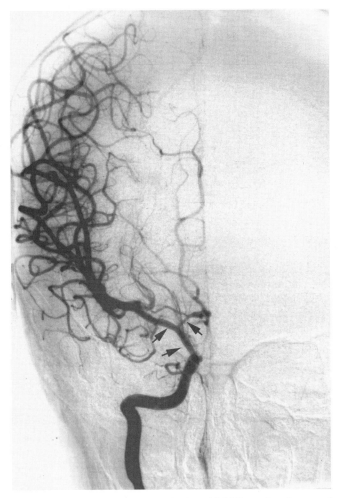

Figure 16.14. Intracranial dissection in a child. Dissections **(arrows)** in children have a predilection for the supraclinoid internal carotid artery. They may be idiopathic or follow trauma. Hemispheric ischemia is the most common presenting event in this age-group.

or diffuse posterior circulation ischemia. The media and adventitia of the intradural vertebral and carotid arteries are thinner than in the extracranial vessels. Therefore, arterial rupture with subarachnoid hemorrhage as a complication of intracranial dissections is more likely to develop than is rupture of extracranial dissections. Intracranial vessels lack an external elastic membrane and have fewer elastic fibers in the media (79). Furthermore, the intracranial arteries are deficient in vasa vasorum (80). Poor healing of intracranial vessels due to the lack of vasa vasorum may be part of the explanation for the greater likelihood of complications in many diseases of these vessels compared with extracranial vessels. In autopsy specimens of intracranial dissection with subarachnoid hemorrhage, extension of clot between the media and adventitia is seen with destruction of all three mural layers (77). Intracranial dissections usually affect the major vessel trunks but have been reported in distal vessels (81).

Dissections in the anterior domain of the circle of Willis are less common than in the posterior, and they may have a predilection for the vessels of children and young adults

(82, 83). Patients may have a variable course after the initial ictus of hemispheric ischemia. Massive infarction and swelling with herniation is the mechanism of death when the deterioration is rapid. When vascular occlusion is only partial, patients can survive with variable deficits.

A dissecting aneurysm is caused by penetration of circulating blood into the wall of the artery with extension between the layers of the arterial wall. An opacified false lumen is contained by the adventitia of the vessel. Rarely, a patent false channel providing distal flow may be seen angiographically lying parallel to the true lumen (76).

A segment of intracranial dissection may measure from 1–5 cm. The patient may present with focal neurologic deficits due to vessel occlusion, thromboembolic occlusions, mass-effect on adjacent structures, or subarachnoid hemorrhage. Once ruptured, intracranial dissecting aneurysms have a high risk of rerupture in the first week after subarachnoid hemorrhage, up to 70%, with a high (46%) rate of mortality (78). A more optimistic outcome was seen in a series of 10 dissecting aneurysms of the basilar artery reported by Pozzati et al. (84), who found that spontaneous improvement or resolution can be seen in some patients.

Intracranial dissections can be recognized angiographically by an irregular tapering of the vessel lumen, a linear filling defect within the lumen, retention of contrast within the wall of the vessel, or by the presence of an irregular aneurysm or pseudoaneurysm associated with focal luminal narrowing or irregularity (86, 87).

The angiographic and MRA appearance of the dissected vessel is sometimes described as a ''pearl and string'' sign referring to the appearance of fusiform dilatation interrupted by segments of string-like narrowing (Figs. 16.15, 16.16). The risk of subarachnoid hemorrhage seems to be much higher with intracranial dissections affecting the posterior fossa than with dissections of the anterior circulation (88).

It is important to distinguish dissecting aneurysms from saccular bifurcation aneurysms as the treatment may be different. Even with good quality angiography, the signs of intracranial dissection may be subtle. The possibility of a dissection as a source for subarachnoid hemorrhage should be borne in mind during aneurysm-search studies. The disease may be bilateral in the vertebro-basilar system in 5–10% of cases (89). Optimal treatment for dissecting extradural and intradural aneurysms involves altering or eliminating, if possible, the flow-pattern in the vessel around the pseudoaneurysm. This hemodynamic alteration will suppress the inflow jet. This can be done by surgical clipping of the vessel or vessel reimplantation (90). Endovascular techniques include trapping the pseudoaneurysm or occluding the parent vessel proximally, if the patient's collateral flow will tolerate such a procedure (Fig. 16.15) (91–94). It is important to perform this occlusion as close as possible to the aneurysm to eliminate the possibility of continued anterograde flow through collateral vessels (73). Without treatment, dissecting aneurysms with

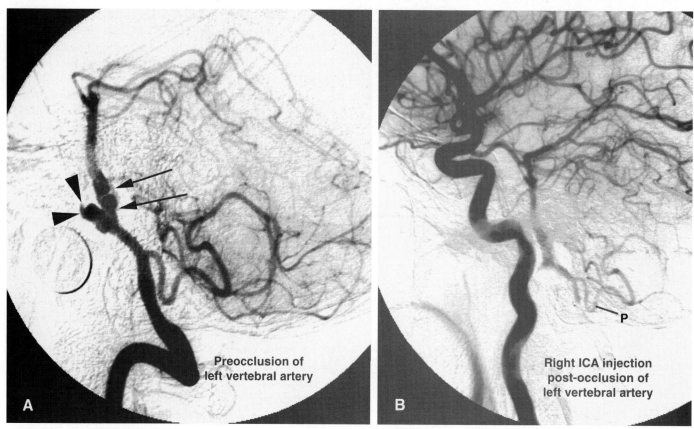

Figure 16.15. *Dissecting aneurysm of the distal left vertebral artery.* A middle-aged male presenting with Grade II subarachnoid hemorrhage was found to have a sharply cornered aneurysm **(arrowheads)** projecting from an irregular segment **(arrows)** of the vertebrobasilar junction, indicating a dissection. The right vertebral artery did not supply flow to the basilar artery. The patient was treated successfully by balloon occlusion of the left vertebral artery. This resulted in reversal of flow down the basilar artery altering the hemodynamic stress on the ruptured dissection. The procedure jeopardized supply to the left posterior inferior cerebellar artery (P). A right carotid injection during placement of the first balloon in the left vertebral artery (prior to detachment) demonstrated adequate filling of the posterior inferior cerebellar artery, and the patient showed no neurologic deficit to suggest posterior fossa ischemia. Consequently balloon occlusion of the left vertebral artery was executed. The patient made an excellent recovery.

subarachnoid hemorrhage have a rebleed-risk reported to be between 30 and 70% (78, 95, 96). Therefore, immediate treatment of intracranial dissecting pseudoaneurysms is advised bearing in mind that ruptured dissecting aneurysms are extremely fragile with a significant risk of intraprocedural rebleeding. The possibility of spasm from subarachnoid hemorrhage related to this disease may affect the efficacy of collateral vessels where vessel occlusion is planned. Dissections without subarachnoid hemorrhage may do well without surgical intervention, although some of these patients may progress to a chronic fusiform dilatation of the vertebrobasilar system (86) and may ultimately need surgical or endovascular treatment. An important discriminator for the clinical effects of the disease seems to be whether extension to the basilar artery from the vertebral artery occurs. When the disease is more confined and there is no subarachnoid hemorrhage, patients have a far more favorable outcome (77).

SACCULAR (BERRY) ANEURYSMS

The cognomen ''berry'' for saccular intracranial aneurysms was introduced in 1931 by Collier (97) because of the fanciful resemblance of these aneurysms with their shining coats to berries hanging from the arterial tree. The perfect berry-shaped aneurysm with a spherical contour and confined neck is uncommon. Many aneurysms have a more complex structure often with more than one distinct compartment or lobule and a neck that can be of variable size. Because of their familial association in some patients, these aneurysms have sometimes been referred to as ''congenital'' to distinguish them from other acquired types of aneurysms. However, the term ''congenital'' is misleading, and most evidence suggests that these aneurysms develop and expand with time. A congenital defect in the arterial media may be one of the explanations for later development of this acquired disease.

Histopathologic examination demonstrates that unruptured small aneurysms have a thin wall measuring 30–150 *m* in thickness, composed of endothelium and adventitia similar to that of the parent vessel (98). As the aneurysm enlarges some portions of the wall become collagenized and thickened with endothelial cells, fibroblasts, and elastic fibers. More attenuated portions become points of potential rupture. When an aneurysm ruptures,

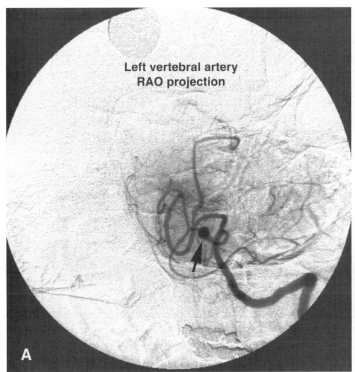

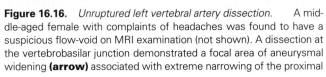

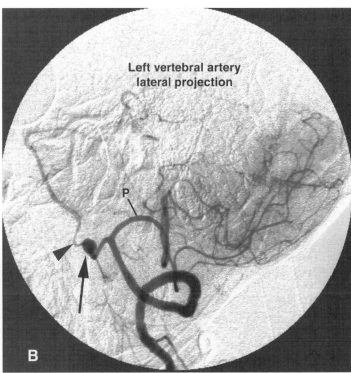

Figure 16.16. *Unruptured left vertebral artery dissection.* A middle-aged female with complaints of headaches was found to have a suspicious flow-void on MRI examination (not shown). A dissection at the vertebrobasilar junction demonstrated a focal area of aneurysmal widening **(arrow)** associated with extreme narrowing of the proximal basilar artery **(arrowhead)** above that level (``string and pearl''). The overlapping posterior inferior cerebellar artery (P) made the standard PA and Townes views difficult to interpret. The anatomy of the vertebro-basilar junction was clarified by these obliqued and skewed images.

it is usually assumed that it is the dome that has given way, but this is not always the case. The wall at the neck may sometimes be the most fragile segment. After the aneurysm ruptures, the wall of the ruptured segment is supported by weak fibrin nets for approximately the first three weeks. This correlates with the clinically observed period of high risk for rerupture. After three weeks the wall becomes infiltrated with capillaries. Stronger collagen is incorporated into the healing wall with a diminishing risk of rerupture (98).

Intracranial saccular aneurysms have a population prevalence between 0.2% and 8.9% based on angiographic and autopsy studies. The higher number refers to more lenient histopathologic definitions of what constitutes an aneurysm. Approximately 15–30% of patients with aneurysms have more than one (99). The majority of all aneurysms remain asymptomatic during life. Aneurysms become symptomatic due to rupture with subarachnoid hemorrhage, expansion with mass-effect on surrounding structures, or development of thrombus and embolic events.

Risk factors for development of intracranial aneurysms include factors such as polycystic kidney disease and hypertension, aortic coarctation, 1-antitrypsin deficiency (100), connective tissue diseases, e.g., Ehlers-Danlos syndrome Type IV (101–103), fibromuscular dysplasia (104, 105), a family history of berry aneurysms.

Some families have been identified with a genetically heterogeneous pattern of inheritance of intracranial aneurysms. Within this group of patients, most will have only one other affected family member, usually a sibling (106). Screening of asymptomatic patients with polycystic kidney disease detects an aneurysm prevalence of approximately 11%, but the prevalence increases to 25% when there is also a family history of intracranial aneurysms (107–109).

Among all patients with aneurysmal subarachnoid hemorrhage, as many as 20% have a first or second degree relative with a similar history. First degree relatives of a patient with aneurysmal subarachnoid hemorrhage have a risk of subarachnoid hemorrhage that is four times that of the general population (109, 110). Ronkainen et al. (111) reported a 10% rate of asymptomatic aneurysms detected by MRA in family members of probands with intracranial aneurysms. In a review of the literature concerning screening for familial aneurysms, Schievink et al. (112) estimated that in families with more than one affected proband, first degree relatives have a 17–44% incidence of aneurysms detectable by screening (113). Therefore, screening of family members with a strong family history of intracranial aneurysms is recommended, at least with magnetic resonance angiography (114). The question of screening of asymptomatic family members is confounded by not knowing the patterns of aneurysm growth and when aneurysms are more likely to bleed. Screening may only detect stable unruptured aneurysms. Dangerous aneurysms that may rupture later in the relative's lifetime may not yet have formed at the time of screening. However, most patients (80–90%) with aneurysms do not fall into this familial category.

Nevertheless familial aneurysms form an important subgroup of aneurysm patients. There is evidence (115–117) that familial aneurysms compared with non-familial aneurysms demonstrate the following features:

They are more likely to rupture at a smaller size.

They are more likely to be multiple.

They show a preponderance in females even greater than is the case for sporadic aneurysms.

They are less likely than sporadically occurring aneurysms to be found with a preponderance at the anterior communicating artery complex.

They are more likely to rupture at a younger age, occur in the same arterial tree, and rupture in the same decade as the proband.

De novo Aneurysm Formation

Another group of patients at risk for intracranial aneurysm formation requiring particular consideration are those who have undergone therapeutic proximal carotid occlusion or ligation for treatment of intracranial aneurysms. It is thought by some authors that altered hemodynamic forces affecting the circle of Willis, and the anterior communicating artery in particular, are responsible for a delayed rate of *de novo* aneurysm formation that may approach 4% or higher in incidence (118–121). In a series of 27 patients who had been treated with surgical occlusion of a carotid artery and followed over a 3–22 year period, Fujiwara et al. (120) reported two complications related to rupture of new aneurysms of the anterior communicating artery and two fatal ruptures of preexisting aneurysms ipsilateral to the remaining carotid artery. A number of reports point to altered hemodynamic forces being responsible for aneurysm development and rupture following therapeutic occlusion of a cephalic vessel (122–124). However, other studies have followed large groups of patients and have detected no major risk of delayed aneurysm formation after a proximal occlusion (125, 126). Considering the known incidence of metachronous formation of multiple aneurysms, this group of patients is at some *a priori* risk for new aneurysm formation even without a ligation or balloon-occlusion procedure. Therefore the additional risk posed by carotid occlusion is unclear.

Rinne and Hernesniemi (127) have estimated that the risk of metachronous aneurysm formation in patients with a previous subarachnoid hemorrhage is approximately two to three times the risk of aneurysm formation in the general population. This risk applies particularly to patients who suffered the initial bleed at an age younger than 40 years. Follow-up neuroradiologic imaging or angiography appears to be warranted in this group of patients after the initial aneurysm has been treated.

Sites of Aneurysm Formation

The most common sites of aneurysm formation are at stress points on the circle of Willis and on the proximal major intracranial vessels where branches bifurcate. Approximately 85% of aneurysms occur in the anterior portion of the circle of Willis as divided by a line transecting the posterior communicating arteries (99). The anterior communicating artery complex represents the single most common site. Between 5–10% of intracranial aneurysms occur in the posterior fossa. When they rupture, they have a considerably poorer prognosis than those of the anterior circulation (128).

Hemodynamic Properties of Aneurysms

All intracranial aneurysms have a capacity to expand with time. This can be demonstrated angiographically in particular patients on sequential angiograms. An uncertain factor is the rate of this expansion. This might be a slow process over months, with a gradual emergence of the aneurysm into the realm of imminent rupture. Alternatively, a critical expansion could occur over hours or days in a previously stable aneurysm.

The risk of rupture is somehow related to aneurysm size. The tensile strength of an aneurysm wall is assumed in some measure to decrease according to Laplace's formula for hollow spheres:

$$P = 2\,T/r$$

where P is the pressure-differential across the aneurysm wall, r is the radius, and T is the tangential tension. However, application of Laplace's law of spheres is an oversimplification of the physical traits of an aneurysm. Factors such as the degree of stasis along the wall of an aneurysm with peripheral thrombus formation are probably important. A larger aneurysm with such mural reinforcement may have greater strength than a much smaller aneurysm with a red, attenuated wall. Some authors argue that the period of maximal risk of aneurysmal rupture is during a phase of acute expansion, implying that a small, expanding aneurysm represents a greater risk than a larger stable one.

The size of the neck of the aneurysm may be a factor in determining the risk of rupture. Pulsatility of flow, turbulence, and inflow-outflow characteristics at the neck may also be important. Pulsatile flow and disturbed flow within the aneurysm probably contribute to mechanical fatigue of the wall. The impact of the inflow pattern on the dome of the aneurysm is probably also important. These theoretical assumptions do not explain, however, why most aneurysms rupture at the dome, while shear forces and flow-turbulence are greatest at the neck adjacent to the inflow path.

In unruptured, stable aneurysms, it is likely that flow is characterized as somewhere between laminar and chaotic. Turbulence and reversed flow within an unruptured aneurysm play a role in dampening the effect of the inflow-jet on the aneurysm wall. However, the characteristics of this pattern change immediately with onset of rupture. In animal experiments, the estimated systolic velocity of the jet from a ruptured aneurysm can reach close to 500 cm per second with an estimated force of 630 to 4,300 dynes (129). The power of a jet from a ruptured aneurysm varies with the cube of velocity, providing an explanation of the immediately destructive effect of some aneurysmal ruptures on surrounding brain parenchyma (129). A frequent observation is aneurysmal rupture with intraparenchymal hematoma formation dissecting into the brain substance or into the intracerebral ventricles. For instance, an anterior communicating artery aneurysm may rupture into the frontal lobes, may perforate the lamina terminalis, or may dissect into the genu of the corpus callosum. This estimate of the velocity and power of a jet probably also explains in part how a subarachnoid aneurysm rupturing can cause a subdural hematoma. Subdural hematoma can be seen after rupture of aneurysms of the anterior communicating artery, posterior communicating artery, middle cerebral artery, and internal carotid artery. German and Black (129) simulated the chain of events after aneurysmal rupture using a model of a ruptured aneurysm, which quickly sliced a path through a gelatin block to a depth of 3 cm.

Biorheology is the study of physiologic fluid-flow in live organisms. Kerber and Liebsch (130, 131) have presented two lucid introductory articles to this field outlining the difficulty of applying deterministic physical principles to the flow of blood in anatomically idiosyncratic vessels. The viscosity of blood changes inversely with the degree of shear forces applied, meaning that blood behaves as a thixotropic, non-Newtonian fluid. The angles encountered in a complex vascular bifurcation in combination with differential slip-streaming or spiraling of blood in the lumen determine the impaction-site of maximal shear forces on the vessel wall. This might explain why aneurysm formation is not always exactly at the carina of a bifurcation.

NATURAL HISTORY OF UNRUPTURED INTRACRANIAL ANEURYSMS

Asymptomatic unruptured aneurysms are discovered incidentally during investigation of unrelated symptoms or during evaluation of other intracranial aneurysms. They represent a particular problem in decision-making with reference to whether they should be treated immediately. It is difficult to predict which asymptomatic aneurysms might be at imminent risk of rupture. The prevalence of aneurysms in the adult population is approximately 1–6% (113, 132), and most of these will not rupture during a particular patient's lifetime. For purposes of clinical decision-making asymptomatic intracranial aneurysms are categorized as follows:

1. Those discovered during evaluation of unrelated problems.
2. Those discovered during evaluation of a different symptomatic aneurysm.

The latter group is thought to be more at risk of rupture and so are subject to more stringent scrutiny than the former. Asymptomatic aneurysms in family members of patients who have ruptured aneurysms are also categorized as being at higher risk than incidental aneurysms.

Precise data on the natural history of asymptomatic aneurysms is scant, but some series suggest that for patients with unruptured aneurysms the most valuable predictors of rupture are patient age and aneurysm size. Asymptomatic aneurysms less than 10 mm in diameter have a small risk of rupture, approximately 2% per year (133). Aneurysms measuring 10–15 mm are thought to have a rupture rate of 3–4% per year, and those measuring 16–25 mm a rupture risk of 5–6% per year, and a 8–9% risk per year for aneurysms 25 mm. Although no patients with aneurysms 10 mm ruptured in the reference series by Wiebers et al. (133), this finding must be reconciled with the observation that 7.5 mm was the average diameter of ruptured aneurysms at the same institution. Many aneurysms may shrink briefly at the time of rupture.

Aneurysms may expand rapidly at the time of initial formation, at which time they are most likely to rupture. Those aneurysms that endure this phase of expansion can then stabilize and fortify their walls. This would explain the observation that most ruptured aneurysms are small (10 mm) in clinical practice and would also explain the epidemiological observation that among more stable larger aneurysms, the risk of rupture appears linked to aneurysm diameter. However, cases of long-standing small aneurysms proceeding to rupture have been well documented (134). Aneurysms as small as 4 mm have enlarged and ruptured (134, 135). In patients with a history of subarachnoid hemorrhage, aneurysm-size has not been as reliable for prediction of aneurysm behavior as it is in other patients. In other words, a patient with a previous subarachnoid hemorrhage may be more likely to bleed again from a small aneurysm than would a patient with no history of aneurysmal rupture. The risk of rupture of asymptomatic aneurysms has been calculated as a function of patient age (years) and aneurysm size (mm) by Wiebers et al. (136). Aneurysms increase in size in the days and weeks after rupture (137). This could represent regrowth to a previously held diameter supported by fibrin and clot with a high risk of rerupture.

Other factors thought to contribute to a risk of aneurysm formation or subarachnoid hemorrhage include atherosclerosis, female sex, smoking, use of oral contraceptives, alcohol consumption, asymmetry of the circle of Willis, viral infections, pituitary tumors, and deficiency of some human leukocyte antigen-associated factors (135, 138–140). Higher rates of subarachnoid hemorrhage are also seen in some geographic areas, e.g., Japan and Finland where an annual incidence of almost 24 per 100,000 is seen (141). The Unruptured Intracranial Aneurysm Study has demonstrated that approximately 80% of enlisted patients are current or former smokers, and that 20% of patients have a family history of aneurysms (136). Factors predisposing to the formation of multiple aneurysms include female gender, smoking, family history, and associated diseases such as polycystic kidney disease, aortic coarctation, brain arteriovenous malformations, or fibromuscular dysplasia.

Elective surgery for unruptured, asymptomatic, intracranial aneurysms is cost-effective if the patient has a life-expectancy of at least 13 years. Consideration is given to whether the patient has a serious decrease in quality of life because of living with the discovery of an unruptured aneurysm. The treating hospital is assumed to have an expected complication rate for morbidity and mortality in line with the published expected rates (142).

For practical purposes, an asymptomatic aneurysm with diameter less than 5 mm does not represent an imminent risk. Using size alone as the single variable to estimate the risk of rupture of an aneurysm is erroneous because aneurysms as small as 2 mm can proceed to fatal rupture. Usually, the risk of rupture of a small asymptomatic aneurysm is presented as a round figure to patients as 2% per year and for unruptured symptomatic aneurysms as 4% per year.

NATURAL HISTORY AND OUTCOME OF RUPTURED INTRACRANIAL ANEURYSMS

The statistics on outcome of patients with subarachnoid hemorrhage depend on whether the data were collected at referral centers or based on population registers. More than 10–17% (143) of patients with subarachnoid hemorrhage in most studies die immediately and do not become part of a hospital based experience. Tertiary centers are also more likely to be referred patients with better grade subarachnoid hemorrhage who have survived the initial triage and who will then be likely to have a better ultimate outcome (144). Of those who make it to a hospital, a further 25% die, and only 42–58% return to a premorbid level of function at 6 months (143, 145). In population studies, aneurysmal subarachnoid hemorrhage has an overall 30-day survival of 40–57% (110, 128). Survival for ruptured posterior fossa aneurysms is considerably poorer in population-based studies, 11% at 30 days (128). This is probably due to devastating mass-effect in the confined space of the infratentorial compartment. For treated patients with anterior circulation aneurysms with Hunt and Hess grades I, II, and III, 30-day survival is approximately 70% and for grades IV and V is less than 20% (146). With modern aggressive management, including use of endovascular techniques for management of cerebral vasospasm, these statistics for anterior circulation aneurysms with good clinical grades are even better. Among patients with Hunt and Hess Grades I–III, 86% return to independent functioning, this figure being 96% for Grade I patients (147).

After the initial rupture, vasospasm and recurrent rupture are the important determinants of outcome (145). Older patients, patients with prior hypertension, and those with intracerebral hematoma have a poorer prognosis, as

Table 16.1.

Hunt and Hess Scale for Clinical Grading of Subarachnoid Hemorrhage (148)

This scale is the most commonly used for initial triage of patients with subarachnoid hemorrhage. In addition to being a shorthand tool for communication during referral conversations, its importance lies in the correlation between the patient's grade and likelihood of a favorable outcome from early intervention. ``Good'' grades are I, II, and III.

Grade I: Asymptomatic, minimal headache, or slight nuchal rigidity.

Grade II: Moderate to severe headache, nuchal rigidity, neurological deficit confined to cranial nerve palsy.

Grade III: Drowsiness, confusion, or mild focal deficit.

Grade IV: Stupor, moderate to severe hemiparesis, possibly early decerebrate rigidity, and vegetative disturbances.

Grade V: Deep coma, decerebrate rigidity, moribund appearance.

do patients with depressed levels of consciousness at presentation, thick layers of subarachnoid clot on CT, preexisting medical conditions and basilar aneurysms (145). In round figures, the risk of immediate rebleeding from an untreated ruptured aneurysm, Grades I–III, is taken as 2–4% per day for the first 10 days, 30% during the first 30 days, and 2–4% per year thereafter (Table 16.1).

The major source of delayed mortality derives from rebleeding. The risk of rerupture is highest immediately after the subarachnoid hemorrhage and declines over the following weeks. It is postulated that subarachnoid clot from the first hemorrhage deflects the new blood towards the brain parenchyma or into the ventricular system. This accounts for the more grave implications and effects of a rebleed, which is less likely to confine itself to the subarachnoid space (149).

Of those who survive the initial rupture, the probability of a favorable outcome depends on the following:

Elimination of risk of rebleeding by treatment of the aneurysm. For instance, among patients presenting to hospital, almost a third present with an initial minor or sentinel leak followed by a more devastating hemorrhage within 24 hours to 4 weeks with a mortality rate of over 50% (150). The question of timing of aneurysm surgery has been a matter of debate for some years (143, 151). Operative risk during the phase of vasospasm after subarachnoid hemorrhage is thought to be higher when the brain is swollen. Therefore, delayed surgery after 7–10 days was previously thought to be safer. However, elimination of intentional delay can approximately double the number of aneurysm patients who undergo surgery (143). In these patients the benefits from having eliminated the risks of rebleeding are thought to outweigh the risks of early surgery (152), and opinion is now more in favor of early therapeutic obliteration of the aneurysm.

Management of vasospasm. Early occlusion of the aneurysm can facilitate aggressive use of hypertension as part of the Triple H therapy for vasospasm: hypertension, hypervolemia, hemodilution, in combination with nimodipine therapy. Without prophylactic and active management, the morbidity of neurologic deficits due to vasospasm becoming evident at days 4–14 after a subarachnoid hemorrhage can approach that related to the hemorrhage itself. The Fisher Scale (153) is occasionally mentioned in reference to the CT appearance of subarachnoid hemorrhage and prediction of the risk of vasospasm. A CT done within 24 hours of the hemorrhage, i.e., before the blood can disperse, which demonstrates large subarachnoid clots in the basal cisterns or extensive blood in the vertically oriented subarachnoid spaces is a helpful predictor of a high risk of vasospasm compared with milder degrees of subarachnoid blood (154).

Management of intracranial pressure. In the absence of focal mass-effect, a cerebral perfusion pressure of 60 mm Hg (mean arterial pressure minus intracranial pressure) is a desirable target to prevent brain ischemia.

Management of hydrocephalus, which can occur in 20–67% of patients following subarachnoid hemorrhage, of whom 13% become symptomatic (155).

Management of other complications such as hyponatremia (10–25%), possibly due to increased secretion of atrial natriuretic factor (156), a condition that can aggravate cerebral ischemia.

Monitoring of EKG abnormalities and myocardial dysfunction, due to coronary artery spasm or catecholamine release (157, 158). This can be complicated by the need for sympathomimetic agents to elevate blood pressure in the treatment of vasospasm.

Giant Aneurysms

Giant aneurysms are defined as those greater than 25 mm in diameter. Ironically, compared with smaller aneurysms, they may have a somewhat diminished risk of rupture if the lumen is surrounded by laminar thrombus. However, the character and thickness of this layer of clot is probably in constant flux, and the possibility of rupture should still be considered as significant. When the aneurysm is almost completely thrombosed, a sinusoidal, residual lumen may be seen. This subtype is sometimes referred to as a giant serpentine aneurysm (159–161). Mass-effect is the typical presentation of such aneurysms and may respond to steroid therapy.

The presence of calcification in the walls of giant aneurysms as well as in smaller saccular aneurysms must be noted as this represents a technical difficulty for satisfactory neurosurgical application of a clip across the neck. Surgical clipping of giant aneurysms is technically impossible in more than half of such cases (162). Without treatment, the 5-year outcome for more than 80% of patients with symptomatic giant aneurysms is poor due to mass-effect, thrombosis of important vessels, or subarachnoid hemorrhage (162–164).

Giant aneurysms are seen most commonly arising from the internal carotid artery (57%) and in the posterior circulation (24%). They are less common in the middle cerebral artery (9%) and anterior cerebral artery (10%) (13). Because of their size, distortion and involvement of surrounding vessels, and overlapping contrast density, they are difficult to study angiographically or during craniot-

omy with respect to defining the afferent and efferent parent vessels.

CEREBRAL ANEURYSMS IN CHILDREN

Intracranial aneurysms in children are rare, accounting for less than 5% of all aneurysms (165). When they are seen in children, aneurysms are less likely to be multiple or to be associated with a family history than is the case in the adult population. Moreover, aneurysms in children are more likely to be associated with an identifiable etiology. Up to 39% of aneurysms in children may be associated with a history of trauma (20). Other etiologies include infection with mycotic aneurysms. HIV infection, with necrotizing vasculitis, may need to be considered (40).

ANGIOGRAPHIC EVALUATION OF CEREBRAL ANEURYSMS AND OF PATIENTS WITH SUBARACHNOID HEMORRHAGE

1. Review the available axial images to discern the distribution of subarachnoid hemorrhage or the location of the suspected abnormality. Decide on which vessels to inject first. With an acutely ill patient a clinical deterioration due to aneurysmal rebleeding or other cause may interrupt the study, precluding completion.
2. Size of the aneurysm will be a concern particularly if endovascular treatment techniques are contemplated. Therefore, bilaterally placed sizing markers help to avoid the inaccuracy of having to guess the size of the discovered lesion.
3. Consideration may need to be given to reducing the rate of injection of contrast compared with elective studies (see Chapter 3). With digital imaging, this should not significantly interfere with the sensitivity of the examination. The main impact of this reduction will be on the degree of venous opacification, which is not a concern in most aneurysm patients.
4. Obliqued magnification runs are essential for complete evaluation of a discovered aneurysm. They are also necessary for thorough evaluation of important high-likelihood sites, which appear normal on the standard orthogonal views. This applies particularly to the anterior and posterior communicating arteries and the posterior fossa (Fig. 16.17).
5. For follow-up studies of a subarachnoid hemorrhage patient with a previous negative angiogram, special care must be taken to look for subtle lesions. Additionally, consideration may be given in such patients to evaluation of the external carotid arteries to exclude dural vascular malformations. This is especially worth considering in patients with systemic illnesses or recent pregnancy, which might lead to dehydration or a hypercoagulable state. In such patients a dural sinus thrombosis might have occurred with establishment of a dural arteriovenous malformation. With repeated angiogram-negative posterior fossa subarachnoid hemorrhages, the spinal cord should be considered as a site of possible hemorrhage from vascular malformation or neoplasm, e.g., ependymoma.
6. An angiogram on a patient with acute sub-arachnoid hemorrhage needs to establish the following points: size of the

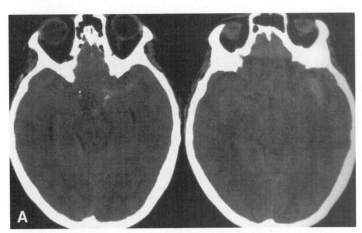

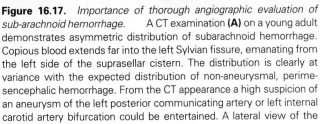

Figure 16.17. *Importance of thorough angiographic evaluation of sub-arachnoid hemorrhage.* A CT examination **(A)** on a young adult demonstrates asymmetric distribution of subarachnoid hemorrhage. Copious blood extends far into the left Sylvian fissure, emanating from the left side of the suprasellar cistern. The distribution is clearly at variance with the expected distribution of non-aneurysmal, perimesencephalic hemorrhage. From the CT appearance a high suspicion of an aneurysm of the left posterior communicating artery or left internal carotid artery bifurcation could be entertained. A lateral view of the left internal carotid artery injection **(B)** was interpreted as demonstrating a loop of the origin of the left posterior communicating artery. The study was thought negative for aneurysm. A follow-up study 10 days later, at which time multiple oblique views were obtained, demonstrated a small aneurysm of the left posterior communicating artery. The double-density **(arrow in B)** projecting over the posterior communicating artery should have been evaluated more closely with oblique views during the initial angiogram, particularly in view of the CT distribution of blood.

aneurysm; the direction in which it points in three planes; its relationship to the parent vessel and to nearby critical structures, especially perforator branches; angiographic or other evidence that the opacified lumen does not correspond with the total size of the aneurysm and that a significant degree of thrombus is present; the presence of one or multiple lobules and the mutual relationship of these lobules; mural calcification; the presence of a daughter-sac or apical teat; size of the aneurysm neck in its most optimal profile with the parent vessel; the status of collateral flow in the circle of Willis in case major vessel occlusion becomes a necessary or inadvertent component of surgical or endovascular aneurysm treatment; the presence/absence of multiple aneurysms, and which aneurysm caused the subarachnoid hemorrhage; a definitive evaluation of all four major vessels. In particular the right posterior inferior cerebellar artery may be problematic either because reflux from the left vertebral artery injection was suboptimal or selection of the non-dominant right vertebral artery itself appears difficult. The possibility of an aneurysm at this site should not be overlooked.

Discerning the Site of Bleeding Among Multiple Aneurysms

Up to 30% of patients with aneurysmal subarachnoid hemorrhage have multiple intracranial aneurysms identifiable

at angiography (166). Because aneurysms in differing locations cannot all be clipped during a single craniotomy, it is important to identify that aneurysm from among many which is most likely to represent the site of current bleeding. Even when multiple aneurysms are present, it is possible angiographically to predict with greater than 95% accuracy which aneurysm has ruptured (167–169). Angiographic features pointing to the offending aneurysm include the following:

Contrast extravasation. This is the only angiographic finding that gives an absolute indication of aneurysmal rupture, but fortunately it is rare.

Size. In more than 90% of subarachnoid hemorrhages in the setting of multiple aneurysms, the largest aneurysm is the culprit.

Contour. Irregularity of the profile of the aneurysm and, in particular, the presence of an apical nipple or teat are highly persuasive findings, probably more discriminating than aneurysm size (167).

Location. In the setting of multiple aneurysms, those of the anterior communicating artery, basilar tip, and of the posterior inferior cerebellar artery are more likely to have ruptured. Moreover, a collation of the CT images with the angiogram is frequently helpful in that the former will demonstrate a preponderance of subarachnoid blood in close proximity to the aneurysm in question (170).

Localization of angiographic signs such as focal spasm, mass-effect, or serial change in appearance of the aneurysm on sequential angiograms.

SUB-ARACHNOID HEMORRHAGE WITH NEGATIVE CEREBRAL ANGIOGRAPHY

Nonaneurysmal Perimesencephalic Subarachnoid Hemorrhage

In approximately 15–30% of patients with spontaneous subarachnoid hemorrhage, no cause of bleeding can be identified on the initial cerebral angiogram (151, 171–174). While patients with negative angiography after a subarachnoid hemorrhage have a benign overall prognosis with a low yield from repeated angiography, it is important to discern between the sub-groups of patients within this population to avoid missing potentially serious or treatable lesions. Within this population of patients with negative cerebral angiography, van Gijn and co-workers in the Netherlands (175) have identified a particular subgroup with a favorable outcome. Within this subgroup hemorrhage is mild and confined to the perimesencephalic area, and the clinical condition is characterized by headache and signs of meningeal irritation only. The clinical entity of ''non-aneurysmal perimesencephalic subarachnoid hemorrhage'' has since been validated in other countries (176, 177). Patients within this group, comprising 50–60% or more of the angiogram-negative population, share the following features:

Onset of subarachnoid hemorrhage is spontaneous and presents with severe headache and meningeal irritation. Focal neurologic deficits, focal signs, and diminished levels of consciousness are not seen.

The CT pattern of hemorrhage is symmetric or virtually so, confined to the perimesencephalic area, the prepontine cistern and interpeduncular fossa, the posterior part of the suprasellar cistern, the posterior part of the interhemispheric fissure, and the medial aspects of the Sylvian fissures (Fig. 16.18). Dense clots of blood are uncharacteristic. Extension into the anterior extent of the interhemispheric fissure, into the lateral aspects of the Sylvian fissures, and into the ventricles, or intraparenchymal hematoma are rarely or never seen with this entity (178). MRI demonstrates that the blood may extend into the premedullary cistern. The CT images used to define this pattern must be obtained within 48 hours of the bleed.

Hydrocephalus may develop in a minority of patients with nonaneurysmal perimesencephalic subarachnoid hemorrhage but is usually mild and resolves spontaneously. Hydrocephalus has been reported in 22–28% of such patients, but many authors report a lower incidence (173, 178).

Hydrocephalus occurs in patients in whom encirclement of the mesencephalon by blood obstructs flow of CSF through the tentorial incisura (179). Occasionally, patients with this pattern of hemorrhage have needed ventriculostomies.

The prognosis for patients with this pattern of hemorrhage

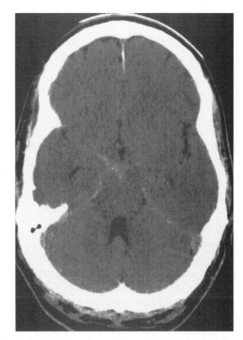

Figure 16.18. *Non-aneurysmal perimesencephalic hemorrhage.* A CT image demonstrates a typical appearance of non-aneurysmal perimesencephalic subarachnoid hemorrhage. The anterior interhemispheric and Sylvian fissure are clear. There is mild dilatation of the temporal horns, indicating hydrocephalus. The development of mild hydrocephalus does not preclude the diagnosis of perimesencephalic hemorrhage.

and with negative cerebral angiography is excellent with a low risk of vasospasm, rehemorrhage, or of neurologic sequelae (175, 176, 180, 181).

It is thought that the source of hemorrhage in this group of patients may be venous, possibly from a ruptured prepontine vein or an angiographically occult vascular malformation at the pial surface. The combination of a typical CT pattern of perimesencephalic subarachnoid hemorrhage and a negative angiogram in a patient with a good clinical grade is very reassuring that the prognosis for the patient is favorable. The likelihood of vasospasm in this group of patients is also very low and rarely of clinical concern. However, reassurance is predicated on the technical and interpretative quality of the cerebral angiogram.

The chance of finding an aneurysm in the setting of this pattern of hemorrhage is less than 3–6%. Fewer than 2% of aneurysms present with this pattern of hemorrhage (182). Rinkel et al. (179) estimated that reliance on the CT scan alone when it demonstrated such a pattern would yield a 5–6% rate of missing an aneurysm, findings similar to those of a consecutive series reported by Van Calenbergh et al. (183). This indicates a need for cerebral angiography even when the initial CT pattern is typical for nonaneurysmal perimesencephalic subarachnoid hemorrhage. Aneurysms presenting with this CT pattern can be found at the tip of the basilar artery (Fig. 16.19); the vertebro-basilar junction possibly associated with a fenestration; the origin of the posterior inferior cerebellar artery contra-

Figure 16.19. *Dysplastic basilar artery aneurysm causing subarachnoid hemorrhage.* In the setting of subarachnoid hemorrhage, one's level of suspicion for subtle abnormalities should be higher than during angiograms performed for other indications. Townes **(A)** and lateral **(B)** views of the posterior circulation in this middle-aged male with recurrent subarachnoid hemorrhage demonstrated a bulbous, dysplastic aneurysm of the basilar artery tip which had been initially dismissed as an irrelevant finding **(arrow in B).** Arrowheads point to the C3 anastomosis from the left vertebral artery to the neuromeningeal trunk.

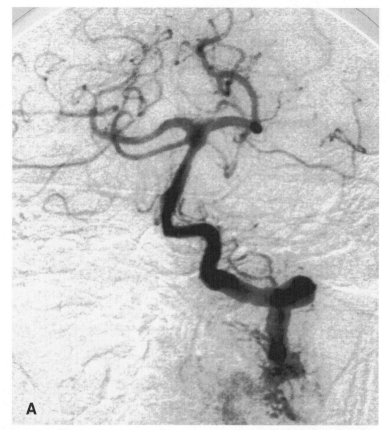

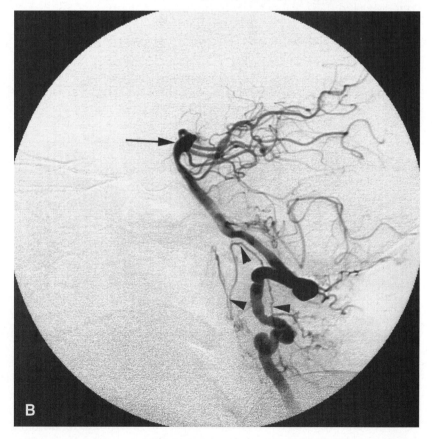

lateral to the side of vertebral artery injection; the distal posterior cerebral artery; or the posterior communicating artery (184).

These sites must be screened perfectly on the initial angiogram to allow discharge of the patient without further investigation. Most authors consider that there is not an indication for repeat cerebral angiography if the clinical appearance of the patient, the CT pattern of hemorrhage, and the technical quality of the angiogram (particularly that of the posterior fossa), are all satisfactory for the diagnosis of perimesencephalic hemorrhage. The final dilemma is a counterbalance between the small risk of an angiogram versus the risk of missing a subtle aneurysm or other lesion in this group of patients.

OTHER CAUSES OF ANGIOGRAPHICALLY NEGATIVE SUBARACHNOID HEMORRHAGE

Undetected Aneurysms

Approximately 30–40% of subarachnoid hemorrhage patients with an initial angiogram which is negative for aneurysm do not fall into the category of nonaneurysmal perimesencephalic subarachnoid hemorrhage. The commonest cause for subarachnoid hemorrhage in this group after trauma has been excluded is probably a subtle undetected aneurysm (Figs. 16.20, 16.21, 16.22). Sensitivity of the initial angiogram may have been impaired by technical factors, vasospasm, thrombosis of the aneurysm, or motion artifact by an agitated patient. A prolonged study of the initial angiogram and a review of the site of maximal hemorrhage on the CT will help in the follow-up angiogram. Repeat angiography at an interval of 2 or more weeks has a positive yield between 2 and 22% for identifying a source of hemorrhage (185–188). Having the previous films hanging in the control-room for purposes of collation during the repeat study will increase one's sensitivity to subtle abnormalities on the original or new studies. Some authors advocate use of cross-compression of the contralateral carotid artery to evaluate the anterior communicating artery. Carotid artery compression during vertebral artery injections may increase sensitivity to abnormalities of the posterior communicating artery. These compression techniques carry definite risks to the patient and risks of increased radiation exposure to the operator, with an unclear efficacy. Magnification and oblique views and use of higher injection-rates will accomplish the same end without these risks.

In a study of 40 patients in whom an initial angiogram was negative, Tatter et al. (188) reported a 6% yield from repeat angiography. Nine of their remaining angiogram-negative patients underwent surgical exploration based on a high index of suspicion derived from the CT appearance of hemorrhage localization. Of these explorations, seven patients were found to have either subtle aneurysms of 4 mm in size or microaneurysms which were treated with coagulation and wrapping. These particular authors' algorithm for subarachnoid hemorrhage and negative an-

giography includes repeat angiography at 2 weeks following the first study and, where necessary, again at 1–6 months, with the admonition that a spinal source for subarachnoid hemorrhage should not be forgotten in the course of evaluation (188).

INFUNDIBULUM

An infundibulum is a funnel-shaped origin of a branch vessel that derives its name from the similarity of its contour to that of a Roman wine bottle. Criteria by Taveras and Wood (189) for infundibular widening of the posterior communicating artery are: round or conical in shape, less than 3 mm in diameter, and the posterior communicating artery should arise from its apex.

Infundibular widening of the origin of the posterior communicating artery is seen in approximately 7% of normal in vivo cerebral angiograms (190) or 13% of postmortem angiograms (191).

It is becoming increasingly recognized that infundibula meeting these criteria cannot always be dismissed as trivial findings. Cases of subarachnoid hemorrhage and death from ruptured infundibula have been verified (192, 193), as has aneurysmal growth from previously documented infundibula (194–198). Histologic evidence of medial and elastic defects in the vessel wall associated with infundibular widening has been reported by Hassler and Saltzmann (199). This suggests that infundibula represent sites of potential weakness of the vessel wall and, by implication, may be viewed as preaneurysmal lesions.

When a conically shaped widening of the posterior communicating artery origin exceeds 3 mm in size or otherwise does not fulfill the criteria stated above, it can be impossible to distinguish angiographically a true aneurysm from infundibular widening (200), particularly in the unruptured state. In a patient with subarachnoid hemorrhage and a suspicious distribution of blood on CT, one's degree of suspicion for aneurysm is much greater. In a series of 34 funnel-shaped, unruptured, posterior communicating artery junctional dilatations exceeding 3 mm in size, Endo et al. (200) found that 10 represented true or forming aneurysms during surgical exploration.

There is some debate over whether posterior communicating artery infundibula represent pre-aneurysmal lesions, but definitive treatment for infundibular type lesions over 3 mm in size is considered prudent, particularly in the setting of a patient with an otherwise unexplained subarachnoid hemorrhage.

DURAL ARTERIOVENOUS MALFORMATIONS AS A CAUSE OF SUBARACHNOID HEMORRHAGE

Subarachnoid bleeding mimicking that related to aneurysmal rupture can occur with dural arteriovenous malformations. The mechanism is usually that of venous hypertension due to restriction of venous outflow from the malformation. As sinuses become obstructed venous flow is diverted retrogradely into subarachnoid and cortical

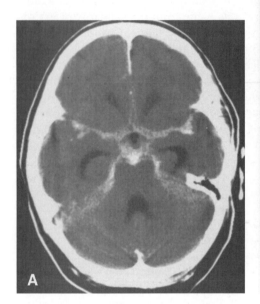

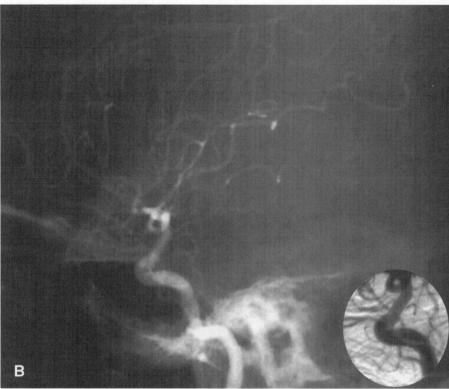

Figure 16.20. Angiographically negative subarachnoid hemorrhage I: importance of obliqued and skewed views. A CT examination in an elderly female with Grade III subarachnoid hemorrhage demonstrates profuse subarachnoid hemorrhage and hydrocephalus. The initial angiogram **(B)** of the left internal carotid artery was performed using cut-film technique and was interpreted as negative (insert of subtracted image of left internal carotid artery siphon). A follow-up angiogram using digital equipment showed an identical appearance on the first lateral view. A skewed view **(C)** of the left siphon demonstrated the aneurysm **(arrow).** On the magnified insert a waist-like constriction of the aneurysm probably represents where this subarachnoid aneurysm enters the dura of the cavernous sinus. This aneurysm could not be seen on any PA or shallow oblique views because of its position directly behind the genu. Looking for a widening of the diameter of the genu (apparent on the initial lateral angiogram) can help to direct one to the presence of such an occult aneurysm. Because this aneurysm extends from the sub-arachnoid space to the extradural cavernous sinus, the term ``transitional'' aneurysm might be invoked. However, transitional aneurysms usually start on the cavernous segment and expand in the other direction.

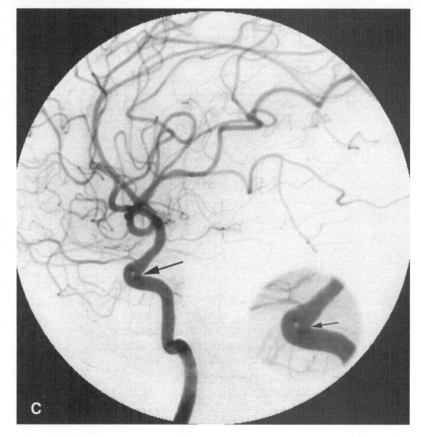

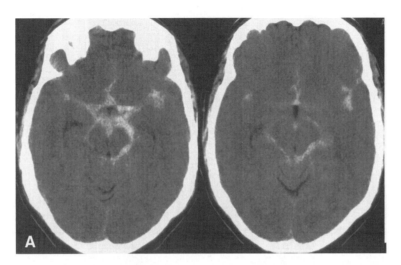

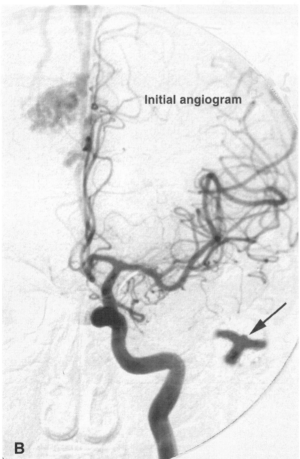

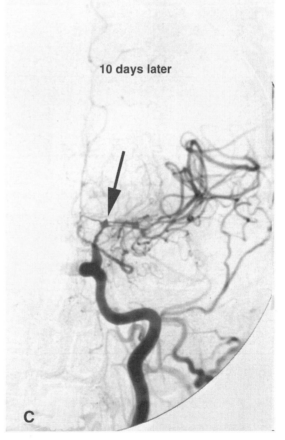

Figure 16.21. Angiographically negative subarachnoid hemorrhage II: importance of follow-up angiography and examining the images very closely. A CT examination **(A)** in a young adult with Grade III subarachnoid hemorrhage and a right hemispheric AVM demonstrates extensive subarachnoid hemorrhage, more profuse on the left side of the suprasellar cistern. The initial angiogram **(B)** was interpreted as negative for the presence of aneurysm. A follow-up angiogram **(C)** demonstrated significant intracranial vasospasm. Serendipitously the vasospasm allowed recognition of a 2-mm aneurysm of the internal carotid artery bifurcation **(arrow)**, which was confirmed at surgery. In retrospect, a very subtle dimple of the internal carotid artery bifurcation was evident on the initial angiogram **(insert on B).**

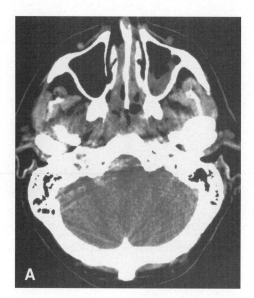

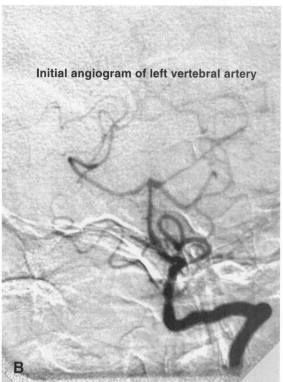

Initial angiogram of left vertebral artery

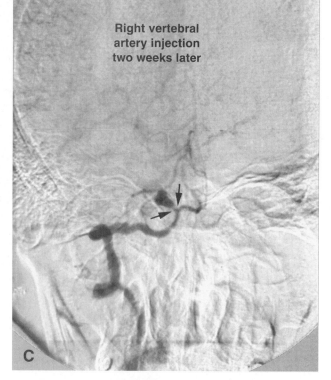

Right vertebral
artery injection
two weeks later

Figure 16.22. Angiographically negative subarachnoid hemorrhage III: importance of the distal right vertebral artery and right posterior inferior cerebellar artery. An elderly male was admitted to hospital with Grade II subarachnoid hemorrhage and a preponderance of blood on the right side of the posterior fossa **(A)**. This CT appearance should prompt particular suspicion about the right posterior inferior cerebellar artery. Its omission from angiographic interrogation constitutes a major, and in this case fatal, oversight. Moreover, in the setting of a posterior fossa hemorrhage in which the right posterior inferior cerebellar artery origin has been seen by reflux, the possibility of a subara- chnoid dissection of the right vertebral artery should not be forgotten, when no other explanation for subarachnoid hemorrhage has been found. The initial angiogram **(B)** of the posterior fossa was performed via the left vertebral artery only, an injection which did not opacify the distal right vertebral artery. The patient made a complete clinical recovery. A follow-up angiogram **(C),** 2 weeks later included an injec- tion of the right vertebral artery. This demonstrated an aneurysm of the origin of the right posterior inferior cerebellar artery **(arrows).** The patient was immediately scheduled for treatment, but the aneurysm ruptured fatally the next day.

veins. Being thin-walled, veins under pressure are at risk of rupture. Therefore, when subarachnoid hemorrhage occurs in this disease there is usually other evidence of subarachnoid venous hypertension. Distended vessels may be evident on the MRI or contrast enhanced CT examination. Venous hypertension may cause signal change on the T2-weighted images, or gadolinium enhancement in the parenchyma of the supratentorial or infratentorial structures. Hemorrhage may also be seen within brain parenchyma. Some of these appearances may mimic the findings of a brain arteriovenous malformation. To exclude the rare possibility of a dural arteriovenous malformation causing isolated subarachnoid hemorrhage, a repeat cerebral angiogram for subarachnoid hemorrhage should include a study of the external carotid artery vessels. The clinical history of the patient may also reveal features that point in this direction, and these include bruit, history of head trauma or skull fractures, or a history of headaches deriving from a pregnancy or an episode of illness characterized by fever and dehydration when a dural sinus may have become thrombosed.

SPINAL TUMORS AND SPINAL VASCULAR MALFORMATIONS AS A CAUSE OF SUBARACHNOID HEMORRHAGE

Subarachnoid hemorrhage is the presenting feature of approximately 10% of patients with a spinal vascular malformation, particularly when the patient is younger than age 20 (201–203). Tumors of the spine such as meningioma or ependymoma may present similarly. These are rare causes for an otherwise indistinguishable presentation with intracranial subarachnoid hemorrhage. However, they must be considered when other avenues of investigation have been exhausted, particularly in a patient with repeated hemorrhages. There may be clinical evidence of a cervical lesion, back or shoulder pain, and spinal symptoms. Sagittal MRI images of the head may reveal clues to the spinal etiology of the bleeding. In patients with repeated hemorrhages siderosis of the upper cervical spine and posterior fossa may be seen on the T2 weighted images (Fig. 16.23). Dural arteriovenous malformations of the cervical region may present with subarachnoid hemorrhage, although this is extremely rare.

COCAINE ABUSE AND SUBARACHNOID HEMORRHAGE

Other causes of subarachnoid hemorrhage with the exception of trauma are rare. Subarachnoid hemorrhage is a recognized complication of cocaine abuse (204, 205) and may recur even in patients who do not demonstrate an aneurysm or arteriovenous malformation at angiography. Neurologic complications including subarachnoid hemorrhage, intracranial vasospasm and vasculitis (Fig. 16.24) have been reported with a variety of drugs of abuse, particularly amphetamine derivatives (206, 207), phenylpropanolamine (208), ephedrine (209), pseudoephedrine (210), and heroin (211).

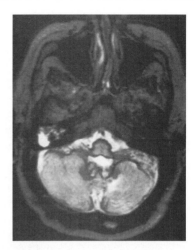

Figure 16.23. *Siderosis of the sub-arachnoid tissues due to a spinal ependymoma.* An axial T2 weighted MRI image in a patient with recurrent angiogram-negative subarachnoid hemorrhage demonstrates outlining of the structures of the posterior fossa by susceptibility artifact due to deposition of hemosiderin. An ependymoma of the spine was subsequently identified as the cause of bleeding.

Cocaine has been demonstrated to have a powerful vasoconstrictive effect on the basilar artery and middle cerebral artery at concentrations seen in drug users (212). Cocaine use has been associated with cerebral hemorrhage (213), cerebral vasculitis (214, 215), and cerebral infarctions (216). A non-necrotizing, hypersensitivity-type vasculitis associated with use of cocaine derivatives affects small peripheral cortical vessels and may not demonstrate the beaded angiographic appearance classically associated with intracranial vasculitis (214). Angiography may demonstrate large vessel occlusions, with or without beading, probably due to vasospasm with secondary thrombus formation (215, 217, 218). However, the angiographic examination is normal in approximately 70% of patients with neurological problems related to cocaine. Angiographic evidence of vasculitis is not common (213). Corticosteroid therapy has been used empirically in some patients with documented vasculitis related to cocaine use.

OTHER CAUSES OF SUBARACHNOID HEMORRHAGE

Rarely subarachnoid hemorrhage may be a complication of cerebrovascular occlusive vasculitis or sickle cell disease in children where fragile leptomeningeal vessels rupture (219). Children with sickle-cell disease are also more prone than the general population to multiple aneurysm formation. Aneurysmal rupture may be the most likely cause of subarachnoid hemorrhage in a child with this disease (220). The possibility of physical abuse also needs to be considered in children who present with subarachnoid hemorrhage. Coagulopathies presenting in isolation with subarachnoid hemorrhage are rare. Pituitary apoplexy presents frequently with the typical clinical features of subarachnoid hemorrhage but also has a high likelihood of impairment of visual acuity and oculoparetic cranial nerve palsies (221). Other diseases that can present

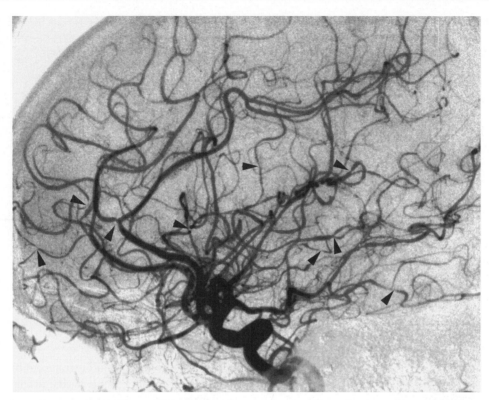

Figure 16.24. Angiographic appearance of intracranial vasculitis. A common carotid arteriogram on a middle-aged female whose neurologic status was improving at the time of this study after empirical treatment with corticosteroids for suspected vasculitis. Multiple focal narrowings and irregularities (**arrowheads**) of the intracranial circulation are seen.

with subarachnoid hemorrhage are discussed in Chapter 19.

REFERENCES

1. Sachdev VP, Drapkin AJ, Hollin SA, et al. Subarachnoid hemorrhage following intranasal procedures. Surg Neurol 1977; 8:122–125.
2. Wakai S, Yoshimasu N, Eguchi T, et al. Traumatic intracavernous aneurysms of the internal carotid artery following surgery for chronic sinusitis. Surg Neurol 1980;13:391–394.
3. Yamaura A, Makino H, Hachisu H, et al. Secondary aneurysm due to arterial injury during surgical procedures. Surg Neurol 1978;10:327–333.
4. Hudgins PA, Browning DG, Gallups J, et al. Endoscopic paranasal sinus surgery: Radiographic evaluations of severe complications. Am J Neuroradiol 1992;13:1161–1167.
5. Ahuja A, Guterman LR, Hopkins LN. Carotid cavernous fistula and false aneurysm of the cavernous carotid artery: complications of transsphenoidal surgery. Neurosurgery 1992;31: 774–779.
6. Cabezudo JM, Carillo R, Vaquero J, et al. Intracavernous aneurysm of the carotid artery following transsphenoidal surgery J Neurosurg 1981;54:118–121.
7. Sahrakar K, Boggan JE, Salamat MS. Traumatic aneurysm: a complication of stereotactic brain biopsy: case report. Neurosurgery 1995;36(4):842–846.
8. Connaughton PN, Williams JP. Iatrogenic intracranial aneurysms. Acta Radiol Suppl 1976;347:59–62.
9. Aarabi B. Management of traumatic aneurysms caused by high-velocity missile head wounds. Neurosurg Clin North Am 1995;6(4):775–797.
10. Loop JW, White LE, Shaw CM. Traumatic occlusion of the basilar artery within a clivus fracture. Radiology 1964;83: 36–40.
11. Overton MC, Casvin TH. Iatrogenic cerebral cortical aneurysm: Case report. J Neurosurg 1966;24:672–675.
12. Lassman LP, Ramani PS, Sengupta RP. Aneurysms of peripheral cerebral arteries due to surgical trauma. Vasc Surg 1974; 8:1-5.
13. Fox AL. Intracranial aneurysms. New York, Berlin, Heidelburg: Springer, 1983:419–431,1453–1463.
14. Buckingham MJ, Crone KR, Ball WS, et al. Traumatic intracranial aneurysms in childhood: two cases and a review of the literature. Neurosurgery 1988;22:398–408.
15. Parkinson D, West M. Traumatic intracranial aneurysms. J Neurosurg 1980;52:11–20.
16. Quintana F, Diez C, Gutierrez A, et al. Traumatic aneurysm of the basilar artery. Am J Neuroradiol 1996;17:283–285.
17. Amirjamshidi A, Rahmat H, Abbassioun K. Traumatic aneurysms and arterio-venous fistulas of intracranial vessels associated with penetrating head injuries occurring during war: principles and pitfalls in diagnosis and management. J Neurosurg 1996; 84:769–780.
18. Holmes B, Harbaugh RE. Traumatic intracranial aneurysms: a contemporary review. J Trauma 1993;35:855–860.
19. Nakstad P, Nornes H, Hauge HN. Traumatic aneurysms of the pericallosal arteries. Neuroradiology 1986;28:335–338.
20. Ventureyra ECG, Higgins MJ. Traumatic intracranial aneurysms in childhood and adolescence. Case reports and review of the literature. Child Ner Syst 1994;10:361–379.
21. Carey ME, Young HF, Rish BL, et al. Follow up study of 103 American soldiers who sustained a brain-wound in Vietnam. J Neurosurg 1974;41:542–549.

22. Ferry DJ, Kempe LG. False aneurysm secondary to penetration of the brain through orbitofacial wounds. Report of two cases. J Neurosurg 1972;36:503–506.

23. Rahimizadeh A, Abtahi H, Daylami MS, et al. Traumatic cerebral aneurysm caused by shell fragments. Report of four cases and review of the literature. Acta Neurochir (Wien) 1987;84: 93–98.

24. Haddad FS. Nature and management of penetrating head injuries during the Civil War in Lebanon. Can J Surg 1978;21: 233–240.

25. Kieck CF, de Villiers JC. Vascular lesions due to transcranial stab wounds. J Neurosurg 1984;60:42–46.

26. Tsubakowa T, Katani A, Suguwara T, et al. Treatment for traumatic aneurysm of the cerebral artery. Identification between deteriorating type and spontaneously disappearing type. Neurol Surg (Tokyo) 1976;3:663–672.

27. Acosta C, Williams PE, Clark K. Traumatic aneurysms of the cerebral vessels. J Neurosurg 1972;36:531–536.

28. Soria ED, Paroski MW, Schamann ME. Traumatic aneurysms of the cerebral vessels: A case study and review of the literature. Angiology 1988;39:609–615.

29. Davis JM, Zimmerman RA. Injury of the carotid and vertebral arteries. Neuroradiology 1983;25:55–69.

30. Davis KR. Embolization of epistaxis and juvenile nasopharyngeal angiofibromas. Am J Neuroradiol AJNR 1986;7:953–962.

31. Du Trevou MD, van Dellen JR. Penetrating stab wounds to the brain: Timing of angiography in patients presenting with the weapon already removed. Neurosurgery 1992;31:905–912.

32. Cohen MM, Hemalatha CP, D'Addario RT, et al. Embolization from a fusiform middle cerebral artery aneurysm. Stroke 1980; 11:158–161.

33. Little JR, St Louis P, Weinstein M, et al. Giant fusiform aneurysm of the cerebral arteries. Stroke 1981;12:183–188.

34. Bederson JB, Zabramski JM, Spetzler RF. Treatment of fusiform intracranial aneurysms by circumferential wrapping with clip reinforcement. J Neurosurg 1992;77:478–480.

35. Wakui K, Kobayashi S, Takemae T, et al. Giant thrombosed vertebral artery aneurysm managed with extracranial-intracranial bypass surgery and aneurysmectomy. Case report. J Neurosurg 1992;77:624–627.

36. Anson JA, Lawton MT, Spetzler RF. Characteristics and surgical treatment of dolichoectatic and fusiform aneurysms. J Neurosurg 1996;84:185–193.

37. Boeri R, Passerini A. The megadolichobasilar anomaly. J Neurol Sci 1964;1:475–484.

38. Mizutani T. A fatal, chronically growing basilar artery: a new type of dissecting aneurysm. J Neurosurg 1996;84:962–971.

39. Sinzobahamvya N, Kalangu K, Hamel-Kalinowski W. Arterial aneurysms associated with human immunodeficiency virus (HIV). Acta Chir Belg. 1989;89(4):185–188.

40. Lang C, Jacobi G, Kreuz W, et al. Rapid development of giant aneurysm at the base of the brain in an 8-year-old boy with perinatal HIV infection. Acta Histochem Suppl. 1992;42: 83–90.

41. Marks C, Kuskov S. Pattern of arterial aneurysms in acquired immunodeficiency disease. World J Surg 1995;19(1):127–132.

42. Roach MR, Drake CG. Ruptured cerebral aneurysms caused by micro-organisms. N Engl J Med 1965;273:240–244.

43. Lerner PI, Weinstein L. Infective endocarditis in the antibiotic era. N Engl J Med 1966;274:199–206, 259–266, 323–331.

44. Radhakrishnan VV, Saraswathy A, Rout D, et al. Mycotic aneurysms of the intracranial vessels. Indian J Med Res 1994;100: 228–231.

45. Corr P, Wright M, Handler LC. Endocarditis-related cerebral aneurysms: Radiologic changes with treatment. Am J Neuroradiol 1995;16:745–748.

46. Bohmfalk GL, Story JL, Wissinger JP, et al. Bacterial intracranial aneurysm. J Neurosurg 1978;48:369–382.

47. Cates JE, Christie RV. Subacute bacterial endocarditis. Q J Med 1951;20:93–120.

48. Pankey GA. Acute bacterial endocarditis at the University of Minnesota Hospitals, 1939–1959. Am Heart J 1962;64: 583–591.

49. Jones HR, Siekert RG, Geraci JE. Neurologic manifestations of bacterial endocarditis. Ann Intern Med 1969;71:21–28.

50. Bingham WF. Treatment of mycotic intracranial aneurysms. J Neurosurg 1977;46:428–437.

51. Morawetz RB, Karp RB. Evolution and resolution of intracranial bacterial (mycotic) aneurysms. Neurosurgery 1984;15: 43–49.

52. Khayata MH, Aymard A, Casasco A, et al. Selective endovascular techniques in the treatment of cerebral mycotic aneurysms. Report of three cases. J Neurosurg 1993;78:661–665.

53. Scotti G, Li MH, Righi C, et al. Endovascular treatment of bacterial intracranial aneurysms. Neuroradiology 1996;38: 186–189.

54. Hove B, Andersen BB, Christiansen TM. Intracranial oncotic aneurysms from choriocarcinoma. Case report and review of the literature. Neuroradiology 1990;32:526–528.

55. Pullar M, Blumbergs PC, Phillips GE, et al. Neoplastic cerebral aneurysm from metastatic gestational choriocarcinoma. J Neurosurg 1985;63:644–647.

56. Ho KL. Neoplastic aneurysms and intracranial hemorrhage. Cancer 1982;50:2935–2940.

57. Kochi N, Tani E, Yokota M, et al. Neoplastic cerebral aneurysm from lung cancer. J Neurosurg 1984;60:640–643.

58. Reina A, Seal RB. False cerebral aneurysm associated with metastatic carcinoma of the brain. J Neurosurg 1974;41:380–382.

59. Barker CS. Peripheral cerebral aneurysm associated with glioma. Neuroradiology 1992;34:30–32.

60. Fujiwara T, Mino S, Nagao S, et al. Metastatic choriocarcinoma with neoplastic aneurysms cured by aneurysm resection and chemotherapy. J Neurosurg 1992;76:148–151.

61. Markel ML, Waller BF, Armstrong WF. Cardiac myxoma. A review. Medicine 1987;66:114–125.

62. Desousa AL, Muller J, Campbell RL, et al. Atrial myxoma: a review of the neurological complications, metastases and recurrences. J. Neurol Neurosurg Psychiatry 1978;41: 1119–1124.

63. Stoane L, Allen JH, Collins HA. Radiologic observations of cerebral embolization from left heart myxomas. Radiology 1966;87:262–266.

64. New PFJ, Price DL, Carter B. Cerebral angiography in cardiac myxoma. Correlation of angiographic and histopathological findings. Radiology 1970;96:335–345.

65. Olmstead WW, McGee TP. The pathogenesis of peripheral aneurysms of the central nervous system: a subject review from the AFIP. Radiology 1977;123:661–666.

66. Furuya K, Sasaki, Yoshimoto Y, et al. Histologically verified cerebral aneurysm formation secondary to embolism from cardiac myxoma. Case report. J Neurosurg 1995;83:170–173.

67. Knepper LE, Biller J, Adams HP. Neurologic manifestations of atrial myxoma. A 12 year experience and review. Stroke 1988;19:1435–1440.

68. Marazuela M, García-Merino A, Yebra M, et al. Magnetic resonance imaging and angiography of the brain in embolic left atrial myxoma. Neuroradiology 1989;31:137–139.

69. Bobo H, Evans OB. Intracranial aneurysms in a child with

recurrent atrial myxoma. Pediatric Neurology 1987;3: 320–322.

70. Schievink WI, Mokri B, Piepgras DG, et al. Recurrent spontaneous arterial dissections. Risk in familial versus nonfamilial disease. Stroke 1996;27:662–624.

71. Mokri B, Sundt TM, Houser OW, et al. Spontaneous dissection of the cervical internal carotid artery. Ann Neurol 1979;19: 126–138.

72. Mokri B, Piepgras DG, Houser OW. Traumatic dissections of the extracranial internal carotid artery. J Neurosurg 1988;68: 189–197.

73. Halbach VV, Higashida RT, Dowd CF, et al. Endovascular treatment of vertebral artery dissections and pseudoaneurysms. J Neurosurg 1993;79: 183–191.

74. Morgan MK, Sekhon LHS. Extracranial-intracranial saphenous vein bypass for carotid or vertebral artery dissections: a report of six cases. J Neurosurg 1994;80:237–246.

75. Berger MS. Wilson CB. Intracranial dissecting aneurysms of the posterior circulation. Report of 6 cases and review of the literature. J Neurosurg 1984;36:882–894.

76. Mizutani T. Middle cerebral artery dissecting aneurysm with persistent patent pseudolumen. Case Report. J Neurosurg 1996;84:267–268.

77. Sasaki O, Ogawa H, Koike T, et al. A clinicopathological study of dissecting aneurysms of the intracranial vertebral artery. J Neurosurg 1991;75:874–882.

78. Mizutani T, Aruga T, Kirino T, et al. Recurrent subarachnoid hemorrhage from untreated ruptured vertebrobasilar dissecting aneurysms. Neurosurgery 1995;36:905–913.

79. Scott GE, Neubuerger KT, Denst J. Dissecting aneurysm of intracranial arteries. Neurology 1960;10:22–27.

80. Clower BR, Sullivan DM, Smith RR. Intracranial vessels lack vasa vasorum. J Neurosurg 1984;61:44–48.

81. Piepgras DG, McGrail KM, Tazelaar HD. Intracranial dissection of the distal middle cerebral artery as an uncommon cause of distal cerebral artery aneurysm. J Neurosurg 1994; 80:909–913.

82. Chang V, Rewcastle NB, Harwood-Nash DCF, et al. Bilateral dissecting aneurysms of the internal carotid arteries in an 8-year-old boy. Neurology 1975;25:573–579.

83. Kitani R, Itouji T, Noda Y, et al. Dissecting aneurysms of the anterior circle of Willis. Report of two cases. J Neurosurg 1987; 67:296–300.

84. Pozzati E, Andreoli A, Padovani R, et al. Dissecting aneurysms of the basilar artery. Neurosurgery 1995;36:254–258.

85. Kitanaka C, Sasaki T, Eguchi T, et al. Intracranial vertebral artery dissections: Clinical, radiological features, and surgical considerations. Neurosurgery 1994;34:620–627.

86. Kitanaka C, Tanaka JI, Kuwahara M, et al. Nonsurgical treatment of unruptured intracranial vertebral artery dissection with serial follow-up angiography. J Neurosurg 1994;80: 667–674.

87. Kitanaka C, Sasaki T, Eguchi T, et al. Intracranial vertebral artery dissections: Clinical, radiological features, and surgical considerations. Neurosurgery 1994;34:620–627.

88. Friedman AH, Drake CG. Subarachnoid hemorrhage from intracranial dissecting aneurysm. J Neurosurg 1984;60: 325–334.

89. Yamaura A, Watanabe Y, Saeki N. Dissecting aneurysms of the intracranial vertebral artery. J Neurosurg 1990;72:183–188.

90. Durward QJ. Treatment of vertebral artery dissecting aneurysm by aneurysm trapping and posterior inferior cerebellar artery reimplantation. J Neurosurg 1995;82:137–139.

91. Higashida RT, Halbach VV, Cahan LD, et al. Detachable balloon embolization therapy of posterior circulation intracranial aneurysms. J Neurosurg 1989;71:512–519.

92. Hodes JE, Aymard A, Gobin P, et al. Endovascular occlusion of intracranial vessels for curative treatment of unclippable aneurysms. Report of 16 cases. J Neurosurg 1991;75:628–633.

93. Steinberg GK, Drake CG, Peerless SJ. Deliberate basilar or vertebral artery occlusion in the treatment of intracranial aneurysms. J Neurosurg 1993;79:161–173.

94. Tsukahara T, Wada H, Satake K, et al. Proximal balloon occlusion for dissecting vertebral aneurysms accompanied by subarachnoid hemorrhage. Neurosurgery 1995;36:914–920.

95. Aoki N, Sakai T. Rebleeding from intracranial dissecting aneurysm in the vertebral artery. Stroke 1990;21:1628–1631.

96. Yamaura A. Diagnosis and treatment of vertebral aneurysms. J Neurosurg 1988;69:345–349.

97. Collier J. Cerebral haemorrhage due to causes other than atherosclerosis. British Medical Journal 1931;2:519.

98. Suzuki J, Ohara H. Clinicopathological study of cerebral aneurysms. Origin, rupture, repair and growth. J Neurosurg 1978; 48:505–514.

99. Stebhens WE. Aneurysms and anatomical variations of cerebral arteries. Archives of Pathology 1963;75: 45–64.

100. Schievink WI, Katzmann JA, Piepgras DG, et al. Alpha-1-antitrypsin phenotypes among patients with intracranial aneurysms. J Neurosurg 1996;84:781–784.

101. Rubinstein MK, Cohen MH. Ehlers-Danlos syndrome associated with multiple intracranial aneurysms. Neurology 1964; 14:125–132.

102. Graf CJ. Spontaneous carotid-cavernous fistula. Ehlers-Danlos syndrome and related conditions. Arch Neurol 1965;13: 662–672.

103. Lach B, Nair SG, Russell NA, et al. Spontaneous carotid-cavernous fistula and multiple arterial dissections in type IV Ehlers-Danlos syndrome. J Neurosurg 1987;66:462–467.

104. Mettinger KL, Ericson K. Fibromuscular dysplasia and the brain. Observations on angiographic, clinical, and genetic characteristics. Stroke 1982;13:46–52.

105. Mettinger KL. Fibromuscular dysplasia and the brain. II. Current concept of the disease. Stroke 1982;13:53–58.

106. Schievink WI, Schaid DJ, Rogers HM, et al. On the inheritance of intracranial aneurysms. Stroke 1994;25:2028–2037.

107. Chapman AB, Rubinstein D, Hughes R, et al. Intracranial aneurysms in autosomal dominant polycystic kidney disease. N Engl J Med 1992;327:916–920.

108. Huston J, Torres VE, Sullivan PP, et al. Value of magnetic resonance angiography for the detection of intracranial aneurysms in autosomal dominant polycystic kidney disease. J Am Soc Nephrol 1993;3:1871–1877.

109. Ruggieri PM, Poulas N, Masaryk TJ, et al. Occult intracranial aneurysms in polycystic kidney disease: screening with MR angiography. Radiology 1994;191:33–39.

110. Schievink WI, Schaid DJ, Michels VV, et al. Familial aneurysmal hemorrhage; a community-based study. J Neurosurg 1995; 83:426–429.

111. Ronkainen A, Hernesniemi J, Ryynänen M, et al. A ten percent prevalence of asymptomatic familial intracranial aneurysms; preliminary report of 110 magnetic resonance angiography studies in members of 21 Finnish familial intracranial aneurysm families. Neurosurgery 1994;35:208–213.

112. Schievink WI, Schaid DJ, Rogers HM, et al. On the inheritance of intracranial aneurysms. Stroke 1994;25:2028–2037.

113. Nakagawa T, Hashi K. The incidence and treatment of asymptomatic, unruptured cerebral aneurysms. J Neurosurg 1994; 80:217–223.

114. Obuchowski NA, Modic MT, Magdinec M. Current implica-

tions for the efficacy of noninvasive screening for occult intracranial aneurysms in patients with a family history of aneurysms. J Neurosurg 1995;83:42–49.

115. Lozano AM, Leblanc R. Familial intracranial aneurysms. J Neurosurg 1987;66:522–528.

116. Leblanc R, Melanson D, Tampieri D, et al. Familial cerebral aneurysms: A study of 13 families. Neurosurgery 1995;37:633–639.

117. Leblanc R. Familial cerebral aneurysms. A bias for women. Stroke 1996;27:1050–1054.

118. Dyste GW, Beck DW. De novo aneurysm formation following carotid ligation: Case report and review of the literature. Neurosurgery 1989;24:88–92.

119. Hassler O. Experimental carotid ligation followed by aneurysmal formation and other morphological changes in the circle of Willis. J Neurosurg 1963;20:1-7.

120. Fujiwara S, Fujii S, Fukui M. De novo aneurysm formation and aneurysm growth following therapeutic carotid occlusion for intracranial internal carotid artery aneurysms. Acta Neurochir 1993;120:20–25.

121. Timperman PE, Tomsick TA, Tew JM, et al. Aneurysm formation after carotid occlusion. Am J Neuroradiol 1995;16:329–331.

122. Somach FM, Shenkin HA. Angiographic end results of carotid ligation in the treatment of carotid aneurysms. J Neurosurg 1966;24:966–974.

123. Klemme WM. Hemorrhage from a previously undemonstrated intracranial aneurysm as a late complications of carotid artery ligation. Case report. J Neurosurg 1977;46:654–658.

124. Salar G, Mingrino S. Development of intracranial saccular aneurysms: Report of two cases. Neurosurgery 1981;8:462–465.

125. Odom GL, Tindall GT. Carotid ligation in the treatment of certain intracranial aneurysm. Clin Neurosurg 1968;15:101–116.

126. Nishioka H. Report on the cooperative study of intracranial aneurysms and subarachnoid hemorrhage. Results of the treatment of intracranial aneurysms by occlusion of the carotid artery in the neck. J Neurosurg 1966;25:660–683.

127. Rinne JK, Hernesniemi JA. De novo aneurysms: Special multiple intracranial aneurysms. Neurosurgery 1993;33:981–985.

128. Schievink WI, Wijdicks EFM, Piepgras DG, et al. The poor prognosis of ruptured intracranial aneurysms of the posterior circulation. J Neurosurg 1995;82:791–795.

129. German WJ, Black SPW. Intraaneurysmal hemodynamics-jet action. Circulation Research 1955;3:463–468.

130. Kerber CW, Liepsch D. Flow dynamics for radiologists. I. Basic principles of fluid flow. AJNR Am J Neuroradiol 1994;15:1065–1075.

131. Kerber CW, Liebsch D. Flow dynamics for radiologists. II. Practical considerations in the live human. Am J Neuroradiol 1994;15:1076–1086.

132. Chason JL, Hindman WM. Berry aneurysms of the circle of Willis. Neurology 1958;8:41–44.

133. Wiebers DO, Whisnant JP, Sundt TM, et al. The significance of unruptured intracranial saccular aneurysms. J Neurosurg 1987;66:23–29.

134. Schievink WI, Piepgras DG, Wirth FP. Rupture of previously documented small asymptomatic saccular intracranial aneurysms. J Neurosurg 1992;76:1019–1024.

135. Juvela S, Porras M, Heiskanen O. Natural history of unruptured intracranial aneurysms: a long-term follow-up study. J Neurosurg 1993;79:174–182.

136. Wiebers DO. Unruptured aneurysms. Risk of hemorrhage for single, multiple, familial. Presented at Cerebral Aneurysms

and Vascular Malformations: 1996 and Beyond. Massachusetts General Hospital Brain Aneurysm/AVM Center. May, 1996.

137. Kassell NF, Torner JC. Size of intracranial aneurysms. Neurosurgery 1983;12:291–297.

138. Sacco RL, Wolf PA, Bharucha NE, et al. Subarachnoid and intracerebral hemorrhage. Natural history, prognosis, and precursive factors in the Framingham Study. Neurology 1984;34:847–854.

139. Bell BA, Symon L. Smoking and subarachnoid hemorrhage. British Medical Journal 1979;1:577–578.

140. Petitti DB, Use of oral contraceptives, cigarettes, and risk of subarachnoid hemorrhage, Lancet 1978;2:234–236.

141. Fogelholm R. Subarachnoid hemorrhage in Middle-Finland: incidence, early prognosis, and indications for neurosurgical treatment. Stroke 1981;12:296–301.

142. King JT, Glick HA, Mason TJ, et al. Elective Surgery for asymptomatic, unruptured, intracranial aneurysms: a cost-effectiveness analysis. J Neurosurg 1995;83:403–412.

143. Ljunggren B, Saveland H, Brandt L, et al. Early operation and overall outcome in aneurysmal subarachnoid hemorrhage. J Neurosurg 1985;62:547–551.

144. Whisnant JP, Sacco SE, O'Fallon M, et al. Referral bias in aneurysmal subarachnoid hemorrhage. J Neurosurg 1993;78:726–732.

145. Kassell NF, Torner JC, Haley EC, et al. The international cooperative study on the timing of aneurysm surgery. Part 1 Overall management results. J Neurosurg 1990;73:18–36.

146. Longstreth WT, Nelson LM, Keopsell TD, et al. Clinical course of spontaneous subarachnoid hemorrhage: A population-based study in King County, Washington. Neurology 1993;43:712–718.

147. Le Roux PD, Elliot JP, Downey L, et al. Improved outcome after rupture of anterior circulation aneurysms: a retrospective 10-year review of 224 good-grade patients. J Neurosurg 1995;83:394–402.

148. Hunt WE, Hess RM. Surgical Risk as related to time of intervention in the repair of intracranial aneurysms. J Neurosurg 1968;28:14–20.

149. Vermeulen M, van Gijn J, Hijdra A, et al. Causes of acute deteriorations in patients with a ruptured intracranial aneurysm. A prospective study with serial CT scanning. J Neurosurg 1984;60: 935–939.

150. Leblanc R. The minor leak preceding subarachnoid hemorrhage. J Neurosurg 1987;66:35–39.

151. Kassell NF, Torner JC, Jane JA, et al. The international cooperative study on the timing of aneurysm surgery. Part 2: Surgical Results. J Neurosurg 1990;73:37–47.

152. Suzuki J, Onuma T, Yoshimoto T. Results of early operations on cerebral aneurysm. Surg Neurol 1979;11:407–412.

153. Fisher CM, Kistler JP, Davis JM. Relation of cerebral vasospasm to subarachnoid hemorrhage visualized by computerized tomographic scanning. Neurosurgery 1980;6:1-9.

154. Kistler JP, Crowell RM, Davis KR, et al. The relation of cerebral vasospasm to the extent and location of subarachnoid blood visualized by CT scan: A prospective study. Neurology 1983;33:424–436.

155. Graff-Radford NR, Torner J, Adams JP, et al. Factors associated with hydrocephalus after subarachnoid hemorrhage. Arch Neurol 1989;46:744–752.

156. Hasan D, Wijdicks EF, Vermeulen M. Hyponatremia is associated with cerebral ischemia in patients with aneurysmal subarachnoid hemorrhage. Ann Neurol 1990;27:106–108.

157. Yuki K, Kodama Y, Onda J, et al. Coronary vasospasm following subarachnoid hemorrhage as a cause of stunned myocardium. Case report. J Neurosurg 1991;75:308–311.

158. Elrifai AM, Bailes JE, Shih SR, et al. Characterization of the cardiac effects of acute subarachnoid hemorrhage in dogs. Stroke 1996;27:737–742.

159. Segal HD, McLaurin RL. Giant serpentine aneurysm. Report of two cases. J Neurosurg 1977;46:115–120.

160. Mawad ME, Klucznik RP. Giant serpentine aneurysms: Radiographic features and endovascular treatment. Am J Neuroradiol 1995;16:1053–1060.

161. Aletich VA, Debrun GM, Monsein LH, et al. Giant serpentine aneurysms. A review and presentation of five cases. Am J Neuroradiol 1995;16:1061–1072.

162. Drake CG. Giant intracranial aneurysms: experience with surgical treatment in 176 patients. Clin Neurosurg 1979;26: 12–95.

163. Ojemann RG, Ogilvy CS, Crowell RM, et al, eds. Surgical Management of Neurovascular Disease. 3rd ed. Baltimore, Williams & Wilkins, 1995.

164. Morley TP, Barr HW. Giant intracranial aneurysms: diagnosis, course, and management. Clin Neurosurg 1969;16:73–94.

165. Ito M, Yoshihara M, Ishii M, et al. Cerebral aneurysms in children. Brain Dev 1992;14:263–268.

166. Rinne J, Hernesniemi J, Puranen M, et al. Multiple intracranial aneurysms in a defined population: Prospective angiographic and clinical study. Neurosurgery 1994;35:803–808.

167. Nehls DG, Flom RA, Carter LP, et al. Multiple intracranial aneurysms: determining the site of rupture. J Neurosurg 1985; 63:342–348.

168. Marttilla I, Heiskanen O. Value of neurological and angiographic signs as indicators of the ruptured aneurysm in patients with multiple intracranial aneurysms. Acta Neurochir 1970;23:95–102.

169. Wood EH. Angiographic identification of the ruptured lesion in patients with multiple cerebral aneurysms. J Neurosurg 1964;21:182–198.

170. Weisberg LA. Computed tomography in aneurysmal subarachnoid hemorrhage. Neurology 1979;29:802–808.

171. West HH, Mani RL, Eisenberg RL, et al. Normal cerebral angiography in patients with spontaneous subarachnoid hemorrhage. Neurology 1977;27:592–594.

172. Shepard RH. Prognosis of spontaneous subarachnoid hemorrhage of unknown cause. A personal series 1958–1980. Lancet 1984; i:777–778.

173. Congia S, Carta S, Coraddu M. Subarachnoid hemorrhage of unknown origin. A 44 cases study. Acta Neurol 1994;16: 177–183.

174. Duong H, Melancon D, Tampieri D, et al. The negative angiogram in subarachnoid hemorrhage. Neuroradiology 1996;38: 15–19.

175. van Gijn J, van Dongen KJ, Vermeulen M, et al. Perimesencephalic hemorrhage: a non-aneurysmal and benign form of subarachnoid hemorrhage. Neurology 1985;35:993–997.

176. Goergen SK, Barrie D, Sacharias N, et al. Perimesencephalic subarachnoid hemorrhage: negative angiography and favourable prognosis. Austral Radiol 1993;37:320–323.

177. Canhao P, Ferro JM, Pinto AN, et al. Perimesencephalic and nonperimesencephalic subarachnoid hemorrhages with negative angiograms. Acta Neurochir (Wien) 1995;132:14–19.

178. Rinkel GJE, Wijdicks EFM, Vermeulen M, et al. Nonaneurysmal perimesencephalic subarachnoid hemorrhage: CT and MR patterns that differ from aneurysmal rupture. Am J Neuroradiol 1991;12:829–834.

179. Rinkel GJE, Wijdicks EFM, Vermeulen M, et al. Acute hydrocephalus in non-aneurysmal perimesencephalic hemorrhage: evidence of cerebro-spinal fluid block at the tentorial hiatus. Neurology 1992;42:1805–1807.

180. Alexander MSM, Dias PS, Yttley D. Spontaneous subarachnoid hemorrhage and negative cerebral panangiography. Review of 140 cases. J Neurosurg 1985;64:537–542.

181. Juul R, Fredriksen TA, Rinkjob R. Prognosis in subarachnoid hemorrhage of unknown etiology. J Neurosurg 1986;64: 359–362.

182. Pinto AN, Ferro JM, Canhao P, et al. How often is a perimesencephalic subarachnoid hemorrhage CT pattern caused by ruptured aneurysms? Acta Neurochir (Wien) 1993;124:79–81.

183. Van Calenbergh F, Plets C, Goffin J, et al. Nonaneurysmal subarachnoid hemorrhage: Prevalence of perimesencephalic hemorrhage in a consecutive series. Surg Neurol 1993;39: 320–323.

184. Schievink WI, Wijdicks EFM, Piepgras DG, et al. Perimesencephalic subarachnoid hemorrhage. Additional perspectives from four cases. Stroke 1994;25:1507–1511.

185. Forster DMC, Steiner L, Hananson S, et al. The value of repeat pan-angiography in cases of unexplained subarachnoid hemorrhage. J Neurosurg 1978;48:712–716.

186. Nishioka H, Torner JC, Graf CJ, et al. Cooperative study of intracranial aneurysms and subarachnoid hemorrhage: A long-term prognostic study-III. Subarachnoid hemorrhage of undetermined etiology. Arch Neurol 1984;41:1147–1151.

187. Suzuki S, Kayama T, Sakurai Y, et al. Subarachnoid hemorrhage of unknown cause. Neurosurgery 1987;21:310–313.

188. Tatter SB, Crowell RM, Ogilvy CS. Aneurysmal and microaneurysmal "angiogram-negative" subarachnoid hemorrhage. Neurosurgery 1995;37:48–55.

189. Taveras JM, Wood EH. Diagnostic Neuroradiology. Baltimore, Williams and Wilkins, 1964.

190. Saltzmann GF. Infundibular widening of the posterior communicating artery studied by carotid angiography. Acta Radiol 1959;51:415–421.

191. Wollschlaeger G, Wollschlaeger PB: The circle of Willis, in Newton TH, Potts DG, eds: Radiology of the Skull and Brain. St. Louis, CV Mosby, 1974, vol 2, book 2:1171–1201.

192. Koike G, Seguchi K, Koshima K, et al. Subarachnoid hemorrhage due to rupture of infundibular dilation of a circumflex branch of the posterior cerebral artery; Case report. Neurosurgery 1994;34:1075–1077.

193. Ohyama T, Ohara S, Momma F. Fatal subarachnoid hemorrhage due to ruptured infundibular widening of the posterior communicating artery-case report. Neurol Med Chir 1994:34: 172–175.

194. Itakura T, Ozaki F, Nakai E, et al. Bilateral aneurysm formation developing from junctional dilatation (infundibulum) of the posterior communicating arteries. J Neurosurg 1983;58: 117–119.

195. Stunz JT, Ojemann GA, Alvord EC. Radiographic and histologic demonstration of an aneurysm developing on the infundibulum of the posterior communicating artery. Case report. J Neurosurg 1970;33:591–595.

196. Waga S, Morikawa A. Aneurysm developing on the infundibular widening of the posterior communicating artery. Surg Neurol 1979:11:125–127.

197. Yoshimoto T, Suzuki J. Surgical treatment of an aneurysm on the funnel-shaped bulge of the posterior communicating artery. Case report. J Neurosurg 1974;41:377–379.

198. Young B, Meacham WF, Allen JH. Documented enlargement and rupture of a small arterial sacculation. Case report. J Neurosurg 1971;34:814–817.

199. Hassler O, Saltzmann GF. Angiographic and histological changes in infundibular widening of the posterior communicating artery. Acta Radiol 1964;1:321–327.

200. Endo S, Furuichi S, Takaba M, et al. Clinical study of enlarged

infundibular dilation of the origin of the posterior communicating artery. J Neurosurg 1995;83:421–425.

201. Caroscio JT, Brannan T, Budabin M, et al. Subarachnoid hemorrhage secondary to spinal arteriovenous malformation and aneurysm: report of a case and a review of the literature. Arch Neurol 1980;37:101–103.

202. Kandel EI. Complete excision of arteriovenous malformations of the cervical spinal cord. Surg Neurol 1980;13:135–139.

203. Rinkel GJE, van Gijn J, Wijdicks EFM. Subarachnoid hemorrhage without detectable aneurysm. A review of the causes. Stroke 1993;24:1403–1409.

204. Wojack JC, Flamm ES. Intracranial hemorrhage and cocaine use. Stroke 1987;18:712–715.

205. Mangiardi JR, Daras M, Geller ME, et al. Cocaine related intracranial hemorrhage; report of nine cases and review. Acta Neurol Scand 1988;77:177–180.

206. Rumbaugh CL, Bergeron RT, Fang HCH, et al. Cerebral angiographic changes in the drug abuse patient. Radiology 1971;101:335–344.

207. Matick H, Anderson D, Brumlik J. Cerebral vasculitis associated with oral amphetamine overdose. Arch Neurol 1983;40:253–254.

208. Fallis RJ, Fisher M. Cerebral vasculitis and hemorrhage associated with phenylpropanolamine. Neurology 1985;35:405–407.

209. Wooten MR, Khangure MS, Murphy MJ. Intracerebral hemorrhage and vasculitis related to ephedrine abuse. Ann Neurol 1983;13:337–340.

210. Loizou LA, Hamilton JG, Tsementzis SA. Intracranial hemorrhage in association with pseudoephedrine overdosage. J Neurol Neurosurg Psychiatry 1982;45:471–472.

211. King J, Richards M, Tress B. Cerebral arteritis associated with heroin abuse. Med J Aust 1978;2:444–445.

212. He GQ, Zhang A, Altura BT, et al. Cocaine-induced cerebrovasospasm and its possible mechanism of action. J Pharmacol Exp Ther 1994;268:1532–1539.

213. Levine SR, Brust JC, Futrell N, et al. Cerebrovascular complications of the "crack" form of alkaloidal cocaine. N Engl J Med 1990;323:699–704.

214. Morrow PPL, McQuillen JB. Cerebral Vasculitis associated with cocaine abuse. J Forensic Sci 1993;38:732–738.

215. Krendel DA, Ditter SM, Frankel MR, et al. Biopsy proven cerebral vasculitis associated with cocaine abuse. Neurology 1990;40:1092–1094.

216. Klonoff DC, Andrews BT, Obana WG. Stroke associated with cocaine use. Arch Neuro 1989;46:989–993.

217. Kaye BR, Fainstat M. Cerebral vasculitis associated with cocaine abuse. JAMA 1987;258:2104–2106.

218. Konzen JP, Levine SR, Garcia JH. Vasospasm and thrombus formation as possible mechanisms of stroke related to alkaloidal cocaine. Stroke 1995;26:1114–1118.

219. Overby MC, Rothman AS. Multiple intracranial aneurysms in sickle cell anemia. J Neurosurg 1985;62:430–434.

220. Anson JA, Koshy M, Ferguson L, et al. Subarachnoid hemorrhage in sickle-cell disease. J Neurosurg 1991;75:552–558.

221. McFadzean RM, Doyle D, Rampling R, et al. Pituitary apoplexy and its effect on vision. Neurosurgery 1991;29:669–675.

CHAPTER 17

Vascular Malformations of the Brain and Spine

Vascular malformations of the intracranial blood vessels are categorized into four types:

    Capillary teleangiectasias

    Cavernous malformations

    Arteriovenous malformations

    Anomalies of venous drainage

Capillary teleangiectasias and cavernous malformations cannot usually be visualized by angiography and are collectively termed "angiographically occult vascular malformations."

TELEANGIECTASIAS (CAPILLARY ANGIOMAS)

These are common, incidental findings at autopsy, found particularly in the pons. They consist of ill-defined areas of thin-walled capillaries without smooth muscle or elastic fibers. Normal brain tissue may be found within the interstices of these areas. When saccular dilatations and surrounding gliosis with abundant mineralization are present, pathologic differentiation from cavernous malformations can be difficult (1). However, they are usually not associated with evidence of surrounding gliosis or pigment deposition. Their exact borders can be difficult to discern, even microscopically (2). Occasional reports of symptomatic capillary teleangiectasias have been published (3, 4), but most studies represent these lesions as incidental curiosities.

CAVERNOUS MALFORMATIONS OF THE BRAIN

Cavernous malformations of the brain are described as hamartomatous lesions that are characterized by the presence of sinusoidal, thin-walled vessels. They have a more circumscribed or defined border than that seen in capillary teleangiectasias and are unlikely to have intervening normal brain tissue (1). The recognition of *de novo* appearance of cavernous malformations in the brain and the dynamic, changing quality of the disease, particularly in familial forms, has brought an understanding that these lesions are not classified easily as hamartomatous or static (5). The gross appearance has been likened to a cluster of mulberries.

They have a prevalence of under 1% in the general population and account for approximately 5–16% of vascular malformations of the nervous system (1, 6, 7). They can be found anywhere in the brain (Figs. 17.1, 17.2), and may also occur in the spinal cord, dura, optic nerve, optic chiasm, and pineal gland. Histologically, they demonstrate a simple endothelial lining and a thin fibrous adventitia, which is devoid of elastin, smooth muscle, or other elements characteristic of mature vascular walls. Although the absence of intervening normal brain tissue is one of the hallmarks of a cavernous malformation, occasionally satellite lesions may give a more complex appearance to their apparent configuration. Foci of maturing thrombosis, hyalinization, calcification, cysts, and cholesterol granules are characteristic, with an absence of large afferent or efferent vessels and of arteriovenous shunting. Surrounding gliosis with ferritin and hemosiderin deposition from repeated hemorrhages or calcification from repeated episodes of thrombosis give the appearance of encapsulation and contribute to the typical MRI ring-appearance.

A vascular lesion may occasionally demonstrate mixed characteristics with angiographic and histologic features of more than one type of abnormality (Figs. 17.1, 17.3). Most often, one of the components will have characteristics of a cavernous malformation associated either with a venous anomaly or with an arteriovenous malformation. In these instances adjacent enlarged vessels will be identified. The possibility of an associated venous anomaly is of particular concern when surgery is planned as it is important not to disturb the pattern of venous flow in the associated anomaly (8, 9). Cavernous malformations associated with a venous malformation can have a more aggressive clinical course (10). Smaller cavernous malformations may resemble petechiae; others can be much larger measuring some centimeters in diameter.

Cavernous malformations are multiple in approximately 33% of sporadic cases and in up to 73% of familial cases (5). Familial cases may also demonstrate an increase in the number of detectable lesions when followed over time (5). A gene associated with familial cavernous malformations has been identified (11). *De novo* genesis of cavernous malformations has been seen in association with capillary teleangiectasis from which they may evolve (12), with venous anomalies (9), at sites of stereotactic biopsy (13), and in patients who have undergone radiation therapy (14).

The natural history of cavernous malformations before they become symptomatic is difficult to evaluate. MR imaging is capable of demonstrating a larger number of asymptomatic cavernous malformations than was previously ap-

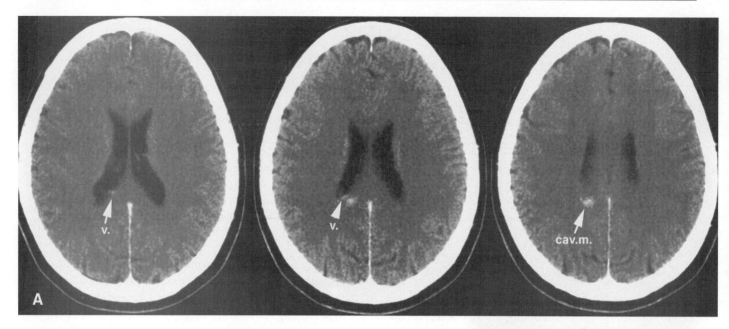

Figure 17.1. *Cavernous malformation associated with anomalous draining vein.* **(A)** Contiguous enhanced CT images in a young female. A cavernous malformation (cav.m.) in the right centrum semiovale drains inferiorly via an anomalous vein (v.), which is directed along the medial wall of the right atrium. **(B)** An axial MRI T2 weighted image of the same patient shows a typical "popcorn" appearance with a surrounding ring of susceptibility. (Same patient as Fig. 14.10)

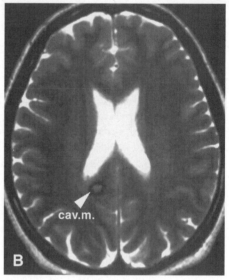

parent. Interpretation of the significance of a cavernous malformation in a patient presenting with headache depends on origins of the reference data. Studies from countries in which patients are stringently screened before being referred for MR imaging will likely deal with patients who are more symptomatic and who have more severe lesions than patients screened in countries where MRI is performed more indulgently. Therefore, cavernous malformations seen on MRI in countries with stringent patient screening are more likely to be significant lesions. This bias may generate the belief that all such lesions seen on MRI are significant.

The natural history of symptomatic and asymptomatic cavernous malformations has been reviewed by Aiba et al. (15) and Kondziolka et al. (16). Cavernous malformations that become symptomatic present with hemorrhage, seizure, or other focal neurologic deficit. Seizures may be simple, complex partial, or generalized, and when found

in the temporal lobes may be medically difficult to manage. Considering their size and location, cavernous malformations are considerably more epileptogenic than are arteriovenous malformations, possibly a reflection of the reactive gliosis and iron deposition, which occur in the periphery of cavernous malformations.

In addition to seizures, bleeding is another common complication of cavernous malformations. A distinction is drawn between the more common, slow, repeated microhemorrhages associated with cavernous malformations and overt or major hemorrhage, which is reported in 8–37% of symptomatic lesions. Significant hemorrhage from a cavernous malformation can be identified by CT or MRI with blood outside the confines of the hemosiderin ring, in the subarachnoid space, or with clinical evidence of apoplectic hemorrhage (17). Hemorrhage may rarely be fulminant and life-threatening, but is usually milder than that associated with arteriovenous malformations.

Hemorrhage from a cavernous malformation is usually associated with onset of severe headache and clinical signs and has a stepwise pattern of worsening deficits according to the location of hemorrhage. Lesions in the brainstem are most likely to present with severe cranial nerve or long tract deficits as they are particularly likely to affect multiple pathways. Intraventricular cavernous malformations can cause obstructive hydrocephalus and hypothalamic symptoms (18, 19). Cerebellar lesions present with nausea, vomiting, nystagmus, ataxia, and diplopia. Exacerbations and prompt remissions can mimic the clinical course of demyelinating diseases (20).

The clinical behavior of particular cavernous malformations changes with time in response to the effects of cumulative intralesional hemorrhage, thrombosis, and mineralization. Age is a significant factor in the natural history of

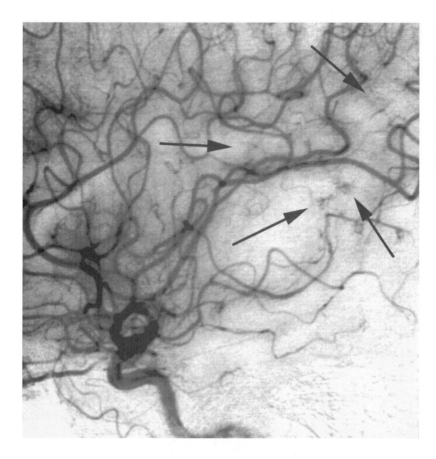

Figure 17.2. *Unusual angiographic evidence of a cavernous malformation.* The majority of cavernous malformations are angiographically occult. In this adult female with a large cavernous malformation of the left hemisphere, there is displacement of the adjacent branches of the left middle cerebral artery. Subtle puddling of contrast within the cavernous malformation is seen **(arrows).** This is seen in only a minority of such lesions. The angiogram was performed to exclude an accompanying arteriovenous malformation following a symptomatic hemorrhage.

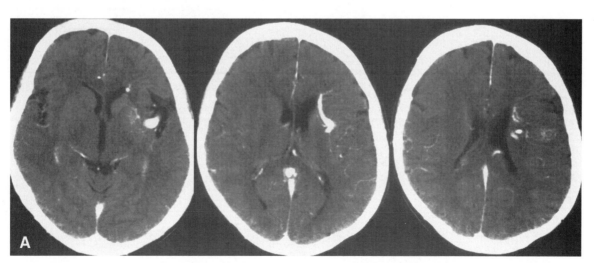

Figure 17.3. *Mixed vascular lesion.* **(A)** A contrast-enhanced CT demonstrates a typical appearance of a venous anomaly of the left frontal lobe draining centrifugally to a sylvian vein. The patient presented with a large subarachnoid hemorrhage in the left sylvian fissure some weeks prior to this CT.

Figure 17.3. *(continued)* **(B)** The venous phase of a left internal carotid artery injection, lateral view, confirms the finding. An extensive anomaly of venous drainage in the left hemisphere drains to an insular vein (ins.v.) and the middle cerebral vein (m.c.v.). The anterior components of the anomaly drain to the cavernous sinus via the ipsilateral sphenoparietal sinus (s.p.s.). The cavernous sinuses drain posteriorly via the inferior petrosal sinuses (ips). The sphenoparietal sinus also drains to the sigmoid sinus via an alternative channel (double arrow) which probably represents a variant dural sinus along the floor of the middle cranial fossa. The posterior aspect of the anomaly drains via an atrial vein (a.v.) to the internal cerebral vein (icv). **(C)** An oblique magnification view of the Sylvian area from the arterial phase of the study (same patient) demonstrates fistulous opacification of a venous structure **(arrows)** directed medially. This represents a micro-avm associated with a larger anomaly of venous drainage. The micro-AVM was almost certainly the source of the patient's sylvian hemorrhage.

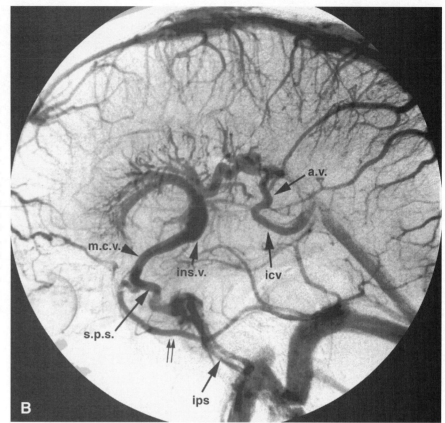

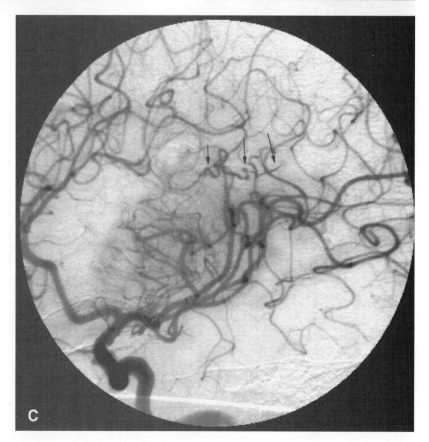

these lesions, with most patients presenting in the 2nd to 4th decades. Children who are symptomatic with such lesions have a greater likelihood of significant hemorrhage and of acute neurologic deficits than young male adults who present with seizures. Female adults become symptomatic predominantly in the 4th to 6th decade. As is the case with symptomatic children, females with a pattern of late presentation tend to demonstrate significant hemorrhage and neurologic deficits (15, 17, 21). The clinical course of cavernous malformations in women is adversely affected during pregnancy (6, 10). Hormonal factors may influence the behavior of cavernous malformations because they are more likely to become hemorrhagic in females. A more aggressive clinical course has been reported also for patients with familial forms of the disease; patients with multiple lesions; patients with previous whole brain or stereotactic radiotherapy; and patients with lesions with an intraventricular location or an associated venous anomaly (10, 19).

The best predictor for bleeding in a particular lesion is a history of bleeding (21). Asymptomatic lesions that have not previously hemorrhaged have an annual hemorrhage rate of less than 1% per year (21, 22). For those lesions with previous bleeding, the annual figure for re-bleeding may be as high as 4.5% (16), with a cumulative risk as high as 20–80% over a period of weeks to years. Patients who present with nonspecific neurologic symptoms have a risk of developing seizures of approximately 1.5% per year (22).

CAVERNOUS MALFORMATIONS OF THE SPINE AND VERTEBRAL HEMANGIOMAS

Cavernous malformations can occur within the intramedullary space of the spinal cord (Fig. 17.4), in the intradural extramedullary space, or within the spinal dura. They are histologically similar to hemangiomas seen in the vertebral column and in the intervening epidural tissues. Their histologic appearance is similar to the cavernous malformations seen in the brain, being composed of thin collagenous walls surrounding sinusoidal vascular spaces without prominent arterial features. Hemosiderin, prominently seen in brain and spinal intramedullary lesions, is less evident in hemangiomas of the dura or vertebral bodies (23, 24). Approximately 3% of cavernous malformations of the vertebral column and spine occur in the intramedullary space; otherwise, the overwhelming majority affect the vertebral bodies. Lesions can occur in an intradural extramedullary location, but these are rare (25, 26).

Harrison et al. (24) have emphasized that vertebral hemangiomas and cavernous malformations of the spine do not necessarily segregate themselves according to tissue-planes; lesions can transgress the dural boundaries in both directions. They are most commonly confined to the vertebral bodies, being seen in 12% of spines at autopsy (23, 27). The great majority of vertebral lesions are asymptomatic incidental findings on MRI or CT. Asymptomatic hemangiomas may be seen at multiple levels of the vertebral column in 30% of cases, extending over 2–5 non-contiguous levels (23). Symptomatic hemangiomas of the

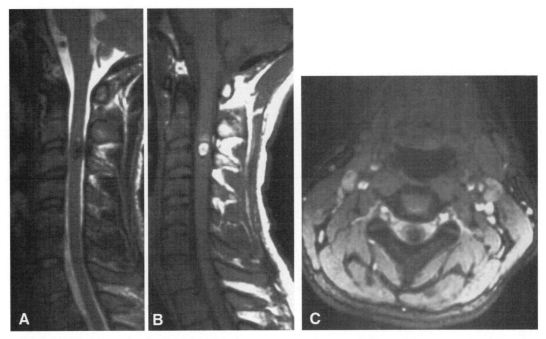

Figure 17.4. *Presumed cavernous malformation of the cervical spine.* A young adult with abrupt onset of long tract signs demonstrates a typical appearance of acute hemorrhage into a cavernous malformation of the upper cervical spine. Sagittal T2 **(A)** and non-enhanced T1 **(B)** images indicate the presence of intracellular methemoglobin with surrounding expansion of the cord. An axial gradient echo sequence **(C)** demonstrates prominent susceptibility artifact within the center of the cord.

vertebral column are most commonly seen in the thoracic area, and they may present with localized or radicular pain. Patients may demonstrate myelopathic signs of paraparesis or sensory loss when there is expansion into or primary involvement of the cord. Similar clinical deficits may be seen with mass-effect and cord-compression from epidural hematomas after lesional hemorrhage or collapse of a vertebral body.

A different angiographic appearance is seen with malformations that involve the vertebral body or extradural space compared with cavernous malformations within the spinal cord. The former are more vascular, particularly in a patient with new symptoms when the lesion is in an "active" phase. They are at risk for high intraoperative blood loss if a fixation or decompressive procedure is planned (28) (Fig. 17.5). Preoperative embolization can help to reduce this degree of blood loss considerably and may also diminish the subjective symptoms of the patient (23, 29–32).

Lesions confined to the intramedullary cord, on the other hand, are angiographically occult, and gadolinium-enhanced MRI is the imaging modality most favored for detection and evaluation of these lesions (33, 34). Intramedullary cavernous malformations are more commonly seen in females and tend to present in the 3rd to 6th dec-

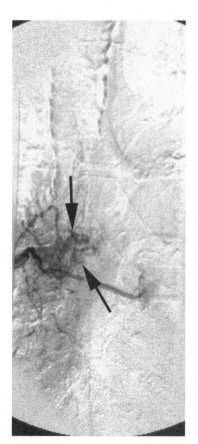

Figure 17.5. *Vertebral hemangioma.* A right T7 injection demonstrates a speckled irregular contrast stain of a vertebral body hemangioma **(arrows).** This differs from the smooth homogeneous contrast stain normally seen in vertebral bodies.

ade (35, 36). The are dark-blue or reddish-brown in gross appearance. Frequently discoloration of the adjacent spinal cord surface can be seen. No abnormal arterial feeders or venous drainage channels are seen. When they bleed into the surrounding cord, they typically present with sensorimotor symptoms and a progressive painful paraparesis. Subarachnoid hemorrhage and hematomyelia have been described (37, 38). They may be associated with syrinx formation.

ANOMALIES OF VENOUS DRAINAGE

The venous angioma, venous malformation, or anomaly of venous drainage represents an innocuous developmental aberration of venous arborization. This is a common finding at autopsy, identified in 2.5% of a large autopsy series (39, 40). Surrounded by normal neural parenchyma, it consists in a converging pattern of abnormally prominent medullary veins draining to a single trunk (Figs. 17.1, 17.3, 17.6). Frequently disposed in a radial or star pattern, the appearance of these prominent veins is likened to the "caput medusae." Occasional instances of this lesion are seen where the draining vein has a particularly distended and indolent aspect, earning the qualification of an "intracerebral varix" (41, 42). Although rare, an intraaxial varix can constitute a diagnostic hazard as it can resemble a cystic mass on CT or MRI (43).

Usually these anomalies appear small on axial imaging, with vessel components extending over an area measuring 2–3 cm or less in maximal dimensions (Fig. 17.1). Although they are so small, such dimensions amplify into considerably larger venous territories paying tribute to a venous anomaly. The significance of this observation is evident in the consequences of extensive venous infarction and hemorrhage which can follow surgical excision of these lesions. Therefore, they are now conceptualized as developmental anomalies. They are thought to involve little if any innate risk and do not warrant any specific treatment in most circumstances (44–48). Some authors believe that venous anomalies of the posterior fossa may be associated with cerebellar symptoms, such as gait disturbance, diplopia, and dizziness, but this is controversial (47, 49).

The clinical significance of venous anomalies is first to recognize them as distinct from arteriovenous malformations and to treat conservatively. Second, the anomaly of venous drainage has a propensity to occur in association with more symptomatic lesions, particularly with cavernous malformations (Fig. 17.1) (50). The latter agent is responsible when venous anomalies are seen in close proximity to small intraparenchymal areas of hemorrhage. If treated surgically, it is important to preserve the integrity of the venous components of the anomaly and to confine the resection procedure to the cavernous malformation.

Venous anomalies are frequently associated with aberrations or deficiencies of adjacent pial veins and dural sinuses, similar to those seen with arteriovenous malformations of the brain. Mullan et al. (51) have suggested that

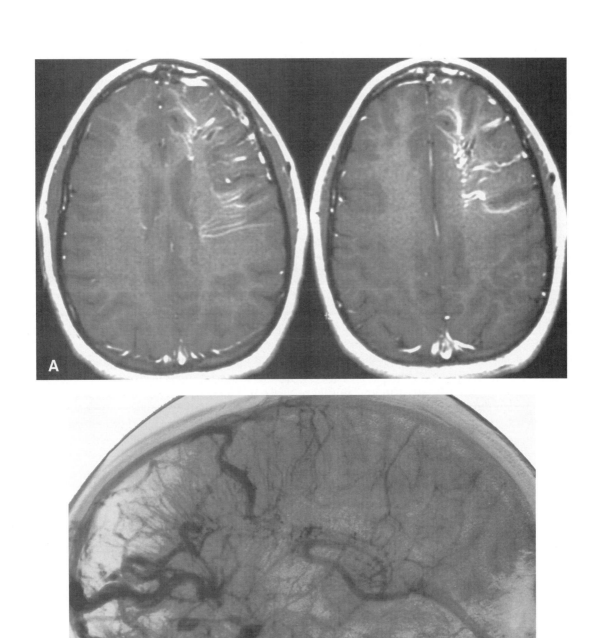

Figure 17.6. *Incidental anomaly of venous drainage.* An inciden- tally discovered anomaly of venous drainage is seen throughout the left frontal lobe. Radially disposed transmedullary veins with a charac- teristic straight appearance are seen on the axial MRI T1 enhanced images **(A).** The disposition of the transmedullary veins is thought to emulate the migration of the primitive germinal layer of the brain. The accompanying angiogram **(B)** illustrates a typical ``caput medusae'' draining anteriorly to the superior sagittal sinus.

cerebral venous malformations and arteriovenous malformations may have a related mechanism of genesis, arguing cogently that an arteriovenous malformation represents a fistulization of a venous anomaly. Venous anomalies can be incorporated into the venous components of arteriovenous malformations. Alternatively, microfistulas can sometimes be seen in association with cerebral venous malformations (Fig. 17.3). Although not common, this is an important consideration because inadvertent surgical obliteration of the venous anomaly can result in severe complications from venous infarction of the involved territory of normal tissue (52). Angiograms of venous anomalies must be studied carefully in the late arterial phases to detect the possibility of abnormal arterio-venous shunting. It is easy to miss such a finding when one's perception is overwhelmed by the subsequent pattern of the venous-phase.

ARTERIOVENOUS MALFORMATIONS OF THE BRAIN

Arteriovenous malformations of the brain are vascular lesions in which an abnormal tangle or nidus of vessels permits pathologic shunting of blood-flow from the arterial to the venous tree without an intervening capillary bed. Whether they are present at birth, are acquired during infancy, or grow in size during childhood are questions of research and debate, but most writings on the subject assume that they are primarily congenital. Vessels within the malformation may be well differentiated into veins and arteries, or they may be malformed, thick or thin-walled, hyalinized vessels (1). An arteriovenous malformation may involve multiple feeding arteries or be confined to a single fistula. They can occasionally present in childhood but are usually seen in early adulthood in the 3rd decade. A second peak of presentation may be observed in the 6th decade. They are thought to be sporadic in occurrence and are not thought to be familial or inherited, with the exception of rare syndromic vascular malformations associated with Sturge-Weber encephalotrigeminal angiomatosis, hereditary hemorrhagic teleangiectasia (Rendu-Osler-Weber syndrome), and other rarer neurooculocutaneous angiomatosis syndromes.

HIGH-FLOW ANGIOPATHY AND ANGIOMATOUS CHANGE

Arteriovenous malformations induce secondary changes in the surrounding vascular architecture over a period of time. Hemodynamic effects due to shunting cause an opening of collateral vessels in territories adjacent to but not primarily involved in the arteriovenous malformation (Figs. 17.7, 17.8). Collateral vessels that are enlarged because of hemodynamic effects can be prominently seen during angiography and can be easily misinterpreted as being part of the nidus. Such collateral vessels are sometimes referred to as areas of "angiomatous change." It is important during angiographic analysis of an arteriovenous malformation to discern the tortuous, often bizarre

appearance of such collateral vessels from the primary nidus.

Second, a dysplastic appearance is frequently seen in the angiographic behavior of feeding pedicles in an AVM. This morphologic change is termed "flow-induced angiopathy." These dysplastic changes can sometimes be reversible in laboratory models or in patients whose AVMs are treated (53). Changes of high-flow angiopathy have been described as variable degrees of luminal dilatation with irregularity of the elastic membrane and endothelium, vacuolization and necrosis of the media muscle, and invasion of adventitia by foreign cells and small blood vessels. Superimposed on these changes, aneurysms of the feeding pedicles or nidus may develop, presumably related to a combination of hemodynamic stress and mural weakness (Fig. 17.9).

Risk of Hemorrhage in Arteriovenous Malformations

Major hemorrhage is the most serious complication of sporadic cerebral arteriovenous malformations. Hemorrhage is the reason for presentation in more than 50% of symptomatic patients. Histologic findings of hemosiderin deposits in arteriovenous malformations suggest that smaller leaks of blood into surrounding tissues without causing clinical presentation may be common. The baseline risk of clinical hemorrhage in adulthood for a previously unruptured arteriovenous malformation is 2–4% per year. The mortality rate is about 10–29% during the first hemorrhage, or more than 50% in instances of posterior fossa hemorrhage (54–57). Pregnancy is not a specific risk factor for hemorrhage. After a hemorrhage, the risk of re-hemorrhage in the first year is high (6–17%), declining thereafter to near baseline with a total lifetime risk of re-hemorrhage as high as 67% (58). Mortality with rehemorrhages is even higher than with initial hemorrhages. Other patients may present with seizure, headache, complications of hydrocephalus, and focal or progressive neurologic deficits.

Characteristics of arteriovenous malformations associated with a higher propensity for bleeding include: a periventricular or intraventricular location; a central location in the basal ganglia or thalamus; arterial aneurysms; intranidal aneurysms; central (deep) venous drainage; a single venous drainage outlet; venous restrictions or stenoses (see Fig. 14.7); delay in venous drainage; feeding by perforator vessels or by the vertebrobasilar artery (59–61). Obviously, these are not all independent variables; for instance, a perforator vessel off the vertebrobasilar system will feed an arteriovenous malformation in a deep location draining to the deep veins. A lower risk of hemorrhage may prevail when there is a prominent network of collateral arterial supply to the surrounding tissue ("angiomatous change") (59). This observation might be a reflection of how the hemodynamics which promote the formation of collateral flow may also have a bearing on decreasing the risk of hemorrhage. Smaller arteriovenous malformations which become symptomatic are most likely to do so by

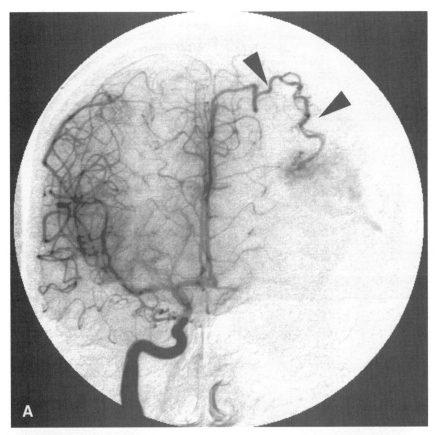

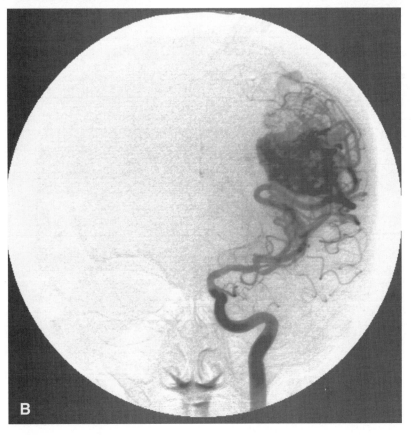

Figure 17.7. *Hemodynamic effects of arteriovenous malformations.* A right internal carotid artery injection **(A)** in a young adult opacifies a left hemispheric arteriovenous malformation via a long meandering vessel **(arrowheads)** supplied by the left anterior cerebral artery. The left internal carotid artery injection **(B)** demonstrates the main nidus of the arteriovenous malformation opacified by branches of the left middle cerebral artery. In certain situations it is important to understand the dynamics of flow surrounding a nidus. In this instance, the meandering vessel draped over the cerebral convexity in A represents ACA-to-MCA pial-pial collateral flow. Therefore, the long branch indicated with arrowheads in A actually represents a branch of the MCA flowing retrogradely to supply the arteriovenous malformation.

Figure 17.8. *Hemodynamic effects of arteriovenous malformations.* Misinterpretation of adjacent collateral or ``angiomatous'' change. An error that is frequently made in angiographic interpretation of brain AVMs is to overestimate the size and extent of the nidus. This is because the vasculature of adjacent normal brain has a bizarre tortuous appearance. This change is a response of normal vessels to an abnormal hemodynamic ``sump'' effect of the arteriovenous malformation. Vessels directly involved with the nidus fail to supply their normal vascular territory adequately, and therefore this function is assumed by other adjacent vessels. Occasionally the sump effect is so great that adjacent normal vessels not only supply this additional territory but also support the nidal supply of the involved direct vessel. However, it is vitally important in surgical and embolization planning to understand the collateral nature of this supply. In this AVM of the posterior right hemisphere, direct supply to the nidus is from the parieto-occipital branch of the right posterior cerebral artery (**arrowheads** in **(A),** a Townes projection of the left vertebral artery injection). Interpretation of the early arterial phase of the right internal carotid artery injection **(B)** must first recognize that the posterior cerebral artery is again opacified on this injection **(arrowheads)** causing the major part of nidal opacification in the late arterial phase **(C).** In treatment planning for this nidus, it is important to realize that the bizarre vascular pattern **(encircled in B and C)** along the lateral aspect of the AVM represents collateral flow only. Contrast reaches the AVM via the right MCA, but it does so only through circulation routes that are supplied more directly by the posterior cerebral artery on the vertebral artery injection. In other words, the MCA is supporting the PCA in supplying the AVM rather than directly supplying the AVM. The implication of this observation is that the lateral aspects of the nidus which are supplied indirectly by the middle cerebral artery, can be embolized directly via the posterior cerebral artery without risk to the middle cerebral artery territory. From the point of view of radiosurgical treatment, limit the treatment window to nidus only. This will avoid radiation injury to normal brain tissue and increase the efficacy of treatment to the nidus.

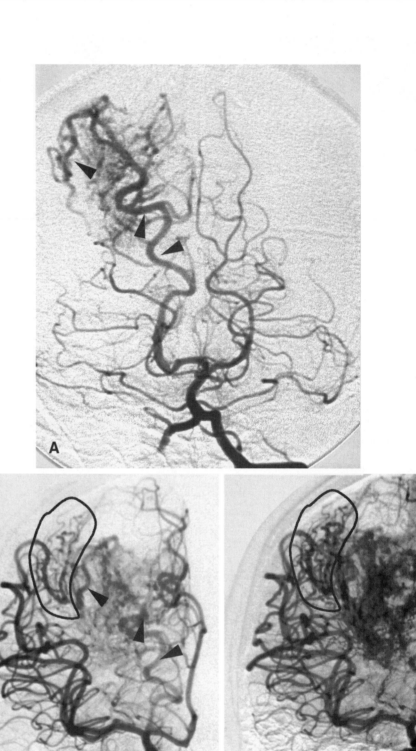

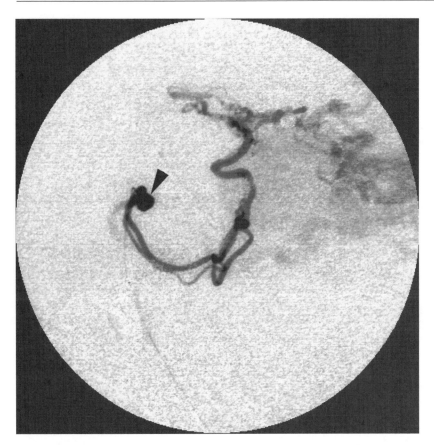

Figure 17.9. *Flow-related aneurysm.* A super-selective microcatheter injection into the left medial posterior choroidal artery, lateral projection, which is supplying an arteriovenous malformation of the velum interpositum. A small aneurysm **(arrowhead)** is present at the origin of the artery from the posterior cerebral artery.

hemorrhage rather than by provoking a non-hemorrhagic neurologic deficit.

Some authors have concluded that smaller arteriovenous malformations represent a higher risk of hemorrhage to a particular patient than would a larger arteriovenous malformation. Kader et al. (62) found that, in a large series of patients with arteriovenous malformations, variables associated with a higher risk of bleeding included: small size of the nidus (2.5 cm); deep venous drainage; and a higher mean arterial pressure of the feeding artery.

Pollock et al. (63) found that a history of bleeding, a single draining vein, and an ill-defined nidus were the most important predictors for risk of bleeding in small arteriovenous malformations.

Aneurysms and Pseudoaneurysms Related to Arteriovenous Malformations

A major focus of angiography in patients with arteriovenous malformations is the presence of aneurysms in the nidus, on the feeding arteries, or in the circle of Willis. Aneurysms of major or feeding vessels are seen in approximately 10% of arteriovenous malformations (64). When one includes small intranidal aneurysms, the incidence increases to more than 20% (65), and as high as 58% (61) with superselective microcatheter injections. Interpretation of superselective angiography of the nidus can be difficult, and therefore what constitutes an intranidal aneurysm can be a matter of subjectivity.

Aneurysms are considered to be a primary site of hemorrhage in the course of the natural history of the disease and during surgery or embolization (66). In certain instances, treatment may be initially directed towards an aneurysm on a feeding pedicle before attention is turned to the arteriovenous malformation. In a patient presenting with hemorrhage, a quandary can arise over whether to treat the arteriovenous malformation or an aneurysm of the feeding pedicle first. It is better to treat the site of hemorrhage first but this can be difficult to determine. When the exact site of hemorrhage is uncertain, part of the argument for treating the aneurysm first is that the risk of immediate rehemorrhage is far greater with a ruptured aneurysm than with a bleeding arteriovenous malformation. Aneurysms on major or accessible vessels can be clipped or can be treated by endovascular coil embolization. When they are close to the nidus they can sometimes be embolized with the nidus by including the aneurysm site in the glue cast.

Arterial or venous pseudoaneurysms are seen with an incidence of approximately 8% in acutely ruptured arteriovenous malformations (67). They are recognized by their irregular contour, development since a previous angiogram, and relationship on axial imaging to the site of hematoma. Endovascular treatment of an arteriovenous malformation with an arterial pseudoaneurysm should focus on the pedicle feeding the pseudoaneurysm first. Initial embolization of other pedicles might cause hemodynamic changes which could rupture the pseudoaneurysm anew.

Grading of Arteriovenous Malformations

Every arteriovenous malformation is unique. Although it is impossible to predict exactly the risk of hemorrhage or other complication, the presence of some of the angiographic features described would prompt more concern towards treatment for a particular patient. A slightly alternative approach used by many neurosurgeons is to predict the perioperative and postsurgical outcome by using a scale or grading system (68, 69). These scales score each arteriovenous malformation based on size, relationship to critical tissue, venous drainage, and surgical accessibility. The Spetzler-Martin scale (68) is one of the most commonly used and correlates with the risk of surgical intervention. Patients are assigned points on three features and categorized into Grades I–VI, based on the total number of points.

Spetzler-Martin Scale for Prediction of Surgical Risk for AVM (68)

Graded Feature	Points
Maximum Diameter of AVM	
Measured from the angiogram and correcting for magnification.	
Small 3 cm	1
Medium 3–6 cm	2
Large 6 cm	3
Eloquence of Adjacent Brain	
Eloquent brain includes primary sensorimotor, language, and visual cortex, hypothalamus, thalamus, internal capsule, brainstem, cerebellar peduncles, and the deep cerebellar nuclei.	
Eloquent	1
Non-eloquent	0
Pattern of Venous Drainage	
Deep veins are considered those which drain to the internal cerebral vein, the basal vein of Rosenthal or the precentral cerebellar vein.	
Superficial	0
Deep	1

Prospective application of the Spetzler-Martin grading scheme demonstrates a strong correlation between the pretreatment grade of an arteriovenous malformation and the risks of surgical excision of the arteriovenous malformation, with or without preoperative embolization (70). Arteriovenous malformations of Grades I to III have extremely low rates of surgically related morbidity and mortality, but these rates rise considerably for higher grade malformations. Patients in Grade VI are considered to be inoperable (70, 71).

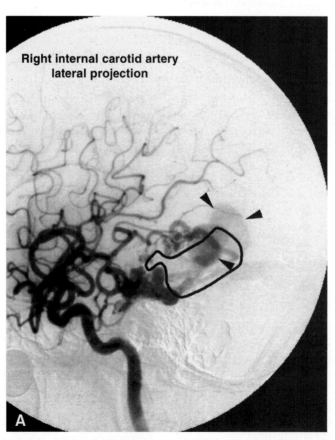

Figure 17.10. External carotid artery supply to arteriovenous malformations: compartments of arteriovenous malformations. A right internal carotid artery injection **(A)** opacifies an unruptured arteriovenous malformation of the posterior aspect of the right inferior temporal gyrus. An anterior and a superior compartment of the arteriovenous malformation are opacified on this injection, between which there is a lucent unopacified portion **(encircled)**.

Figure 17.10. *(continued)* The major part of this remaining section of the arteriovenous malformation is opacified on the left vertebral artery injection **(B).** The venous patterns from the compartments seen in A and B were distinct. The right external carotid artery injection **(C)** opacifies the periphery of the compartment not seen in the internal carotid artery injection. Although this compartment of the AVM overlaps with that seen on B, it shares the venous routes of the compartments seen on A **(small arrowheads on A and C).**

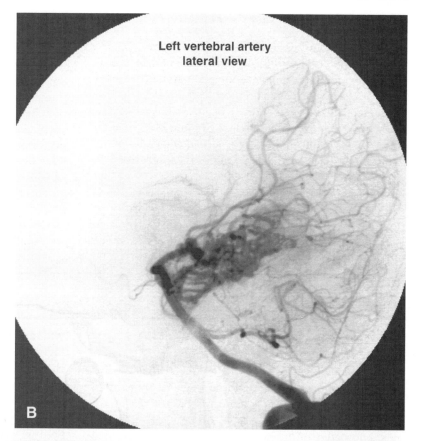

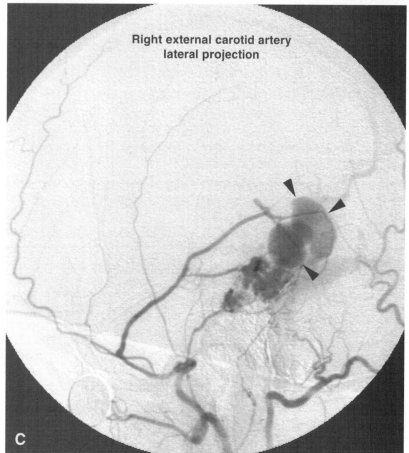

Angiography of Arteriovenous Malformations

Due to the resolution and sensitivity of CT and MRI, it is more common for cerebral angiography to play an analytic rather than a diagnostic role in the evaluation of arteriovenous malformations. Usually the diagnosis of arteriovenous malformation has already been established before the study. Therefore, a cerebral angiogram is expected to supply specific information on the characteristics of the malformation not available through other imaging techniques. Particular features in question concern any bearing on the immediate and long term prognosis of the patient, choice of therapeutic methods, and evaluation of risks of treatment and of non-treatment. Omission of these considerations or inadequate modification of one's technique in performing the angiogram may result in the patient having to undergo a second study.

TECHNICAL MODIFICATIONS

The single most common technical difficulty in interpreting cerebral angiograms of arteriovenous malformations is inadequate opacification of the lesion, particularly with cut-film technique. Before performing the run, a hand injection to check catheter position and cerebral run-off will reveal the abnormality if it is of substantial size. With *a priori* knowledge of the presence of an arteriovenous malformation, the following modifications may be considered.

Selective internal carotid artery and distal vertebral artery catheterization will improve the study quality.

Increase the rate and volume of injection (see Table 2.5).

Increase the filming rate from a standard of 2 fps (frames per second) to 3 fps or higher.

Use higher density contrast (see Table 2.2). Cut-film technique, in particular, will require higher volumes and higher density contrast than will digital imaging.

Specify small focal spot filming. Otherwise, the technologist may choose a large focal spot in response to a request for faster filming-rates.

Continue filming later than standard until the venous system has been adequately visualized.

Use sizing markers to improve estimation of nidus size and to correct for magnification. Some radiosurgical series have demonstrated that radiation therapy for lesions greater than 10 cm^3 in volume is less effective or slower in its effect than for those measuring less than 10 cm^3. Therefore, an accurate estimation of the size of the nidus in three planes is an important item of data to gather from the study.

The external carotid artery may have to be injected bilaterally if not previously done to evaluate the possibility of dural-pial supply to the arteriovenous malformation. This may be considered particularly in patients with previous craniotomy in whom the dura has been breached and who are thus more likely to have these anastomoses. Dural supply to arteriovenous malformations is seen in approximately 10–15% of cases (Figs. 17.10, 17.11).

Due to high flow in the arterial and venous structures, it may be difficult to interpret the abnormal vascular anatomy, particularly on the venous side. Therefore, head positioning for the runs must be meticulous. Magnification oblique views as a supplement to standard projections are particularly useful for arteriovenous malformations of the posterior fossa. Oblique views for the cerebral hemispheres are helpful in cases where the presence or absence of shunting is in question or where clarification of the angioarchitecture of the arteriovenous malformation is required.

Oblique, magnification views of the brain are particularly important for patients undergoing a repeat or postoperative angiogram in whom there is suspicion of an occult or subtle arteriovenous malformation remnant.

DO NOT INTERPRET ANGIOMATOUS CHANGE AS PART OF THE NIDUS

When an arteriovenous malformation of the brain has a high-flow state involving multiple feeders, adaptive changes can occur in the vasculature of the adjacent normal tissue. As the pedicles involved with the arteriovenous malformation become more dedicated to an exclusive, or almost exclusive, supply to the malformation, collateral pathways open to maintain supply to the normal tissue. Extended over the lifetime of a patient, these adaptive "angiomatous "changes can bring about the formation of distinctly enlarged collateral vessels in the immediate vicinity of an arteriovenous malformation. The bizarre appearance of the collateral vessels can provoke the erroneous interpretation that they constitute part of the malformation nidus (Figs. 17.7, 17.8).

An overestimation of the extent of the arteriovenous malformation nidus can have deleterious effects on the patient in terms of treatment recommendation, surgical planning, etc. Radiosurgical treatment for the arteriovenous malformation under these circumstances will be less effective and carries a greater risk due to unnecessary irradiation of normal brain tissue.

To distinguish between primary nidal opacification and epiphenomenal collateral vascular changes, rapid sequence filming is necessary, followed by careful serial review of the images on the viewing board or video monitor. Features that help to distinguish these vessels include: the phase or time at which they are seen; the sources from which they fill; the venous opacification pattern or absence thereof which derives from their filling; and the timing of their wash-out.

Occasionally, it can be difficult to be certain where exactly the margin of the nidus stops, but the velocity of flow within collateralized channels is of a pace with other normal branches on the angiogram, in contrast to the higher velocity of the direct feeders of the arteriovenous malformation. Sometimes, collateral vessels to the penumbra of an arteriovenous malformation result in reconstitu-

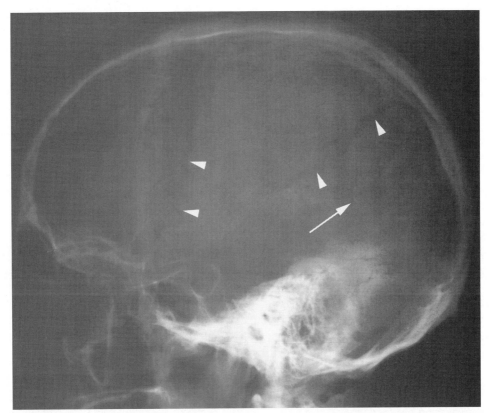

Figure 17.11. *Enlarged dural vessels in a large hemispheric arteriovenous malformation.* A lateral view of the skull in a patient with a long standing untreatable arteriovenous malformation of the right hemisphere with mixed pial and dural supply. Prominent grooves on the inner table of the skull **(arrowheads)** have been etched by the massively enlarged middle meningeal arteries. Calcification within the arteriovenous malformation is marked with a long arrow, probably reflecting a site of previous thrombosis within the arteriovenous malformation.

tion of distal vessels of the involved arterial tree. These reconstituted branches can be identified flowing antegrade to the brain parenchyma or retrograde towards the malformation. Absence of early venous opacification is strong evidence that the vessels in question are hypertrophied normal branches.

The same questions and sequential analytic evaluation of phase and of venous opacification are necessary to avoid erroneous diagnosis of persistent malformation in postoperative angiograms that are done immediately after surgery. In these patients, the enlarged collateral vessels have not yet had time to regress, and there is frequently a hyperemic blush seen on the angiogram in the site of surgical manipulation.

VASCULAR MALFORMATIONS INVOLVING THE VEIN OF GALEN

The term "Vein of Galen aneurysm" describes a group of high flow vascular malformations of the brain in which there is marked dilatation of the Galenic venous system. Two major categories of vascular malformation are included: Vein of Galen Aneurysmal Malformation (VGAM) and Vein of Galen Aneurysmal Dilatation (VGAD) (72, 73). These two disorders have different angiographic and clinical patterns of presentation.

Vein of Galen Aneurysmal Malformations

Vein of Galen aneurysmal malformations are congenital lesions in which a deep arteriovenous fistulous system in the region of the velum interpositum is established in early embryological life (50 mm). The venous receptacle of the shunt is the median vein of the prosencephalon. The median vein of the prosencephalon is the unpaired midline precursor of the internal cerebral veins and Galenic vein. Because the venous system of the brain is still in evolution (see Chapter 5), the presence of a high flow malformation at such an early stage results in a thwarting of the subsequent maturation of the intracranial venous system. Therefore, the venous system of these patients becomes "arrested" in a primitive configuration. The basal vein, the vein of Galen, and the straight sinus do not form in a recognizable pattern. In this condition the median vein of the prosencephalon maintains a persistent pattern of drainage through primitive falcine and tentorial channels which would normally otherwise regress with formation of the straight sinus. Other venous territories of normal brain which are usually collected by the deep venous and galenic systems must find alternative routes of drainage.

Therefore it is common in patients with VGAMs to find that the malformation is drained by a system of falcine and tentorial sinuses to the superior sagittal and transverse sinuses, while there is hypoplasia or absence of the straight sinus (74). Moreover, territories usually drained by the deep venous system are drained by alternative venous channels through circuitous routes. Some circuitous routes of normal brain venous drainage result in distention of the cavernous sinus, ophthalmic veins, and facial veins which can be prominent from an early stage in children with this disorder. The early development of these diverting channels and their relative insulation from the high flow varix of the prosencephalic vein may also explain the low rate of spontaneous venous hemorrhage in VGAM patients compared with the VGAD type lesions.

VGAMs are classified into two types, depending on the relationship of the arterial feeders to the prosencephalic vein (75):

1. Choroidal VGAMs are located in the cistern of the velum interpositum. The arterial feeders are usually from bilateral sources including thalamoperforator arteries, choroidal arteries, and the pericallosal branches of the anterior cerebral arteries. The arterial network is more complex

and the rate of flow more torrential in this group of patients than in mural type VGAMs. These patients present in neonatal life or early infancy with cardiac failure, failure to thrive, and hydrocephalus.

2. Mural VGAMs demonstrate a fistula in the wall of the prosencephalic vein. The arterial complex is usually less extensive than in the Choroidal type. Unilateral or bilateral arterial feeders from the collicular, posterior choroidal, or pineal region arteries are most commonly involved. The rate of flow is less severe than in choroidal types. Children with mural VGAMs present in later infancy or childhood with hydrocephalus, cardiomegaly, mild cardiac failure, and neuropsychological delay or retardation.

Hydrocephalus is a common finding with both types of VGAM. The enormously distended prosencephalic vein on sagittal MRI scans frequently gives the appearance of compressing the aqueduct of Sylvius. However, hydrocephalus is probably almost always due to the effects of venous hypertension in these patients. Therefore placement of a VP shunt for hydrocephalus without treating the malformation itself is usually ineffective. In some patients placement

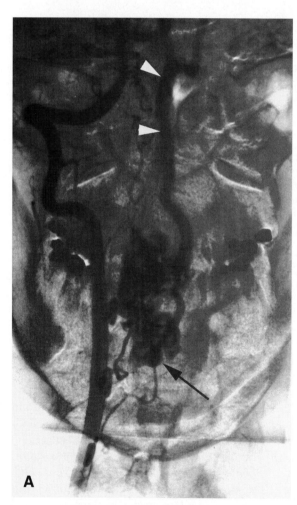

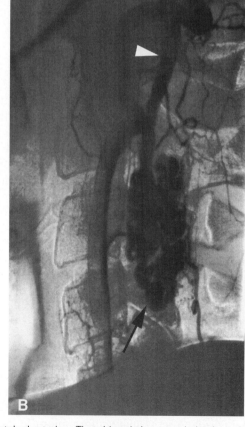

Figure 17.12. Intramedullary arteriovenous malformation of the spinal cord. PA **(A)** and lateral **(B)** views of a right vertebral artery injection in a young adult demonstrate a large arteriovenous malformation of the C2-C4 level supplied by multiple branches of both vertebral arteries. The nidus drains superiorly via a single dominant anterior spinal vein **(white arrowheads)** to the posterior fossa. At least one intranidal aneurysm is seen **(arrow).**

of a VP shunt can be more detrimental because it facilitates an enlargement of the already distended venous structures.

Vein of Galen Aneurysmal Dilatation

Sub-pial arteriovenous malformations of brain adjacent to the velum interpositum can cause massive distention of the internal cerebral vein as a secondary phenomenon. The effect of sub-pial vascular malformations that cause varicose distention of the internal cerebral vein or vein of Galen in this manner is termed vein of Galen aneurysmal dilatation (VGAD).

Arteriovenous malformations of brain occur later in the process of embryologic maturation of the venous system than do VGAMs. Therefore, the degree of absence or hypoplasia of venous sinuses in VGADs is variable, but not as prominent as that seen in VGAMs. Furthermore, the venous components of VGADs communicate with venous structures emanating from normal brain. VGADs are thought to be more at risk for spontaneous hemorrhage than are VGAMs. VGADs present in later childhood or adulthood. The natural history of VGADs is similar to other deeply located brain arteriovenous malformations.

ARTERIOVENOUS MALFORMATIONS OF THE SPINE

Arteriovenous malformations of the spine are divided into two distinct categories.

Intradural, intramedullary vascular malformations are supplied by medullary arterial feeders or branches (i.e., from the anterior or posterior spinal arteries) and are seen in adolescents or young adults (30 years). They are high-flow lesions that have a propensity to rupture and cause subarachnoid hemorrhage. They can affect upper spinal function and can cause acute catastrophic neurologic decline.

Dural or peridural arteriovenous fistulas, on the other hand, are tiny, slow-flow lesions which represent an acquired disease of later adulthood (40 years). They are supplied by dural arteries and typically affect the lower spine and lower extremities. They cause a more progressive slow decline compared with intramedullary vascular malformations. They do not typically cause subarachnoid hemorrhage (76). They are discussed in Chapter 18.

Intradural Spinal Arteriovenous Malformations

Intradural, intramedullary spinal arteriovenous malformations occur most commonly in the cervical or thoracic cord and are classified into three types.

JUVENILE TYPE SPINAL ARTERIOVENOUS MALFORMATION

The juvenile type of spinal arteriovenous malformation occupies the entire spinal canal at the involved level(s) and can have normal spinal parenchyma present within the interstices of its components. There may be multiple medullary arterial feeders, most prominently the anterior

spinal artery, which like the arterial feeders to arteriovenous malformations in the brain, may have a dysplastic appearance. Feeding pedicle or intranidal aneurysms may be seen in approximately 20% of intramedullary arteriovenous malformations (76, 77), as can venous ectasia or venous aneurysms (Fig. 17.12). A minority of patients show a widened interpedicular distance, and an audible spinal bruit has been present in a few cases. They can present with gradual or abrupt onset of motor and sensory symptoms related to the level of involvement, or with spinal subarachnoid hemorrhage.

GLOMUS TYPE SPINAL ARTERIOVENOUS MALFORMATION

Glomus type spinal arteriovenous malformations are more compact and defined than the juvenile type. They do not have intermingled normal spinal tissue, are confined to a shorter segment of cord and are usually fed by a single arterial pedicle (Fig. 17.13). They have a risk of subarachnoid hemorrhage higher than that of other types of intradural vascular malformations. Hemorrhage was seen in 85% of symptomatic patients in a series by Rosenblum et al. (76).

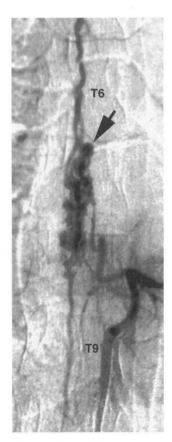

Figure 17.13. *Intramedullary arteriovenous malformation of the spinal cord.* A PA view of a left T8 injection in a young adult who presented with back pain and gait disturbance demonstrates an intramedullary arteriovenous malformation supplied by a single posterior spinal artery. An intranidal aneurysm projects from the upper aspect of the nidus **(arrow).** Draining veins ascend and descend in the midline.

Figure 17.14. *Perimedullary spinal arteriovenous malformation.* An elderly male presented with a clinical history of gait disturbance and urinary incontinence. MRI and myelographic findings (not shown) suggested spinal venous hypertension. A left T12 injection demonstrates an enlarged posterior spinal artery **(arrowheads)** supplying a perimedullary arteriovenous malformation of the surface of the cord. The early venous phase of the PA view **(B)** shows drainage of the arteriovenous malformation superiorly through the tortuous coronal plexus of the spine. An oblique magnification view of the same pedicle (C early, D late) helps to clarify the surgical anatomy. The posterior spinal artery **(arrowheads in C)** behind the cord makes a hairpin-turn on the posterior surface to supply the perimedullary nidus. A slightly later image **(D),** taken when the posterior spinal artery is almost washed out, demonstrates the most prominent vein **(double arrow in D)** draining along the surface of the cord. (Case courtesy of F. Huang-Hellinger, MD, PhD, Boston, MA.)

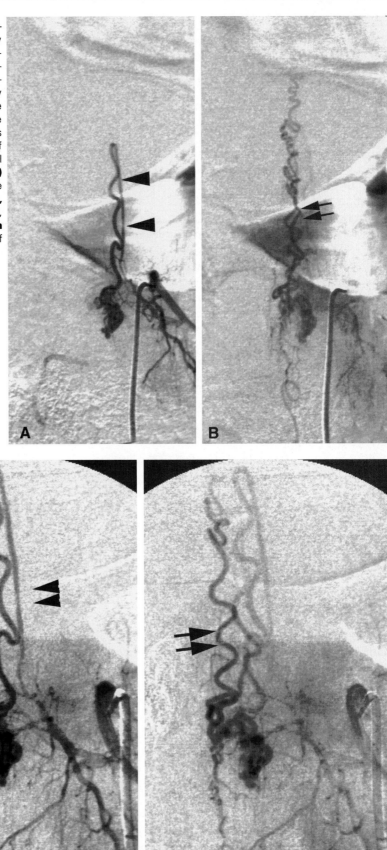

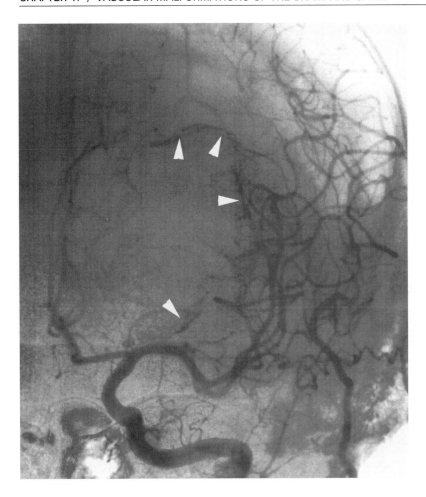

Figure 17.15. *Hypervascular glioblastoma multiforme.* A left common carotid artery injection demonstrates the hypervascular periphery of a glioblastoma in the left hemisphere. An arteriovenous malformation which has recently hemorrhaged with compression of peripheral vessels might be considered in the differential diagnosis for such a lesion. However, AV shunting is not clearly seen in this patient. On later images centripetal progression of contrast was evident, a pattern not likely to be seen with an arteriovenous malformation.

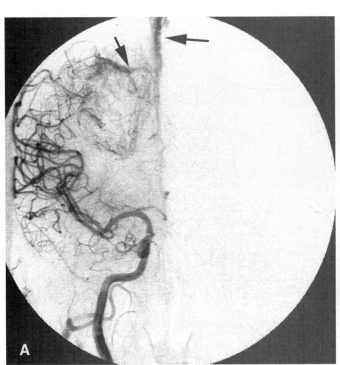

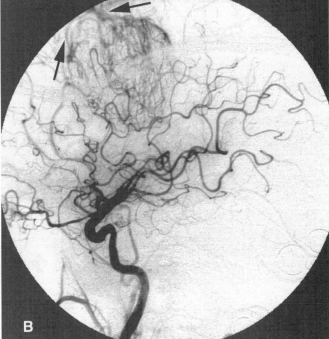

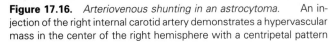

Figure 17.16. *Arteriovenous shunting in an astrocytoma.* An injection of the right internal carotid artery demonstrates a hypervascular mass in the center of the right hemisphere with a centripetal pattern of opacification. Early venous opacification due to shunting **(arrows in A and B)** is present, but the angiographic appearance is dominated by a mass-like arrangement of radially arranged vessels.

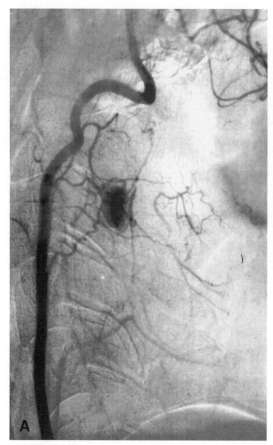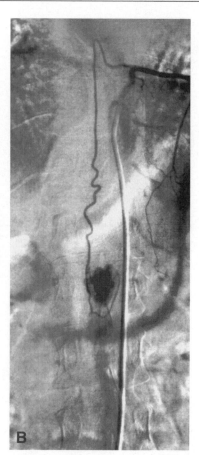

Figure 17.17. *Spinal hemangioblastomas.* Two patients with Von Hippel Lindau syndrome and known hemangioblastomas of the posterior fossa. Opacification of hemangioblastomas in the cervical spine **(A)** lateral view of right vertebral artery injection and lumbar spine **(B)** PA view of left T8 injection is demonstrated. Hemangioblastomas typically give a dense immediate blush which reaches prominence during the early arterial phase of an injection. Therefore, the timing of the blush of hemangioblastoma is earlier than that of most other hypervascular tumors. Among vascular tumors, the opacification of hemangioblastomas is that most likely to be confused with an arteriovenous malformation.

INTRAMEDULLARY AND PERIMEDULLARY ARTERIOVENOUS FISTULAS

Fistulas of the spinal cord may be intramedullary or perimedullary. Flow is usually from a medullary artery which connects directly to a vein without an identifiable nidus. Flow is usually faster than that seen in dural arteriovenous fistulas. They can present with intramedullary or subarachnoid hemorrhage, but this appears to be a minority of cases. As is the case for dural arterio-venous fistulas, venous hypertension with cord edema appears to be an important pathophysiological mechanism for symptoms of intradural arteriovenous shunts (78). Aneurysms of the feeding pedicles are not as likely to be present with perimedullary fistulas compared with intramedullary arteriovenous malformations (77) (Fig. 17.14).

HYPERVASCULAR TUMORS SIMULATING ARTERIOVENOUS MALFORMATIONS

Arteriovenous shunting or early venous opacification can be seen with vascular intraaxial tumors such as glioblastoma multiforme (Figs. 17.15, 17.16) or hemangioblas-

toma (see Fig. 13.17). Extraaxial vascular tumors, such as hemangiopericytoma (see Fig. 2.25) and extraaxial or spinal hemangioblastoma (Fig. 17.17), may also give an appearance that could be confused with that of an arteriovenous malformation. Usually the vascularity of such tumors is easily recognized as subordinate in prominence to other evidence of a mass-lesion. Arteriovenous shunting is rarely as fast in a tumor as that seen in arteriovenous malformations. A parenchymal blush characteristically seen in vascular tumors is not seen in arteriovenous malformations.

REFERENCES

1. McCormick WF. The pathology of vascular ("arteriovenous") malformations. J Neurosurg 1966;24:807–816.
2. Challa VR, Moody DM, Brown WR. Vascular malformations of the central nervous system. J Neuropath Exp Neurol 1995;54: 609–621
3. Farrell DF, Forno LS. Symptomatic capillary telangiectasis of the brainstem without hemorrhage. Report of an unusual case. Neurology 1960;20:341–360.
4. Teilmann K. Hemangiomas of the pons. Arch Neurol 1953;69: 208–223.

5. Zabramski JM, Wascher TM, Spetzler RF, et al. The natural history of familial cavernous malformations: Results of an ongoing study. J Neurosurg 1994;80:422–432.

6. Sage MR, Brophy BP, Sweeney C, et al. Cavernous haemangiomas (angiomas) of the brain: Clinically significant lesions. Austral Radiol 1994;37:147–155.

7. Simard JM, Garcia-Bengochea F, Ballinger WE, et al. Cavernous angioma: a review of 126 collected and 12 new clinical cases. Neurosurgery 1986;18:162–172.

8. Zimmerman RS, Spetzler RF, Lee KS, et al. Cavernous malformations of the brainstem. J Neurosurg 1991;75: 32–39.

9. Rigamonti D, Spetzler RF. The associations of venous and cavernous malformations. Report of four cases and discussion of the pathophysiological, diagnostic and therapeutic implications. Acta Neurochir (Wien) 1988;92:100–105.

10. Pozzati E, Acciarri N, Tognetti F, et al. Growth, subsequent bleeding, and de novo appearance of cerebral cavernous angiomas. Neurosurgery 1996;38:662–670.

11. Gunel M, Awad IA, Anson J, et al. Mapping of a gene causing cerebral cavernous malformations to 7q 11.2-q21. Proc Natl Acad Sci USA 1995;92:6620–6624.

12. Rigamonti D, Johnson PC, Spetzler RF, et al. Cavernous malformations and capillary telangiectasia: A spectrum within a single pathological entity. Neurosurgery 1991;28:60–64.

13. Ogilvy CS, Moayeri N, Golden JA. Appearance of a cavernous hemangioma in the cerebral cortex after a biopsy of a deeper lesion. Neurosurgery 1993;33:307–309.

14. Wilson CB. Cryptic vascular malformations. Clin Neurosurg 1992;38:49–84.

15. Aiba T, Tanaka R, Koike T, et al. Natural history of intracranial cavernous malformations. J Neurosurg 1995;83:56–59.

16. Kondziolka D, Lunsford LD, Kestle JRW. The natural history of cerebral cavernous malformations. J Neurosurg 1995;83: 820–824.

17. Robinson JR, Awad IA, Little JR. Natural history of the cavernous angioma. J Neurosurg 1991;75:709–714.

18. Sinson G, Zager EL, Grossman RI, et al. Cavernous malformations of the third ventricle. Neurosurgery 1995;37:37–42.

19. Katayama T, Tsubokawa T, Maeda T, et al. Surgical management of cavernous malformations of the third ventricle. J Neurosurg 1994;80:64–72.

20. Maraire JN, Awad IA. Intracranial cavernous malformations. Lesion behavior and management strategies. Neurosurgery 1995;37:591–605.

21. Robinson JR, Awad IA, Magdinec M, et al. Factors predisposing to clinical disability in patients with cavernous malformations of the brain. Neurosurgery 1993;32:730–736.

22. Del Curling O, Kelly DL, Elster AD, et al. An analysis of the natural history of cavernous angiomas. J Neurosurg 1991;75: 702–708.

23. Fox MW, Onofrio BM. The natural history and management of symptomatic and asymptomatic vertebral hemangiomas. J Neurosurg 1993;78:36–45.

24. Harrison MJ, Eisenberg MB, Ullman JS, et al. Symptomatic cavernous malformations affecting the spine and spinal cord. Neurosurgery 1995;37:195–205.

25. Mastronardi L, Ferrante L, Scarpinati M, et al. Intradural extramedullary cavernous angioma. Case report. Neurosurgery 1991;29:924–926.

26. Pagni CA, Canavero S, Forni M. Report of a cavernoma of the cauda equina and review of the literature. Surg Neurol 1990; 33:124–131.

27. Topfer D. Über en infiltrierend wachsendes Hemangiom der Haut und multipel Kapillarektasien der Haut und unneren Organae: II Zur Kenntnis der Wirbelangiome. Z Pathol 1928;36: 337–345.

28. Feuerman T, Dwan PS, Yound RF. Vertebrectomy for treatment of vertebral hemangioma without preoperative embolization. Case report. J Neurosurg 1986;65:404–406.

29. Hekster REM, Luyendijk W, Tan TI. Spinal-cord compression caused by vertebral haemangioma relieved by percutaneous catheter embolisation: 15 years later. Neuroradiology 1972;3: 160–164.

30. Hekster REM, Endtz LJ. Spinal-cord compression caused by vertebral haemangioma relieved by percutaneous catheter embolisation: 15 years later. Neuroradiology 1987;29:101.

31. Raco A, Ciappetta P, Artico M, et al. Vertebral hemangiomas with cord compression: The role of embolization in five cases. Surg Neurol 1990;34:164–168.

32. Djindjian M, Nguyen JP, Gaston A, et al. Multiple vertebral hemangiomas with neurological signs. Case report. J Neurosurg 1992;76:1025–1028.

33. Fontaine S, Melanson D, Cosgrove R, et al. Cavernous hemangiomas of the spinal cord. MR imaging. Radiology 1988;166: 839–841.

34. Barnwell SL, Dowd CF, Davis RL, et al. Cryptic vascular malformations of the spinal cord. Diagnosis by magnetic resonance imaging and outcome of surgery. J Neurosurg 1990;72: 403–407.

35. Cosgrove GR, Bertrand G, Fontaine S, et al. Cavernous angiomas of the spinal cord. J Neurosurg 1988;68:31–36.

36. Anson JA, Spetzler RF. Surgical resection of intramedullary spinal cord cavernous malformations. J Neurosurg 1993;78: 446–451.

37. Heimberger K, Schnaberth G, Koos W, et al. Spinal cavernous haemangioma (intradural-extramedullary) underlying repeated subarachnoid hemorrhage. J Neurol 1982;226:289–293.

38. Ueda S, Saito A, Inomori S, et al. Cavernous angioma of the cauda equina producing subarachnoid hemorrhage. Case report. J Neurosurg 1987;66:134–136.

39. McCormick WF, Hardman JM, Boulter TR. Vascular malformation (angiomas) of the brain, with special reference to their occurring in the posterior fossa. J Neurosurg 1968;28:241–251.

40. Sarwar M, McCormick WF. Intracerebral venous angioma. Case report and review. Arch Neurol 1978;35:323–325.

41. Handa J, Suda K, Sato M. Cerebral venous angioma associated with a varix. Surg Neurol 1984;21:436–440.

42. Kelly KJ, Rockwell BH, Raji R, et al. Isolated cerebral intraaxial varix. Am J Neuroradiol 1995;16:1633–1635.

43. Uchino A, Hasuo K, Matsumoto S, et al. Varix occurring with cerebral venous angioma: a case report and review of the literature. Neuroradiology 1995;37:29–31.

44. Garner TB, Curling OD, Kelly DL, et al. The natural history of intracranial venous angiomas. J Neurosurg 1991;75:715–722.

45. Senegor M, Dohrmann GJ, Wollman RL. Venous angiomas of the posterior fossa should be considered an anomalous venous drainage. Surg Neurol 1983;19:26–32.

46. Numaguchi Y, Kitamura K, Fukui M, et al. Intracranial venous angiomas. Surg Neurol 1982:18:193–202.

47. Rigamonti D, Spetzler RF, Medina M, et al. Cerebral venous malformations. J Neurosurg 1990;73:560–564.

48. Kondziolka D, Dempsey PK, Lunsford LD. The case for conservative management of venous angiomas. Can J Neurol Sci 1991; 18:295–299.

49. Moritake K, Handa H, Mori K, et al. Venous angiomas of the brain. Surg Neurol 1980;14:95–105.

50. Wilms G, Bleus E, Demaerel P, et al. Simultaneous occurrence of developmental venous anomalies and cavernous angiomas. Am J Neuroradiol 1994;15.

51. Mullan S, Mojtahedi S, Johnson DL, et al. Cerebral venous malformation-arteriovenous malformation transition forms. J Neurosurg 1996; 85:9-13.

52. Meyer B, Stangl AP, Schramm J. Association of venous and true arteriovenous malformation: a rare entity among mixed vascular malformations of the brain. J Neurosurg 1995;83:141–144.

53. Pile-Spellman JMD, Baker KF, Liszczak TM, et al. High-Flow angiopathy: cerebral blood vessel changes in chronic arteriovenous fistula. Am J Neuroradiol 1986;7:811–815.

54. Ondra SL, Troupp H, George ED, et al. The natural history of symptomatic arteriovenous malformations of the brain: a 24-year follow-up assessment. J Neurosurg 1990;73:387–391.

55. Brown RD, Wiebers DO, Forbes G, et al. The natural history of unruptured intracranial arteriovenous malformations. J Neurosurg 1988;68:352–357.

56. Wilkins RH. Natural history of intracranial vascular malformations: a review. Neurosurgery 1885;16:421–430.

57. Graf CJ, Perret GE, Torner JC. Bleeding from cerebral arteriovenous malformations as part of their natural history. J Neurosurg 1983;58:331–337.

58. Fults D, Kelly DL. Natural history of arteriovenous malformations of the brain: A clinical study. Neurosurgery 1984;15:658–662.

59. Marks MP, Lane B, Steinberg GK, et al. Hemorrhage in intracerebral arteriovenous malformation: angiographic determinants. Radiology 1990;176:807–813.

60. Miyasaka Y, Yada K, Ohwada T, et al. An analysis of the venous drainage system as a factor in hemorrhage from arteriovenous malformations. J Neurosurg 1992;76:239–243.

61. Turjman F, Massoud TF, Viñuela F, et al. Correlation of the angioarchitectural features of cerebral arteriovenous malformations with clinical presentation of hemorrhage. Neurosurgery 1995;37:856–862.

62. Kader A, Yound WL, Pile-Spellman J, et al. The influence of hemodynamic and anatomic factors on hemorrhage from cerebral arteriovenous malformations. Neurosurgery 1994;34:801–808.

63. Pollock BE, Flickinger JC, Lunsford LD, et al. Factors that predict the bleeding risk of cerebral arteriovenous malformations. Stroke 1996;27:1-6.

64. Cunha e Sa MJ, Stein BM, Solomon RA, et al. The treatment of associated intracranial aneurysms and arteriovenous malformations. J Neurosurg 1992;77:853–859.

65. Lasjaunias P, Piske R, Terbrugge K, et al. Cerebral arteriovenous malformations and associated arterial aneurysms. Analysis of 101 AVM cases with 37 AA in 23 patients. Acta Neurochir (Wien) 1988;91:29–36.

66. Abe T, Nemoto S, Iwata T, et al. Rupture of a cerebral aneurysm during embolization for a cerebral arteriovenous malformation. Am J Neuroradiol 1996;16:1818–1820.

67. Garcia-Monaco R, Rodesch G, Alvarez H, et al. Pseudoaneurysms within ruptured intracranial arteriovenous malformations: diagnosis and early endovascular management. Am J Neuroradiol 1993;14:315–321.

68. Spetzler RF, Martin NA. A proposed grading system for arteriovenous malformations. J Neurosurg 1986;65:476–483.

69. Shi YQ, Chen XC. A proposed scheme for grading intracranial arteriovenous malformations. J Neurosurg 1986;65:484–489.

70. Hamilton MG, Spetzler RF. The prospective application of a grading system for arteriovenous malformations. Neurosurgery 1994;34:2–7.

71. Heros RC, Korosue K, Diebold PM. Surgical excision of cerebral arteriovenous malformations: late results. Neurosurgery 1990;26:570–578.

72. Berenstein A, Lasjaunias P. Surgical Neuroangiography, Endovascular Treatment of Cerebral Lesions. Vol.4. Springer-Verlag, New York, Berlin, Heidelberg, 1992: 270–317.

73. Morris PP, Choi IS, Berenstein A, et al. Vein of Galen Aneurysms. In: Ojemann RG, Ogilvy CS, Crowell RM, Heros RC, eds. Surgical Management of Neurovascular Disease. 3rd ed. Baltimore: Williams & Wilkins, 1995:482–488.

74. Lasjaunias P, Garcia-Monaco R, Rodesch G, et al. Deep Venous drainage in great cerebral vein (vein of Galen) absence and malformations. Neuroradiology 1991:33:234–38.

75. Seidenwurm D, Berenstein A, Hyman A, et al. Vein of Galen malformation: Correlation of clinical presentation, arteriography, and MR imaging. Am J Neuroradiol 1991;12:347–54.

76. Rosenblum B, Oldfield EH, Doppman JL, et al. Spinal arteriovenous malformations: a comparison of dural arteriovenous fistulas and intradural AVMs in 81 patients. J Neurosurg 1987;67:795–802.

77. Biondi A, Merland JJ, Hodes JE, et al. Aneurysms of spinal arteries associated with intramedullary arteriovenous malformations. I. Angiographic and clinical aspects. Am J Neuroradiol 1992;13:913–922.

78. Tomlinson FH, Rüfenacht DA, Sundt TM, et al. Arterio-venous fistulas of the brain and spinal cord. J Neurosurg 1993;79:16–27.

CHAPTER 18

Dural Vascular Disease of the Brain and Spine

CRANIAL DURAL ARTERIOVENOUS FISTULAS AND MALFORMATIONS

Vascular malformations or fistulas of the dura are uncommon diseases, but they are potentially serious with the capacity to develop irreversible complications. They account for 10–15% of intracranial arteriovenous malformations of all types. They can occur in the brain or spine with characteristic patterns of pathophysiology in both locations.

The cranial dura consists of two tightly apposed layers, an outer periosteal layer and an inner meningeal layer, separated by a rich vascular layer of meningeal or dural veins and arterioles. Where the two layers of dura become separated, a larger venous space forms the dural sinuses. In the spine, the epidural plexus represents the layer of interdural vasculature separating the spinal dura from the periosteum of the spinal canal. In the cranial and spinal dura any meningeal artery which perforates the dura usually does so in close relationship to surrounding venous plexuses. The artery penetrates the dura through or may run for a while within such a venous structure or sinus. Venous thrombosis or other injury, including surgery (1–3), may occasion a process of inflammation, neovascularization, and angiogenesis (4). The adjacent arterioles are thought to become involved with the formation of pathologic shunts to venous channels (5). Alternatively, the fistulous connection could be the initiating event. Arterialized flow, changes in the venous wall, and turbulent conditions may make thrombus formation more likely. In most patients an acquired etiology is certain, in view of well-documented cases of such lesions soon after surgery, trauma, or mastoid air-cell infection. Metachronous formation of dural arteriovenous malformations has been seen, supporting the assumption of an acquired etiology (6). Patients with systemic syndromes involving abnormalities of vascular fragility, such as neurofibromatosis type I, fibromuscular dysplasia, and Ehlers-Danlos syndrome are reported to be slightly more prone to develop these disorders of the cranial dura or spine.

An acquired dural fistula may be single, multifocal, or complex. Some debate exists over whether to term these acquired lesions "dural arteriovenous malformations" or "dural arteriovenous fistulas." The latter term is favored by those who want to stress the acquired nature of the disease, as is the case for most adults. Fistulous malformations of the dura can be seen in young children also. In children, long-standing changes suggest that some rare instances of congenital dural arteriovenous malformations occur. Therefore, the compromise term "dural arteriovenous fistulous malformation" has been proposed by some authors.

In the cranial dura, the pathophysiology and significance of these lesions derive from their effects on venous flow. Various classification schemes have been proposed to categorize these lesions (7–9). The quintessence of all of these schemes is an analysis of the state of disruption of venous outflow from the malformation, and the patency and direction of flow in adjacent dural sinuses, dural veins, and subarachnoid veins. The particular arterial feeders involved with a dural vascular malformation are usually not of primary importance for analysis of risks or treatment options (Figs. 18.1, 18.2).

Uncomplicated dural arteriovenous malformations are occasionally seen as incidental findings (Fig. 18.3). They may be single or multiple, resulting in arterialization of flow in an orthograde fashion in a major dural sinus. Symptomatic patients present with pulsatile tinnitus, audible bruit, or cranial nerve deficits depending on location of the lesion. Pulsatile tinnitus may be reported in 20–70% of patients, some of whom will volunteer a history of being able to suppress the bruit by manual compression of the neck. Visual symptoms and headache are also common (10). Hydrocephalus due to impaired resorbtion of CSF in more advanced cases can be seen, progressing in extreme instances to a state of dementia, which can be reversible (11–13).

Dural arteriovenous fistulas are most commonly seen in the cavernous (Fig. 18.4), sigmoid, and transverse sinuses (Fig. 18.5). Dural arteriovenous fistulas in the early stages may undergo spontaneous remission, although the likelihood of this in a well-established lesion is low (8, 14, 15). The dural sinus in early or uncomplicated cases may be completely normal in appearance or may show evidence of only partial thrombosis at the time of presentation. Depending on the patient's tolerance of symptoms, expectant management of patients with uncomplicated dural arteriovenous malformations may be reasonable. Training the patient to perform manual contralateral carotid compression at home can occasionally help to eliminate smaller lesions over a few weeks.

The venous pattern changes as the pressure in the venous system increases due to intimal flow-related changes in the main venous channels or recruitment of arterial feeders. Diversion of cortical venous flow away from the

Figure 18.1. *Dural AVM of right sigmoid sinus.*
An elderly patient presented with a 3-month history of pulsatile tinnitus. Angiography demonstrated a dural arteriovenous malformation of the right sigmoid sinus supplied by the ipsilateral occipital **(A)** and vertebral **(B)** arteries. All avenues of fistulous flow converge on a single venous channel **(arrow)** which empties into the sigmoid sinus. Although this dural arteriovenous malformation is confined and simple on its arterial side, there is constriction **(arrowhead)** in the sigmoid sinus (S) with bidirectional flow to the jugular bulb and transverse sinus (T). This suggests that the dural arteriovenous malformation has passed the early stages of evolution and is developing signs of sinus hypertension.

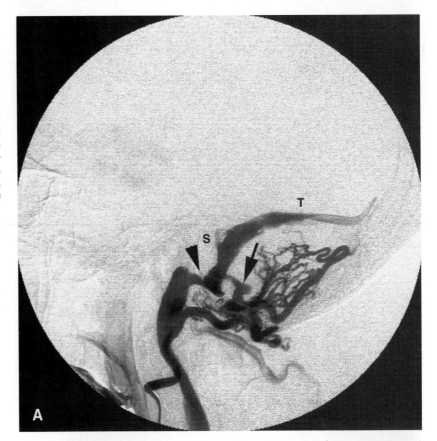

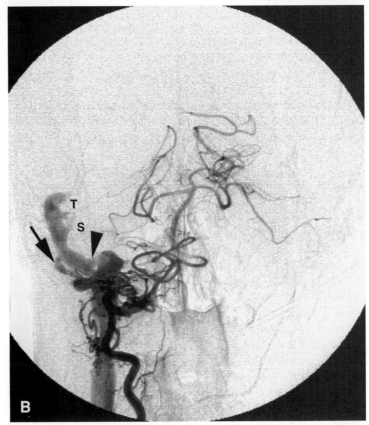

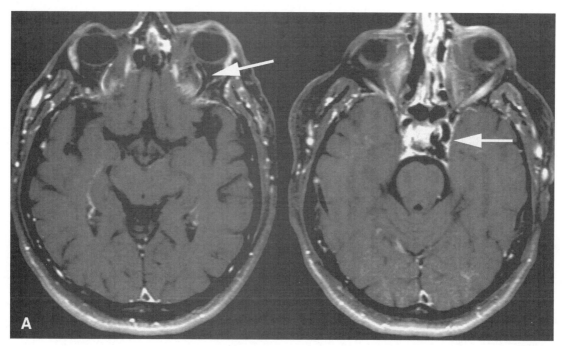

Figure 18.2. Postsurgical dural arteriovenous malformation of the cavernous sinus. A middle-aged male presented with left-sided proptosis and an audible bruit after surgery for chronic ethmoid sinusitis. A contrast-enhanced MRI **(A)** demonstrates prominent paracaver- nous vessels and distention of the left superior ophthalmic vein **(arrows)**. These findings were not seen on the preoperative MRI. Because of worsening proptosis, endovascular treatment was recommended.

involved sinus is seen angiographically with retrograde flow in the dural sinuses. It can be difficult to identify the presence of incipient cortical venous hypertension unless a careful examination of the entire angiogram is performed. For example, an internal carotid arteriogram in which opacification of the dAVM is not seen may still demonstrate very ominous signs in the patterns of flow in the venous stages. In other words, a cerebral arteriogram in a patient with a dAVM is not simply a matter of identifying the vessels that do or do not opacify the malformation.

With increasing venous and sinus hypertension, retrograde flow of contrast from the sinuses into leptomeningeal (cortical) veins becomes evident. With elevation of venous pressure in the cortical veins new symptoms related to seizure, headache, venous hemorrhage, elevated intracranial pressure, and focal neurologic deficits are seen (Fig. 18.6). Depending on the venous territory involved, patients may present with focal hemispheric symptoms, motor weakness, and brainstem or cerebellar symptoms. Cranial nerve deficits may also be seen, particularly ophthalmoplegia in the setting of a cavernous sinus dural arteriovenous malformation. Interestingly, it is during this stage of diversion of flow away from the sinuses into cortical veins, perhaps with progressive occlusion of the main sinus, that patients may experience a subjective improvement in tinnitus. Thus, such a report from a patient with a known dural arteriovenous malformation is concerning as it may bode an ominous turn of events. Immediate treatment is indicated when complications appear imminent.

Urgent treatment is required also for patients with dural arteriovenous malformations near the cavernous sinus who are developing complications of exophthalmos, secondary glaucoma, or visual deterioration.

The most grave progression of the disease occurs when venous outflow is completely restricted to cortical veins due to complete occlusion of the sinuses. In these instances, the arterial flow may be directed exclusively into the subarachnoid veins or into an isolated segment of sinus which drains only through cortical veins. These patients present with severe neurologic deficits, extensive cortical venous hypertension (Fig. 18.6), venous hemorrhages or infarcts, and hydrocephalus. Dural arteriovenous malformations of the anterior cranial fossa or of the tentorium represent a particular risk of sudden massive frontal lobe or subarachnoid hemorrhage, which may be the presenting symptom in more than 70–80% of cases (Fig. 18.7) (16–20). Dural arteriovenous malformations in the anterior cranial fossa are usually close to the cribriform plate and have a propensity to develop venous aneurysms or varices adjacent to the site of fistulous flow from the ethmoidal branches of the ophthalmic arteries (21, 22). Prompt surgical clipping of the dural arteriovenous malformation is the treatment of choice for this particular subgroup of patients. Embolization has little or no therapeutic role in this location, given the risks and difficulties involved in catheterization and embolization of ophthalmic artery branches.

The natural history of dural arteriovenous malforma-

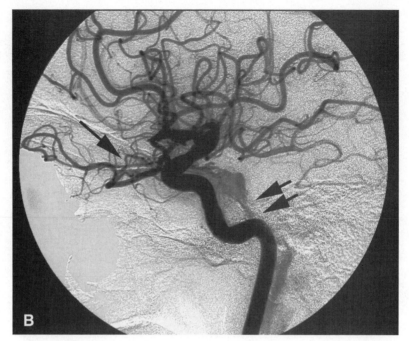

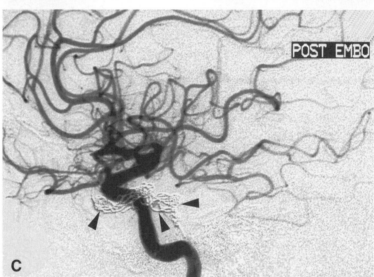

Figure 18.2. *(continued)* An angiogram of the left internal carotid artery **(B)** demonstrates a large recurrent meningeal artery **(arrow)** from the ophthalmic artery opacifying the cavernous sinus and inferior petrosal sinus **(double arrow)**. Identification of the inferior petrosal sinus on pre-embolization angiography points to the most accessible route of transvenous access to a dural arteriovenous malformation in this region. Multiple external carotid artery branches were also involved in the fistulous lesion. The cavernous sinus was embolized **(C)** via the left inferior petrosal sinus with thrombogenic coils **(arrowheads)** causing an immediate normalization of flow in the previously involved vessels.

tions is variable. Certain anatomic locations are typically more likely to develop serious complications. The presence of venous aneurysms at angiography, and a location close to the tentorial incisura, or venous drainage to the Galenic system, the superior petrosal sinus, or straight sinus should prompt concern for an unfavorable disease progression (18, 23). Patients with these features seem particularly prone to severe neurological complications and intracranial hemorrhage. The location of the shunt and pattern of venous flow have a far greater bearing on the significance of the lesion than the particular arterial feeders involved or the volume of flow.

Treatment of Cranial Dural Arteriovenous Malformations

Surgical treatment of cranial dural arteriovenous malformations is accomplished by techniques such as clipping of the malformation, surgical isolation (skeletonization) of the involved sinus, or cauterization of involved vessels. Endovascular transarterial or transvenous embolization may

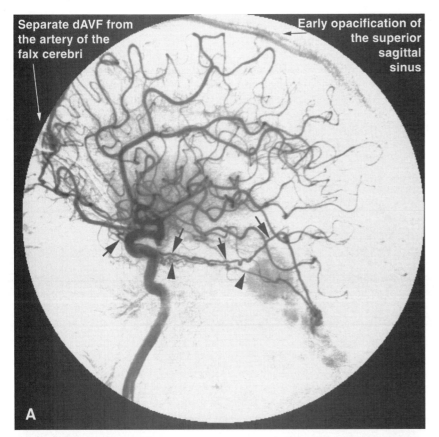

Separate dAVF from the artery of the falx cerebri

Early opacification of the superior sagittal sinus

A

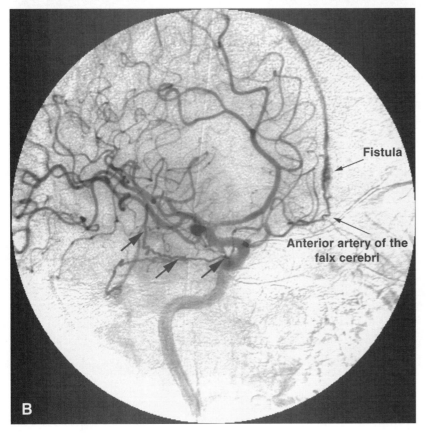

Fistula

Anterior artery of the falx cerebri

B

Figure 18.3. *Synchronous dural arteriovenous malformations.* An elderly male presented with headaches. Two separate dural arteriovenous malformations were demonstrated on lateral **(A)** and oblique **(B)** images of the right internal carotid artery. A dural arteriovenous malformation of the tentorium causing the patient's symptoms opacifies greatly distended veins in the posterior fossa. It is supplied by the marginal tentorial artery **(arrows)** arising from the ophthalmic artery, and tentorial arteries **(arrowheads)** from the cavernous internal carotid artery. A separate fistula of the superior sagittal sinus is supplied by the anterior artery of the falx cerebri.

Figure 18.4. *Dural AVM of the cavernous sinus.* A lateral view of a left internal maxillary artery injection demonstrates opacification of a distended and tense cavernous sinus **(arrow)** via the accessary meningeal artery (ama) and artery of the foramen rotundum (fr). The cavernous sinus drains anteriorly to the superior ophthalmic vein (sov), and subsequently to the facial vein (fv). In contrast to the patient in Figure 18.2, the inferior petrosal sinus is not seen in this patient, which implies that transvenous access to the lesion through that route may not be possible. In a patient with a lesion such as this, urgency of treatment is guided primarily by concerns for the patient's vision. An ophthalmologist's involvement to monitor the intraocular pressure and visual acuity is imperative. The likelihood of such complications depend in part on the anastomoses of the ophthalmic veins with other drainage routes.

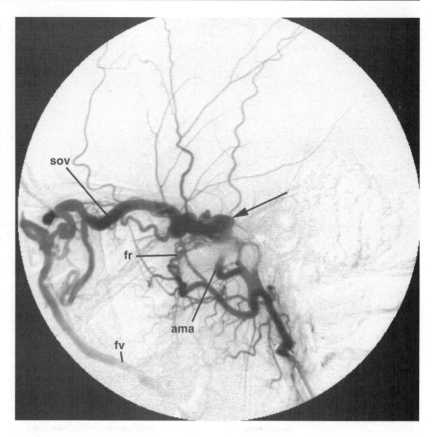

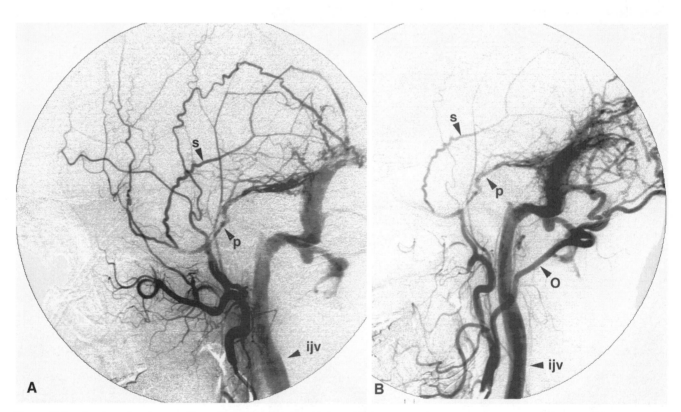

Figure 18.5. *Dural arteriovenous malformation of the transverse and sigmoid sinus.* **(A)** Lateral view of a distal external carotid artery injection. **(B)** Lateral view of the proximal external carotid artery. A dural arteriovenous malformation in a prolonged segment of the transverse and sigmoid sinuses is opacified by squamous (s) and petrosal (p) branches of the middle meningeal artery and transosseous branches of the occipital artery (O). Flow is antegrade into the internal jugular vein (ijv). The transverse sinus is occluded between the dural arteriovenous malformation and the Torcular.

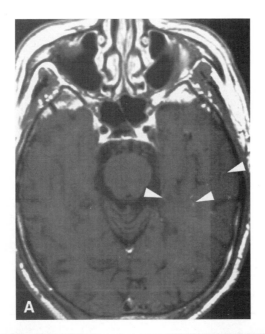

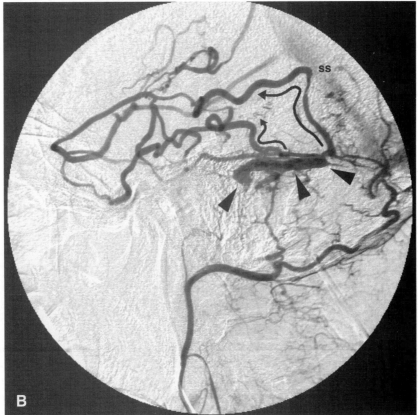

Figure 18.6. *Venous hypertension due to a dural arteriovenous malformation.* An elderly male presented with sudden loss of consciousness and seizure. A CT scan (not shown) demonstrated a small intraparenchymal bleed of the left occipital lobe. An axial image from a T1-weighted contrast-enhanced MRI sequence **(A)** shows a profusion of enhancing vessel-like structures **(arrowheads)** through the left hemisphere. A dural arteriovenous malformation of the left transverse sinus was found by angiography. A lateral view of the left occipital artery injection **(B)** shows that the involved segment of transverse sinus **(arrowheads)** is isolated from the remainder of the sinus. Therefore, this segment of transverse sinus decompresses via cortical veins to the occipital and temporal lobes **(curved arrows indicating direction of flow)**. This causes an extreme elevation of venous pressure throughout the left cerebral hemisphere. This resulted in the patient's condition of venous infarction and hemorrhage. ss, straight sinus.

Figure 18.7. *Dural arteriovenous malformation of the anterior cranial fossa.* A middle-aged patient presented with headaches. A dural arteriovenous malformation of the cribriform plate is opacified by ethmoidal branches of the left ophthalmic artery. Venous drainage from this malformation is posteriorly to the lesser wing of the sphenoid bone. In this patient, most of the subsequent drainage was via the cavernous sinuses.

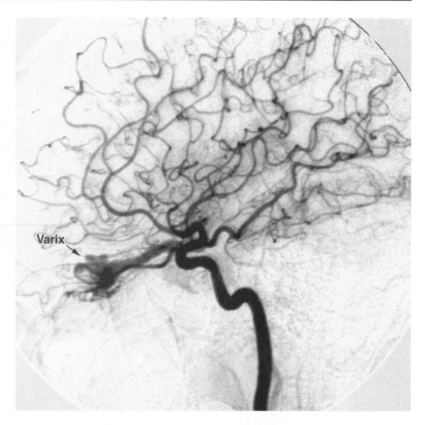

Varix

be effective too, either alone or in combination with surgical techniques. For some lesions, such as dural arteriovenous malformations of the anterior fossa, treatment is exclusively surgical due to the easy accessibility of the ethmoidal vessels by craniotomy. Other dural arteriovenous malformations, particularly of the cavernous, transverse and sigmoid sinuses, lend themselves exclusively to endovascular treatment (24–26). In instances of isolated sinus involvement, surgical exposure of the sinus combined with intra-operative packing of the sinus using endovascular techniques can be effective.

The utility of transvenous endovascular treatment of dural arteriovenous malformations derives from the observation that obliteration of the venous component of dural arteriovenous malformations results in a regression of the arterial feeders. This is in contrast to arteriovenous malformations of the brain where (inadvertent) selective venous occlusion carries an enormously high risk of nidal rupture and disastrous bleeding.

The degree of necessity and mode of treatment of dural arteriovenous malformations depends largely on the pattern of venous drainage and imminence of complications. In asymptomatic patients in whom a dural arteriovenous malformation has been discovered incidentally, a period of conservative management can be pursued while the patient practices contralateral carotid compression. Spontaneous thrombosis and remission can be seen occasionally with this technique. However, most patients are symptomatic by the time of presentation. Rather than run the risk of developing the complications outlined, treatment is

usually recommended. Because the treatment of dural arteriovenous malformations can be difficult and fraught with some hazards, it is usually prudent to have a diagnostic angiogram performed initially to allow time for careful analysis of the findings. The pretreatment angiogram must be performed diligently. In particular, the risks of treatment in this disorder relate to the possibility of misunderstanding the venous anatomy. This can result in an interventional procedure that makes the abnormality worse by directing more flow into the cortical veins. This can happen particularly when an unrecognized cortical vein drains into a segment of sinus involved with the dural arteriovenous malformation. Occluding this segment of sinus could obstruct and reverse flow in this unseen vein with disastrous results.

Transarterial embolization may have a place in selected instances, but it is usually difficult to accomplish a complete cure of the lesion by this technique. Usually the dural arteriovenous malformation will persist or recur due to formation of tiny collateral channels and the impossibility of occluding each one (Fig. 18.8). Transarterial treatment has a role to play in palliative management of malformations, which cannot be embolized transvenously. In most instances, the precise identity of the arterial feeders will be of secondary importance. The angiographic questions to answer are the following:

1. What segment of sinus is involved? In which direction is it flowing? Is there evidence of established or impending restriction of venous flow in those sinuses?

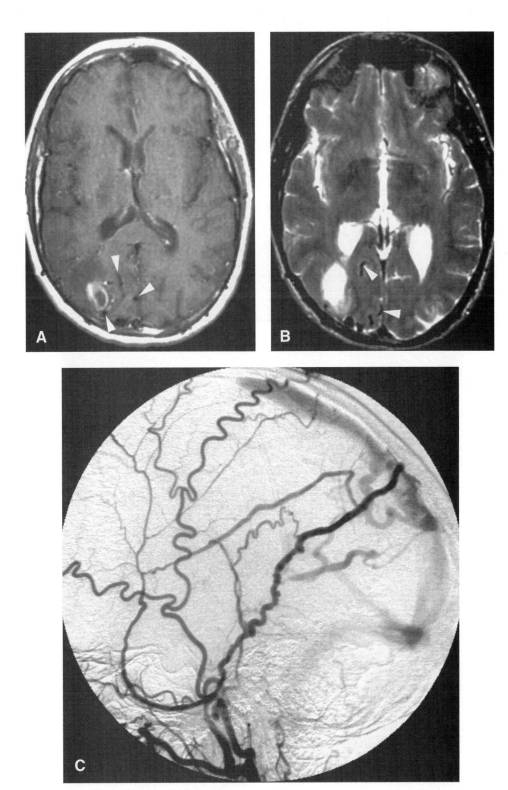

Figure 18.8. *Dural arteriovenous malformation of the cerebral convexity.* A middle-aged patient presented with sudden onset of seizures and headaches. MRI demonstrated a right parieto-occipital parenchymal hematoma with mass-effect, edema, and prominent surrounding flow-voids **(arrowheads in A and B)**. A diagnosis of a dural arteriovenous malformation of the right parasagittal convexity was confirmed with angiography of the external carotid arteries **(C)**. Transarterial embolization of the external carotid artery feeders was performed before surgical resection of the dural arteriovenous malformation. Unfortunately the parenchymal signs of complications from the dural arteriovenous malformation masked signs that the patient had a coexistent glioblastoma multiforme in the same location.

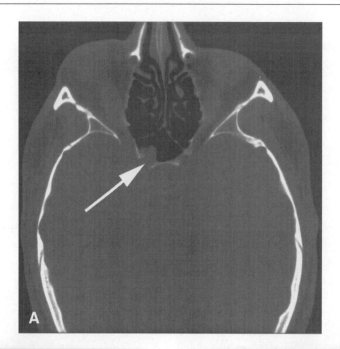

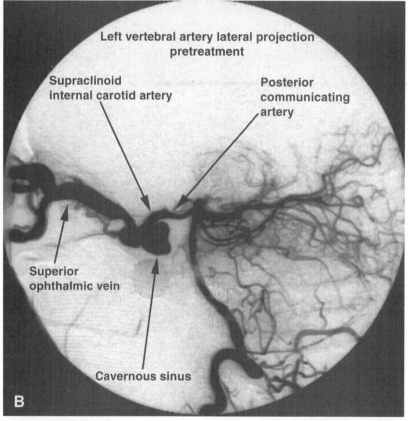

Figure 18.9. *Post-traumatic carotid cavernous fistula with ipsilateral carotid dissection.*   A young adult male presented with history of mild right-sided proptosis and a pulsatile bruit following an assault with a lead pipe. A CT examination demonstrated prominent vascular structures in the region of the right cavernous sinus. A most significant finding on the bone-windows was a breach **(arrow in A)** in the bony wall of the sphenoid sinus with protrusion of a soft tissue density from the cavernous sinus. With a history of trauma and a diagnosis of carotid cavernous fistula, the possibility of a pseudoaneurysm or tense venous pouch expanding into the sphenoid sinus must be considered, raising the risk of life-threatening epistaxis from that site. The right common carotid artery arteriogram (not shown) demonstrated complete occlusion of the right internal carotid artery. The carotid cavernous fistula filled via the right posterior communicating artery from the left vertebral artery injection **(B)**. Contrast flows from the right posterior cerebral artery to the supraclinoid internal carotid artery. A distended cavernous sinus drains exclusively to a massively distended superior ophthalmic vein. Despite the torrential rate of flow in the superior ophthalmic vein, the patient's proptosis was mild.

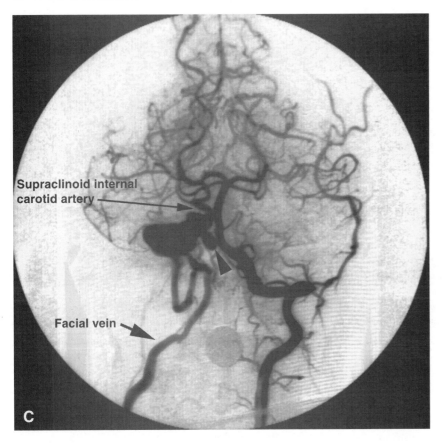

Figure 18.9. *(continued)* This was because of prompt drainage to the facial vein, seen on the Townes view **(C)**. On this view, a medially projecting pouch **(arrowhead)** from the genu of the internal carotid artery is seen, correlating with the CT appearance in A. Because of the possibility of massive epistaxis from the pouch or pseudoaneurysm, urgent embolization was undertaken. The first treatment was deployment of thrombogenic coils in the cavernous sinus and cavernous internal carotid artery via the posterior communicating artery. This resulted in occlusion of the fistula. However, an anterior pocket of the fistula recanalized 2 weeks later. Access to the recurrent pocket was gained by surgical exposure of the superior ophthalmic vein. The superior ophthalmic vein was catheterized retrogradely, and the remaining fistula was occluded with more coils. The patient made a complete recovery.

2. What is the status of the remainder of that sinus and the other sinuses? Remember that to see these sinuses, injections of vessels not involved with the dural arteriovenous malformation will be necessary. For instance, injection of the contralateral internal carotid artery may provide crucial information about direction of flow in venous fields remote from, but affected by, a distant dural arteriovenous malformation. Similarly, complete opacification of the posterior fossa, including injection of the non-dominant vertebral artery, if necessary, is required to assure that all of the cerebellar cortical veins and petrosal veins of the posterior fossa have been visualized.

3. What is the status of adjacent cortical veins and are any veins draining into the diseased sinus?

4. What is the status of the deep venous drainage system?

5. Is there evidence of retrograde or stagnant flow in cortical veins?

Where transvenous occlusion of the involved sinus appears safe, this can be performed as the most effective endovascular approach by deploying fibered thrombogenic coils and occasionally balloons in a tightly packed configuration in the sinus lumen. In keeping with the understanding of the disease as one related to abnormal venous pressures, it is important to take stock of the anatomy before treatment so as not to exacerbate the flow pattern even temporarily during coil deployment.

For instance, consider a cavernous sinus dural arteriovenous malformation that is draining anteriorly to a superior ophthalmic vein in combination with drainage laterally to a sphenoparietal sinus or centrally to an uncal vein. Transarterial embolization of ophthalmic artery meningeal branches and of internal carotid artery branches would probably be ineffective and unsafe. Endovascular treatment could involve transvenous catheterization of the inferior petrosal sinus and packing of the cavernous sinus with thrombogenic coils. However, this particular dural arteriovenous malformation may develop serious intraprocedural complications if the cavernous sinus is packed in a standard anterior to posterior manner. After occlusion of flow to the anteriorly located superior ophthalmic vein, the pressure on the alternative drainage route, a cortical vein, may increase raising the possibility of a venous infarction before there is time to occlude the malformation completely.

Therefore, where faced with the possibility of diversion of flow into critical vessels, it is important to modify one's therapeutic approach to reduce this risk by eliminating flow to the critical vein first. This assumes a centrifugal flow away from the dural arteriovenous malformation in this vein. Pretreatment flow in a critical vein towards the dural arteriovenous malformation precludes this approach completely.

CAROTID-CAVERNOUS FISTULAS

Dural arteriovenous malformations of the cavernous sinus and carotid-cavernous fistulas may present with similar clinical symptoms and signs of bruit, chemosis, exophthalmos, headache, ophthalmoplegia, or antecedent history of head trauma. At a glance, the angiographic appearance of a common carotid angiogram in both conditions may appear similar. Therefore, these two disorders are frequently subclassified into one category, as two subtypes of a common entity. However, it is probably more enlightening to dissociate the two. A dural arteriovenous malformation of the cavernous sinus is most easily understood as are dural arteriovenous malformations elsewhere in the cranial dura. A carotid-cavernous fistula, on the other hand, represents a rent in the wall of the cavernous internal carotid artery, which has established a direct arteriovenous fistula between the internal carotid artery and the venous spaces of the cavernous sinus.

An arteriovenous fistula between the cavernous internal carotid artery and the venous spaces of the cavernous sinus can result from a traumatic laceration of the artery or from rupture of a carotid cavernous aneurysm into the surrounding venous sacs. Post-traumatic carotid cavernous fistulas are particularly seen in young adult males for whom road accidents or physical battery are typical antecedent events (Figs. 18.9, 18.10, 18.11). Ruptured cavernous aneurysms are more likely to be seen in elderly or middle aged patients, more commonly seen in females than in males (27). Onset of symptoms is usually abrupt. The pattern and gravity of symptoms is determined by the venous anatomy of the compartment of the cavernous sinus into which the fistula has access. Commonly the ipsilateral cavernous sinus has free communication throughout its domain. Flow across the midline to the contralateral side through the intercavernous sinuses is common, such that fistulous flow commonly drains via the superior ophthalmic veins and inferior petrosal sinuses bilaterally. The clinical impact of a fistula is most commonly related to changes in flow in the superior ophthalmic vein. Venous hypertension in the orbit, proptosis and stretching of the optic nerve, chemosis and abrasion of the cornea, and retinal hemorrhages can make treatment of a carotid cavernous fistula an emergency. Less commonly, but also implying the most severe consequences, egress of arterialized venous blood from the cavernous sinus may be restricted such that all or most of the venous flow is directed into a cortical (uncal) vein or other venous structure which drains normal brain, e.g., the spheno-parietal sinus (28). The capacitance of the cortical venous channels thus involved cannot cope with the torrential flow-rates typically associated with a carotid-cavernous fistula. Therefore, complications such as venous hypertension of the deep venous system or venous infarcts may become the presenting signs (29).

In performing angiography in the setting of abnormal arterio-venous flow in the region of the cavernous sinus, the most important questions to answer include the following:

1. Establishing the correct diagnosis. A fistula from the internal carotid artery to the cavernous sinus ("direct type carotid cavernous fistula") must be distinguished from a dural arteriovenous malformation in the region of the cavernous sinus. Both disorders can give a similar clinical and venous appearance. Selective internal carotid artery and external carotid artery injections are necessary bilaterally. A high rate of filming may be necessary to study the fistula site. Sometimes, the most instructive images are those acquired by an indirect route, from the contralateral internal carotid artery or from the vertebral artery injections. These injections sometimes allow a glimpse of the fistula site by retrograde opacification of the supraclinoid internal carotid artery. The opacification of the cavernous sinus through this route is not so fulminant as to obscure visualization of the precise fistula site, as is frequently the case with ipsilateral internal carotid injections. A vertebral injection is necessary to evaluate collateral flow through the circle of Willis via the posterior communicating arteries, lest carotid occlusion should become a component of endovascular balloon-treatment of a fistula.

2. What is the status of the intracranial venous structures and is there evidence of transmission of venous hypertension to the deep venous system of the brain or to the sphenoparietal sinus?

3. Delayed venous images are helpful to study the status of the inferior petrosal sinuses and ophthalmic veins because transvenous endovascular therapy frequently uses these routes for treatment of dural arteriovenous malformations or carotid cavernous fistulas.

Treatment of Carotid-Cavernous Fistulas

Imaging and clinical features of carotid cavernous fistulas that indicate a need for urgent treatment include: evidence of venous hypertension affecting the intracranial venous system; increasing proptosis or diminishing visual acuity; increasing intraocular pressure; elevated intracranial pressure; rupture into the subarachnoid space; extension of a pseudoaneurysm or venous varix from the cavernous sinus into the subarachnoid space (30).

The treatment of choice for carotid cavernous fistulas is endovascular occlusion of the fistula with a detachable balloon device, while preserving flow in the internal carotid artery. Balloons are most commonly placed by a transarterial route. More than one balloon may be necessary on occasion. Transvenous balloon placement can be performed too, but is technically more difficult because the balloon advancement is against the direction of blood-flow (28). Transarterial or transvenous coil therapy is an alternative possibility, the latter being most commonly used for treatment of dural arteriovenous malformations adjacent to the cavernous sinus.

After endovascular balloon occlusion of a carotid cavernous fistula, spontaneous deflation of the balloon device is to be expected with most such balloons, over a period of weeks to months. Therefore, recanalization of a carotid cavernous fistula can occur. More commonly, deflation of the balloon sitting in the fistulous breach occasions delayed formation of a pouch or pseudoaneurysm at the site of the treated fistula, possibly in as many as 30% of cases (31).

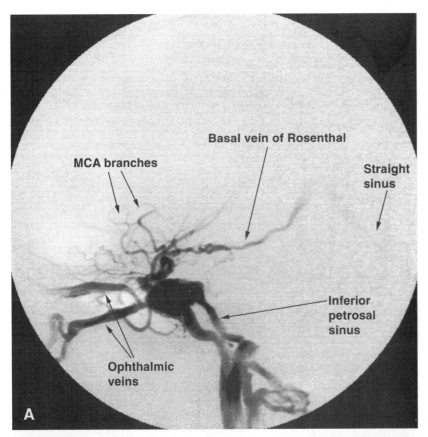

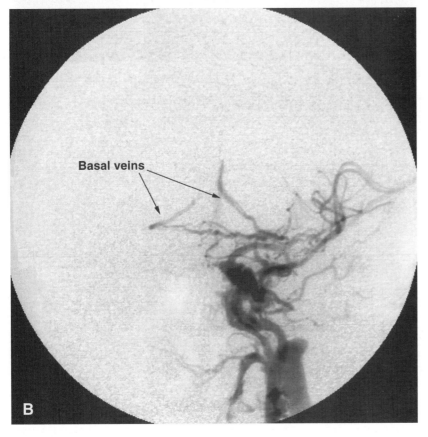

Figure 18.10. *Carotid-cavernous fistula after a motor vehicle accident.* A carotid cavernous fistula of the right internal carotid artery in a young adult after severe head trauma. In contrast to the case of Figure 18.9, this patient demonstrates opacification of the subarachnoid basal veins of Rosenthal, an alarming finding because of its implications for the risks of complications from venous hypertension and hemorhage. The inferior petrosal sinus is also opacified. Antegrade flow to the middle cerebral artery branches is diminished. A carotid cavernous fistula such as this is best treated by balloon occlusion of the fistula placed by an internal carotid approach.

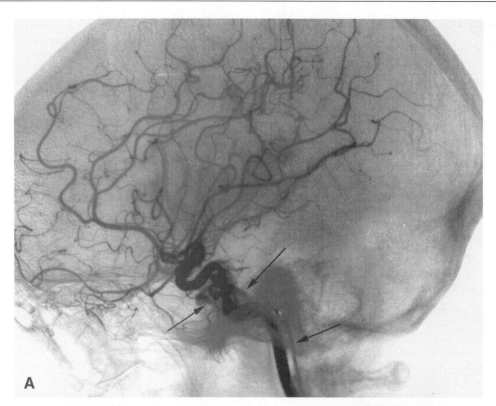

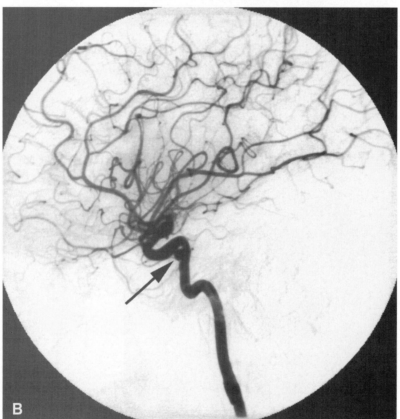

Figure 18.11. *Spontaneous regression of a carotid cavernous fistula.* A left internal carotid artery angiogram **(A)** in an elderly female with bruit and headaches after head trauma. A fistula from the precavernous internal carotid artery to the paracavernous veins and inferior petrosal sinus was present **(arrows in A)**. Three weeks later **(B)** the fistula had closed spontaneously leaving a residual pseudoaneurysm **(arrow in B)** at the site of traumatic tear in the internal carotid artery. A small pouch or pseudoaneurysm of this appearance is thought to be a common long-term event after balloon-occlusion of a carotid cavernous fistula because most balloons undergo a slow deflation over time.

INDIRECT OPACIFICATION OF HIGH FLOW LESIONS

When performing an angiographic study of a high-flow lesion such as a fistula, visual examination of the images is frequently frustrated by the immediacy and density of superimposed, distended venous structures. It can be difficult to see where exactly a fistulous rent might be or which vein is opacified first, etc. To circumvent this problem, it is frequently more informative to examine the *indirect* routes of arterial flow to the fistula.

The indirect route probably does not have as high a rate of flow and will often demonstrate a segment of the parent vessel not well seen on the direct images. For instance, when studying a carotid cavernous fistula of such a high rate of flow that all of the ipsilateral arterial flow is draining to the cavernous veins, then the likelihood of seeing the fistula itself is not high. However, flow through the ipsilateral posterior communicating artery or from the anterior communicating artery will opacify the supraclinoid internal carotid artery and drain retrogradely to the exact point of the fistula. Similarly, the exact site of an arterial laceration, such as with vertebro-venous fistulas, can frequently be most precisely located by a *contralateral refluxing* vertebral artery injection.

SPINAL DURAL ARTERIOVENOUS MALFORMATIONS

Various types of vascular malformations of the spine or related dura result in a myelographic appearance of distention of the coronal spinal venous plexus and of the medullary veins. However, this is the final common pathway or outcome of a variety of disparate processes. To understand these diseases, it is necessary to discern clearly between arteriovenous fistulas of the dura and intradural vascular malformations of the spinal cord itself. The pathophysiology, epidemiology, mechanism of cord injury, and treatment of these disorders differ substantially. Although both categories are rare diseases, dural vascular fistulas are probably more common than intradural vascular malformations (32, 33).

Pathophysiology of Spinal Dural Vascular Disease

The pathophysiology of dural or peridural arteriovenous malformations along the spine is similar to those of the cranial dura mater. The cranial dural layers separate at the foramen magnum to become the spinal dura and the periosteal dura of the spinal canal separated by the epidural space. Within the subarachnoid space, a venous retic-

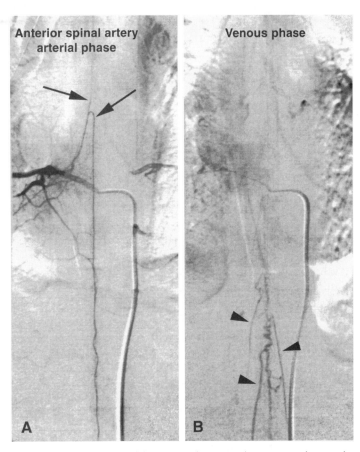

Figure 18.12. *Centrifugal medullary veins.* A young adult was studied to exclude the possibility of a spinal dural arteriovenous fistula as a cause for atypical back pain. An injection into a lower thoracic pedicle opacifies the anterior spinal artery **(arrows in A)**. Unusually prominent and tortuous veins around the conus **(B)** were eventually interpreted as representing a variant of normal because they opacified in normal phase with the remainder of venous structures of the injection. Drainage via the centrifugal medullary veins **(arrowheads in B)** was normal in timing and duration.

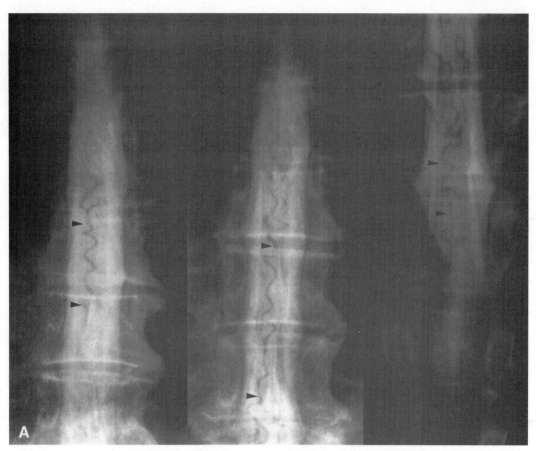

Figure 18.13. *Spinal dural AVF: myelographic and MRI appearance.* An elderly patient with a 6-month history of gait disturbance and lower extremity weakness, rapidly progressing in the weeks prior to diagnosis. Supine myelographic images **(A)** demonstrate distended serpentine subarachnoid veins covering the length of the cord **(arrowheads)**.

ulum called the coronary plexus covers the medullary surface of the spinal cord. In the normal state the coronary venous plexus of the spinal cord is protected against reflux from the epidural venous plexus so there is no connection between the arterial supply of the spinal dura or dura covered nerve roots on the one hand, and the medullary veins of the cord on the other. In other words, the venous territory of the spinal cord normally derives its supply only from the radiculomedullary (anterior spinal) or radiculopial (posterior spinal) arteries. A valve-mechanism has been proposed as an explanation for the insulation of the coronary plexus from pressure fluctuations in the epidural plexus (34).

The venous system of the spinal cord consists of posterior and anterior median longitudinal veins and a circumferential periphery of veins called the coronary plexus. Normal venous drainage away from these structures is via medullary veins, running in association with nerve roots, which drain normally in a centrifugal fashion to the epidural venous plexus (Fig. 18.12). Medullary veins are more common on the posterior aspect of the cord, and the posterior longitudinal vein is usually larger than its anterior counterpart (35, 36). Myelographic examinations are, therefore, more sensitive to abnormalities of these veins when performed in the *supine* position (Fig. 18.13).

Dural-related vascular malformations or fistulas result in an abnormal state of slow arteriovenous shunting into the medullary veins and coronary venous plexus of the cord. This results in venous hypertension in the cord. There is enlargement of the perimedullary veins, cord edema, and myelomalacia. The MRI appearance is one of prominently enlarged, enhancing intrathecal vessels, cord T2 hyperintensity, cord enhancement, and a variable appearance of mass-effect within the cord (Figs. 18.13, 18.14) (37).

Although most spinal dural arteriovenous fistulas are centered primarily within the spinal dura, epidural and intradural variants are seen occasionally (33, 38, 39). Fistulas form at the points where arterioles pierce the dura mater in close relation to dural veins, and can occur at any level from the foramen magnum to the sacrum (40). The malformation or fistula forms most commonly near the intervertebral foramen along the dural sleeve of a nerve root. The fistula is most commonly, but not always, located on the dorsal aspect of the nerve root near the axilla of the dural sleeve.

Intracranial dural arteriovenous malformations with restricted venous egress draining to the spinal veins can give an identical clinical presentation due to venous hypertension and edema of the spinal cord. Therefore, the intracranial vessels are included in the evaluation of patients with

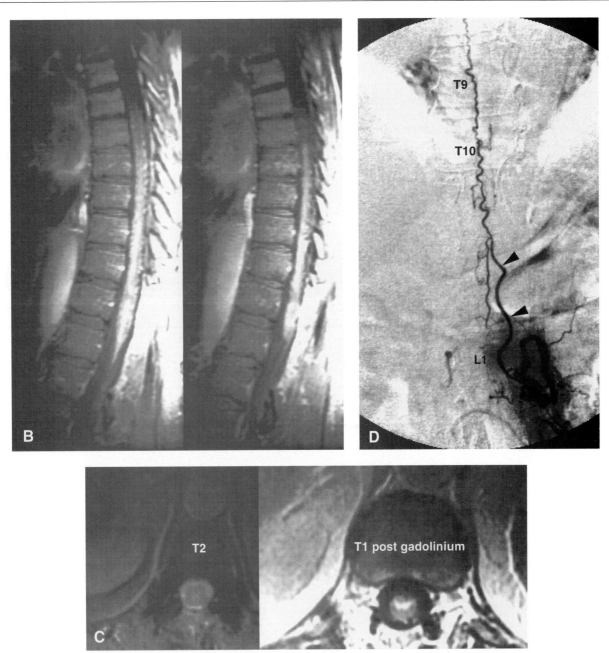

Figure 18.13. *(continued)* Sagittal T1-weighted MRI images **(B)** post-gadolinium demonstrate diffuse cord expansion and enhancement. Enhancing vessels are seen studding the surface of the cord, more prominent posteriorly. Axial images **(C)**, T2-weighted and enhanced T1 weighted, demonstrate characteristic expansion of the cord with central T2 bright signal and gadolinium enhancement. The spinal dural arteriovenous fistula was found on injection of the left L1 pedicle **(D)**. Contrast flows cephalad in the left L1 medullary vein **(arrowheads)** until it meets the coronary plexus of the spine. The veins seen on the myelographic images then become slowly opacified.

suspected spinal dural arteriovenous malformations (Fig. 18.15) (41, 42). Similarly, the internal iliac arteries are included to evaluate the sacral nerve roots (42).

Microangiographic studies of the most common type of dural arteriovenous malformation by McCutcheon et al. (43) demonstrate that the lesion is a usually a true arteriovenous fistula with one or two arterial feeders and a single draining medullary vein. Occasionally, the site of the shunt may be intradural or extradural (44). Venous drainage may also involve the epidural venous plexus in

a supplementary or exclusive manner (45–47). Paravertebral or pelvic vascular tumors, post traumatic fistulous injuries, and other conditions with arteriovenous shunting or high flow may connect to the medullary veins causing a radiographic and clinical presentation similar to that seen with dural vascular malformations (9, 48, 49).

The arteriolar rete or complex connected to the final fistulous arterial feeders can frequently draw from multiple adjacent or contralateral segmental pedicles. Therefore, treatment must allow for a propensity for ready recan-

Figure 18.14. *Epidural variant of spinal dural arteriovenous fistula.* An elderly patient presented with a 9-month history of progressive lower extremity weakness. Like many patients with this disease he underwent surgery with the assumption that his complaints were related to degenerative disc disease. Sagittal T2 and T1 **(A)** weighted images demonstrate expansion of the cord with elevated T2 signal. Flow-voids are seen along the surfaces of the cord, particularly in the upper thoracic region. A right L4 injection **(B)** demonstrates opacification of the coronary plexus of the spine via a fistulous malformation composed of a number of varicose pouches in the epidural space. The venous varix decompresses into the intradural space via the contralateral L4 medullary vein. A magnified oblique view **(C)** of the pedicle demonstrates the typical speckled angiographic appearance **(arrowhead)** of such small fistulas.

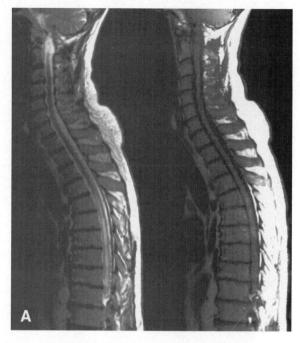

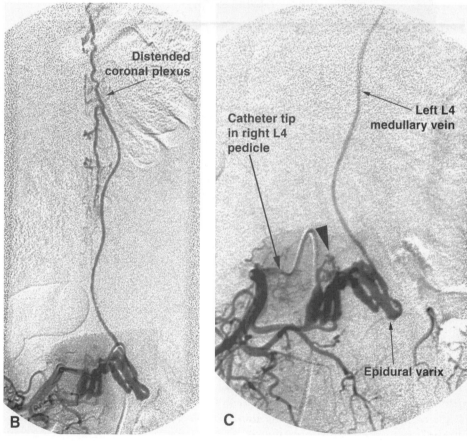

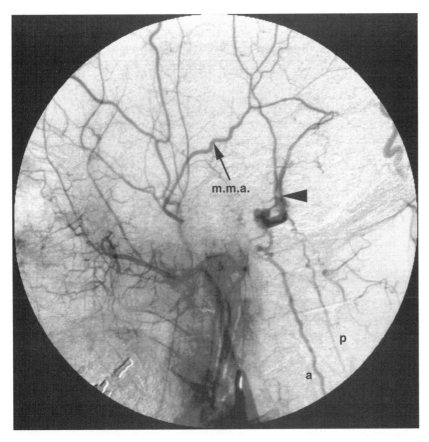

Figure 18.15. *Intracranial dural arteriovenous malformation presenting with a myelopathic syndrome.* A lateral view of the right external carotid artery injection performed at the end of a complete spinal angiogram in a middle-aged patient complaining of lower extremity weakness and MRI findings suggesting venous hypertension of the cord. A tiny dural fistula **(arrowhead)** from the distal middle meningeal artery (m.m.a.) is seen along the right sigmoid sinus draining into a restricted venous compartment. This results in distention of the anterior (a) and posterior spinal vein (p) causing the patient's symptoms.

alization. Surgical or endovascular treatment of spinal dural arteriovenous fistulas must aim to obliterate the arterial and venous components of the fistulas either by dural resection or permanent embolic occlusion. This usually includes cauterization, division, or sclerosis of the proximal segment of the draining medullary vein.

Clinical Manifestations of Spinal Dural Vascular Disease

Spinal dural arteriovenous fistulas are the most common vascular malformations of the spine. In contrast to the cranial variant of dural vascular malformation, most spinal dural arteriovenous fistulas drain directly into the subarachnoid vein(s) without initial opacification of the equivalent of the cranial dural venous sinus. However, epidural lakes or varices can be seen in some instances in which filling of the subarachnoid veins is secondary (Fig. 18.14).

It is a singular observation how minuscule and slow spinal dural fistulas may be in relation to the advanced incapacitation of the patient. The potential for clinical deterioration with such a small fistula rests in the relative physiologic restriction of venous outflow from the coronary plexus. This restriction limits the ability of the system to adapt to the pathologically increased state of venous flow. The veins of the spine normally drain out of the dural sac by a limited number of medullary centrifugal veins.

These are more common along the dorsal aspect of the spine than on the ventral aspect.

With increasing pressure and distention of the spinal veins, a decrease in the arteriovenous gradient of the spinal circulation takes place. Circulation time becomes prolonged. The effects of such an altered gradient are maximal at the farthest reach of the circulation, and in the case of the spine this occurs at the distal end of the spinal axis, i.e., the conus. Therefore patients will present with symptoms of a conal syndrome, although their fistulas may be remote from the conus.

Rare cases of paravertebral fistulas with exclusively epidural venous drainage have been described in which the coronary plexus is of normal pressure and caliber. In these instances, the symptoms of the fistula may be caused by compression of the cord or nerve roots by distended, tense epidural vessels (47, 50).

A shared feature of both dural and intradural arteriovenous malformations is the presence of distended draining subarachnoid veins on myelographic images. Publications describing spinal vascular diseases before the advent of selective spinal arteriography were therefore imprecise in terminology (compare the venous phases of Figs. 17.14 and 18.13). Spinal dural arteriovenous malformations are epidemiologically, pathophysiologically, anatomically, and clinically distinguishable from parenchymal arteriovenous malformations of the spine. Patients with spinal dural arteriovenous fistulas present in late middle-age or older (

40 years) and are more often male. They frequently have a history of progressive decline in gait, sensory function, strength, and loss of bladder and bowel control. Paresthesiae and subjective sensations of spasm in affected limbs are common, and muscle wasting with fasciculation is frequently seen (33). Hemorrhage into the epidural or subarachnoid spaces from a spinal dural arteriovenous fistula is rare. Symptoms may be aggravated by activity although this is not constant. The period of decline can range from a few months to 2–3 years. They can have a more rapid deterioration over some weeks, but it usually does not have the saltatory, episodic quality seen with intranidal hemorrhage of parenchymal arteriovenous malformations (51). Frequently, patients with advanced symptoms may spontaneously report a sensory level below which sensation is dulled. Hyperesthesia may be experienced as the disease process ascends along the trunk. Formerly such a subacute myelopathy would have been termed Foix-Alajouanine syndrome. This syndrome was described as a progressive myelopathy and was thought to be due to vascular thrombosis. However, in this context the term is imprecise and not commonly used.

Because the MRI and myelographic signs can be subtle and symptoms of dural vascular disease can be similar to more common conditions such as degenerative disc disease or spinal stenosis, these patients frequently are misdiagnosed. By the time of final angiographic diagnosis they often have had multiple imaging studies, myelograms, and even surgical procedures for symptoms of presumed spinal stenosis, disc compression, or spinal tumor. Myelography is sometimes insensitive to the presence of the serpentine intrathecal vessels which are the hallmark of this disease. MRI is the most sensitive noninvasive test for this disease. MRI demonstrates high T2 signal and patchy gadolinium enhancement in the conus, ascending in the cord. Gadolinium enhancement also accentuates the conspicuousness of distended venous structures. T2-weighted images and gadolinium-enhanced images demonstrate a characteristic pattern of serpentine vessels more numerous along the posterior aspect of the cord. However, motion artifact or too large a field of view will reduce the sensitivity of MRI to this disease.

Treatment of Spinal Dural Arteriovenous Malformations

Early surgical techniques for patients with spinal dural arteriovenous fistulas sometimes involved stripping an extended segment of vein from the spinal cord. This technique inherently involved a risk of depriving the cord of its normal venous drainage. Therefore the results were sometimes not favorable. Selective surgical clipping or cauterization of the single draining medullary vein identified at spinal angiography is the current treatment of choice (51). Depending on the degree and duration of preoperative decline, patients have variable prospects for recovery of premorbid function.

Given the tedious and protracted nature of spinal arteri-

Table 18.1.

Specific Surgical Information Required from Spinal Arteriography for Dural Vascular Fistulas

1. Location of the fistula, feeding pedicle, and neighboring vertebral body
2. Side of the fistula
3. How the vertebrae were counted
4. Presence of internal markers, e.g., coils, glue casts, etc.
5. Type of fistulaÐdural, epidural, perimedullary
6. Locations of the anterior and posterior spinal arteries

ography needed to identify a single tiny offending fistula, there is a strong desire to derive a double benefit from this procedure by combining it with therapeutic embolization (Table 18.1). If successful this can avoid the need for surgery and its attendant morbidity. However, to be effective the embolization needs to be permanent, and to be safe it needs to accomplish its effect without occluding the anterior or posterior spinal arteries. Early embolization techniques of spinal dural arteriovenous malformations using particulate matter such as polyvinyl alcohol, muscle fragments, or collagen were effective only in the short term. After initial clinical improvement patients experienced relapse after 2 to 8 months. Recanalization was seen at repeat angiography in most cases following use of these agents. Embolization with liquid acrylate carries the possibility of permanent sclerosis of the draining medullary vein. Propinquity of spinal arteries precluding embolization or capricious behavior of the acrylate gives a success rate for embolization somewhat less than that of surgery. However, when appended to a planned diagnostic procedure or as an interventional procedure with surgery as a fallback in the event of failure, it is a worthwhile undertaking. In situations where embolization is avoided due to the presence of dangerous connections, a radiographically dense coil can be placed in the feeding pedicle as a fluoroscopic landmark for subsequent surgery.

Concern about recanalization of the fistula should be prompted when a patient does not improve clinically after embolization or surgery. Transient improvement followed by relapse may also indicate that recanalization has taken place. Prompt repeat angiography is indicated for these patients. Rare cases of synchronous or metachronous anatomically separate lesions have been described (52).

REFERENCES

1. Nabors MW, Azzam CJ, Albanna FJ, et al. Delayed postoperative dural arteriovenous malformations. Report of two cases. J Neurosurg 1987;66:768–772.
2. Watanabe A, Takahara Y, Ibuchi Y, et al. Two cases of dural arteriovenous malformation occurring after intracranial surgery. Neuroradiology 1984;26:375–380.
3. Sakaki T, Morimoto T, Nakase H, et al. Dural arterio-venous fistula of the posterior fossa developing after surgical occlusion of the sigmoid sinus. J Neurosurg 1996;84:113–118.

4. Sundt TM, Piepgras DG. The surgical approach to arteriovenous malformations of the lateral and sigmoid dural sinuses. J Neurosurg 1983;59:32–39.

5. Mullan S. Reflections upon the nature and management of intracranial and intraspinal vascular malformations and fistulas. J Neurosurg 1994;80:606–616.

6. Yamashita K, Taki W, Nakahara I, et al. Development of sigmoid dural arterio-venous fistulas after transvenous embolization of cavernous dural arterio-venous fistulas. Am J Neuroradiol 1993; 14:1106–1108.

7. Djindjian R, Merland JJ. Superselective Arteriography of the External Carotid Artery. Berlin: Springer-Verlag, 1978.

8. Lalwani AK, Dowd CF, Halbach VV. Grading venous restrictive disease in patients with dural arteriovenous fistulas of the transverse/sigmoid sinus. J Neurosurg 1993;79:11–15.

9. Cognard C, Gobin YP, Pierot L, et al. Cerebral dural arteriovenous fistulas: clinical and angiographic correlation with a revised classification of venous drainage. Radiology 1995;194: 671–680.

10. Lasjaunias P, Chiu M, Ter Brugge K, et al. Neurological manifestations of intracranial dural arteriovenous malformations. J Neurosurg 1986;64:724–730.

11. Zeitman SM, Monsein LH, Arosarena O, et al. Reversibility of white matter changes and dementia after treatment of dural fistulas. Am J Neuroradiol 1995;16:1080–1083.

12. Ito M, Sonokawa T, Mishina H, et al. Reversible dural arteriovenous malformation-induced venous ischemia as a cause of dementia; treatment by surgical occlusion of draining dural sinus: case report. Neurosurgery 1995;37:1191–1192.

13. Nencini P, Inzitari G, Gibbs J, et al. Dementia with leukoaraiosis and dural arteriovenous malformation: clinical and PET case study. J Neurol Neurosurg Psychiatry 1993;56:929–931.

14. Bitoh S, Sasaki S. Spontaneous cure of dural arteriovenous malformation in the posterior fossa. Surg Neurol 1979;12:111–114.

15. Magidson MA, Weinberg PE. Spontaneous closure of a dural arteriovenous malformation. Surg Neurol 1976;6:107–110.

16. Baskaya MK, Suzuki Y, Seki Y, et al. Dural arteriovenous malformations in the anterior cranial fossa. Acta Neurochir (Wien) 1994;129:146–151.

17. Grisoli F, Vincentelli F, Fuchs S, et al. Surgical treatment of tentorial arteriovenous malformations draining into the subarachnoid space; report of four cases. J Neurosurg 1984;60: 1059–1066.

18. Awad IA, Little JR, Akarawi WP, et al. Intracranial dural arteriovenous malformations: factors predisposing to an aggressive neurological outcome. J Neurosurg 1990;72: 839–850.

19. Kikuchi K, Kowada M. Anterior fossa dural arteriovenous malformation supplied by bilateral ethmoidal arteries. Surg Neurol 1994;41:56–64.

20. Kobayashi H, Hayashi M, Noguchi Y, et al. Dural arteriovenous malformations in the anterior cranial fossa. Surg Neurol 1988; 30:396–401.

21. Espinosa JA, Mohr G, Robert F. Dural arteriovenous malformation of the ethmoidal region. British J Neurosurg 1993;7: 431–435.

22. Kaplan SS, Ogilvy CS, Crowell RM. Incidentally discovered arteriovenous malformation of the anterior fossa dura. Br J Neurosurg 1994;8:755–759.

23. Brown RD, Wiebers DO, Nichols DA. Intracranial dural arteriovenous fistulae: angiographic predictors of intracranial hemorrhage and clinical outcome in nonsurgical patients. J Neurosurg: 1994;81: 531–538.

24. Halbach VV, Higashida RT, Hieshima GB, et al. Transvenous embolization of dural fistulas involving cavernous sinus. Am J Neuroradiol 1989;10:377–383.

25. Halbach VV, Higashida RT, Hieshima GB, et al. Transvenous embolization of dural fistulas involving transverse and sigmoid sinuses. Am J Neuroradiol 1989;10:385–392.

26. Halbach VV, Higashida RT, Hieshima GB, et al. Treatment of dural fistulas involving the deep cerebral venous system. Am J Neuroradiol 1989;10:393–399.

27. Lewis AI, Tomsick TA, Tew JM. Management of 100 consecutive direct carotid cavernous fistulas: results of treatment with detachable balloons. Neurosurgery 1995;36:239–245.

28. Halbach VV, Higashida RT, Hieshima GB, et al. Transvenous embolization of direct carotid cavernous fistulas. Am J Neuroradiol 1988;9:741–747.

29. Lin TK, Chang CN, Wai YY. Spontaneous intracerebral hematoma from occult carotid cavernous fistula during pregnancy and puerperium. J Neurosurg 1992;76:714–717.

30. Halbach VV, Hieshima GB, Higashida RT, et al. Carotid cavernous fistulas: indications for urgent treatment. Am J Neuroradiol 1987;8:627–633.

31. Moret J. Commentary on: Lewis AI, Tomsick TA, Tew JM. Management of 100 consecutive direct carotid cavernous fistulas: results of treatment with detachable balloons. Neurosurgery 1995;36:239–245.

32. Kendall BE, Logue V. Spinal epidural angiomatous malformations draining into intrathecal veins. Neuroradiology 1977;13: 181–189.

33. Rosenblum B, Oldfield EH, Doppman JL, et al. Spinal arteriovenous malformations: a comparison of dural arteriovenous fistulas and intradural AVMs in 81 patients. J Neurosurg 1987;67: 795–802.

34. Tadie M, Hermet J, Aaron CL, et al. Le dispositif protecteur antireflux des veines de la moelle. Neurochirurgie 1979;25; 28–30.

35. Fried LC, Doppman JL, DiChiro G. Venous phase in spinal cord angiography. Acta Radiol 1971;11:393–401.

36. Thron AK. Vascular Anatomy of the Spinal Cord: Neuroradiological Investigations and Clinical Syndromes. New York, NY: Springer-Verlag, 1988;7:13–64.

37. Gilbertson JR, Miller GM, Goldman MS, et al. Spinal dural arterio-venous fistulas: MR and Myelographic appearance. Am J Neuroradiol 1995;16:2049–2057.

38. Oldfield EH, DiChiro G, Quindlen EA, et al. Successful treatment of a group of spinal cord arteriovenous malformations by interruption of dural fistula. J Neurosurg 1983;59:1019–1030.

39. Oldfield EH, Doppman JL. Spinal arteriovenous malformations. Clin Neurosurg 1988;34:161–183.

40. Gaensler EHL, Jackson DE, Halbach VV. Arterio-venous fistula of the cervicomedullary junction as a cause of myelopathy: radiographic findings in two cases. Am J Neuroradiol 1990;11: 518–521.

41. Gobin YP, Rogopoulos A, Aymard A, et al. Endovascular treatment of intracranial dural arterio-venous fistulas with spinal perimedullary venous drainage. J Neurosurg 1992;77:718–723.

42. Partington MD, Rüfenacht DA, Marsh WR, et al. Cranial and sacral dural arterio-venous fistulas as a cause of myelopathy. J Neurosurg 1992;76:615–622.

43. McCutcheon IE, Doppman JL, Oldfield EH. Microvascular anatomy of dural arteriovenous abnormalities of the spine: a microangiographic study. J Neurosurg 1996;84:214–220.

44. Arnaud O, Bille F, Pouget J, et al. Epidural arterio-venous fistula with perimedullary venous drainage: case report. Neuroradiology 1994;36:490–491.

45. Heier LA, Lee BCP. A dural spinal arteriovenous malformation with epidural venous drainage: a case report. Am J Neuroradiol 1987;8:561–563.

46. Cahan LD, Higashida RT, Halbach VV, et al. Variants of radiculomeningeal vascular malformations of the spine. J Neurosurg 1987;66:333–337.

47. Willinsky R, Terbrugge K, Montanera W, et al. Spinal epidural arterio-venous fistulas: Arterial and venous approaches to embolization. Am J Neuroradiol 1993;14:812–817.

48. Han S, Love M, Simeone F. Diagnosis and treatment of a lumbar extradural arteriovenous malformations. Am J Neuroradiol 1987;8:1129–1130.

49. Kim DI, Choi IS, Berenstein A. A sacral dural arterio-venous fistula presenting with intermittent myelopathy aggravated by menstruation. J Neurosurg 1991;75:947–949.

50. Kohno M, Takahashi H, Ide K, et al. A cervical dural arterio-venous fistula in a patient presenting with radiculopathy. J Neurosurg 1996;84:119–123.

51. Symon L, Kuyama H, Kendall B. Dural arteriovenous malformations of the spine. Clinical features and surgical results in 55 cases. J Neurosurg 1984;60:238–247.

52. Pierot L, Vlachopoulos T, Attal N, et al. Double spinal dural arterio-venous fistulas. Report of two cases. Am J Neuroradiol 1993;14:1109–1112.

CHAPTER 19

Other Vascular Diseases

FIBROMUSCULAR DYSPLASIA

Fibromuscular dysplasia is a segmental, non-atheromatous disease of intermediate sized vessels that may affect the extracranial or intracranial cerebral vasculature. Disease-related changes in the fibrous and smooth muscle components of arterial walls have been divided into three histopathologic subtypes. Medial fibromuscular dysplasia (80–90%) is characterized by a fibroblastic proliferation or thickening of fibrous tissue and smooth muscle with destruction of the elastic lamina. Intimal fibroplasia (5–15%) involves elastic lamina destruction and thickening of the vessel intima. Periadventitial or periarterial fibroplasia (1–5%) affects only the adventitial layer (1).

Fibromuscular dysplasia is a disease that characteristically affects middle-age females, particularly in its medial form, but it can be seen in males, children, or adolescents. An autosomal dominant inheritance with incomplete penetrance in males has been suggested as likely in many patients (2). When it affects the cephalic circulation, it may be seen as an incidental finding at angiography, or it may present with hypertension, subarachnoid hemorrhage, or ischemic complications. Ischemic symptoms are related either to emboli from cervical disease or to direct involvement of the intracranial vessels. Large institutional series of cerebral angiograms have demonstrated an incidence of fibromuscular dysplasia of less than 1% (2–4). The disease may be progressive in some patients, but most patients seem to do well with medical rather than surgical management of arterial lesions (5).

Fibromuscular dysplasia of the extracranial vessels is much more common than intradural disease. Intracranial disease may be limited to the petrosal segment of the internal carotid artery or to the siphon. However, a high predilection for intracranial aneurysm formation and subarachnoid hemorrhage is a serious concern in these patients. The angiographic appearance of fibromuscular dysplasia in the cephalic vessels has been described by a number of authors (2, 3, 6). Extracranial fibromuscular dysplasia of the cephalic vessels has three typical appearances (6). Medial fibroplasia, the most common variant, typically affects the internal carotid artery at the C1-C2 level with sparing of the vessel proximally. More than 60% have bilateral internal carotid artery involvement, and 10% demonstrate involvement of the vertebral arteries. Medial fibroplasia is most commonly associated with an angiographic pattern of irregularly spaced concentric narrowings separated by segments of normal luminal diameter or by segments dem-

onstrating post-stenotic dilatation (Figs. 19.1, 19.2). This appearance is termed ''a string of beads'' or ''chaussettes en accordéon'' (baggy stockings) (7). Such an appearance is thought to be virtually pathognomonic of fibromuscular dysplasia (Fig. 19.3) and is seen in up to 80% of cases (6). Unifocal or multifocal tubular stenosis in which a smooth concentric narrowing extends over a longer segment of vessel is a less common angiographic appearance. It may be associated with post-stenotic dilatation. This is thought to be a less specific appearance that can be seen with other angiopathic diseases such as Takayasu's arteritis, tumor encasement, or arterial hypoplasia. Atypical or uncommon aspects of fibromuscular dysplasia in the cephalic vessels include eccentric, focal corrugations with or without diverticulum formation (8). Unifocal webs or septa near the carotid bifurcation may also be seen in the relative absence of other evidence of the disease. Webs may be either asymptomatic or become the site of thromboembolic complications (3, 9–11). Carotid webs usually respond well to surgery.

Intracranial arterial disease from fibromuscular dysplasia is less common than extracranial disease. It is seen in both the anterior and posterior circulations (6, 12), most commonly affecting the middle cerebral artery. Intracranial lesions have an angiographic appearance similar to that seen in the cervical vessels, including vessel occlusion and narrowing.

A more concerning association or complication of fibromuscular dysplasia in the intracranial circulation is the development of saccular aneurysms and subarachnoid hemorrhage. The incidence of intracranial aneurysms in this population has been estimated as between 20% and 50% of those patients with CNS symptoms (2, 6), with a high rate of multiple aneurysms in affected patients. There is a particular tendency for aneurysmal involvement of the middle cerebral artery in female patients. Arterial wall dissection is most likely the mechanism for subarachnoid hemorrhage in the absence of a saccular aneurysm in some of these patients. Subarachnoid hemorrhage was the presenting symptom in 15% of a series of patients reported by So et al. (3).

Mural dissection or aneurysm rupture undoubtedly also explain the recognized incidence of spontaneous arteriovenous fistulas in this disease affecting the carotid and vertebral arteries. This complication may present with carotid-cavernous fistulas or vertebro-venous fistulas (13–16). Some patients may have multiple mural dissec-

361

dition, such as fibromuscular dysplasia. The latter group had a greater likelihood of developing bilateral disease and complications of the disease such as dissecting aneurysms, which were less likely to resolve spontaneously.

EHLERS-DANLOS SYNDROME TYPE IV

Because of the considerable danger of a severe or fatal complication from angiography in patients with Ehlers-Danlos Syndrome Type IV, this condition, although rare, warrants a specific reference. Ehlers-Danlos syndrome, of which there are at least nine subtypes, is one of the most frequently inherited disorders of connective tissue. Approximately 4% of these patients belong to a heterogeneous group or subtype (Type IV), which is thought to have autosomal dominant and autosomal recessive modes of inheritance. The definitive diagnosis depends on demonstrating a deficiency of Type III collagen or procollagen in fibroblast cultures (18). Of the Ehlers-Danlos subtypes,

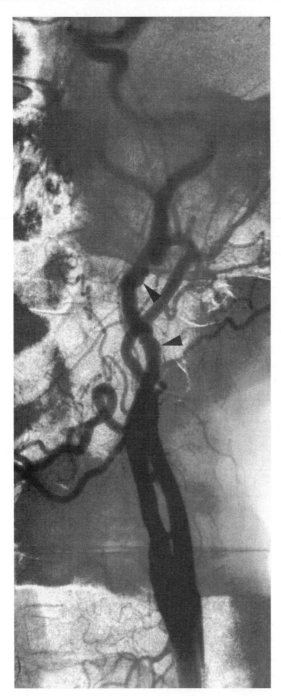

Figure 19.1. *Detection of asymptomatic fibromuscular dysplasia on common carotid arteriography.* An oblique view of the right common carotid artery injection in a middle-aged male being studied for other reasons. It demonstrates mild irregularity **(arrowheads)** of the internal carotid artery at the C1-C2 level characteristic of the changes seen in fibromuscular dysplasia.

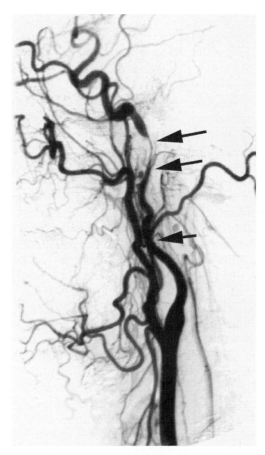

Figure 19.2. Fibromuscular dysplasia associated with dissection of the right internal carotid artery A middle-aged male presented with malignant hypertension. Visceral angiography demonstrated finding of fibromuscular dysplasia of the renal arteries with renal infarction. Subsequent development of a Wallenberg's syndrome prompted a cerebral angiogram which demonstrated further evidence of vessel irregularities. The right internal carotid artery has a corrugated appearance **(lowest arrow)** in the mid-cervical region, above which it tapers to a narrow dissection **(upper arrows)**. It resumes a normal caliber in the petrous segment. Both vertebral arteries also demonstrated dissections.

tions affecting many arteries; some care is warranted in puncture technique to avoid severe or fatal procedural complications such as retroperitoneal aortic rupture and iliac arterial occlusion (16). In a study of dissections of the cervical carotid arteries, Friedman et al. (17) drew a clinical distinction between patients with spontaneous unilateral carotid dissection and those with a predisposing con-

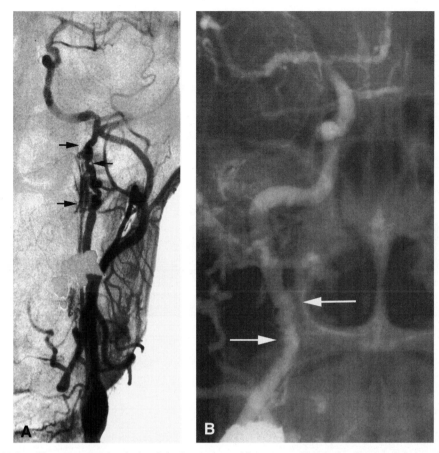

Figure 19.3. *Fibromuscular dysplasia of the internal carotid artery.* Notice the characteristic location of the diseased segments **(arrows)** in both examples at the C1-C2 level with sparing of the vessel more proximally.

only Type IV is a concern for arterial disease and angiographic complications, although multiple intracranial aneurysm formation in the setting of radiation therapy has been reported with other sub-types (19).

The peripheral stigmata in Type IV ("arterial-ecchymotic type") may be subtle or absent so that the individual may be completely unaware of the condition until the onset of a vascular complication. Peripheral signs, if present, in this subgroup of patients include slight hypermobility of the digits, thin elastic skin, and prominent visibility of the subcutaneous vasculature with easy bruisability. There may be a family history available, which would spark suspicion of such a disorder. The patient may have a medical history of spontaneously resolving past aneurysms elsewhere, such as the radial artery, tibial artery, superficial temporal artery, etc. (Fig. 19.4).

With disease complications involving major vessels, the prognosis is poor with a high preoperative or perioperative mortality of more than 60% (20, 21). In a review of the literature Cikrit et al. (21) reported that mortality before the age of 40 years was more than 50% and was related to spontaneous arterial perforations, bowel perforations, or other catastrophic vascular events. Angiography is best avoided if at all possible in this condition due to the risk of vessel rupture at the site of puncture, or at any arterial

site of wire or catheter navigation. Cikrit et al. (21) reported a complication rate of almost 70%, including some fatalities, in this group of patients during angiography.

Ehlers-Danlos Type IV patients may be referred for neuroangiography because of the high rate of spontaneous complications involving the cerebral vasculature in this population. These complications include multiple intracranial aneurysms, dissections and pseudoaneurysms of the cervical vessels, and spontaneous carotid cavernous fistulas (22, 23).

MOYA-MOYA

Moya-Moya disease is a progressive bilateral occlusive state of the distal internal carotid artery and of the proximal segments of the middle cerebral and anterior cerebral arteries. In its primary form it is bilateral but asymmetric and is characterized late in its course by a profusion of collateral vascular pathways around the basal ganglia and brainstem (Figs. 19.5, 19.6) (24). Multiple, enlarged and chaotic appearing thalamoperforator and lenticulo-striate vessels are typically seen, as are transdural external carotid-internal carotid and pial-pial collateral vessels.

Cases of unilateral disease are more commonly seen when a cause can be identified. These include cases after inflammatory arteritis and tuberculous meningitis (25),

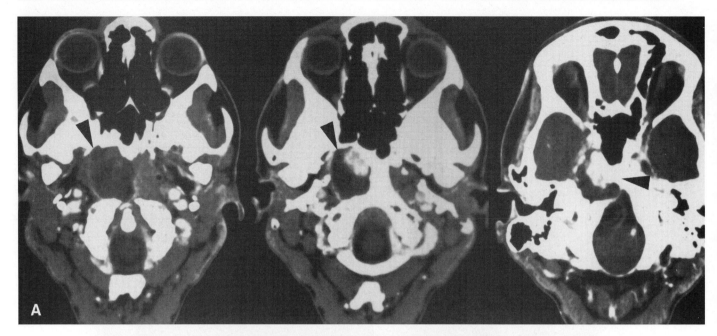

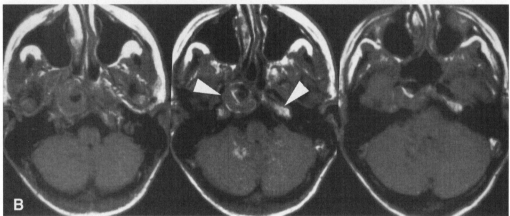

Figure 19.4.   *Multiple spontaneous dissections and aneurysms.* A middle-aged female with a presumed variant of Ehlers-Danlos Type IV Disease. She had a strong family history of aneurysms and sudden death at a young age. She presented with severe headache related to an expanding aneurysm of the right internal carotid artery. A contrast-enhanced CT **(A)** of the skull-base demonstrates remodeling of the floor of the middle cranial fossa by a centrally enhancing aneurysm **(arrowheads)** with surrounding low density thrombus. Gadolinium-enhanced axial T1-weighted MRI images **(B)** demonstrate T1 bright signal within the petrous segments of the left and right internal carotid arteries **(arrowheads).**

thromboembolic or occlusive events (26), and childhood irradiation of the base of brain for tumors in the region of the sella and other neoplasms (27).

Two peaks of incidence are described, in the first decade and in the fourth decade (28). Children are prone to focal hemispheric deficits due to ischemia; adults are more vulnerable to hemorrhagic complications. Bleeding may be subarachnoid or intraparenchymal. Vascular epiphenomena associated with Moya-Moya include formation of saccular aneurysms (29), dissections (30), and arteriovenous malformations (31).

CEREBRAL SINUS AND VENOUS THROMBOSIS

Since the advent of MRI, conventional angiography has had a lesser role in the diagnosis of cerebral venous throm-

bosis. This is an uncommon disease that can present with headache, elevated intracranial pressure, venous infarcts and hemorrhage, seizure, and other focal deficits (Fig. 19.7). The nature of etiologic factors causing predisposing hypercoagulability varies among populations. Puerperal cerebral venous thrombosis is an important cause of maternal mortality in some countries such as India (32). Behçet's disease is an important predisposing condition in Saudia Arabia (33). Screening for protein S, protein C, antithrombin III deficiency, and for antiphospholipid antibodies is routinely pursued in most cases. Recent series have estimated an acute mortality rate ranging between 5 and 30% (34–6), but in general for those patients treated with anticoagulation, mortality is mostly related to the underlying predisposing disease. Long-term follow-up of patients presenting with cerebral venous thrombosis reveals

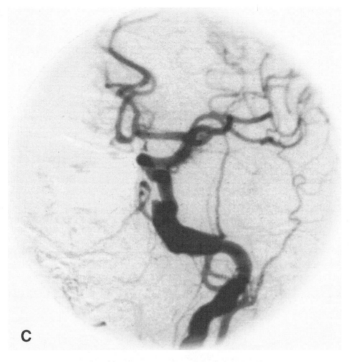

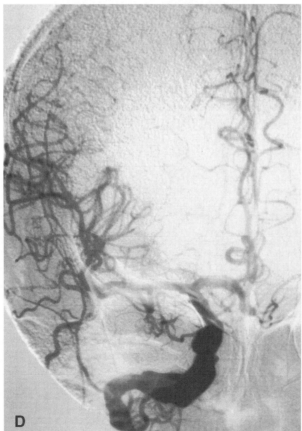

Figure 19.4. *(continued)* AP views of the left **(C)** and right **(D)** internal carotid artery show the patent lumen of the aneurysms of the cervical and petrous segments. Within a few weeks of these studies, the patient died unexpectedly from spontaneous cardiac tamponade.

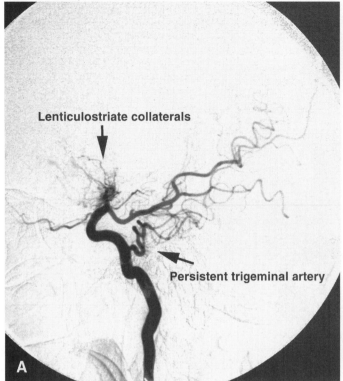

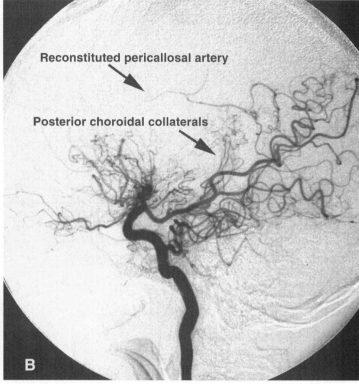

Figure 19.5. *Moya-Moya disease.* A young adult patient with ischemic hemispheric symptoms was found to have an occlusive Moya-Moya pattern of the supraclinoid right internal carotid artery. Tortuous collateral enlargement of lenticulostriate and choroidal vessels is seen on these sequential lateral views. Reconstitution of the distal anterior cerebral artery via the perisplenial branch of the posterior cerebral artery is well demonstrated in **(B).** A persistent trigeminal artery contributes to the posterior fossa **(A).** (see Fig. 13.16 for PA view).

Figure 19.6. *Moya-Moya occlusive pattern in a patient with sickle-cell disease.* A Moya-Moya pattern is seen in the lenticulostriate branches on the lateral view of the right internal carotid artery in a young adult male with severe sickle-cell disease and a right hemispheric arteriovenous malformation. Dural-pial collaterals from the ophthalmic artery and middle meningeal artery are prominently seen **(arrowheads)** contributing to collateral flow to the hemisphere.

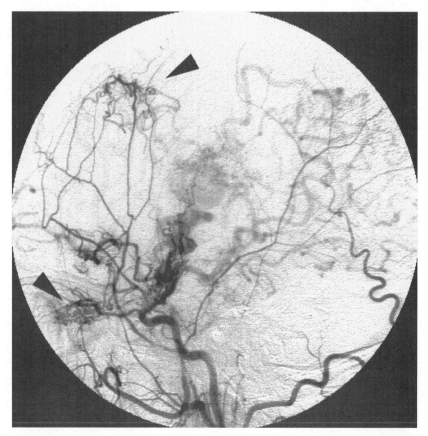

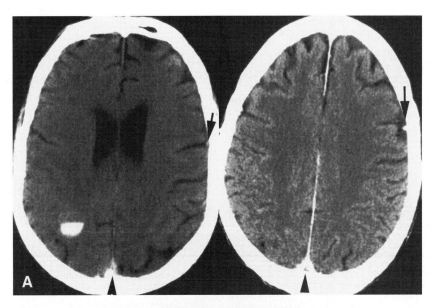

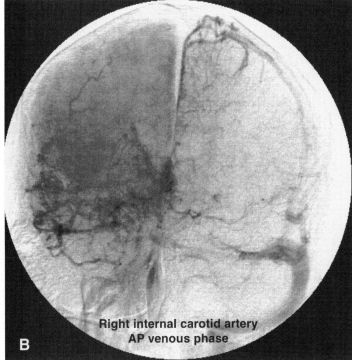

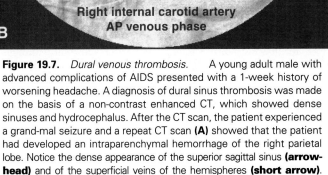

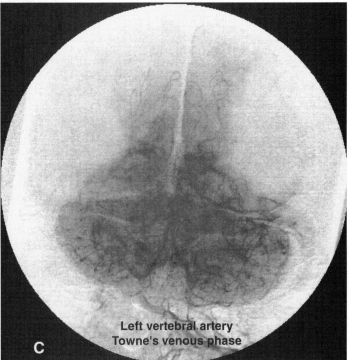

Figure 19.7. *Dural venous thrombosis.* A young adult male with advanced complications of AIDS presented with a 1-week history of worsening headache. A diagnosis of dural sinus thrombosis was made on the basis of a non-contrast enhanced CT, which showed dense sinuses and hydrocephalus. After the CT scan, the patient experienced a grand-mal seizure and a repeat CT scan **(A)** showed that the patient had developed an intraparenchymal hemorrhage of the right parietal lobe. Notice the dense appearance of the superior sagittal sinus **(arrowhead)** and of the superficial veins of the hemispheres **(short arrow)**.

Angiography of the carotid **(B)** and vertebral arteries **(C)** demonstrated that there was complete thrombosis of virtually all of the dural sinuses and no filling of the superficial veins of the right hemisphere. Superficial veins of the left hemisphere are present but stagnant. Because of his worsening condition, a decision was made to thrombolyze the sinuses. This was accomplished transvenously with 1 million units of urokinase (see Chapter 21). The patient made a satisfactory recovery from this particular complication of his underlying condition.

a 15% incidence of neurologic morbidity due to persistent seizures, optic atrophy after elevated intracranial pressure, development of dural arteriovenous malformations, or recurrent thrombosis (37).

Transvenous thrombolysis of the sinuses can be accomplished in cases in which medical treatment is failing. Dose regimens may be either an acute infusion similar to cerebral arterial thrombolysis or prolonged over hours or days similar to peripheral arterial thrombolysis. Although the angiographic results are satisfactory in both instances, the influence of this procedure on patient outcome compared with conservative medical therapy is not established (38, 39).

REFERENCES

1. Sato S, Hata J. Fibromuscular dysplasia. Its occurrence with a dissecting aneurysm of the interior carotid artery. Arch Pathol Lab Med 1982;106:332–335.

2. Mettinger KL, Ericson K. Fibromuscular dysplasia and the brain. Observations on angiographic, clinical, and genetic characteristics. Stroke 1982;13:46–52.

3. So EL, Toole JF, Dalal P, et al. Cephalic fibromuscular dysplasia in 32 patients. Clinical findings and radiologic features. Arch Neurol 1981;38:619–622.

4. Corrin LS, Sandok BA, Houser OW. Cerebral ischemic events in patients with carotid artery fibromuscular dysplasia. Arch Neurol 1981;38:616–618.

5. Mettinger KL. Fibromuscular dysplasia and the brain. II. Current concept of the disease. Stroke 1982;13:53–58.

6. Osborn AG, Anderson RE. Angiographic spectrum of cervical and intracranial fibromuscular dysplasia. Stroke 1977;8: 617–626.

7. Manelfe C, Clarisse J, Fredy D, et al. Dysplasie fibromusculaire des artères cervico-céphaliques à propos de 70 cas. J Neuroradiol 1974;1:149–321.

8. Houser OW, Baker HL. Cephalic arterial fibromuscular dysplasia. Radiology 1971;101:605–611.

9. Rainer WG, Cramer GG, Newby JP, et al. Fibromuscular dysplasia of the carotid artery causing positional cerebral ischemia. Ann Surg 1968;167:444–446.

10. So EL, Toole JF, Moody DM, et al. Cerebral embolism from septal fibromuscular dysplasia of the common carotid artery. Ann Neurol 1976;6:75–78.

11. Morgenlander JC, Goldstein LB. Recurrent transient ischemic attacks and stroke in association with an internal carotid artery web. Stroke 1991;22:94–98.

12. Frens DB, Petajan JH, Anderson R, et al. Fibromuscular dysplasia of the posterior cerebral artery: Report of a case and review of the literature. Stroke 1974;5:161–166.

13. Hieshima GB, Cahan LD, Mehringer CM, et al. Spontaneous arteriovenous fistulas of cerebral vessels in association with fibromuscular dysplasia. Neurosurgery 1986;18:454–458.

14. Bonduelle M, Ruscalleda J, Zalgal P. Dysplasie fibromusculaire avec fistule arterio-veineuse de l'artère vertébrale extra-crânienne. Rev Neurol (Paris) 1973;128:203–206.

15. Geraud J, Manelfe C, Caussanel JP, et al. Fistule artério-veineuse spontanée de l'artère vértébrale. Rôle éventuel de la dysplasie fibro-musculaire dans sa pathogénie. Rev Neurol (Paris) 1973; 128:206–213.

16. Bellot J, Gherardi R, Poirier J, et al. Fibromuscular dysplasia of cervico-cephalic arteries with multiple dissections and a carotid-

17. Friedman WA, Day AL, Quisling RG, et al. Cervical carotid dissecting aneurysms. Neurosurgery 1980;7:207–214.

18. Dunmore PJ, Roach MR. The effects of age, vessel size, and Ehlers-Danlos type IV on the waviness index of arteries. Clin Invest Med 1990;13:67–70.

19. Holodny AI, Deck M, Petito CK. Induction and subsequent rupture of aneurysms of the circle of Willis after radiation therapy in Ehlers-Danlos Syndrome: A plausible hypothesis. Am J Neuroradiol 1996;17:226–232.

20. Krog M, Almgren B, Eriksson I, et al. Vascular complications in the Ehlers-Danlos Syndrome. Acta Chir Scand 1983;149: 279–282.

21. Cikrit DF, Miles JH, Silver D. Spontaneous arterial perforation: The Ehlers-Danlos specter. J Vasc Surg 1987;5:248–255.

22. Rubinstein MK, Cohen MH. Ehlers-Danlos syndrome associated with multiple intracranial aneurysms. Neurology 1964;14: 125–132.

23. Imahori S, Bannerman RM, Graf CJ, et al. Ehlers-Danlos syndrome with multiple arterial lesions. Am J Med 1969;47: 967–977.

24. Suzuki J, Takaku A. Cerebro-vascular "moya-moya" disease. Disease showing abnormal net-like vessels in the base of brain. Arch Neurol 1969;20:288–299.

25. Mathew NT, Abraham J, Chandy J. Cerebral angiographic features of tuberculous meningitis. Neurology 1970;20: 1015–1023.

26. Zulch KJ, Dreesbach HA, Eschbach O. Occlusion of the middle cerebral artery with the formation of an abnormal arterial collateral system—moyamoya type—23 months later. Neuroradiology 1974;7:19–24.

27. Bitzer M, Topka H. Progressive cerebral occlusive disease after radiation therapy. Stroke 1995;26:131–136.

28. Hardy RC, Williams RG. Moyamoya disease and cerebral hemorrhage. Surg Neurol 1984;21:507–510.

29. Yabumoto M, Funahashi K, Fujii T, et al. Moyamoya disease associated with intracranial aneurysms. Surg Neurol 1983;20: 20–24.

30. Yamashita M, Tanaka K, Matsuo T, et al. Cerebral dissecting aneurysms in patients with moyamoya disease. J Neurosurg 1983;58:120–125.

31. Lichtor T, Mullan S. Arteriovenous malformation in moyamoya syndrome. J Neurosurg 1987;67:603–608.

32. Srinavasan K. Ischemic cerebrovascular disease in the young: two common causes in India. Stroke 1984;15:733–735.

33. Daif A, Awada A, Al-Rajeh S, et al. Cerebral venous thrombosis in adults. A study of 40 cases from Saudia Arabia. Stroke 1995; 26:1193–1195.

34. Bousser MG, Chiras J, Bories J, et al. Cerebral venous thrombosis: a review of 38 cases. Stroke 1985;16:199–213.

35. Thron A, Wessel K, Linden D, et al. Superior sagittal sinus thrombosis: neuroradiological evaluation and clinical findings. J Neurol 1986;233:283–288.

36. Ameri A, Bousser MG. Cerebral venous thrombosis. Neurol Clin 1992;10:87–111.

37. Preter M, Tzourio C, Ameri A, et al. Long-term prognosis in cerebral venous thrombosis. Stroke 1996;27:243–246.

38. Scott JA, Pascuzzi RM, Hall PV, et al. Treatment of dural sinus thrombosis with local urokinase infusion. Case report. J Neurosurg 1988;68:284–287.

39. Smith TP, Higashida RT, Barnwell SL, et al. Treatment of dural sinus thrombosis by urokinase infusion. Am J Neuroradiol 1994; 15:801–807.

cavernous fistula. A pathological study. Stroke 1985;16: 255–261.

PART IV / INTRODUCTION TO INTERVENTIONAL NEURORADIOLOGY AND EMERGENCY PROCEDURES

CHAPTER 20

Interventional Techniques, Devices, and Materials

MICROCATHETERS

There are two categories of microcatheters available for interventional neuroradiologic procedures, discrimination of which is determined by their principles of navigation. Flow-directed catheters are manufactured such that the distal section of the catheter is made of a polymer blend so supple that its progress within the intracranial circulation is determined by the drag of blood-flow. Wire-directed microcatheters are also of a pliable composition with a soft tip to prevent endothelial damage. They are stiffer than flow-directed microcatheters, and for intracranial navigation are advanced over a steerable microwire. Hybrid microcatheters that combine some advantages of the two categories are available.

Hydrophilically Coated Microcatheters

Hydrophilic coating of both types of microcatheters is available. Hydrophilically coated materials adsorb surrounding fluid with a reduction of friction or drag during manipulation. They must be kept soaked with saline when not in use, or they become sticky and difficult to manage. Hydrophilic coating has a discernible impact on microcatheter performance in navigating distal curves and loops. This is an advantage while en route to the desired target, but by virtue of the reduction of friction with the surrounding vessel, the attitude of the microcatheter in its final position can be extremely unstable. Therefore, the microcatheter might easily be dislodged from position if the shaft becomes stuck to one's glove during manipulation, for instance, or by the jet-effect of a contrast injection. Alternatively, forward tension within the microcatheter may spontaneously expend itself and cause a surge in the position of the microcatheter. This is a dangerous event if the microcatheter tip is close to or in a subarachnoid aneurysm. A compromise is reached by some manufacturers who apply hydrophilic coating to the distal part only of the catheter. Hydrophilic coating may also reduce the likelihood of a microcatheter tip becoming resolutely fixed within an embolus of acrylate, compared with non-hydrophilic varieties.

Some proprietary variations of hydrophilic coating cause an expansion of the diameter of the device with prolonged service. This can be a problem with hydrophilic wires, in particular, which have a tendency to swell and drag within the microcatheter. This effect can damage the inner surface of the microcatheter, causing problems with particle injection. Many microcatheters are of a multi-layered composition, which begins to disintegrate under prolonged duress. These layers may heap on one another like an accordion if dragged upon by an adherent or damaged wire. When this happens proximally within the introducer catheter, it is unlikely to cause harm if the whole system is removed immediately. However, similar damage to the microcatheter within an intracranial vessel could be disastrous.

Flow-Directed Microcatheters

Flow-directed microcatheters are used almost exclusively for embolization of brain arteriovenous malformations with acrylate material. Wire-directed microcatheters can be used for the same purpose but do not have the facility of flow-directed devices to gain extreme distal access. A fresh microcatheter is needed for each injection of glue in either instance. Flow-directed microcatheters are manufactured in a number of sizes between 1.5 Fr and 2 Fr outer diameter, and have a radioopaque distal marker. Occasionally, flow-directed microcatheters can be used to inject particles, but this is usually in the smaller range below 250–350 m.

Because the distal tip of a flow-directed microcatheter is so pliable its shape does not resist gravity. Therefore flow-directed microcatheters must by advanced within the introducing catheter on a supporting or navigation wire. With catheters advanced on a supporting wire not designed for intracranial use, it is important to halt the advance of the wire before the wire-tip exits the introducing catheter. Otherwise the possibility of vessel dissection or perforation might be countenanced.

Once the stiffer proximal shaft of the microcatheter is advanced out of the main catheter, the wire can be withdrawn completely. The microcatheter is then irrigated, cleaned, and injected with contrast. By steam-shaping a curve on the microcatheter before mounting it on the wire, more flexibility can be obtained in vessel-selection, once in the brain. The flow-guided microcatheter is advanced and allowed to select its own route by force of flow. Should it select an undesired route, jets of contrast from the microcatheter can be timed to force it to buckle and flow into an alternative channel.

Wire-Directed Microcatheters

Arteriovenous malformations apart, wire-directed microcatheters are the most commonly used for interventional procedures. A variety of designs, profiles, and sizes is available. They are all supplied with a radioopaque distal tip for visualization. It is extremely important, however, during embolization cases with Guglielmi detachable coils (GDC®) to start with a two-tip or double-marker microcatheter, which is required for this type of case. The proximal marker is used as a guide for halting the advancement of the coils.

Wire-guided microcatheters for intracranial use are usually 150 cm or longer in length, and the associated wires are 175–190 cm long. Two size ranges predominate, those with a 0.010″ ID and those with a 0.018″ ID. The 0.018″ variety is the most commonly used because it is the most steerable and allows a greater variety of embolic materials, particle sizes, and coils to be placed. PVA particles up to 1,000 m can be embolized through 0.018″ microcatheters. They may also be used to place Tracker 10 GDC coils, although there is some risk of the smaller caliber GDC coil bunching on itself within the 0.018″ lumen. The 0.018″ series of microcatheters is steered by a range of wires of 0.014–0.016″ caliber.

The 0.010″ microcatheters are limited to a smaller range of push-coils, GDC® coils of the Tracker 10 series, acrylate embolization, or particles of approximately 250 m. They are technically more difficult to control and steer. Because of the restricted lumen-size they give a less satisfactory injection-bolus for angiographic runs. However, they are considered by many interventionalists to be more gentle on the wall of subarachnoid aneurysms. The Tracker 10 GDC series of coils is considered safer for the same reason. They are steered with 0.010″ microwires, but for extra support and dirigibility, some larger wires up to 0.014″ will usually fit.

LOADING A WIRE-DIRECTED MICROCATHETER

Managing the loading of a microcatheter is invariably a two-person task. Bearing in mind that the total volume of most microcatheters is in the range of 0.4–0.6 mL, it is important to realize the potential for clot formation of significant dimensions or bubble embolization from microcatheters during the process of loading. Therefore, they must be flushed with heparinized saline before use and advanced with an eye towards preventing thrombus formation by undue delay.

Wire-directed microcatheters can be loaded through the Tuohy-Borst system without the support of a wire (see Fig. 2.18). Some interventionalists load these microcatheters on a navigation wire; others prefer to advance them to the end of the guiding catheter in a flushed state, with an assistant advancing saline or contrast from a 1 mL syringe mounted on the microcatheter.

Outside the body, microcatheters and microwires appear so delicate and slight of construction that it is difficult to presuppose a potential for harm. However, when confined within a guiding catheter and a narrow distal blood vessel, the axial loading of tension onto the tip of a microcatheter or wire can be considerable. Intracranial dissections and perforations do occur from these devices with

alarming ease and they should not be used intracranially without experienced guidance.

Furthermore, it is easy during intense periods of concentration on wire navigation to neglect how long the wire may have been in the microcatheter without a forward flush system running. Upon removal of the wire from an 0.018″ microcatheter, there should be slow blood return. If not evident as a rising meniscus within 5–10 seconds, a 1-ml syringe may be applied and aspirated gently. If there is not easy return from the intracranial circulation, remove the microcatheter. After what may have been a tedious navigation to get the microcatheter to its present position, there is a tremendous temptation to think that the microcatheter "only needs a little flush to get it going again." One must resist this lure. Frequently, when microcatheters are withdrawn from the body and injected forcefully after such an occlusion, a chastening yarn of thrombus will eject from the tip. This usually happens in association with a kink in the microcatheter. If the presence of a kink is confirmed, a new microcatheter should be unpacked. Kinks are difficult to see and are usually found distally by curving the microcatheter-tip between one's fingers.

Extended-tip Microcatheters

A microcatheter that sometimes causes misunderstandings and appears identical, at a glance, to a standard microcatheter is the extended-tip microcatheter. The difference is that the distal radioopaque marker is placed 5 mm proximally on the distal shaft. This is to allow the distal tip to be used for mounting a valve or ligature balloon, without interference from the extra bulk associated with the radioopaque marker.

The extended-tip microcatheter allows the retention of a shaped wire within the microcatheter during navigation of a balloon. In tortuous vessels, this has considerable advantages over other systems of balloon insertion.

Nycomed® Coaxial Microcatheter System

The alternative to an extended-tip microcatheter for balloon placement is a coaxial 2 Fr/3 Fr system of microcatheters, which is supplied on a supporting wire. The balloon is mounted on the red inner 2 Fr microcatheter, and the wire is removed rendering the inner 2 Fr catheter so flexible that it becomes effectively flow-directed. This is advanced into position, and the balloon is inflated. The black outer 3 Fr catheter is then advanced like a sleeve over the 2 Fr catheter until its tip abuts the balloon. The outer 3 Fr catheter is thus used to apply a counterforce to the balloon to prevent a shift in position as the inner microcatheter is pulled from the valve, leaving the balloon in position.

MICROWIRES

Neurointerventional microwires are manufactured in sizes from 0.010″ to 0.016″ in caliber. Some are hydrophilically coated. Like hydrophilically coated microcatheters, they must be kept wet while out of the body. The behavior of microwires differs by virtue of their metallic composition and their grind profile. Stainless steel wires are the standard, being rendered radiographically dense distally with a leader of platinum or other metal. Nitinol wires are more expensive and are more difficult to curve by hand, but have the advantage of not becoming deformed by the tortuosity of the distal arterial tree, as happens with stainless steel wires. Wires differ also by virtue of the profile of the distal grind, which usually means trading responsiveness and dirigibility for flexibility.

Other wires are supplied for specific purposes. The ''valve wire'' of the Stealth® angioplasty balloon system, for instance, is designed with a segment that occludes the distal orifice of the balloon catheter, allowing the more proximal balloon to be inflated.

MICROCATHETER ANGIOGRAPHIC RUNS

A digital angiographic run through the microcatheter is imperative before all embolizations to evaluate the anatomy and possible anastomoses with greater resolution than one can obtain on fluoroscopic images. Extracranial microcatheter injections can be made with a power-injector. To obtain a technically satisfactory injection, it is necessary to set the injector at 300–450 psi.. This is far in excess of the recommended limits of tolerance for microcatheters. Power injections through microcatheters should be performed in the external carotid system only, and at that only when the microcatheter is free of any wedging or spasm. Kinking or obstruction of the microcatheter with the force of a 450 psi injection will cause microcatheter rupture. Microcatheter injections in the intraaxial compartment should always be done by hand.

EMBOLIC MATERIALS

Polyvinyl Alcohol

Polyvinyl alcohol (PVA) particles are the staple of tumor and mass preoperative embolization in the head and neck. They are also used occasionally for transarterial embolization of arteriovenous malformations of the brain and dura.

Various commercial preparations of PVA are available, which are supplied in sizes between 45 and 1,000 m. PVA particles of 50–150 m have a more effective histopathologic outcome for inducing tumor necrosis than larger particles (1). However, this size-range probably carries a greater risk of cranial neuropathy should inadvertent embolization of vasa nervorum occur. Particles of this range could also cause skin necrosis. Particle sizes of 150–250 m are most commonly used in head and neck embolization because they constitute an adequate compromise between the need to penetrate the vascular bed of a preoperative tumor, on the one hand, and the need to avoid ischemic necrosis of target tissue and possible delay of healing in the surgical bed, on the other hand.

Particles are prepared as a dilute suspension in radio-graphic contrast and injected as punctuated mini-boluses that are monitored on a fluoroscopic roadmap while being carried to their destination by antegrade arterial flow. Careful monitoring of the pattern of flow is maintained throughout the embolization to avoid reflux of particles and to identify the development of vasospasm or opening of potentially dangerous anastomoses.

In situations in which small anastomoses are suspected or arteriovenous shunting is evident on the angiogram, larger particles may be preferred. The chances of obstructing a microcatheter with clumps of particles are greater with bigger particles. Microcatheters of the 0.010″ series are usually limited to PVA particles up to 250 m.

Biological Effect of PVA

Polyvinyl alcohol particles impair blood flow by adherence to the vessel wall in clumps, with preservation of some luminal flow in many vessels (2, 3). They also provoke variable degrees of acute inflammatory reaction. Foreign body giant-cell reaction, mural angionecrosis, and necrotizing vasculitis can be seen in the acute phase (days) after embolization of arteriovenous malformations and other lesions (4). However, the behavior of PVA is still relatively inert compared with other embolic agents, particularly compared with acrylate materials (5).

After PVA embolization of an arteriovenous malformation there is usually preservation of some flow in large and medium sized vessels, and a tendency of embolized territories to recanalize slowly, over a period of weeks to months (4). This has suggested to some authors that PVA embolization of brain arteriovenous malformations provides only a temporary improvement in the angiographic appearance. The size of an AVM nidus may be underestimated after PVA embolization. Radiotherapy planning based on this angiographic appearance runs the risk of recurrence of the AVM in those regions not included in the radiation port (6).

Gelfoam®

Gelfoam is a pliable, water-insoluble embolic agent prepared from purified pork-skin gelatin granules. It is supplied in the form of a white powder or as a sponge that can be cut to required sizes. Its utility lies in a physical hemostatic effect due to its ability to hold up to 45 times its weight of blood within its interstices. It is resorbed by the body within 2–6 weeks and does not have a significant sclerosing effect.

Gelfoam sponge can be cut easily with a scissors into small pledgets that can be injected via a microcatheter to occlude a small vessel, usually after the distal field has been embolized with PVA. Once should err on the small side in cutting pledgets to avoid obstructing the microcatheter. They are injected in a bolus of contrast. A reduction in resistance in the microcatheter confirms delivery of the gelfoam. Gelfoam pledgets are useful in situations in which ultimate recanalization of the vessel might be acceptable or desired, e.g., post-traumatic small vessel bleeding or epistaxis embolization.

Due to the small quantity of force needed to deliver the pledget via a microcatheter, pledgets should be used in safe situations only, i.e., where a degree of inadvertent reflux would not have disastrous complications. Gelfoam pledgets are typically used in a distal branch of the external carotid artery. Use of gelfoam pledgets close to the origin of the external carotid artery would threaten the internal carotid artery.

Gelfoam powder has particle dimensions of 40–60 m. Mixed with radiographic contrast for fluoroscopic visualization, it has the ability to penetrate an arterial field to the level of the distal arterioles. Therefore, in contrast to embolization with larger PVA particles, in which preservation of distal tissue or mucosa is maintained through small vessel collateral flow, gelfoam powder embolization produces a powerful, ischemic lysis of the targeted tissue. It is used in safe situations for preoperative tumor embolization, where the possibility of reflux or of dangerous anastomoses is not present, and where flow from the microcatheter is directed exclusively towards the tumor.

Glue

TECHNIQUE

Because it is such an effective embolic agent, the risk of inadvertent glue embolization of normal tissue can make the use of this agent extremely dangerous. Acrylate glue, NBCA (N-butyl-cyanoacrylate), is supplied in a liquid form. It is diluted with Ethiodol® to render it radiographically visible and occasionally with tungsten or tantalum powder. When it comes in contact with an ionic solution of alkali pH, NBCA solidifies quickly into a hard paste by an exothermic reaction. To prevent this from happening within the delivery system or too quickly within the body, the bolus of glue is preceded by a low pH, non-ionic flush solution such as 5% dextrose or glacial acetic acid. The approximate angiographic point at which the glue solidifies is ideally controlled by altering the mixture and dilution of the glue. More Ethiodol is added when more distal migration of the glue is desired. Two techniques of glue injection are used.

Continuous Column Technique

After the microcatheter has been injected with 5% dextrose, a continuous injection of glue is performed to penetrate the nidus and spill into desired alternative pedicles. Often it is desirable for the glue to back into the catheterized pedicle and fill it to precisely the desired point. This is monitored closely on a fluoroscopy roadmap or with a digital angiographic run. It calls for decision-making on the spot while the column advances. Undesired developments, e.g., premature setting of the glue with threatened reflux much earlier than expected, may require an immediate cessation of the injection. On the other hand, an undesirable appearance of the developing glue cast, e.g., fistulous shooting of the glue into an already compromised venous channel, might require the interventionalist to avoid momentary panic and continue or even accelerate the injection with the intention of closing the fistula. There are certain situations during continuous column technique in which early withdrawal would represent a great danger.

Because of the potential for danger by virtue of compromising the veins, or even embolizing the pulmonary arteries, the column technique is thought to be hazardous but the more effective technique in certain situations. It is usually performed with systemic hypotension, in an effort to reduce the velocity of flow in the pedicle. At the end of the injection, a pause is observed to allow the last drop of viscous glue to extrude itself. This can, alternatively, be avoided by withdrawing on the syringe.

At the end of the injection, the whole catheter-system, including the main catheter, is pulled sharply of a piece together. This is done to avoid shaving any remaining clump of glue on the microcatheter by the tip of the main catheter. The carotid or vertebral artery in question is quickly selected again and an angiographic run performed immediately, lest any ominous change in the appearance of the arteriovenous malformation should require urgent attention.

"Sandwich" or "Push" Technique

A mini-bolus of glue is injected from the microcatheter, preceded and followed by inert dextrose flush. The bolus of glue, usually 0.05–0.1 mL is injected more sharply and with less control than is a continuous column. This technique is used when the microcatheter is somewhat remote from the desired target, or when one wishes to embolize multiple small vessels together in a large field. It has the additional advantage of allowing a number of injections to be made through one catheter placement, although the catheter ultimately clogs with glue after a few rounds.

THEORY OF EMBOLIZATION OF AVMs

Embolization of an arteriovenous malformation or of an arterio-venous fistula may be considered for a number of reasons:

Complete elimination of an AVM such that subsequent surgery is unnecessary. It is uncommon to achieve a complete cure with embolization alone. Complete cure of a brain AVM by embolization is seen in 5–14% of all cases (7, 8). This figure could be as high as 70% if one considers small AVMs only (9).

Reduction of size of an AVM to bring it into a size range where radiotherapy may be more successful (8).

Reduction of overall flow in an AVM such that subsequent surgery can be safer, more effective, and more complete.

Elimination of intranidal or arterial aneurysms in an otherwise untreatable AVM to reduce the risk of bleeding.

CHOICE OF EMBOLIC AGENTS FOR AVM EMBOLIZATION

The difficulty in embolization of arteriovenous malformations is how to inject a stable, non-toxic, permanent matter into a rapidly flowing stream of blood so that it lodges in precisely the correct location. There are a number of embolic agents available which have been used by interventional neuroradiologists for AVM embolization. The most commonly used are coils, PVA particles (polyvinyl alcohol), and cyano-acrylate glues (iso-butyl-cyano-acrylate IBCA or n-butyl-2-cyanoacrylate NBCA).

Use of IBCA and NBCA in the United States has become more restricted since the 1980s when concern was raised over an experimental observation in rats that had been given large doses of intraperitoneal IBCA (10). Supplies of NBCA are available from sources outside of the US where it is approved as a tissue adhesive and suture substitute. Although opinions vary, there is a strong consensus that acrylate glue is an important option in the therapeutic approach to dealing with AVMs. This derives from the following evidence:

> Despite many years of use in hundreds of children and thousands of adults, there is no evidence of carcinogenesis related to the acrylate glues (11–13).

> Histopathologic evaluation of the effects of acrylate use in vivo in animals and humans demonstrates it to be a powerful sclerosing agent, even in small quantities, capable of instantly shutting down arterial feeders to AVMs. It is effective without any evidence of tissue neoplastic change (12, 14, 15). Studies demonstrate that the effect of cyanoacrylates is mediated by an intense foreign body giant-cell granulomatous arteritis (16), which effectively fibroses the vessel. This inflammatory response is similar to but more intense and enduring than that seen with PVA.

> Revascularization of a completely eliminated AVM after acrylate embolization can happen but is rare (7, 8, 17). On the other hand, revascularization after PVA embolization begins within 2–14 days (4). This is a major concern if the purpose of embolization is to reduce AVM size for radiosurgical planning. An AVM immediately after PVA embolization will have a deceptively small appearance causing the radiosurgical target to omit parts of the AVM, which may later recanalize (6). A similar phenomenon could possibly happen with presurgical embolization, resulting in a recurrence of the AVM.

> Acrylate embolization of an AVM feeding pedicle carries the additional advantage of being able to fill the entire pedicle and with it, any aneurysms along the pedicle, which could rupture and cause bleeding (18). This is a particular concern for AVMs because the feeding pedicles prior to treatment carry blood at higher velocity but at substantially lower pressures than uninvolved equivalent cerebral vessels. After embolization, the pressure rises rapidly in these pedicles causing a theoretical risk of severe bleeding in these pedicles from weak points or aneurysms (19). PVA particle embolization does not have the ability to occlude such aneurysms, leading some interventionalists to believe that PVA embolization carries a higher risk of intraprocedural pedicle rupture.

Acrylate is the most powerful and permanent of the currently available embolic agents (5). Angiographic follow-up of arteriovenous malformations treated with N-butyl-cyanoacrylate demonstrates a very small incidence of recurrence or recanalization (8, 20), relative to recanalization rates after particulate embolization (6). Emergence of collateral flow from dural and pial sources can be seen after partial acrylate embolization of arteriovenous malformations (7, 8).

A study by Jordan et al. (21) analyzed the cost of combined endovascular embolization (NBCA) with surgery versus surgery alone for treatment of AVMs. Their methods, in contrast to some previous studies, make allowance for the long-term costs of increased morbidity and mortality associated with treatment without embolization. Their conclusion was that the net effective treatment cost per cure was less when surgery was used in combination with embolization. Costs that take into account life expectancy, expected economic productivity of the patient, and other longer term hidden costs of morbidity indicated savings as high as 34% with combined surgery-embolization compared with surgery alone.

Dehydrated Alcohol

Dehydrated alcohol consists of 98% by volume ethyl alcohol. It is supplied as a clear, colorless fluid. When used as an embolic agent, it has a powerful sclerosing and lytic effect. It produces injury by cell dehydration and precipitation of protoplasm. Its toxic effect on neural tissue makes it a suitable agent for nerve blocking procedures. In the domain of interventional neuroradiologic procedures, the possibility of inadvertent cranial nerve, spine, or brain injury must be considered carefully before this agent is used. It has an acutely painful effect on the injected tissue, and for this reason is most frequently used under general anesthesia. In combination with metrizamide (as a radiographic marker), it is used for percutaneous sclerosis of peripheral venous malformations or tumors. Transarterial or percutaneous embolization with alcohol preparations is used in situations in which an aggressive lytic effect is required, e.g., malignant tumors, and where there is a margin of safety for avoiding embolization of normal or critical structures.

Ethiodol®

Ethiodol is an amber-colored, oily fluid used for lymphangiography and hysterosalpingography. It contains 37% iodine (475 mg/mL) organically combined with ethyl monoiodostearate and ethyl diiodostearate, fatty acids from poppyseed oil. A combination of its high radiographic density and oily composition makes it a useful marking and diluting agent for acrylate glue embolization. Additional radiographic density can be achieved by use of tantalum or tungsten powder in the embolic preparation. Ethiodol functions as a retardant for the polymerization of glue by limiting anion availability to the glue (12).

Metrizamide

Metrizamide (Amipaque®) is a nonionic water-soluble contrast for use in myelography. It is supplied as a white powder that is reformulated in an aqueous solution as 3.75

g/20 mL (1.81 g organically bound iodine) or 6.75 g/50 mL (3.26 g organically bound iodine). When reformulated with dehydrated alcohol, it provides a means of rendering the alcohol radiographically dense without diluting its sclerosant effect during percutaneous injection of venous malformations or tumors.

Urokinase

Urokinase is refrigerated during storage as a sterile white powder and reconstituted in aliquots of 250,000 units in 5 mL of sterile water. When reconstituted in sterile water, it is a straw-colored translucent fluid. Because of its proteinaceous composition, it can froth considerably if agitated during reconstitution. Therefore, during mixing, the urokinase bottle is rolled smoothly and then decanted with a large bore needle by running it down the side of a glass beaker or other receptacle. Up to 1.2 million units can be used acutely over a period of 1–2 hours for cerebral arterial thrombolysis.

Urokinase is an proteolytic enzyme that functions as a plasminogen activator causing rapid lysis of thrombus. It has a half-life of 16 minutes. The low molecular weight form, most commonly used, is degraded by the liver, having a prolonged half-life in the setting of hepatic disease. Although the serum half-life is short, its biologic effectiveness is thought to continue for some hours, with reduced plasma levels of plasminogen and fibrinogen and elevated levels of fibrin degradation products persisting for up to 24 hours.

In the setting of a disease such as basilar artery thrombosis with a high mortality, contraindications to use of urokinase or other forms of thrombolysis are relative. The possibility of provoking hemorrhage in sites of recent surgery (10 days), diabetic retinopathy, recent myocardial infarction, or recent trauma must all be considered, as must the risk of dislodging emboli from cardiac sites of thrombus formation or endocarditis related vegetations.

Wada Testing and Superselective Provocative Testing

Wada testing is used for preoperative evaluation of the laterality of language and memory, the better to estimate potential surgical morbidity from lesions located in the dominant hemisphere (22). A variety of disease states may be referred for testing, requiring some important modification of technique under certain circumstances.

Patients are studied angiographically in a standard manner without prior administration of sedating agents, which might adversely affect test performance. Therefore, a little more local anesthesia than usual in the groin may be worthwhile. In cases of tumors or hippocampal sclerosis, the hemisphere ipsilateral to the lesion is studied angiographically and tested with amobarbital first. The normal hemisphere is studied last. However, in the situation of an arteriovenous malformation, rapid shunting of the amobarbital through the arteriovenous malformation may re-

quire that a higher dose be given for full effectiveness. This could cause a prolonged systemic effect of the amobarbital, influencing psychological performance for some time. Therefore, in the setting of an arteriovenous malformation during Wada testing, the normal hemisphere is studied first.

There are a number of features of the angiographic examination that warrant consideration before amobarbital infusion. The presence of carotid-basilar anastomoses, such as a persistent trigeminal artery, could cause a serious complication if the posterior fossa were infused with barbiturate. In these instances, the patient must be heparinized and the carotid-basilar anastomosis bypassed with a microcatheter. Secondly, the flow pattern of the internal carotid artery angiogram must be studied to ensure that when the hand-injection of amobarbital is made that it is done with verve sufficient to perfuse the whole hemisphere but to avoid cross-flow via the anterior communicating artery. Hand-injections of contrast can be made to practice technique and speed of injection.

During Wada testing, to facilitate psychological evaluation, the patient table is usually removed from under the fluoroscopy unit, baseline testing is performed, the amobarbital injection given, and the catheter pulled down while post-amobarbital testing is conducted. It is possible for the catheter to be unknowingly pulled down into the common or external carotid artery before the amobarbital is administered, thus rendering the subsequent injection ineffective. Therefore, it is important to catheterize the internal carotid artery in a stable position and to be extremely careful not to tug or pull on the catheter or related tubing while moving the fluoroscopic equipment. While the initial bolus of 80–100 mg of amobarbital in 5 mL of solution is administered, the contralateral arm is tested for strength by an unscrubbed neurologist. The infusion is discontinued when he/she is satisfied that the patient is completely plegic on that side. If plegia is not complete, the infusion is continued for another 30–80 mg. After a 20–30 minute rest period after testing, the contralateral internal carotid artery is catheterized, studied angiographically, and tested.

SUPERSELECTIVE FUNCTIONAL TESTING

For superselective testing of arterial pedicles related to an arteriovenous malformation during embolization, doses of amobarbital of approximately 30 mg injected via a microcatheter are used in conjunction with tailored neurological testing. For testing of external carotid branches during a potentially dangerous embolization, two concerns exist: embolization via collateral channels to the internal carotid artery circulation, and embolization of the vasa nervorum of local cranial nerves, which could result in a permanent deficit.

Testing for internal carotid artery collateral flow is done using amobarbital in doses of 30–70 mg, injected by hand in a solution of 50 mg/mL with sterile water. The injection is made at speeds similar to the anticipated embolization to avoid reflux and to emulate the vascular territory of the proposed embolization. Dilution with equal parts of non-ionic contrast can be used for visualization of the injection.

Amobarbital is less effective for testing cranial nerve function than is lidocaine. Therefore, when concern for possible cranial nerve deficits exists, pre-embolization testing with injections of 20—70 mg of lidocaine is used (23, 24). Cardiac preparations of 2% lidocaine are usually used for this purpose. Lidocaine can be buffered with six drops of 4.2% bicarbonate per 10 mL of lidocaine to reduce patient discomfort during the procedure (23). Positive results from provocative testing with lidocaine and amobarbital are short in duration, most recovering within 15 minutes. Lidocaine has been used successfully for provocative testing of the central retinal artery also, where amobarbital may give a false-negative result (25).

Coils

Coils are made from radiographically dense metal, usually platinum, and are mostly made by labor intensive production techniques. They are therefore extremely expensive. Coils are divided into two categories: the Guglielmi detachable coil system or similar systems for aneurysm embolization, and push-coils that are placed by being advanced through a catheter or microcatheter with a wire or pusher.

GUGLIELMI DETACHABLE COILS (GDC®)

Guglielmi detachable coils are constructed of fine, soft platinum wire. They are designed to fill an intracranial aneurysm gently to obliterate the aneurysm and eliminate the risk of bleeding, while preserving the parent artery. They are supplied in a plastic coil holder, which straightens them so they can be advanced into the microcatheter. The coils are soldered at their proximal end to a stainless steel pusher. They are advanced into a satisfactory position and detached from the stainless steel pusher by dissolving the soldered segment with a 9V current from a standard battery. A coil of similar design but with an interlocking mechanism instead of a solder is used in some countries.

The welded segment must be exposed at the microcatheter tip in order for the detachment electrolysis to occur. The precise position of the coil and steel pusher is controlled by aligning markers on the steel pusher with markers on the microcatheter. Microcatheters for GDC procedures must have two markers; one is at the end of the microcatheter to indicate the tip during navigation, the other is more proximal for alignment with the coil-marker during coil-placement.

Guglielmi detachable coils are manufactured in two size categories corresponding with the Tracker® 0.010" and 0.018" series of microcatheters. Their construction is based on a platinum wire wound into a 0.010" or 0.016" helix. This first helix, in its turn, is then wound into a larger helix with a variety of diameters and of varying total lengths. These measurements are specified in choosing coils for placement within aneurysms.

PUSH COILS

Push-coils are manufactured for placement via a microcatheter, i.e., 0.010–0.016" construction, or via a standard catheter, up to 0.038" or larger in caliber. They may be impregnated with dacron or other fibers to increase thrombogenicity. They are used in situations where for reasons of expense or otherwise, the precision of GDC technology is unsuitable or not necessary. They are used to occlude flow in an artery or vein. This can be done to eliminate pathologic flow when other agents are unsuitable, such as in a fistula or in a laceration after trauma. Alternatively, a coil may be placed proximally in a non-diseased pedicle to protect it from a subsequent potentially dangerous embolization agent or procedure. For example, during middle meningeal artery embolization a coil might be placed in the meningo-orbital branch to prevent flow of emboli to the orbit, thus protecting the orbit from subsequent embolization.

Push-coils for microcatheters are supplied in various lengths and shapes, from straight 2 mm coils to 50–60 mm complex helical, conical, and flower-shaped coils. Care is needed with placement because they have a strong tendency to push the microcatheter back as they emerge from the distal tip. Therefore, the measurement of the curve diameter of the coils should correspond with the lumen of the targeted vessel to allow the coil to assume its shape.

Balloons

Detachable balloons for intravascular use are supplied in two varieties, silicone and latex. Detachable balloons are used to occlude a large vessel, or to close a large hole in an artery which is causing a large arteriovenous fistula or life-threatening exsanguination. When properly used, they allow safe and fast treatment in circumstances in which surgery cannot be performed with the same speed or with as low a risk. Detachable balloons have been used for over 20 years in Europe and the United States. Efficacy has been demonstrated in various situations including (26):

> Major vessel occlusion for tumor encasement, pseudoaneurysm, laceration, or dissection complicated by embolic events to the brain (27).
>
> Fistula occlusion, e.g., carotid-cavernous fistula, where surgical techniques are difficult and risky.
>
> Major vessel trauma.
>
> Major vessel occlusion for treatment of distal aneurysms that cannot be surgically approached directly. Such treatment aims to alter the hemodynamics around an aneurysm and diminish the risk of rupture (28–31).
>
> Major vessel occlusion distal to and proximal to an aneurysm, i.e., "trapping" of an aneurysm.

Vasospasm during Interventional Procedures

External carotid artery branches may be particularly prone to spasm from the minimal trauma of wire and catheter navigation during angiographic procedures. This is usually of little immediate consequence to the patient as long as it is recognized promptly and the catheter is withdrawn. However, it can impede progress with a case significantly. Catheter-related vasospasm within the internal carotid artery during a prolonged procedure may be more hazardous, especially if it is not detected immediately. Spasm may have deleterious hemodynamic effects or expose the intima to a greater degree of abrasive trauma at the catheter tip, possibly inducing a dissection. To prevent or treat the onset of procedure related extracranial vasospasm, sublingual nifedipine 10–20 mg or 2–4 inches of nitropaste applied to non–hair-bearing skin have been used successfully (32).

REFERENCES

1. Wakhloo AK, Juengling FD, Van Velthoven V, et al. Extended preoperative polyvinyl alcohol microembolization of intracranial meningiomas: assessment of two embolization techniques. Am J Neuroradiol 1993;14:571–582.
2. Davidson GS, Terbrugge KG. Histologic long-term follow-up after embolization with polyvinyl alcohol particles. Am J Neuroradiol 1995; 16:843–846.
3. Quisling RJ, Mickle JP, Ballinger WB, et al. Histopathologic analysis of intraarterial polyvinyl alcohol microemboli in rat cerebral cortex. Am J Neuroradiol 1984;5:101–104.
4. Germano IM, Davis RL, Wilson CB, et al. Histopathological follow-up study of 66 cerebral arteriovenous malformations after therapeutic embolization with polyvinyl alcohol. J Neurosurg 1992;76:607–614.
5. White RI, Strandberg JV, Gross GS, et al. Therapeutic embolization with long-term occluding agents and their effects on embolized tissues. Radiology 1977;125:677–687.
6. Mathis JA, Barr JD, Horton JA, et al. The efficacy of particulate embolization combined with stereotactic radiosurgery of large arteriovenous malformations of the brain. Am J Neuroradiol 1995;16:299–306.
7. Fournier D, TerBrugge KG, Willinsky R, et al. Endovascular treatment of intracerebral arteriovenous malformations: experience in 49 cases. J Neurosurg 1991;75:228–233.
8. Gobin YP, Laurent A, Merienne L, et al. Treatment of brain arteriovenous malformations by embolization and radiosurgery. J Neurosurg 1996;85:19–28.
9. Vinuela F, Dion JE, Duckwiler G, et al. Combined endovascular embolization and surgery in the management of cerebral arteriovenous malformations: experience with 101 cases. J Neurosurg 1991;75:856–864.
10. Samson D, Marshall D. Carcinogenic potential of isobutyl-2-cyanoacrylate (letter). J Neurosurg 1986;65:571–572.
11. Berenstein A, Hieshima G. Clinical versus experimental use of iso-butyl-2 cyanoacrylate (letter). J Neurosurg 1987;67:318–319.
12. Brothers MF, Kaufmann JCE, Fox AJ, et al. N-Butyl 2-cyanoacrylate. Substitute for IBCA in interventional neuroradiology: histopathologic and polymerization time studies. Am J Neuroradiol 1989;10:777–786.
13. Lasjaunias P, Hui F, Zerah M, et al. Cerebral arteriovenous malformations in children. Management of 179 consecutive case and review of the literature. Child Nerv Syst 1995; 1166–1179.
14. Cromwell LD, Freeny PC, Kerber CW, et al. Histologic analysis of tissue response to bucrylate-pantopaque mixture. Am J Neuroradiol 1986;147:627–631.
15. Schweitzer JS, Chang BS, Madsen P, et al. The pathology of arteriovenous malformations of the brain treated by embolotherapy. II. Results of embolization with multiple agents. Neuroradiology 1993;35:468–474.
16. Lylyk P, Vinuela F, Vinters HV, et al. Use of a new mixture for embolization of intracranial vascular malformations. Neuroradiology 1990;32:304–310.
17. Rao VRL, Ravi Madalam K, Gupta AKI, et al. Dissolution of isobutyl 2 cyanoacrylate on long term follow up. Am J Neuroradiol 1989;10;135–141.
18. Perata HJ, Tomsick TA, Tew JM. Feeding artery pedicle aneurysms: association with parenchymal hemorrhage and arteriovenous malformation in the brain. J Neurosurg 1994;80:631–634.
19. Sorimachi T, Takeuchi S, Koike T, et al. Blood pressure monitoring in feeding arteries of cerebral arteriovenous malformations during embolization. A preventive role in hemodynamic complications. Neurosurgery 1995;37:1041–1048.
20. Wikholm G. Occlusion of cerebral arteriovenous malformations with N-butyl-cyanoacrylate is permanent. Am J Neuroradiol 1995;16:479–482.
21. Jordan JE, Marks MP, Lane B, et al. Cost-effectiveness of endovascular therapy in the surgical management of cerebral arteriovenous malformations. Am J Neuroradiol 1996;17:247–254.
22. Wada J, Rasmussen T. Intracarotid injection of sodium amytal for the lateralization of cerebral speech and dominance. J Neurosurg 1960;17:266–282.
23. Deveikis JP. Sequential injections of amobarbital sodium and lidocaine for provocative neurologic testing in the external carotid circulation. Am J Neuroradiol 1996;17:1143–1147.
24. Horton JA, Kerber CW. Lidocaine injection into external carotid branches: provocative testing to preserve cranial nerve function in therapeutic embolization. Am J Neuroradiol 1986; 7:105–108.
25. Horton JA, Dawson RC. Retinal Wada test. Am J Neuroradiol 1988;9:1167–1168.
26. Lewis AI, Tomsick TA, Tew JM. Management of 100 consecutive direct carotid cavernous fistulas: results of treatment with detachable balloons. Neurosurgery 1995;36:239–245.
27. Halbach VV, Higashida RT, Dowd CF, et al. Endovascular treatment of vertebral artery dissections and pseudoaneurysms. J Neurosurg 1993;79: 183–191.
28. Higashida RT, Halbach VV, Cahan LD, et al. Detachable balloon embolization therapy of posterior circulation intracranial aneurysms. J Neurosurg 1989;71:512–519.
29. Hodes JE, Aymard A, Gobin P, et al. Endovascular occlusion of intracranial vessels for curative treatment of unclippable aneurysms. Report of 16 cases. J Neurosurg 1991;75:628–633.
30. Steinberg GK, Drake CG, Peerless SJ. Deliberate basilar or vertebral artery occlusion in the treatment of intracranial aneurysms. J Neurosurg 1993;79:161–173.
31. Tsukahara T, Wada H, Satake K, et al. Proximal balloon occlusion for dissecting vertebral aneurysms accompanied by subarachnoid hemorrhage. Neurosurgery 1995;36:914–920.
32. Erba M, Jungreis CA, Horton JA. Nitropaste for prevention and relief of vascular spasm. Am J Neuroradiol 1989;10:155–156.

CHAPTER 21

Emergency Interventional Procedures

ARTERIAL THROMBOLYSIS

Direct infusion of urokinase or similar thrombolytic agents into sites of acute intracranial occlusion, if performed in a timely manner, can facilitate reperfusion of ischemic brain and prevent infarction. In certain circumstances, this treatment can have dramatic effects (Figs. 21.1, 21.2). In other circumstances, the treatment can severely complicate the effects of the stroke (Figs. 21.3, 21.4). The question concerning direct intra-arterial thrombolysis of the intracerebral circulation is not whether the agent and technique are effective, but instead which patients should be treated in this manner.

Acute occlusions in the anterior circulation are most commonly related to emboli. In the vertebro-basilar circulation, acute occlusions are more likely to be related to thrombosis in situ due to the effects of critical stenosis and atherosclerotic narrowing. If a complete occlusion in the anterior circulation can be reopened quickly after onset, the risks of thrombolytic therapy are low enough to justify interventional treatment (1–3). Three hours of complete occlusion in the middle cerebral artery territory is usually taken as the time-limit. Beyond this limit, infarction is established to a degree at which risks of hemorrhagic transformation after thrombolysis preempt direct intra-arterial infusion. Approximately 6 hours of complete occlusion in the posterior circulation is taken as an equivalent guide. However, the degree of occlusion, partial or complete, and the state of collateral flow can greatly impact the time at which infarction is established, potentially prolonging these limits.

Pretreatment Evaluation

Patients with anterior circulation hemispheric ischemia present with abrupt onset of asymmetric motor or sensory dysfunction, language deficits, or dyspraxias. The clinical presentation of posterior fossa acute ischemia depends on the rapidity with which the narrowed vessel occludes. Abrupt basilar artery occlusions present with sudden loss of consciousness and loss of brainstem function. A more stuttering course of intermittent crescendo basilar artery occlusion will present with a history of alternating cranial nerve deficits and fluctuating levels of consciousness. Therefore, consent for an interventional thrombolytic procedure must usually be obtained from a family member. The risks specific to intracranial arterial thrombolysis include rupture or perforation of an intracranial vessel, intracranial intimal dissection, and aggravation of the dis-

ease state through reperfusion injury in an established infarct. Hemorrhagic transformation and hematoma formation in an infarct may follow. Systemic complications of thrombolysis include bleeding at recent post-surgical sites, bleeding into infarcted myocardium with tamponade, or bleeding in the retroperitoneum and groin due to trauma at time of placement of the vascular sheath. In the setting of a life-threatening disease, such as acute occlusion of the basilar artery, contraindications to thrombolysis are relative but include diabetic retinopathy from which hemorrhage could cause permanent blindness; pregnancy; surgery within the past 10 days; coagulopathic diseases; and a small established infarct on CT scan.

Even with a small established infarct, reperfusion by thrombolysis may prevent other areas at risk from becoming ischemic or infarcted, but carries the risk of hemorrhagic transformation in an established infarction. For this reason, a CT scan of the head to evaluate for evidence of hemorrhage and infarction is necessary before (Fig. 21.5) and after (Fig. 21.6) each thrombolysis procedure. The initial CT scan may also demonstrate evidence of intraluminal dense thrombus or mural calcification. The latter is a particular concern should angioplasty of a stenotic area be contemplated at the time of the procedure or thereafter.

Procedural Preparation

Emergency thrombolysis procedures are most safely and effectively performed with deep sedation under monitored anesthesia care or under general anesthesia, if an anesthesiology team is available. A central venous line, a radial arterial line, and a urinary catheter will also contribute enormously to the quality of care. With a cooperative team-effort these prefatory steps can be accomplished smoothly with minimal if any delay.

Procedural Techniques

There are a number of advantages to choosing a 7 French sheath as a standard issue for thrombolysis cases. First, patients are older, hypertensive, and liable to have diffuse atherosclerotic disease. Being that time is of the essence, minimal delay in vessel selection from the aortic arch can be achieved with the maneuverability and responsiveness of a 7 French or 6 French catheter. Furthermore, with a 6 French catheter inside a 7 French sheath, a transducer line from the sheath can be attached for blood-pressure monitoring, thus eliminating the need for a radial line.

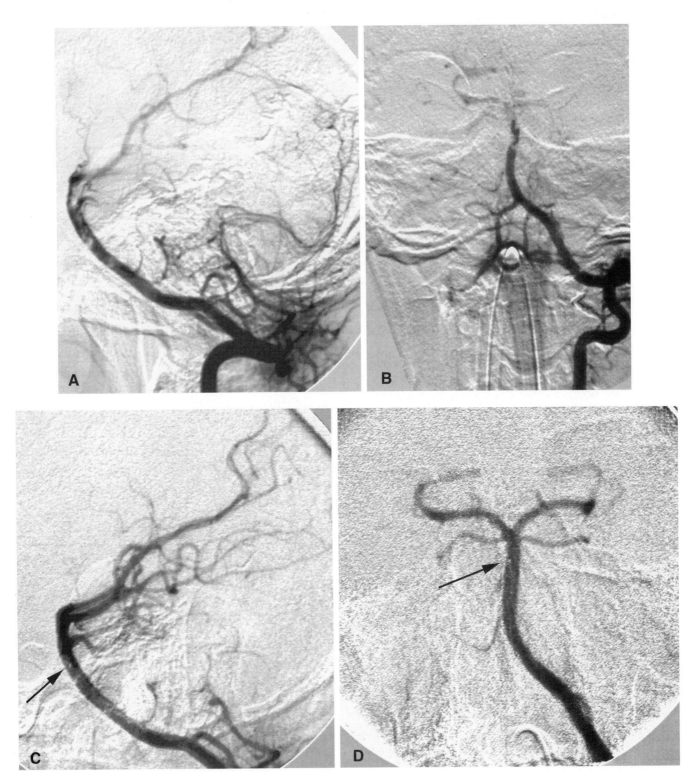

Figure 21.1. *Acute basilar artery thrombosis during pregnancy.* A 28-year-old female who was 8 weeks pregnant presented following a long air-flight with signs of posterior fossa ischemia. Her MRA demonstrated attenuation of flow-signal in the basilar artery. She responded well to heparin at first but after approximately 18 hours became suddenly obtunded and hemiparetic. Left vertebral angiography, lateral **(A)** and PA **(B)** views, demonstrated an elongated filling defect in the upper two thirds of the basilar artery with poor filling of the left posterior cerebral artery and superior cerebellar arteries. Thrombolysis was performed at various points within the thrombus through a microcatheter using a total of 600,000 units of urokinase. Lateral **(C)** and PA **(D)** views after urokinase show complete filling of the previously non-visualized branches. The microcatheter tip is indicated with an arrow; the injection of contrast was made through the introducer catheter. The patient left hospital with a residual deficit of a mild VIth palsy. Her pregnancy was apparently unaffected. Pregnancy is mentioned as a contraindication to the use of urokinase, but under circumstances such as these all contraindications are relative.

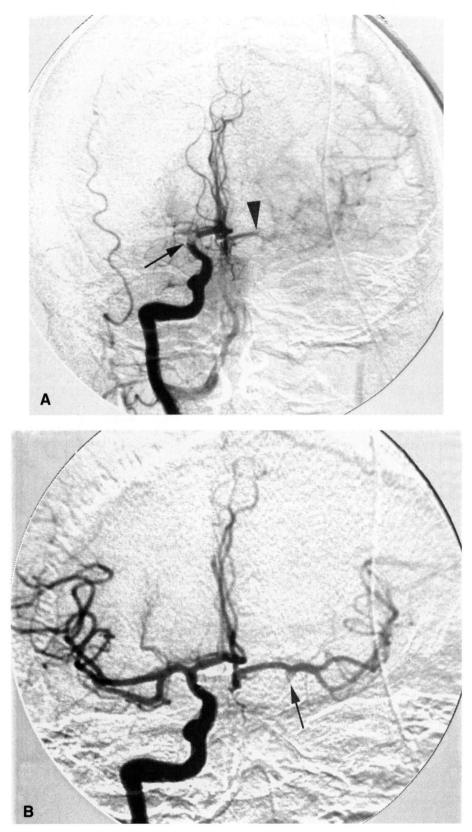

Figure 21.2. *Thrombolysis of acute internal carotid embolus.* An elderly male presented with an acute embolus to the right internal carotid artery. The left internal carotid artery was occluded. Injection of the right common carotid artery **(A)** demonstrates a filling defect **(arrow)** at the top of the internal carotid. Cross-filling to the left hemisphere is diluted by inflow from the left posterior communicating artery **(arrowhead).** After thrombolysis with 1,000,000 units of urokinase in the right internal carotid artery, an injection **(B)** demonstrates complete filling of both hemispheres. The supraclinoid segment of the occluded left internal carotid artery is opacified **(arrow).** The patient made an excellent clinical recovery.

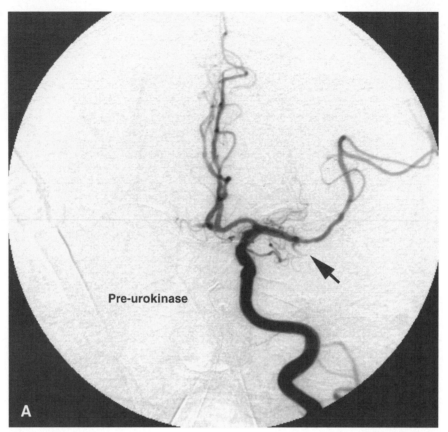

Pre-urokinase

A

Figure 21.3. *Complications of thrombolysis of the middle cerebral artery.* An elderly female presented with sudden aphasia and right hemiparesis. Thrombolysis was performed approximately 4 hours after the onset of stroke. The initial angiogram **(A)** of the left internal carotid artery demonstrates complete occlusion of a division of the middle cerebral artery with a tapered appearance **(arrow).** The left middle cerebral artery and its occluded division were cannulated with a micro-catheter **(B)**. Following a total of 800,000 units of urokinase, the angiographic appearance is very promising, with complete opening of the occluded branch **(arrow).** A CT scan done immediately after the procedure showed early hemorrhagic conversion of the left middle cerebral artery infarction. A second CT **(C)** done 12 hours later shows massive hemorrhage within the left hemisphere. The patient died soon afterwards from brain herniation.

Full heparinization of a patient before placement of the femoral arterial sheath carries some risk of excessive bleeding at the puncture-site, although this is not commonly seen. When delay is foreseen with preprocedural preparations, a femoral arterial line or sheath can be placed in the emergency room. This allows full dosage with heparin before transport to angiography.

The initial vessel of choice is that which allows confirmation of the diagnosis of occlusion and identification of the site. In certain circumstances, injections of other vessels to evaluate collateral flow are necessary to gather more information on the risks of thrombolysis for a particular patient. For instance, a patient with a basilar artery occlusion or near total occlusion seen from a vertebral artery injection, may have begun to recover clinically while on the angiographic table. Evidence of excellent collateral flow to the upper basilar artery via the posterior communicating arteries in such a patient might prompt one to hesitate from superselective injection of urokinase. Similarly, a total internal carotid artery thrombosis might be best left alone if the contralateral internal carotid artery or vertebral artery injections show good collateral flow distal to the internal carotid artery occlusion, particularly if a clinical response to hypertensive therapy is seen during angiography.

It is thought that maximal efficacy of thrombolytic agents is achieved by infusion directly into clot. The presence of this clot and stagnation of blood in occluded vessels preclude roadmap acquisition. Therefore, the process of microwire and microcatheter navigation into unopacified thrombus is based on blind probing of the expected vessel course. To reduce the trauma of this procedure, a generously rounded curve on the wire tip will often cleave the thrombus and find the vessel lumen of its own accord. A hydrophilically coated microcatheter can be of enormous advantage where vessels are tortuous. Hydrophilically coated microcatheters are also very useful when one is working from a position where the guiding catheter is being retained low in the neck because of impassable atherosclerotic obstacles or loops.

When the microcatheter is embedded in thrombus, blood return may not be seen from the microcatheter after wire withdrawal. To establish the location of the microcatheter and to exclude the possibility of wedging in a

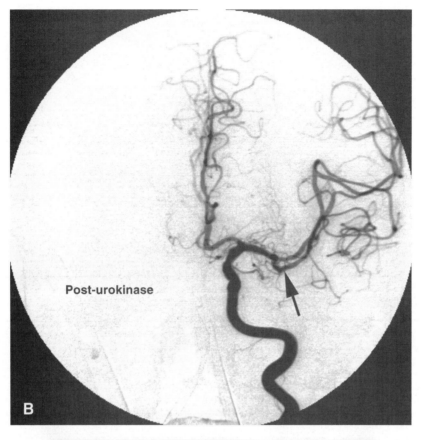

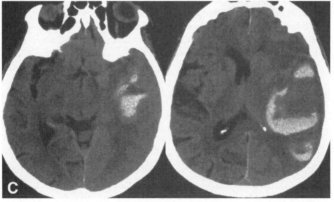

Figure 21.3. *(continued)*

small vessel such as a perforator or choroidal artery, a small injection of contrast is made slowly on a mask image.

Urokinase is formulated as 250,000 units in 5 mL of water, i.e., 50,000 units per mL. Being proteinaceous it is prone to froth during mixing if it is agitated excessively (Figs. 21.7, 21.8). This solution may be used as the thrombolytic infusion or may be further diluted in normal saline to make a higher volume. A very slow rate of urokinase infusion is desirable, e.g., 50,000 units infused over a few minutes.

At regular intervals, the microcatheter position and status of the surrounding vessels are checked with contrast injections. Gentle probing with the curved tip of the microwire and catheter repositioning can help to accelerate

lysis of the thrombus. It may be necessary to chase distal emboli individually in the event that fragments travel distally and occlude major branches. A total of 1–1.2 million units of urokinase can be infused over 1–2 hours. Periodic monitoring of the ACT during the procedure, hydration, and maintenance of blood pressure are important for the ultimate outcome.

A CT scan after the procedure will allow an update on the possibility of intracranial hemorrhage during or as a result of the procedure, and gives an indication of the risks of high dose heparinization. Because patients are coagulopathic after a thrombolysis procedure, sheath-removal is best deferred to a later time. Some days later if the patient is doing exceptionally well, it may be pos-

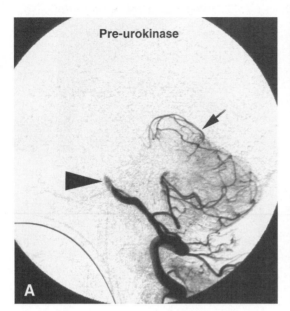 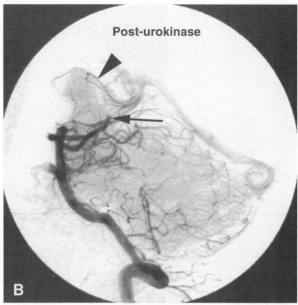

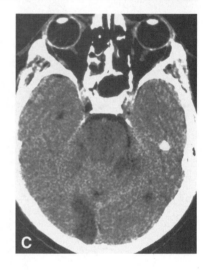

Figure 21.4. *Basilar artery thrombolysis.* An elderly male presented with a mid-basilar artery occlusion. In spite of a good angiographic result of thrombolysis performed approximately 6 hours after the occlusion, his clinical status afterwards was one of neurologic debilitation. A lateral vertebral angiogram **(A)** demonstrates a mid-basilar tapered occlusion **(arrowhead).** Reconstitution of superior vermian branches of the superior cerebellar arteries **(arrow)** is seen along the superior surface of the cerebellum. Collateral flow from the posterior communicating arteries on the carotid injection was not evident. Following infusion of 1,200,000 units of urokinase **(B),** the basilar artery is completely open. Distal emboli in the posterior cerebral arteries **(arrow)** were not pursued due to dose-limitations and the hope that middle cerebral to posterior cerebral artery collateral vessels would assist the distal cortical territories. Early venous opacification of the internal cerebral vein **(arrowhead)** is an angiographic indication that infarction of the thalamus is probably already established. Although the angiographic result was good, the patient developed multiple infarctions of the brain-stem, thalami, and posterior circulation **(C)**.

sible to suspend heparinization for a brief time to allow manual compression of the artery. With larger sheaths and a critical need for full heparinization, sheath removal with arterial repair under local anesthesia in the operating room may be safer.

VENOUS THROMBOLYSIS

The indications for using interventional thrombolysis in the treatment of dural sinus thrombosis versus systemic heparinization alone are not clear (4, 5). However, it seems cogent that with extensive disease and a rapidly deteriorating clinical course, a more immediately effective form of therapy may be warranted in some patients. This condition is unusual among neurological illnesses because intracranial hemorrhagic complications do not contraindicate anticoagulant therapy. Similarly, the presence of hemorrhagic infarcts or subarachnoid hemorrhage may not necessarily contraindicate use of thrombolytic therapy.

Similar to arterial thrombolysis procedures, hepariniza-

tion may be withheld or used in measured form until vascular sheaths have been placed. A 5 French arterial sheath and a 6 or 7 French venous sheath are placed. An arteriogram is performed to confirm the diagnosis and to evaluate the patency of sinuses and state of venous hypertension. A prolonged venous phase is needed to identify which, if any, of the sigmoid and transverse sinuses are patent.

After removing the arterial catheter, the venous guiding catheter is placed in the more patent of the jugular bulbs. Statistically the right jugular bulb is a better route because the right transverse sinus is more likely to have a large connection with the superior sagittal sinus. The dural coverings of the sinuses are robust and impervious to perforation by standard micro-wire maneuvers. However, as the navigation process is one of blind probing of thrombus, a danger of perforation into the subarachnoid space exists through inadvertent and forceful selection of a cortical vein. Therefore, a wide prolapsed curve on the microwire as the leading edge gives a margin of safety in this regard.

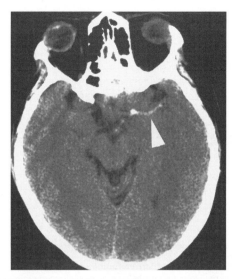

Figure 21.5. *Dense middle cerebral artery.* A pre-angiographic CT in a patient with a thromboembolic stroke demonstrates density of the left middle cerebral artery **(arrowhead)** compared with the normal right side.

Biplane fluoroscopic imaging to ensure that the wire hugs the inner surface of the calvarium and follows the course of the unopacified sinus is essential to avoid catheterization of unopacified cortical veins (Fig. 21.9).

There is only limited interventional neuroradiologic experience with this disease. Two infusion regimens have been used. A rapid infusion over 1–2 hours of 1–1.2 million units of urokinase can be made, similar to the arterial thrombolysis protocol. Alternatively, a prolonged infusion has been attempted over hours to days at a lower rate similar to that used in peripheral thrombolysis.

INTRAARTERIAL PAPAVERINE FOR TREATMENT OF CEREBRAL VASOSPASM

Cerebral vasospasm after subarachnoid hemorrhage is a major cause of delayed neurological morbidity after rupture of an aneurysm. A peak of vasospasm is seen at a 7–10 day interval after the hemorrhage (6, 7). There may also be a brief phase of hyperacute vasospasm in the hours immediately after subarachnoid hemorrhage, similar to that seen in experimental animals. This is occasionally seen during angiography (8). Delayed vasospasm beyond

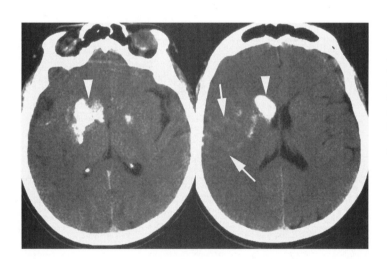

Figure 21.6. *CT following right middle cerebral artery thrombolysis.* After right middle cerebral artery thrombolysis in an elderly female with an unsatisfactory angiographic result, a CT scan was performed. Dense staining of the basal ganglia **(arrowheads)** with contrast is present. This is a common finding after thrombolysis and microcatheter injections with contrast into areas of impending or established infarction. Usually it is not so pronounced as in this patient who has developed an extensive infarction of the right hemisphere. Petechial or hemorrhagic conversion **(arrow)** of the opercular cortex is present.

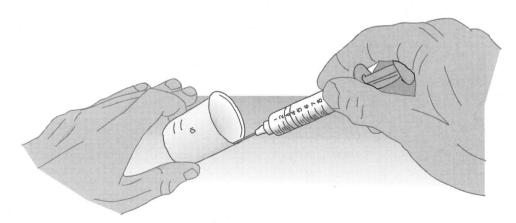

Figure 21.7. *Urokinase.* Urokinase has the capacity to froth if reconstituted with much agitation or shaking. When reformulating it, roll the bottle smoothly from side to side. When decanting it, run the stream of urokinase slowly down the inside of the jar.

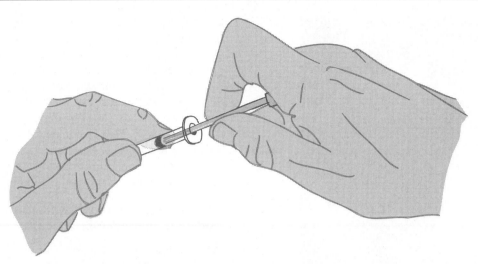

Figure 21.8. *Control of injection rate.* When injecting emboli, it is important not to inject too forcefully. Resistance within the microcatheter may suddenly drop, causing a sustained pressure on the syringe to inject more volume than desirable. To prevent this, a tight grip on the stem of the plunger of the syringe with the right thumb and forefinger, as illustrated, will function as a brake should the resistance change suddenly. This precautionary technique is particularly important for injecting Gelfoam plugs or PVA particles which may clump within the microcatheter.

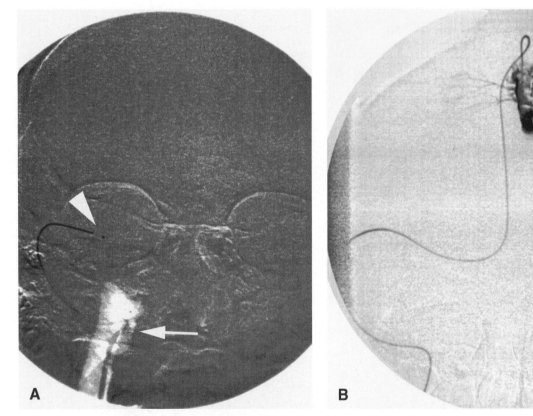

Figure 21.9. *Thrombolysis of dural sinus thrombosis.* Because of rapidly worsening headaches and nosebleeds, a young adult male presented to hospital and was diagnosed with idiopathic dural sinus thrombosis. An AP roadmap image **(A)** of the right jugular bulb demonstrates the position of the main catheter **(arrow).** A hydrophilic microcatheter was advanced through the ipsilateral transverse sinus (arrowhead). The wire (black line) has been withdrawn into the microcatheter.The microcatheter was advanced into the anterior part of the superior sagittal sinus. Angiographic PA **(B)** and lateral **(C)** images demonstrate an extensive filling defect within the sinus **(arrow in B),** with retrograde flow into superficial cortical veins **(arrowheads in C).** A total of 1,200,000 units of urokinase were infused in various locations through the superior sagittal and transverse sinuses. Towards the end of the procedure a PA roadmap image **(D)** shows the microcatheter **(arrow)** in the right transverse sinus with patency of the sinuses from the superior sagittal sinus to the jugular bulb. The patient made a quick recovery.

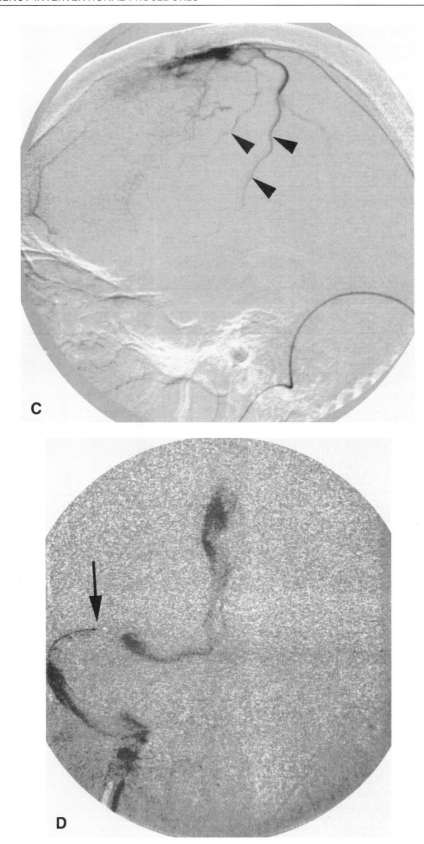

Figure 21.9. *(continued)*

the peak-period can be seen also. The incidence of long-term ischemic deficits in patients with subarachnoid hemorrhage is estimated to be between 1 and 14% (9–11). In the time immediately after the subarachnoid hemorrhage, however, 40–70% of subarachnoid hemorrhage patients have angiographic evidence of narrowing of one or more components of the circle of Willis. Among these patients, less than half will have associated neurologic deficits. Therefore, to discern those patients in need of active therapy for vasospasm, clinical monitoring and serial Doppler measurements are more useful than angiographic studies (7). Treatment measures include hemodilution, hypertension, and hypervolemia ("Triple H therapy") (11), calcium antagonists (12), and early surgery to remove or lyse the subarachnoid clot and to secure the aneurysmal rupture (13).

When these measures do not prevent clinical deterioration of the patient, and transcranial Doppler studies suggest that clinically significant vasospasm is established, interventional procedures for reversal of spasm can be used successfully. Intraarterial papaverine therapy, either alone (14) or as a supplement to balloon angioplasty (15), is an effective (80–95% success) and fairly safe means of increasing cerebral perfusion in patients with critical vasospasm (Fig. 21.10) (16, 17). It has also been used for subarachnoid hemorrhage after trauma (18). Intraarterial papaverine is particularly useful for distal intracranial vessels that are inaccessible to balloon angioplasty techniques. It can be used for vasospasm from other causes, such as for microcatheter induced vasospasm of intracranial vessels (19). Systemic administration of intravenous papaverine is thought to be ineffective for cerebral vasospasm due to the high dose required and the severity of hypotensive complications related to such high doses (20).

Papaverine is an opium alkaloid that causes relaxation of vascular smooth muscle by inhibition of cAMP and cGMP phosphodiesterases in the smooth muscle cell. Commercially papaverine is supplied as a 10 mL vial containing 300 mg of papaverine hydrochloride with 0.5% chlorbutanol, a preservative, and edetate disodium. Papaverine hydrochloride can elute from solution as crystals, particularly when mixed in high concentration. Precipitation may occur also if the preparation is brought into contact with serum, Lactated Ringer's solution, heparin, radiographic contrast, or if exposed to a pH greater than 5.3 (21–23). Crystals formed under these circumstances measuring 50–150 m could be responsible for some of the transient neurologic problems associated with use of papaverine. Providing that the concentration of papaverine at the time of delivery is approximately 300 mg in 100 mL solution or weaker, precipitates formed in contact with human serum probably are dissolved quickly (21).

Preparation

Patients in need of intraarterial papaverine therapy are invariably critically ill, and they have to be monitored closely during and after treatment. An initial CT scan of

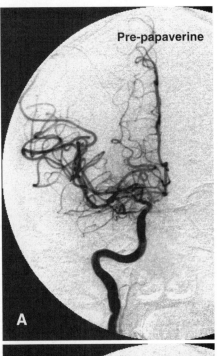

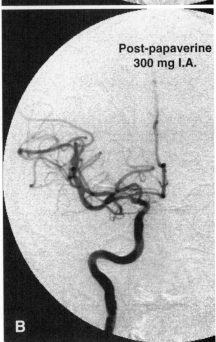

Figure 21.10. *Papaverine infusion for vasospasm.* PA images before **(A)** and after **(B)** infusion of 300 mg of papaverine in the right internal carotid artery in a late middle-age female with complications of subarachnoid hemorrhage. The infusion was made via a microcatheter in the supraclinoid internal carotid artery. Typically, as in this case, the papaverine infusion does not completely reverse the vasospasm. However, it allows dilatation sufficient to improve flow significantly.

the head is essential to eliminate the possibility of infusing papaverine into an infarcted arterial territory that may then become hemorrhagic due to reperfusion effects. Because the papaverine infusion is given over a 30–90 minute period, during which time the guiding catheter and microcatheter create a significant risk for thrombus formation or intimal dissection, the risks and necessity of heparinization must be discussed in advance with the referring neurosurgeon. Previous angiographic images must be available in the angiography suite as a reference with which to evaluate changes on the current study.

Technique

In patients who are immediately post-craniotomy, the heparin dose may be restricted to a bolus of 2,000 units IV. A bolus of 3,000–5,000 units is given otherwise. Hourly checks of the activated clotting time (ACT) and booster doses of 1,000 units, if necessary, are routine.

Papaverine hydrochloride is prepared in solutions of nonheparinized normal saline and delivered in doses as high as 300–450 mg per arterial territory. Up to three territories per treatment session can be perfused. It can be delivered into the internal carotid artery or vertebral artery through standard 4–7 Fr catheters, or through coaxially placed intracranial microcatheters. The infusion should proceed at a rate of approximately 6–9 mg/min. A solution of 300 mg of papaverine hydrochloride in 100 mL total volume requires that a 3 mL syringe (9 mg) be delivered every minute. Contact between papaverine and heparin solutions or contrast within the delivery catheter should be avoided.

Because the rate of delivery of papaverine is so slow, a constant infusion at this slow rate would likely be ineffective. At such a slow constant rate of delivery, slip-streaming of papaverine within the main body of luminal blood flow would probably occur. Therefore, a pulsatile infusion technique is advised.

Risk of respiratory arrest or brainstem depression exists with infusion of papaverine into the posterior circulation. Therefore, these procedures are probably best performed under general anesthesia or under the supervision of an anesthesiologist.

Complications of Papaverine Treatment of Vasospasm

A CT scan of the head is obtained before each papaverine treatment. Use of papaverine in a hemisphere with an established infarct of significant size is avoided because of the risk of reperfusion injury or hemorrhage.

Provided that thromboembolic phenomena or dissections can be avoided and the rate of papaverine delivery is slow, severe complications from this procedure are uncommon. Special caution is advised when using papaverine in patients with documented atrioventricular conduction defects or glaucoma. Mydriasis is seen frequently when the infusion is made below the ophthalmic artery, but it is transient and thought to be of little consequence (24). However, monocular blindness after papaverine infusion below the ophthalmic artery has been reported. For this reason infusions are safer when made in the supraclinoid internal carotid artery or higher (17).

Infusion into the posterior circulation can induce transient neurologic signs such as pupillary asymmetry, nystagmus, etc. These may be related to transient perforator vessel occlusion or hyperperfusion. These signs are usually evanescent and respond well to a lull in the infusion and delayed resumption at a lower rate of delivery. More severe loss of brainstem function with respiratory arrest and fixed, dilated pupils has been described, again of a transient nature with a favorable outcome (25, 26). Systemic circulatory and autonomic side effects of papaverine can be seen occasionally, but, if detected early, most of these are of a transient and inconsequential nature. Such transient effects include systemic hypertension or hypotension, hyperventilation, tachycardia, bradycardia, diaphoresis, pupillary mydriasis, and nausea. The infusion can usually be resumed at a slower rate when the autonomic effect has subsided.

The intracranial pressure (ICP) must be monitored closely during the procedure to avoid prolonged elevation. When the patient does not have a ventriculostomy in place to monitor intracranial pressure during the procedure, the papaverine infusion should be given at an even slower pace with even more intensive clinical monitoring of the patient. Prolonged delivery of papaverine in an undetected situation of rising intracranial pressure can cause transtentorial herniation and irreversible ischemia. Usually, if the ICP rises above 20 mm Hg during a papaverine infusion, discontinuing the infusion and administration of mannitol facilitate prompt normalization of the pressure. Depending on the degree of angiographic response to the dose already delivered, resumption of the infusion at a slower rate may then be attempted (27). In the setting of autonomic instability, use of pressor agents, and the superimposed systemic side-effects of papaverine, an overarching concern must be retained for the cerebral perfusion pressure (mean arterial pressure minus intracranial pressure). The cerebral perfusion pressure should be kept above 60 mm Hg. Below this level, cerebral perfusion may be globally impaired. McAuliffe et al. (27) reported that this was a particular concern when the infusion was made into the common carotid artery, with direct perfusion of the carotid body. Infusion of papaverine in this location is associated with bradycardia, hypotension, and diminished cerebral perfusion pressure.

Severe thrombocytopenia has also been reported after papaverine administration (28). Catheter-induced dissections in the cervical internal carotid artery are a consideration in any prolonged interventional procedure. With a hyperdynamic cardiac cycle in many of these patients, due to the effects of pressors, an exaggerated up-down excursion of the catheter tip in the neck is frequently seen. This probably raises the risk of intimal trauma and flap-formation considerably.

HEAD AND NECK BLEEDING

Catastrophic bleeding from the head and neck may be related to a recent surgical or traumatic event with wound

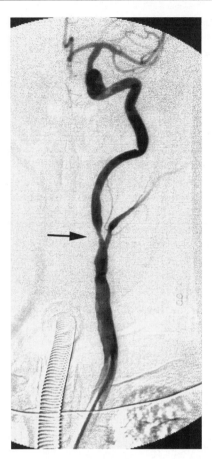

Figure 21.11. *Tumor encasement of the carotid bifurcation.*   An AP image of a left common carotid artery injection in an elderly male with extensive squamous carcinoma of the larynx and bleeding from the tracheostomy site. There is irregular, concentric narrowing **(arrow)** of the origins of the internal carotid artery and external carotid trunk representing tumor encasement of the vessel.

dehiscence and pseudoaneurysm formation (Figs. 21.11, 21.12, 21.13). A typical clinical example is post-tonsillectomy bleeding occurring 7–10 days post resection, but it may follow a number of procedures (Figs. 21.14, 21.15, 21.16, 21.17, 21.18). Stabbing injuries or gun-shot wounds may also be associated with acute or delayed bleeding from a number of sites (Fig. 21.19). Such penetrating wounds may also cause other vascular injuries including major vessel occlusion, arteriovenous fistulas, and intimal dissections (29). Clinical findings such as an expanding hematoma, new bruit, or obvious bleeding may not be present in all patients. Clinical or radiographic definition of the trajectory close to a major vessel can serve to identify those patients in whom angiography is warranted.

Life-threatening epistaxis related to rupture of a pseudoaneurysm or aneurysm of the cavernous internal carotid artery into the sphenoid sinus can occasionally be seen and requires urgent therapy. The presentation of epistaxis may be delayed after the episode of trauma. When massive epistaxis is related to a preexisting non-traumatic cavernous aneurysm, the aneurysm has probably expanded medially causing erosion of the bony sphenoid wall.

Alternatively, in patients undergoing treatment for malignancies of the head and neck, delayed catastrophic bleeding may occur due to progressive weakening of the arterial wall from the effects of surgical cicatrization, external beam radiation, brachytherapy, radical neck dissection, wound infection, erosion by an adjacent sinus or fistula tract, or persistent tumor.

The bleeding site may involve the internal carotid artery, common carotid artery, or external carotid artery. Some patients may have multiple sites of potential bleed-

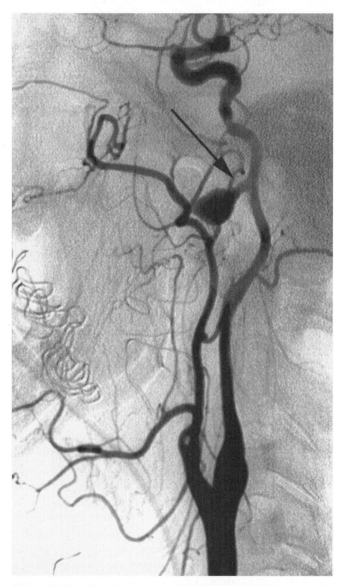

Figure 21.12. *Pseudoaneurysm of the internal carotid artery.*   A lateral view of the left common carotid artery in a middle-aged male who presented with sudden and massive hemorrhage from the pharynx. A large pseudoaneurysm of the internal carotid artery is filling from a defect in the vessel wall at the level of the skull base **(arrow).** The bleeding was controlled by tight packing of the mouth and placement of a balloon-occlusion catheter in the internal carotid artery by the neuroradiologist. The artery was occluded by placement of detachable balloons. Further investigation of the patient revealed that the pseudoaneurysm was related to an occult tumor of the nasopharynx.

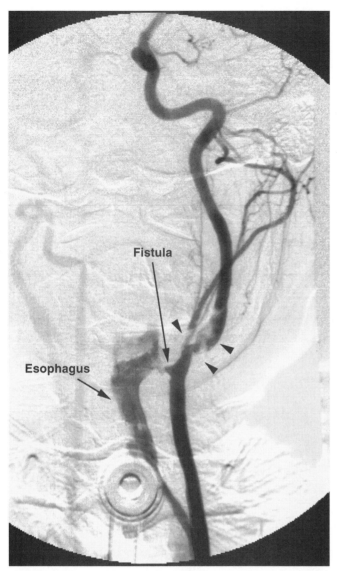

Figure 21.13. *Carotid-esophageal fistula.* An elderly female with laryngeal carcinoma was referred for treatment of massive pharyngeal hemorrhage. She resumed bleeding during the case. A left common carotid arteriogram opacifies the fistula between the common carotid artery and the esophagus. Tumor encasement of the internal carotid artery and external carotid artery is present **(arrowheads).** The bleeding was successfully treated by detachable balloon occlusion of the internal carotid artery and common carotid artery. Despite being resuscitated from cardiac arrest twice during the case, the patient recovered quickly from her ordeal. Two days later while reading a newspaper, she expectorated one of the arterial balloons, which had migrated into the esophagus through the fistula. (Case courtesy of F. Huang-Hellinger, MD, PhD, Boston, MA.)

ing. The phenomenon of such massive carotid bleeding in diverse circumstances has been termed the "carotid blowout syndrome" (30–32). Most frequently, there is a history of radiation therapy. Often the surgical site has become indurated or dehiscent. A repeat surgical procedure to identify and repair the site of bleeding is often a difficult undertaking. Without therapy, however, these patients have mortality rates of 60–100% (33, 34).

Preliminary Preparations

Patients referred for endovascular management of severe bleeding may be hemodynamically stable or unstable. For those who are unstable, the emergent nature of their condition and need for treatment is self-evident, prompting mobilization of assistance from medical, surgical, and anesthesiology teams. Intubation or emergency tracheostomy to protect the airway, placement of large bore intravenous catheters, cross-matching blood units at the blood bank, etc., become obvious necessities.

Head and neck bleeds frequently present with an initial "sentinel" bleed of variable magnitude, which acts as the harbinger of more massive subsequent bleeding. Therefore, when a hemodynamically stable patient is referred for endovascular management of a bleed that has now ceased, all of the precautions and sense of urgency that one might use with an unstable patient should still be exercised. The airway should be protected in advance, because intubation will not be successful if the pharynx fills with blood in a draped patient under the fluoroscopy unit.

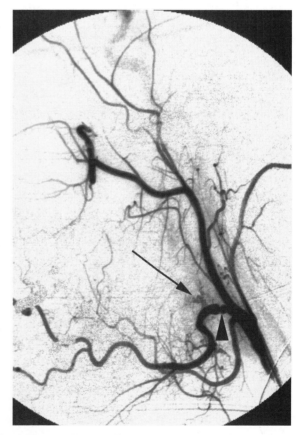

Figure 21.14. *Post-tonsillectomy bleeding I.* A young adult female developed recurrent severe bleeding 2 weeks after a routine tonsillectomy. A left external carotid artery injection demonstrates irregularity of the proximal facial artery **(arrowhead).** At the same level, a small palatine or tonsillar branch **(arrow)** of the facial artery has a cut-off appearance. It was assumed that the tonsillar artery represented the most likely site of bleeding. It was occluded with coils placed through a microcatheter.

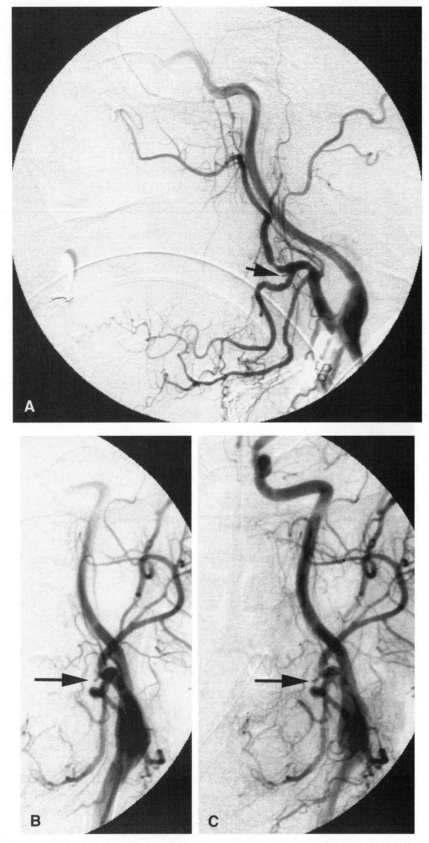

Figure 21.15. *Post-tonsillectomy bleeding II.*   A young adult male developed severe bleeding 4 days after a tonsillectomy. Left common carotid arteriography **(A and B)** demonstrates subtle extravasation from a rent or torn vessel between the external carotid artery and the facial artery **(arrow A and B).** The blush of extravasation becomes more prominent in the late arterial phase **(C).** Above this level, there is spasm of the external carotid artery, best seen on the lateral view **(A).** The area of extravasation was cannulated with a microcatheter and occluded with a push-coil.

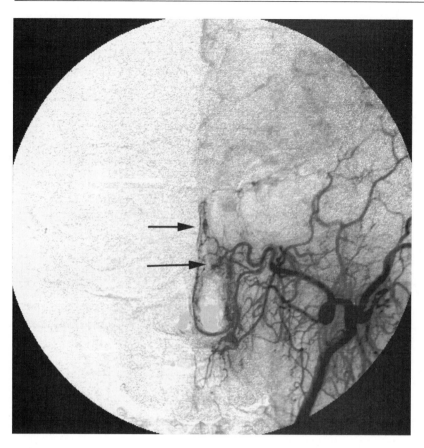

Figure 21.16. *Nasal bleeding post endoscopic nasal surgery.* In cases of bleeding after endoscopic nasal procedures, the first objective is to evaluate the internal carotid artery for injury. Internal carotid artery injuries are more likely to bleed massively and are more difficult to treat. In this patient, even though the visible rate of bleeding was severe, a left external carotid artery injection demonstrates only subtle beading and extravasation of contrast in the territory of the long and short sphenopalatine vessels **(arrows).** These were successfully embolized with PVA particles and Gelfoam.

Therefore, involvement of an anesthesiology team is necessary for safe management.

Consent for the procedure, whether from the patient or family, must anticipate a number of possible necessary treatments, including use of particles, coils, and detachable balloons. If one has to sacrifice a major vessel, physiologic test-occlusion of the vessel in question may not be possible under the circumstances. Although, one would not sacrifice such a vessel without at least evaluating the collateral circulation, the risks of stroke and ischemia must be considered in advance.

Heavy bleeding can occur in the interventional suite. Where the bleeding appears to be worsening and resuscitative measures of a more desperate extreme may be imminent, placement of a 5 French venous sheath in the common femoral vein for rapid fluid administration can be performed quickly during the procedure.

MARK THE SITE OF BLEEDING BEFORE STARTING THE CASE

The speed and efficiency with which a case is conducted depend to a great degree on knowing exactly where to look. Therefore, in patients who have already had packing placed in the oropharynx or nasopharynx, it is important to learn from the referring physician what he/she saw as the packing was being done, and from where the blood appeared most likely to flow. It is often surprisingly difficult, especially under harried circumstances, to correlate the precise location of angiographic findings with the sur-

face anatomy of the patient's head and neck. Therefore, when the patient has a known site of bleeding, such as a skin wound or ostium of a sinus, a metallic marker on that site placed at the beginning of the case can be of enormous assistance. It allows one to center quickly while setting up the image for the initial run. It also helps one to be assured that a subtle irregularity or blush adjacent to the marker represents the significant finding. In the absence of positive findings, the metallic marker also acts as a visible affirmation on the films for the referring physicians that the area of bleeding has been adequately studied.

Procedural Techniques

Without knowing in advance the precise nature of the bleeding abnormality, one's options can be kept open by using a 7 French sheath system. This allows placement of virtually all potentially necessary devices including balloon-catheters.

Even in situations in which there is a reasonable assurance that the bleeding vessel is in the distal external carotid artery tree, a common carotid arterial injection is always a good idea to avoid missing important proximal pathology or proceeding on the basis of misinformed premises concerning the internal carotid artery. When a bleeding site, laceration, or pseudoaneurysm is seen on the initial run, this site is targeted with due speed. When the site involves the internal carotid artery, remember that surgical repair of that artery is possible in certain situa-

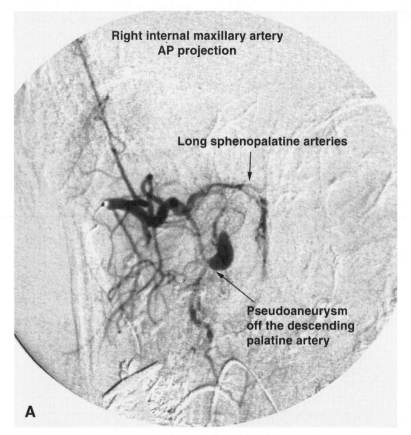

Figure 21.17. Bleeding after LeFort osteotomy: Case I. A young adult developed severe bleeding 8 days after a LeFort osteotomy performed for a congenital facial deformity and dental malocclusion. A right external carotid arteriogram, AP projection **(A),** and lateral projection **(B),** demonstrates a pseudoaneurysm of the descending palatine artery, along the plane cut by the osteotomy saw. A microcatheter was navigated into the descending palatine artery and steered past the pseudoaneurysm. Fibered coils were then laid down distal to, across, and proximal to the neck of the pseudoaneurysm. A post-embolization injection of the ascending palatine artery **(C, lateral projection)** demonstrates the necessity of occluding the torn vessel on both sides of the pseudoaneurysm. There is immediate reconstitution of the descending palatine artery along its horizontal segment **(arrows).** This could potentially fill the pseudoaneurysm from below if an incomplete occlusion had been performed. Notice other vessels **(arrowheads)** of the ascending palatine region, which have been severed by the saw.

tions. If this is not possible, evaluation of the internal carotid artery circulation distal to the laceration gives an idea of how much function remains in that internal carotid artery. Evaluation of the contralateral internal carotid artery and vertebral arteries will reveal to what degree collateral circulation in the circle of Willis can be assumed.

Trapping a Pseudoaneurysm or Laceration Site

The propensity of the external carotid artery to reconstitute itself after an occlusion of any type implies that a pseudoaneurysm or laceration must be controlled by embolization both distally and proximally along its parent vessel. In the major branches of the external carotid artery, this is accomplished more effectively by using coils, preferably of a thrombogenic, fibered construction. Coils are deployed through a catheter distal to the pseudoaneurysm. Ideally, coils placed across the neck of the pseudoaneurysm are desirable too (Fig. 21.17). The catheter is pulled back, and the vessel is occluded proximally with more coils. This means that there is a need to bypass the pseudoaneurysm with a wire or microwire early in the procedure, pos-

ing a risk of perforating the laceration site. For this reason, the main catheter is kept close to the laceration site, so that in the event of severe bleeding, the catheter can be wedged quickly into the compromised segment of vessel to stem the bleeding, while a packing maneuver is quickly undertaken through the microcatheter.

Within the major branches of the external carotid artery, it takes a deceptively large number of microcoils (0.018″) to occlude a vessel lumen completely. Therefore 0.038″ coils introduced directly through the main catheter are more effective, cheaper, and quicker. For mid-size branches of the external carotid artery, coils of the 0.018″ dimension are very helpful. For more distal branches, inaccessible to direct catheterization, PVA particles or Gelfoam pledgets (not powder) are the agents of choice. Occasionally, distal pseudoaneurysms of the external carotid artery can be embolized effectively with superselective embolization using cyanoacrylate (32).

After embolization, a corroborating or control angiogram is necessary to confirm the efficacy of the procedure. Arteries with the potential to supply collateral pathways to

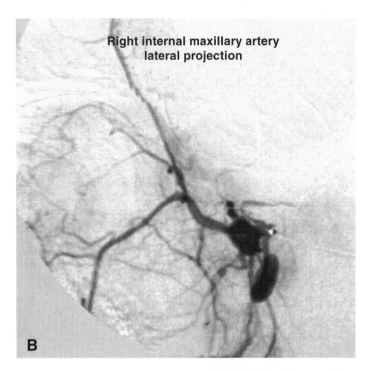

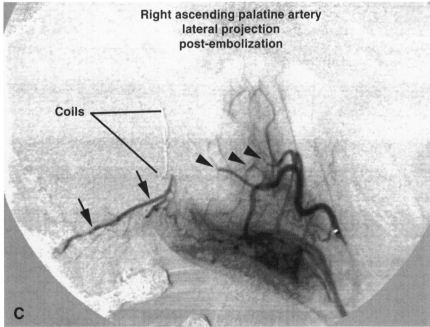

Figure 21.17. *(continued)*

Figure 21.18. *Bleeding after LeFort osteotomy: Case II.* This middle-aged patient had a LeFort osteotomy and maxillary reconstruction for intractable airway obstruction. Ten days after surgery he developed severe bleeding. A lateral external carotid artery **(A)** injection demonstrates a pseudoaneurysm **(arrowhead)** of the external carotid artery at the level of the origin of the internal maxillary artery (i.m.a.). The internal maxillary artery is occluded proximally and fills via the buccal artery (buc.a.) from the facial artery. The transverse facial artery (tr.f.a.) and ascending palatine artery (asc.pal.a.) are labeled. The external carotid artery was occluded with fibered coils along the lacerated segment. A post-embolization lateral projection of the facial artery **(B)** demonstrates filling of the internal maxillary artery via the buccal artery, but no evidence of opacification of the pseudoaneurysm.

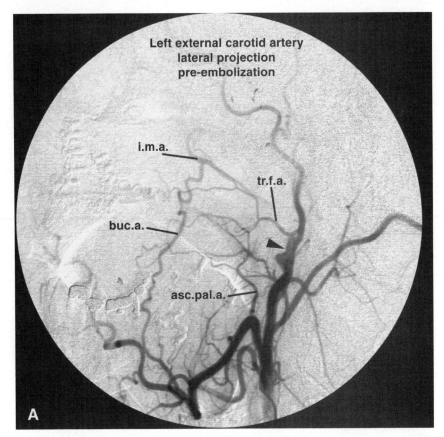

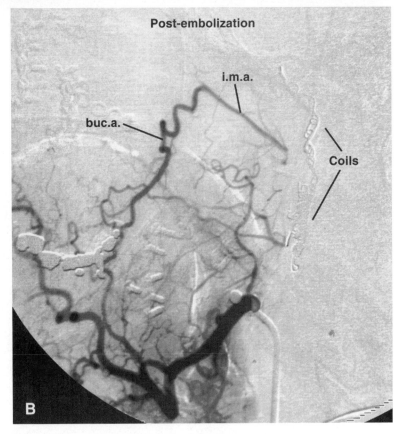

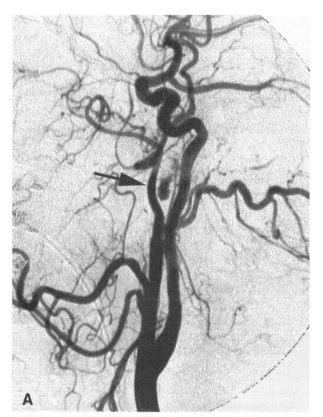

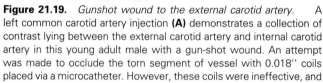

Figure 21.19. *Gunshot wound to the external carotid artery.* A left common carotid artery injection **(A)** demonstrates a collection of contrast lying between the external carotid artery and internal carotid artery in this young adult male with a gun-shot wound. An attempt was made to occlude the torn segment of vessel with 0.018'' coils placed via a microcatheter. However, these coils were ineffective, and the vessel was closed using 0.038'' coils placed via the introducer 5 French catheter. A post-embolization image **(B)** shows how quickly the distal external carotid artery can reconstitute after a proximal occlusion. Collateral vessels, including the buccal artery, ascending palatine artery, and ascending pharyngeal artery, are prominently seen.

the distal territory of the embolized vessel must be studied ipsilaterally and contralaterally.

Neck Bleeding

Cases of intermittent small vessel bleeding in the neck can be among the most frustrating angiographic studies. Labeling the suspected site of bleeding externally with a metallic marker can help to narrow one's search, but frequently the offending vessel is elusive. Potential oversights arise by forgetting to study the collateral vessels adequately, e.g., the contralateral cervical vessels, the contralateral thyroidal arteries, etc. One may start a case with misinformed premises as to where the lesion lies (see Fig. 15.16). Furthermore, embolization in the costocervical and thyrocervical trunks carries the added concern of needing to be vigilant for the presence of the artery of cervical enlargement (anterior spinal artery).

REFERENCES

1. Brandt T, von Kummer R, Müller-Küppers M, et al. Thrombolytic therapy for acute basilar artery occlusion. Variables affecting recanalization and outcome. Stroke 1996;27:875–881.
2. Hacke W, Zeumer H, Ferbert A, et al. Intra-arterial thrombolytic therapy improves outcome in patients with acute vertebrobasilar occlusive disease. Stroke 1988;19:1216–1222.
3. Von Kummer R, Holle R, Rosin L, et al. Does arterial recanalization improve outcome in carotid territory stroke? Stroke 1995; 26:581–587.
4. Scott JA, Pascuzzi RM, Hall PV, et al. Treatment of dural sinus thrombosis with local urokinase infusion. Case report. J Neurosurg 1988;68:284–287.
5. Smith TP, Higashida RT, Barnwell SL, et al. Treatment of dural sinus thrombosis by urokinase infusion. Am J Neuroradiol 1994; 15:801–807.
6. Heros RC, Zervas NT, Varsos V. Cerebral vasospasm after subarachnoid hemorrhage: an update. Ann Neurol 1983;14: 599–608.
7. Kassell NF, Sasaki T, Colohan ART, et al. Cerebral vasospasm following aneurysmal subarachnoid hemorrhage. Stroke 1985; 16:562–572.
8. Taneda M, Otsuki H, Kumura E, et al. Angiographic demonstration of acute phase of intracranial arterial spasm following aneurysm rupture. J Neurosurg 1990;73:958–961.
9. Proust F, Hannequin D, Langlois O, et al. Causes of morbidity and mortality after ruptured aneurysm surgery in a series of 230 patients. The importance of control angiography. Stroke 1995;26:1553–1557.
10. Auer LM. Unfavorable outcome following early surgical repair of ruptured cerebral aneurysms-a critical review of 238 patients. Surg Neurol 1991;35:152–158.
11. Awad IA, Carter LP, Spetzler RF, et al. Clinical vasospasm after subarachnoid hemorrhage: response to hypervolemic hemodilution and arterial hypertension. Stroke 1987;18:365–372.

12. Pickard JD, Murray GD, Illingworth R, et al. Effects of oral nimodipine on cerebral infarction and outcome after subarachnoid hemorrhage: British aneurysm nimodipine study. Br Med J 1989;298:636–642.

13. Handa Y, Weir BK, Nosko M, et al. The effect of timing of clot removal on chronic vasospasm in a primate model. J Neurosurg 1987;67:558–564.

14. Marks MP, Steinberg GK, Lane B. Intraarterial papaverine for the treatment of vasospasm. Am J Neuroradiol 1993;14:822–826

15. Livingston K, Hopkins LN. Intraarterial papaverine as an adjunct to transluminal angioplasty for vasospasm induced by subarachnoid hemorrhage. Am J Neuroradiol 1993;14:346–347.

16. Kassell NF, Helm G, Simmons N, et al. Treatment of cerebral vasospasm with intra-arterial papaverine. J Neurosurg 1992;77:848–852.

17. Clouston JE, Numaguchi Y, Zoarski GH, et al. Intraarterial papaverine infusion for cerebral vasospasm after subarachnoid hemorrhage. Am J Neuroradiol 1995;16:27–38.

18. Vardiman AB, Kopitnik TA, Purdy PD, et al. Treatment of traumatic arterial vasospasm with intraarterial papaverine infusion. Am J Neuroradiol 1995;16:319–321.

19. Eckard DA, Purdy PD, Girson MS, et al. Intraarterial papaverine for relief of catheter-induced intracranial vasospasm. Am J Roentgenol 1992;158:883–884.

20. Kaku Y, Yonekawa Y, Tsukahara T, et al. Superselective intraarterial infusion of papaverine for the treatment of cerebral vasospasm from subarachnoid hemorrhage. J Neurosurg 1992;77:842–847.

21. Mathis JM, DeNardo AJ, Thibault L, et al. In vitro evaluation of papaverine hydrochloride incompatibilities: a simulation of intraarterial infusion for cerebral vasospasm. Am J Neuroradiol 1994;14:1665–1670.

22. Pallan TM, Wulkan IA, Abadir AR, et al. Incompatibility of isovue 370 and papaverine in peripheral angiography. Radiology 1993;87:257–259.

23. Shah SJ, Gerlock AJ. Incompatibility of hexabrix and papaverine in peripheral arteriography. Radiology 1987:162:619–620.

24. Hendrix LE, Dion JE, Jensen ME, et al. Papaverine-induced mydriasis. Am J Neuroradiol 1994;15:716–718.

25. Barr JD, Mathis JM, Horton JA. Transient severe brainstem depression during intraarterial papaverine infusion for cerebral vasospasm. Am J Neuroradiol 1994;15:719–723.

26. Mathis JM, DeNardo A, Jensen ME, et al. Transient neurologic events associated with intraarterial papaverine infusion for subarachnoid hemorrhage-vasospasm. Am J Neuroradiol 1994;15:1671–1674.

27. McAuliffe A, Townsend M, Eskridge JM, et al. Intracranial pressure changes induced during papaverine infusion for treatment of vasospasm. J Neurosurg 1995;83:430–431.

28. Miller JA, Cross DT, Moran CJ, et al. Severe thrombocytopenia following intraarterial papaverine administration for treatment of vasospasm. J Neurosurg 1995;83:435–437.

29. Nemzek WR, Hecht ST, Donald PJ, et al. Prediction of major vascular injury in patients with gunshot wounds to the neck. Am J Neuroradiol 1996;17:161–167.

30. Citardi MJ, Chaloupka JC, Son YH, et al. Management of carotid artery rupture by monitored endovascular therapeutic occlusion (1988–1994). Laryngoscope 1995;105:1086–1092.

31. Borsany SJ. Rupture of the carotids following radical neck surgery in irradiated patients. Ear Nose Throat J 1962;41:531–533.

32. Chaloupka JC, Putman CM, Citardi MJ, et al. Endovascular therapy for the carotid blowout syndrome in head and neck surgical patients: diagnostic and managerial considerations. Am J Neuroradiol AJNR 1996;17:843–852.

33. Stell PM. Catastrophic haemorrhage after major neck surgery. Br J Surg 1969;56:525–527.

34. Maran AGD, Amin M, Wilson JA. Radical neck dissection: a 19 year experience. J Laryngol Otol 1989;103:760–764.

Index

Page numbers in *italics* denote figures; those followed by ''t'' denote tables.

Related Resources for Your Practice

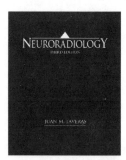

NEURORADIOLOGY, THIRD EDITION

Juan M. Taveras, MD

Learn from the master in this encyclopedic reference on neuroradiology. The foremost authority in the field covers all modalities used in neuroradiologic diagnosis, including: interventional neuroradiology, MR and CT in diagnosis, spectroscopy, and more. It provides superb, comprehensive coverage.

1996/1190 pages/2966 illustrations/08112-8

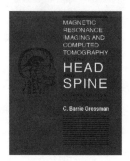

MAGNETIC RESONANCE IMAGING AND COMPUTED TOMOGRAPHY OF THE HEAD AND SPINE, SECOND EDITION

C. Barrie Grossman, MD

Extravagant illustrations make this an indispensable imaging reference. It's completely revised and includes thorough coverage of both head and spine imaging along with full discussions of the most advanced techniques. The excellent text and pictures are augmented by extensive use of detailed charts and gamuts.

1996/810 pages/580 illustrations/03769-2

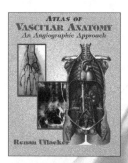

ATLAS OF VASCULAR ANATOMY: AN ANGIOGRAPHIC APPROACH

Renan Uflacker, MD, MSc

The beauty of this volume is surpassed only by its practicality. Each topic is covered in a 2-page spread that details each region in-depth, and is followed by a sequence of correlated 4-color illustrations—all for fast information, eliminating the need to flip from page to page.

1997/811 pages/18110-6

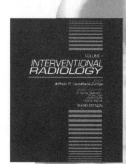

INTERVENTIONAL RADIOLOGY, THIRD EDITION

Wilfrido R. Castaneda-Zuniga, MD, MSc, and S. Murthy Tadavarthy, MD

Some call it the "bible" of Interventional Radiology. You'll call on it daily for its brilliant technical descriptions. This comprehensive reference takes you on a trip through all the organs and system. It covers the latest effective applications of interventional techniques, emphasizing indications, contraindications, approaches, and quality instrumentation.

1996/1816 pages 2 vols./3060 illustrations/01477-3